Nano Drug Delivery Systems for Biomedical Applications

This edited book provides a comprehensive exploration of cutting-edge nanomedicine, bringing together leading research on the design and application of nanoparticles and nanomaterials across a wide spectrum of biomedical fields. Covering topics from tissue engineering, drug delivery, and biomedical implants to cancer therapeutics and precision medicine, the volume highlights how nanotechnology is revolutionizing diagnostics, therapies, and the management of complex diseases. Chapters also examine innovative developments in quantum dots, gene therapy, and strategies for tackling neglected tropical diseases, alongside critical assessments of biocompatibility, toxicity, and the regulatory landscape shaping the future of nanomedicine. This book serves as an essential reference for researchers, clinicians, and policymakers interested in emerging trends, challenges, and translational breakthroughs at the intersection of nanoscience and healthcare.

Nano Drug Delivery Systems for Biomedical Applications

Edited by
Manashjit Gogoi and Sanjukta Patra

CRC Press
Taylor & Francis Group
Boca Raton London New York

CRC Press is an imprint of the
Taylor & Francis Group, an informa business

Designed cover image: Sanjukta Patra and Manashjit Gogoi

First edition published 2026
by CRC Press
2385 NW Executive Center Drive, Suite 320, Boca Raton FL 33431

and by CRC Press
4 Park Square, Milton Park, Abingdon, Oxon, OX14 4RN

CRC Press is an imprint of Taylor & Francis Group, LLC

ISBN: 9781032752327 (hbk)
ISBN: 9781032752334 (pbk)
ISBN: 9781003473015 (ebk)

DOI: 10.1201/9781003473015

Typeset in Times
by codeMantra

Contents

Preface

The convergence of nanotechnology and medicine has ushered in a transformative era in the biomedical sciences, particularly in the field of drug delivery systems. The capacity of nanomaterials to interact with biological systems at the molecular and cellular level has opened new frontiers for targeted therapies, precision medicine, and regenerative healthcare. With their exceptional physicochemical properties, nanoparticles and nanostructures are poised to overcome the limitations of conventional drug delivery systems by enhancing bioavailability, reducing systemic toxicity, improving controlled release, and enabling site-specific action.

This edited volume, *Nano Drug Delivery Systems for Biomedical Applications*, brings together critical insights from leading researchers exploring the multifaceted integration of nanotechnology with contemporary medicine. The chapters span a spectrum of applications, covering both foundational principles and advanced therapeutic strategies.

This book begins with an Introduction to Nanomedicines, setting the stage for understanding the core principles that underpin nanoscale therapeutic interventions. This is followed by discussions on the application of Nanoparticles for Tissue Engineering and Regenerative Medicines and the utilization of Nanomaterials in Biomedical Implants, establishing the role of nanostructures in enhancing tissue repair and implant compatibility.

The exploration of novel materials continues with Organic–Inorganic Hybrid Nanomedicine for Drug Delivery, highlighting the synergistic benefits of hybrid formulations, and extends into unique domains such as Nanoparticles in Nuclear Medicines, underscoring their diagnostic and therapeutic utilities. The contribution on Quantum Dots for Biosensing and Bioimaging Applications emphasizes the growing importance of nanosystems in precise diagnostics and real-time monitoring.

On the therapeutic front, cutting-edge strategies are examined in chapters such as Gene Therapy Using Polymeric Nanocarriers and Cancer Nanotherapeutics: Trends and Challenges, which deal with some of the most pressing challenges in modern medicine. At the same time, chapters like Engineered Nanomaterials for the Treatment of Neglected Tropical Diseases and Nanotechnology-Based Approaches for Diabetes Management broaden the scope of nanomedicine to address global healthcare priorities.

This book further bridges advanced science with clinical practice through chapters like Nanomedicine in Precision Medicine, illustrating patient-specific strategies, and Evaluation of Biocompatibility and Toxicity of Nanoparticles In Vitro and In Vivo, which underscores the indispensable aspect of safety and efficacy studies. Finally, the concluding discussion on Nanomedicine's Potential Through Regulatory and Translational Breakthroughs provides critical reflections on how scientific progress can be effectively channeled into clinical and commercial realities.

This collection aims to serve both as a reference for researchers and practitioners, and as a guide for students and academics seeking to understand the dynamic intersections of nanoscience and medicine. By compiling diverse approaches and emerging trends, this book underscores not only the scientific potential of nano drug delivery systems but also their translational promise in shaping the future of healthcare.

We hope that this volume contributes meaningfully to advancing knowledge, sparking innovation, and inspiring interdisciplinary collaboration in the pursuit of next-generation biomedical solutions.

The Editors

Manashjit Gogoi is an Assistant Professor in the Department of Biomedical Engineering at North-Eastern Hill University (NEHU), Shillong. He obtained his Ph.D. in Biomedical Engineering from the Indian Institute of Technology Bombay, M.Tech. in Bioelectronics from Tezpur University, and B.E. in Chemical Engineering from Gauhati University. His areas of research interest are nanomedicine, biosensors, microfluidics, point-of-care devices, cancer drug delivery, magnetic nanoparticles, and hyperthermia. Dr. Gogoi has led and collaborated on several research and development projects, including work on biosensors for early cancer detection and nanocomposite films for pesticide sensing. Based on his research, he has published three Indian patents, gotten two designs registered, contributed 33 research articles and 22 book chapters, and edited two books on biosensors and a number of conference papers. He also contributes to academic leadership at NEHU through departmental coordination, curriculum development, and laboratory establishment.

Sanjukta Patra is a faculty member in the Department of Medical Sciences and Technology at the Indian Institute of Technology Madras. Prior to this, she was at the Department of Biosciences and Bioengineering at the Indian Institute of Technology Guwahati for a period of more than 17 years. Her research interests include diagnostics and therapeutics, enzyme and microbial technologies, and biomolecules for biomedical applications. Dr. Sanjukta has led and collaborated on several research and development projects, including sensor development for tuberculosis and candida, and whole cell biosensors for small molecules on various platforms. She has to her credit five Indian patents, and has contributed 70 research articles and 30 book chapters, and edited three books and 75 conference papers.

Acknowledgments

The editors would like to thank the Almighty God for providing them with the motivation and strength to complete the endeavor of editing this book.

They sincerely thank Dr. Bhavik Sawhney, Senior Editor (Life Sciences), CRC Press, Taylor & Francis, and all the editorial board members for their approval and for granting them the opportunity to edit this book. They would like to express their sincere gratitude to the editorial team of Taylor & Francis for constantly following up on the editing process, and helping them to complete this assignment.

The editors gratefully acknowledge all the contributors for their valuable chapters and insights, as well as for their patience throughout the process of completing this edited book. Their commitment and cooperation have been vital in bringing this volume to fruition.

Dr. Manashjit Gogoi expresses his thankfulness to his beloved sons, Adityavardhan and Atanu, and wife, Mayuri, who sacrificed a lot and kept him inspired to finish this task. He is also thankful to his sister-in-law, Hewali, and his parents, brothers, and in-laws for their constant support, unconditional love, and blessings.

Dr. Sanjukta Patra expresses her heartfelt thankfulness to little Paridhi. It's her shared time which has brought this book in black and white. She is thankful to all her family members for their constant support and blessings.

Editors
Manashjit Gogoi
Sanjukta Patra

1 Introduction to Nanomedicines

Reshmi Bhattacharjee[1] *and Romesh Borgohain*[2]
[1]Department of Zoology, Birjhora Mahavidyalaya, Bongaigaon, India
[2]Department of Chemistry, Birjhora Mahavidyalaya, Bongaigaon, India

1.1 INTRODUCTION

Nanomaterials or nanoparticles (NPs) are particles ranging in size between 1 and 100 nm. They represent a significant aspect of nanotechnology, which has gained much importance due to possible applications in various aspects of human life and environment. Research on nanomaterials in the current scenario is more focused on recent advances in synthesis, classification, and characterization of nanomaterials (Mageswari et al. 2016), as basic scientific research on micro-sized and nanomaterials has reached a saturation point.

Nanomaterials due to their higher surface area, reactivity, and strength have the ability to be integrated into matrixes, thereby ensuring the possibility of enhancing the physical, mechanical, and chemical properties of their resulting composites. These characteristics have led to a surge in studies on NPs and their applications in various fields such as energetic materials, biomedical, and microelectronics (Velu et al. 2019).

Advances in the fields of nanotechnology and biotechnology have led to the development of nanobiomaterials, which in turn had a high impact on medicine. Such nanobiomaterials are being used for a wide range of biological and biomedical applications, ranging from drug delivery, medical imaging, to artificial implants, among others. As compared to materials with micron or larger level microstructures, nanoscale materials and their structures provide some advantages to a biomaterial. Firstly, it makes them comparable to biological systems and natural tissues, both in terms of structure and chemistry. Secondly, since the size of nanoscale materials is similar to biomolecules, it makes it easier for researchers to detect, work on, and mediate these biomolecules. Thirdly, such nanostructured biomaterials can be modified to utilize their variations in surface properties to make tailored scaffolds, mimicking biological systems (Yang et al. 2011).

There are numerous applications of nanobiomaterials in various fields highlighting the importance of this class of material. Some of them are briefly discussed below:

a. *Cosmetics*: In recent years, the use of nanobiomaterials in the cosmetics industry has increased to a great extent. They are widely used in the synthesis of various deodorants, sunscreens, eye shadows, shampoos, conditioners, lipsticks, moisturizers, aftershave products, and fragrances in which the nanomaterials enhance the value or activity of these products. Nanomaterials consisting of alumina, silver, silicon dioxide, calcium fluoride, copper, titanium dioxide, zinc oxide, etc. are some examples of leading nanomaterials used in the cosmetics industry (Singh & Sharma 2016).
b. *Agriculture*: In agriculture, nanobiomaterials are basically used for the purpose of production and protection of plants, detection of pathogen and residues of pesticides, etc. The use of nanobiomaterials is a very much effective as well as environmentally benign approach in enhancing plant production and in the protection of plants. Furthermore, the application of nanosensors is a useful way for the detection of pathogens and the residues

DOI: 10.1201/9781003473015-1

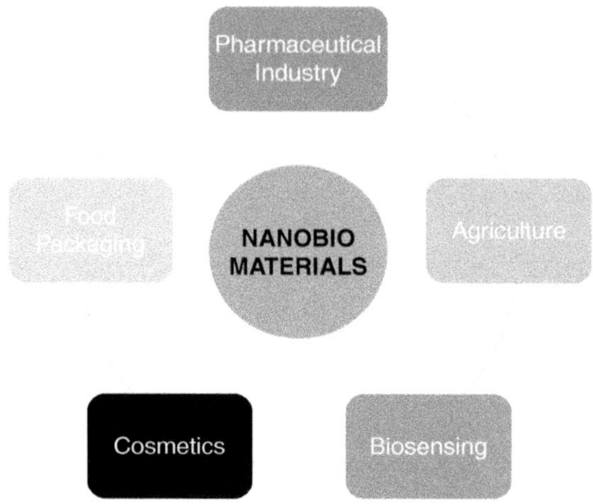

FIGURE 1.1 Applications of nanobiomaterials in different sectors.

of pesticides in plants. Magnetic carbon-coated NPs, inorganic Zn-Al-layered double hydroxide, porous hollow silica nanoparticles (PHSNPs), carbon nanotube (CNT) conjugated with INF24 oligonucleotides, Ag NPs, sodium dodecyl sulphate (SDS)-modified photocatalytic TiO_2/Ag nanomaterial, etc. are some examples of nanomaterials commonly used in the field of agriculture (Khot et al. 2012).

c. *Food Packaging*: Nanobiomaterials also have notable potential as packaging material for food. It has various advantages over the traditional packaging materials such as being lightweight, offers greater protection, and helps in preservation of the food, in addition to being safer for humans and the environment (Bradley et al. 2011).
d. *Biosensing*: Biosensors are used for receiving signals of specific biological analytes such as those originating from bacteria or viruses and other substances produced by the immune system of an infected living organism. The use of nanobiomaterials as bioreceptor units in biosensors has various advantages such as increase of sensitivities, lowering of detection limit even up to individual molecules, and enhanced quantity of the biosensor materials at reduced volumes. NPs consisting of gold, polymer, CNTs, graphene, nanodiamonds, etc. are some leading nanomaterials which are widely used as receptors in biosensors (Holzinger et al. 2014).

Besides these applications, nanobiomaterials also have tremendous importance in the field of pharmaceutical industry such as in medicine and drug delivery which will be discussed later in this chapter (Figure 1.1).

1.2 SOURCES OF NANOBIOMATERIALS

The nanobiomaterials can be basically classified into two categories depending upon their origin, i.e., synthetic or natural origin. They are briefly discussed below:

a. *Nanobiomaterials of Natural Origin:* Most of the natural-based and biologically derived nanobiomaterials include polysaccharide-, protein-, and carbon-based nanomaterials. Among these, polysaccharide-based nanobiomaterials include nanomaterials which are derived from chitin, chitosan, and cellulose. These materials have been effectively used in nanomedicine and drug delivery due to their cost-effectiveness and biocompatible nature. The protein-based nanobiomaterials include nanomaterials derived from naturally occurring protein molecules. They have been getting immense attention in the field of nanomedicine and drug delivery due to their biodegradability and abundant sources. Similarly, carbon-based nanobiomaterials mostly include the carbon nanomaterials such as CNT and graphene. The carbon-based nanomaterials have various effective properties such as their hollow structure, high surface area/volume ratio, thermal conductivity, electrical conductance, and mechanical stiffness, which make them a potential candidate in the competition for developing effective nanobiomaterials (Razavi et al. 2017).

b. *Nanobiomaterials of Synthetic Origin:* Nanobiomaterials can also be obtained synthetically which may involve both metallic and non-metallic sources. Among various metallic nanobiomaterials, gold, silver, iron oxide, TiO_2, ZnO_2 NPs, etc. are some promising examples which have wide applications in the fields of drug delivery, biosensors, cancer treatment, wound healing, textile for ultraviolet protection coating, etc. Ceramic biomaterials are another class of important synthetic nanobiomaterials which also have various applications in the area of analytical tools, drug delivery system, development of nano devices, and in the treatment of bone, teeth, and other medical applications (Gomathi et al. 2023).

1.3 APPLICATIONS OF NANOBIOMATERIALS IN NANOMEDICINE

Nanobiomaterials have become an important precursor for the synthesis of nanomedicine. The advantages of using nanobiomaterials in nanomedicine are that they can be used for easy and accurate diagnosis and they can also treat effectively without any side effects. By using nanomedicine, different characteristics of drugs such as solubility, blood pool retention time, controlled release over short or long durations, environmentally triggered controlled release, or highly specific site-targeted delivery can be controlled according to the requirement. The increased functional surface area of the NPs also gives the opportunity to explore them in other areas (Singh et al. 2013).

The various applications of nanobiomaterials in nanomedicine can be discussed as follows:

I. *Use of Nanobiomaterials as Therapeutic Drugs:* The nanobiomaterials can be used as therapeutic drugs such as antibacterial drugs, antiviral drugs, and analgesic and anti-inflammatory drugs. These uses of nanobiomaterials are briefly discussed below:

   a. *Antibacterial Drugs*: Metal-based NPs act as antibacterial drugs over a wide range of gram-positive and gram-negative bacteria. NPs such as that of Ag, gold, gold-supported cerium oxide, ZnO, and TiO_2 nanotubes are more efficient in comparison to different metal NPs due to their increased functional surface area. The mechanism of their antibacterial activity is believed to be their ability to enter the pathogens due to their nanosize. This allows them to enter and readily combine with the bacterial protein enzymes, resulting in death of the bacteria. Many studies revealed that Ag NPs are one of the most promising antibacterial agents. However, it may be cytotoxic when it is used alone; therefore, these NPs are embedded in the surface of some other materials like titanium, zeolite, etc. or embedded in polymer matrix to increase their cytocompatibility. Thus, these metal NPs may act as potential antibacterial drugs in the near future. However, clinical experiments must be conducted in order to check for any side effects or possible toxicity, and to make them suitable for human usage (Ge et al. 2014, Rai et al. 2009, Mehmood et al. 2015).

   b. *Antiviral Drugs*: In recent years, nanobiomaterials have been getting immense attention in nanomedicine due to their stability, solubility, synthetic accessibility, release pattern, and efficacy in cell penetration. Metal NPs such as Ag and gold act as promising antiviral drugs used for the diagnosis, treatment, prevention, and mitigation of the spread of different viral diseases such as HIV, HSV, HCV, SARS-CoV-1, MERS-CoV, and the recent SARS-CoV-2 pandemic. Recent research indicates that they follow multiple mechanisms of action. These include inhibition of viral DNA/RNA, photocatalysis, photothermal effects, disruptive mimicry of viral structures due to similarity in structures, etc. AuNP-M2e peptide vaccine, AgNP of cinnamon bark extract, AgNP of oseltamivir, AuNPs of Allium sativum, and AgNPs of ribavirin are some examples of nanomaterials that show excellent antiviral activities against a number of viruses (Campos et al. 2020, Ellah et al. 2019).

c. *Analgesic and Anti-Inflammatory Drugs*: Although a number of analgesics and non-steroidal anti-inflammatory drugs (NSAIDs) such as ibuprofen, diflunisal, aspirin, celecoxib, and naproxen sodium are known, they have adverse effects on the human body. However, use of nanobiomaterials can increase the efficacy of the drug and also reduce the adverse effects. They also have other advantages over normal analgesic and anti-inflammatory drugs, such as increase of solubility, stability, and therapeutic index. Chitosan-dexamethasone NPs, hyaluronic-gold-tocilizumab NPs, arginine-glycine aspartic acid attached with gold nano half-shells conjugated with methotrexate, solid lipid NPs, surface-engineered liposomes, nano emulsions, etc. are some examples of potential nanomaterials with analgesic and anti-inflammatory properties (Manzano et al. 2020, Schiavi et al. 2020).

d. *Anticancer Drugs*: Nanomaterials are also getting importance as anticancer drugs because of their efficacy and selectivity. For example, surface-modified gold NPs are capable of killing the tumour cells selectively without affecting the normal cells significantly. Similarly, nanophase selenium on titanium and stainless steel implants can be incorporated to prevent cancerous bone cell functions, thereby promoting healthy bone growth. Poly(lactic-co-glycolic acid), i.e., PLGA NPs, are also known to be an effective anticancer drug which can be used for the treatment of lung cancer (Tran et al. 2010, Zhang et al. 2010).

In addition to these, nanobiomaterials have also received immense attention as NPs encapsulating hormone drugs, nanometre-sized polypeptide and protein drugs, nano traditional Chinese medicine, etc.

II. *Use of Nanobiomaterials in Tissue Engineering*: Nanobiomaterials are widely used in both soft and hard tissue engineering. Some of them are briefly discussed below:

a. *Application in Cardiology:* Naturally, nano-dimensional collagen and elastin forms the extracellular matrix layer of the cardiovascular tissues. Research attempting to mimic the structure of these nanomaterials has been going on in order to improve the vascular cell functions and to prevent inflammation and thrombosis on stents. It is observed that several nanostructured surfaces such as that of titanium, NiTi, CoCrMo, poly(dimethylsiloxane), and PLGA increase the functioning of vascular cells to a great extent. In addition to these nanostructured surfaces, nanoscaffolds are also used in cardiovascular tissue engineering. Polyhedral oligomeric silsesquioxane onto urethane segments, nanofibrous scaffolds by electrospinning collagen, elastin, poly(L-lactic acid), and poly(L-lactic-co-ε-caprolactone) copolymer scaffolds are some examples which act effectively in the treatment of cardiovascular diseases (Choudhary et al. 2007, Ranjan & Webster 2009, Lee et al. 2007).

b. *Application in Neural Tissue Engineering*: Nanobiomaterials are also useful in repairing and recovering damaged nerves. Nanosized ZnO is one such material used for increasing the excitability of neurons. CNTs with their excellent electrical conductivity and mechanical properties are very efficient for repairing damaged nerves. The modified carbon nanomaterials are also useful for growing of neurons and have inhibitory effect on astrocyte functions. Furthermore, nanobiometric scaffolds like hydrogen-terminated ultra-nanocrystalline diamond (NCD) are also known for their capability to support neural stem cells and repairing of central nervous system (Zhao et al. 2009, Mattson et al. 2000).

c. *Application in Bladder Tissue Engineering*: Due to increased surface energy and selectivity towards protein adsorption, nanobiomaterials are promising agents in the regeneration of bladder tissues. For example, polymeric nanometre scaffold comprising of PLGA and polyurethane enhances the functioning of bladder smooth muscle cells. It also increases the production of proteins like elastin and collagen. Similarly, electrospun polystyrene scaffold with aligned nanofibres supports the formation of actin filaments of smooth muscle cells of bladder in a way similar to that of native tissue. Poly(glycolic acid) scaffolds are another example which work efficiently in bladder tissue engineering and increase the adhesion of bladder smooth muscle cell (Thapa et al. 2003, Baker et al. 2006).

d. *Application in Orthopaedic Implants*: Nanobiomaterials are biocompatible and possess mechanical properties such as proper toughness and high strength, and they are stable under severe conditions allowing them to survive for long periods. Therefore, nanobiomaterials are promising candidates for orthopaedic implants. Anodized nanotubular Titania (TiO_2) is one such example which enhances bone cell adhesion and proliferation. Similarly, coating of nanostructured diamond-like carbon (DLC) on metallic implant surfaces enhances bone cell attachment and also lowers friction. The NCD coating is another example of nanobiomaterial which has low friction coefficients and exhibits high chemical resistance, high fracture toughness, and high bonding strength to various implant materials. CNT-based nanocomposites have also been used to improve fracture toughness and anti-wear properties of implant coatings due to the extremely high tensile strength and stiffness (Yang et al. 2009, Sua et al. 2018, Kim et al. 2006).

e. *Application in Bone Tissue Engineering*: Nanostructured scaffolds comprising of polymers such as poly(glycolic acid), PLGA, polyurethane, collagen, chitosan, and silk are some examples of nanobiomaterials that are widely used in bone tissue engineering. They have improved bone cell attachment and osteogenic functions, as well as enhanced adsorption property for bone cell adhesive proteins. Nanostructures comprising of polymer, ceramics, and carbon nanocomposites resemble the natural structure and properties of bone, and hence, they are one of the most efficient coatings for the bone tissue engineering scaffolds. In addition to these, various injectable nanoscaffolds are also known which are used for treatment of cavitary defects in bone (Liu et al. 2006, Hosseinkhani et al. 2007).

f. *Dental Application*: Nanobiomaterials are used in both dental implants and dental adhesives. Nanostructured coatings of Titania, calcium phosphate, silver, gelatin nanogold, calcium phosphate-coated zirconia, etc., are examples of such materials used in the area of dental implants. Similarly, colloidal platinum NPs and poly(methyl methacrylate)-grafted nanoclays are examples of nanobiomaterials used for dental adhesive purposes (Nagano et al. 2009).

Thus, nanobiomaterials have wide and diverse applications in the area of bone engineering and are recognized as promising candidates in this field.

III. *Application of Nanobiomaterials in Nanovaccine*: Nanovaccine consists of biodegradable polymers which are capable of inducing both cell-mediated and humoral immune responses, and it involves a no-pain delivery system since it can be administered through oral or nasal routes. Furthermore, the delivery of a particular antigen in a specific location can be controlled for a long period in the case of nanovaccine. Thus, the immune system of human body can be stimulated using nanovaccines that will prevent infections and spreading of diseases and will also help in curing diseases (Zaman et al. 2013).

IV. *Applications in Medical Instruments*: Nanobiomaterials are widely used in the manufacturing of various medical instruments that enable diagnosis and treatment of diseases at micro levels. Among them, nanoprobes are one of the important developments in this area. They can be transported into different parts of the body through circulation via the bloodstream and can be localized in a targeted location, where the diagnosis can be carried out based on a magnetic interaction. Nanorobot is another development in this field which can

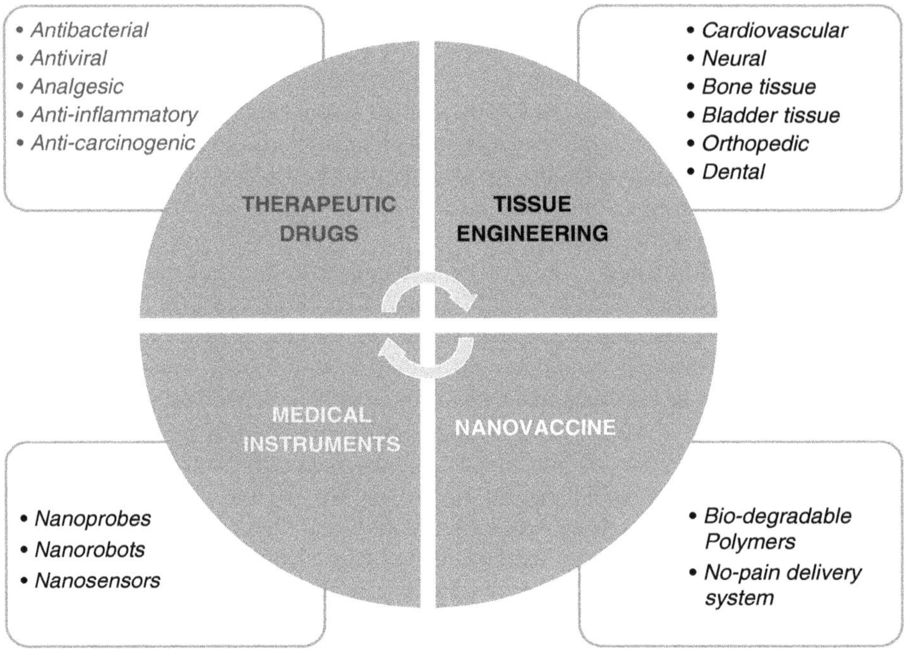

FIGURE 1.2 Application of nanobiomaterials in nanomedicine.

be administered to the human body through the bloodstream for diagnosis of diseases as well as for various other purposes such as cosmetic surgery and installing normal DNA/removal of harmful DNA from genes. It can also be used for the removal of blood clots and kidney stones, wound cleaning, dispel parasites, etc. Similarly, nanobiomaterials are also used as nanosensors that can be used for examining cell pressure, temperature, volume, and concentration and also for differentiating between normal and cancerous cells at the molecular level (Li et al. 2011, 2014, Toumey 2013).

In addition to the above-mentioned areas of medicine, nanobiomaterials are also extensively used in nanogene medicine, radiosensitizer in radiation therapy, skin regeneration, cartilage regeneration, etc. Thus, nanobiomaterials can be considered as a rising potential material in the field of nanomedicine and can be considered as an alternate for many toxic traditional materials (Figure 1.2).

1.4 NANOBIOMATERIALS IN DRUG DELIVERY

Drug-related research has long focused on the discovery of natural products for treating diseases and the synthesis of pharmacologically active, potent agents to replicate natural substances which can help manage and cure diseases. However, in recent decades, it has become apparent that the efficacy of traditional drugs is dependent on methods of drug formulation and delivery within the human body. Conventionally used natural and synthetic compounds are limited by biological barriers at the surface of living cells, drug resistance, and drug clearance by natural processes. The use of large-sized molecules for drug delivery also poses challenges such as poor solubility, non-specific delivery, in vivo instability, and degradation due to patient-specific factors such as temperature, pH, moisture, cellular uptake and metabolism, probable toxicity, excretion and clearance, and short circulating half-lives, among others. As the pharmaceutical and biotechnology industries continue to develop new classes of biopharmaceuticals, improved understanding of the drug delivery barriers in vivo and challenges related to drug delivery and absorption has given rise to research efforts focused on the design, implementation, and translation of biomaterials for drug delivery (Patra et al. 2018).

Along with the development of new classes of biopharmaceuticals and new delivery technologies, improved fundamental understanding of how drug delivery affects safety and efficacy is needed. Drug delivery remains a prominent challenge, including our limited understanding of biological barriers that limit drug delivery. These unmet needs and limitations have given rise to considerable research efforts focused on the design, implementation, and translation of biomaterials for drug delivery (Fenton et al. 2018). Nanotechnology thus plays a significant role in advanced medicine, by helping design new drug delivery systems for targeted drug delivery and controlled drug release (Stoicea et al. 2017).

1.4.1 Advantages of NP Drug Carriers

Over the past decade, advances in nanotechnology, organic and synthetic chemistry, and biotechnology have driven the development of drug delivery systems. The first NPs were developed at the end of the 20th century. These served as carriers for vaccines and cancer chemotherapeutic agents (Boyan et al. 1999). Nowadays, nanobioparticles are approved by the US Food and Drug Administration (FDA) and are used for a wide range of biological and biomedical applications, from artificial implants to drug delivery to medical imaging (Yang et al. 2011). Use of nanobiomaterials has also improved the delivery and efficiency of various pharmaceutical compounds including drugs, enzymes, vaccines, antibodies, and peptides, among others (Afzal et al. 2022).

The various advantages of using nanobiomaterials for drug delivery are as follows:

i. They can circumvent the natural barriers faced by drugs during movement from their site of introduction to the molecular site of action. The polymeric nanostructures of nanobiomaterials can be used to guide them through biological barriers at the surface of living cells and to escape drug resistance and drug clearance by natural processes.
ii. They can be designed to release therapeutics for extended periods of time, therefore avoiding the number of required dosages.
iii. By decreasing the number of required doses nanobiomaterials can help improve patient adherence, which ranges around 50% even in developed nations (Traverso & Langer 2015).
iv. Specific locations inside the body can be targeted, which helps reduce the amount of drug required for therapeutic effect. This in turn helps lower probability of toxicity for the patient (Langer 1998).
v. For targeting drugs to specific tissues and cells within the body, ligands that bind to surface molecules or receptors overexpressed in diseased cells and tissues are selected for and conjugated to the nanobiomaterials. This helps to ensure retention and uptake of the drugs by specific diseased cells and tissues and avoid off-target effects (Afzal et al. 2022, Langer 1998).
vi. Nanobiomaterials can be directly implanted or injected to specific diseased tissue location, which ensures controlled drug release over days to years, and such targeted long therapeutic windows also help limit off-target effects, thereby increasing potency.
vii. Controlled release systems also help to avoid rise and fall in concentration of drug dosage in the body; this helps reduce the total amount of drug required for attaining the required therapeutic effect and ideally protects drugs from clearance and degradation within the body by staying in circulation for too long (Afzal et al. 2022, Schneider et al. 2017).
viii. Different routes of administration can be selected to maximize therapeutic benefits, and the physicochemical properties of nanobiomaterials can be tailored accordingly. Nanobiomaterials have enhanced drug delivery, via various intended routes, including oral, transdermal, pulmonary, transdermal, ocular, and also nasal routes, where each route has its own advantages (Fenton et al. 2018).
ix. 3D nanostructured scaffolds can bio-mimic native biological systems, serving as structural and/or mechanical support for cellular function and tissue regeneration. They can also

be modified to carry and deliver specific drugs, and suppress microbial infection after implantation (Yang et al. 2011).

x. The nanobiomaterials themselves and their degradation products can be tailored to minimize or avoid patient discomfort, by being biocompatible within the body and being non-toxic (Fenton et al. 2018).

1.4.2 Ways of Drug Delivery by Nanomaterials

Targeted drug delivery by NPs is one of the major advantages, and this can be achieved in the following ways:

i. *Passive Targeting*: Diseased tissues display altered physiology, characterized by enhanced permeability and retention (EPR) effect. Passive targeting uses this EPR effect to deliver drugs to specific diseased tissues, whose anatomy varies from normal tissues. Localized delivery is another sub-approach where direct intratumour delivery of anticancer agents is achieved using nanobiomaterials. This method is used in the treatment of local cancers, such as head and neck, and prostate cancers (Parveen et al. 2012).
ii. *Active Targeting*: This method relies on molecular recognition of the diseased cells by various signature molecules. Diseased sites have an overexpression of such molecules and it is recognized via antigen-antibody interactions, ligand-receptor complex, or by aptamers. The size of NPs and their ability to conjugate different ligands helps to break physiological barriers and access different targeted sites in the body. The nanosized carrier can also be coupled with a ligand specific to particular cell or tissue, which allows for accumulation of the drug at the targeted diseased site, while aptamers are either DNA or RNA oligonucleotide sequences that can selectively bind to targets with high specificity and affinity (Parveen et al. 2012).

Besides these methods, there are some other generalized methods of drug delivery for NPs. Some of such methods are briefly discussed below:

a. *Encapsulation and Covalent Bond Mechanism*: The NPs may transport and deliver the drug through encapsulating it or holding it in a stabilizing pocket. In the other mechanism, the NPs may form covalent bond with the drug and transport it to the target. The release of the drug occurs after the breakdown of the covalent bond.
b. The drug can also be transported and delivered at the target site by holding it in some hydrophobic pockets on the surface of NPs. This method is found to be very efficient and compatible to use.
c. Different nanomaterials are sensitive towards different factors such as pH, temperature, and light. Due to this characteristic of nanomaterials, they are widely used for controlled drug delivery induced by light, pH, or temperature (Doane et al. 2012).

1.4.3 Biomaterials Used for Drug Delivery System

The selection of nanobiomaterials for drug delivery purpose depends upon different factors such as the physiochemical properties of the drug and the material as well as on the route through which it is administered. There are mainly two types of polymeric nanobiomaterials commonly used in drug delivery system which are briefly discussed as follows:

a. *Natural-Based Polymeric Biomaterials*: Chitosan, a natural polymer found in the exoskeleton of crustacean and fungal cell walls, is extensively used for drug delivery due to its better solubility, biocompatibility, enhanced permeability, and stronger mucoadhesive properties. Chitosan-based delivery systems range from microparticles to NP composites and films. The poor solubility of chitosan at physiological pH is a major drawback in the use of chitosan for drug delivery systems. But to overcome this and other inherent drawbacks, various derivatives of chitosan are used. Along with the parental compound, chitosan modified through hydroxylation, acylation, and sulphonation shows higher efficacy in the drug delivery system (Elgadir et al. 2015). Another promising material of this group is hyaluronic acid which is known for its better solubility and biocompatibility. It is also naturally found in vitreous humour, extracellular matrix, and in synovial fluid of vertebrates. Due to its capability to bind cancer cells, it is widely used in the drug delivery system for targeted tumour delivery and imaging (Yu et al. 2013). Albumin, which is naturally found in blood, is also used as a drug carrier and it owes its popularity in this field due to its high solubility, beneficial charge, and physiological transport mechanism (Mariam et al. 2016). In addition to these materials, phospholipids, alginate, and cellulose are some examples of natural polymeric biomaterials used in drug delivery.

b. *Synthetic-Based Polymeric Biomaterials*: Synthetic polymeric biomaterials are placed one step ahead of natural polymeric biomaterials because of their better reproducibility, homogeneous composition, and better controllable mechanical properties and degradation rates. PLGA is one such polymeric biomaterial which can be synthesized from lactic and glycolic acid or from their diesters. It is also comparatively easier to process PLGA into different device morphologies as compared to other polymers and these PLGA particles in the form of microcapsules, nanocapsules, nanospheres, nanofibres, nanomesh, etc. can be utilized for controlled release of drugs. Drug molecules are variously released from this polymeric matrix, using different mechanism such as by diffusion through the matrix, desorption from surface, erosion, and also combined erosion diffusion processes. Because of its biocompatibility, biodegradability, and sustained release properties, PLGA has been approved by the US FDA for several therapeutic applications. It is used for controlled drug release in surgical implants, various small molecule drugs, anti-inflammatory drugs, chemotherapeutics, antibiotics, insulin, and vaccines and also for various peptides and proteins such as steroid hormones and fertility hormones (Kapoor et al. 2015). Poly(glutamic acid) is another such material which owes the potentiality in this field due to its biocompatible and biodegradable nature, non-toxicity, and water solubility. It is a preferable material for delivering drug in the human body because of its non-susceptibility to proteases. Biobased capsules formulated from poly(glutamic acid) were found to be ideal for self-regulated release of insulin in the body. The capsules could be triggered to release insulin based on external glucose concentrations, providing good stability and synchronized glucose response in the body (Shi et al. 2016).

Polymeric biomaterials are used for preparation of nanocarriers that will carry the drug into the human body. Depending upon the targeted location and the administered route of the drug, the selection of the polymeric biomaterials as nanocarrier may be different. For example, liposomes which are composed of a lipid or phospholipid are used to deliver many drugs such as anticancer and antimicrobial agents, peptide hormones, vaccines, genetic materials, enzymes, and proteins to the target tissues. Liposome-based drug delivery systems offer a range of advantages including controlled and sustained release of drugs, while also protecting the drugs from degradation and being cleared from the biological system, specific site targeting, better therapeutic effects combined with lower toxic side effects. Doxorubicin-loaded liposome has already been approved by the FDA and is used for the treatment of various cancers. But efficiency of such liposome-based drug vesicles is affected by various factors, such as internal and external stimuli, the microenvironment at the target site, and intracellular uptake. In studies done with doxorubicin-loaded liposomes, cytotoxicity and release rates were found to be affected by intracellular uptake and variation in lipid composition (Sakai-Kato et al. 2015). Albumin and PLGA-based nanobiomaterials are mostly used to deliver anticancer drugs because of their stability and controlled drug release capacity near tumour site. Similarly, NPs of doxorubicin-loaded hyaluronic acid-glycyrrhetinic acid succinate were found to have higher tumour and liver targeting efficiency. Design and construction of such liver-targeted NPs are necessary for the targeted treatment of hepatocytes, as liver cancer becomes a growing problem due to high mortality and morbidity globally. Such NP-based drug delivery systems are also useful in prolonging blood circulation time of associated drugs, reducing toxicity and also enhancing cell targeting efficiency. Furthermore, chitosan-based nanomaterials are also being used in the delivery of anticancer agents, proteins, peptides, and as nanocarriers for gene therapy (Wang et al. 2018). Polymer micelles are also useful as nanocarriers for delivering a number of drugs in the human body such as cytostatic agents and nucleic acids, due to their enhanced mechanical and colloidal properties and better stability (Ohya et al. 2011).

All these nanobiomaterials exhibit excellent efficacy as carriers in drug delivery system which in turn helps overcome a number of difficulties in drug delivery system, which are encountered with traditional approaches. Due to the low molecular size of NPs, they are capable of drug delivery to previously inaccessible body sites. In addition to these, they allow targeted drug delivery to the desired destination, with consequent minimal systemic toxicity and side effects.

1.5 FUTURE PROSPECTS OF NANOBIOMATERIALS IN NANOMEDICINE AND DRUG DELIVERY

It is established that nanobiomaterials are one of the significant milestones in the advancement of nanomedicine and drug delivery. They have established themselves as one of the potential stakeholders in this field within a short period of time. Researchers have been continuing to explore and trying to remove the limitations of these nanobiomaterials and there is a diverse possible trend of development for these materials in the near future. Although nanobiomaterials have achieved a revolutionary development in the field of nanomedicine and drug delivery, the safety and toxicity of these materials towards human body are still major concerns. Therefore, it is very necessary to further investigate the safety and adverse effects of nanobiomaterials on both human body and the environment from all aspects. It is also observed that most of the synthesized nanobiomaterials are made for a specific single-use purpose. Thus, research is needed to focus on the development of nanobiomaterials with multi-functional capability. Furthermore, it is very necessary to investigate the mechanism of action of these materials in detail, i.e., the mechanisms of their interaction with the biological system of human body which will help to remove the limitations and to improvise the materials for making them fully biocompatible.

1.6 CONCLUSION

Nanobiomaterials have achieved a significant growth in both nanomedicine and drug delivery for their efficiency and better compatibility. They are also specific and selective to a great extent because of their stability over long periods and also their small size. They have significantly contributed towards improving the quality of human life by effectively treating patients within a short period of time in comparison to the traditional approaches. However, efforts must be given for making these materials fully biocompatible and for revealing the mechanism of actions of these materials in the human body. Thus, nanobiomaterials can be an alternative pathway for the treatment of various diseases and for the overall development of the pharmaceutical industry over the traditional approaches.

REFERENCES

Afzal, O., Altamimi, A.S., Nadeem, M.S., Alzarea, S.I., Almalki, W.H., Tariq, A., Mubeen, B., Murtaza, B.N., Iftikhar, S., Riaz, N. and Kazmi, I., 2022. Nanoparticles in drug delivery: From history to therapeutic applications. *Nanomaterials* 12(24):4494.

Baker, S.C., Atkin, N., Gunning, P.A., Granville, N., Wilson, K., Wilson, D. and Southgate, J. 2006. Characterisation of electrospun polystyrene scaffolds for three-dimensional in vitro biological studies. *Biomaterials* 27:3136–3146.

Boyan, B.D., Sylvia, V.L., Liu, Y., Sagun, R., Cochran, D.L., Lohmann, C.H., Dean, D.D. and Schwartz, Z., 1999. Surface roughness mediates its effects on osteoblasts via protein kinase A and phospholipase A_2. *Biomaterials* 20(23–24):2305–2310.

Bradley, E.L., Castle, L. and Chaudhry, Q., 2011. Applications of nanomaterials in food packaging with a consideration of opportunities for developing countries. *Trends Food Sci. Technol.* 22(11):604–610.

Campos, E.V.R., Pereira, A.E.S., De Oliveira, J.L., Carvalho, L.B., Guilger-Casagrande, M., De Lima, R. and Fraceto, L.F., 2020. How can nanotechnology help to combat COVID-19? Opportunities and urgent need. *J. Nanobiotechnol.* 18:1–23.

Choudhary, S., Haberstroh, K.M, and Webster, T.J. 2007. Enhanced functions of vascular cells on nanostructured Ti for improved stent applications. *Tissue Eng.* 13:1421–1430.

Doane, T.L. and Burda, C. 2012. The unique role of nanoparticles in nanomedicine: Imaging, drug delivery and therapy. *Chem. Soc. Rev.* 41(7):2885–2911.

Elgadir, M.A., Uddin, M.S., Ferdosh, S., Adam, A., Chowdhury, A.J.K. and Sarker, M.Z.I. 2015. Impact of chitosan composites and chitosan nanoparticle composites on various drug delivery systems: A review. *J. Food Drug Anal.* 23:619–629.

Ellah, N.H.A., Tawfeek, H.M., John, J. and Hetta, H.F., 2019. Nanomedicine as a future therapeutic approach for hepatitis C virus. *Nanomedicine* 14:1471–1491.

Fenton, O.S., Olafson, K.N., Pillai, P.S., Mitchell, M.J. and Langer, R. 2018. Advances in biomaterials for drug delivery. *Adv. Mater.* 30(29):1705328.

Ge, L., Li, Q., Wang, M., Ouyang, J., Li, X. and Xing, M.M. 2014. Nanosilver particles in medical applications: Synthesis, performance, and toxicity. *Int. J. Nanomed.* 9:2399–2407.

Gomathi, T., Sudha, P.N. and Thomas, S. eds., 2023. Nanobiomaterials*: Research Trends and Applications.* CRC Press/Taylor & Francis Group, Boca Raton.

Holzinger, M., Le Goff, A. and Cosnier, S., 2014. Nanomaterials for biosensing applications: A review. *Front. Chem.* 2:63–73.

Hosseinkhani, H., Hosseinkhani, M., Khademhosseini, A. and Kobayashi, H. 2007. Bone regeneration through controlled release of bone morphogeneticprotein-2 from 3-D tissue engineered nano-scaffold. *J. Control Release* 117:380–386.

Kapoor, D.N., Bhatia, A., Kaur, R., Sharma, R., Kaur, G. and Dhawan, S. 2015. PLGA: A unique polymer for drug delivery. *Ther Deliv* 6:41–58.

Khot, L.R., Sankaran, S., Maja, J.M., Ehsani, R. and Schuster, E.W., 2012. Applications of nanomaterials in agricultural production and crop protection: A review. *Crop Prot.* 35:64–70.

Kim, K.-H., Kwon, T.-Y., Kim, S.-Y., Kang, I.-K., Kim, S., Yang, Y. and Ong, J.L. 2006. Preparation and characterization of anodized titanium surfaces and their effect on osteoblast responses. *J. Oral Implantol.* 32:8–13.

Langer, R., 1998. Drug delivery and targeting. *Nature* 392(6679 Suppl):5–10.

Lee, S.J., Yoo, J.J., Lim, G.J., Atala, A. and Stitze, J. 2007. In vitro evaluation of electrospun nanofiber scaffolds for vascular graft application. *J. Biomed. Mater. Res. A* 83A:999–1008.

Li, H., Mu, Y., Lu, J., Wei, W., Wan, Y. and Liu, S. 2014. Target-cell-specific fluorescence silica nanoprobes for imaging and theranostics of cancer cells. *Anal. Chem.* 86:3602–3609.

Li, M., Li, R., Li, C.M. and Wu, N. 2011. Electrochemical and optical biosensors based on nanomaterials and nanostructures: A review. *Front. Biosci. (Schol. Ed.)* 3:1308–1331.

Liu, H., Slamovich, E.B. and Webster, T.J. 2006. Increased osteoblast functions among nanophase titania/poly(lactide-co-glycolide) composites of the highest nanometer surface roughness. *J. Biomed. Mater. Res. A* 798:807.

Mageswari, A., Srinivasan, R., Subramanian, P., Ramesh, N. and Gothandam, K.M. 2016. Nanomaterials: Classification, biological synthesis and characterization. In Ranjan, S., Dasgupta, N., Lichtfouse, E. (eds) *Nanoscience in Food and Agriculture 3. Sustainable Agriculture Reviews*, vol. 23. Springer, Cham.

Manzano, M. and Vallet-Regí, M. 2020. Mesoporous silica nanoparticles for drug delivery. *Adv. Funct. Mater.* 30:1902634.

Mariam, J., Sivakami, S. and Dongre, P.M. 2016. Albumin corona on nanoparticles - a strategic approach in drug delivery. *Drug Deliv* 23:2668–2676.

Mattson, M.P., Haddon, R.C. and Rao, A.M. 2000. Molecular functionalization of carbon nanotubes and use as substrates for neuronal growth. *J. Mol.* Neurosci. 14:175–182.

Mehmood, S., Rehman, M.A., Ismail, H., Mirza, B. and Bhatti, A.S. 2015. Significance of postgrowth processing of ZnO nanostructures on antibacterial activity against gram-positive and gram-negative bacteria. *Int. J. Nanomedicine* 10:4521–4533.

Nagano, F., Selimovic, D., Noda, M., Ikeda, T., Tanaka, T., Miyamoto, Y., Koshiro, K. and Sano, H. 2009. Improved bond performance of a dental adhesive system using nano-technology. *Bio.-Med. Mater.* Eng. 19:249–257.

Ohya, Y., Takeda, S., Shibata, Y., Ouchi, T., Kano, A., Iwata, T., Mochizuki, S., Taniwaki, Y. and Maruyama, A. 2011. Evaluation of polyanion-coated biodegradable polymeric micelles as drug delivery vehicles. *J Control Release* 155:104–110.

Parveen, S., Misra, R. and Sahoo, S.K. 2012. Nanoparticles: A boon to drug delivery, therapeutics, diagnostics and imaging. *Nanomed.: Nanotechnol. Biol. Med.* 8(2):147–166.

Patra, J.K., Das, G., Fraceto, L.F., Campos, E.V.R., Rodriguez-Torres, M.D.P., Acosta-Torres, L.S., Diaz-Torres, L.A., Grillo, R., Swamy, M.K., Sharma, S. and Habtemariam, S. 2018. Nano based drug delivery systems: Recent developments and future prospects. *J. Nanobiotechnol.* 16(1):71.

Rai, M., Yadav, A. and Gade, A. 2009. Silver nanoparticles as a new generation of antimicrobials. *Biotechnol. Adv.* 27:76–83.

Ranjan, A. and Webster, T.J. 2009. Increased endothelial cell adhesion and elongation on micron-patterned nano-rough poly(dimethylsiloxane) films. *Nanotechnology* 20:305102.

Razavi, M., Zhu, K. and Zhang, Y. S. 2017. Naturally based and biologically derived nanobiomaterials. In *Nanobiomaterials Science, Development and Evaluation* (pp. 61–86). Woodhead Publishing, Sawston, UK.

Sakai-Kato, K., Nanjo, K., Kawanishi, T., Okuda, H. and Goda, Y. 2015. Effects of lipid composition on the properties of doxorubicin-loaded liposomes. *Ther Deliv* 6:785–794.

Schiavi, S., Ocampo-Pineda, M., Barakovic, M.; Petit, L., Descoteaux, M., Thiran, J.-P. and Daducci, A. 2020. A new method for accurate in vivo mapping of human brain connections using microstructural and anatomical information. *Sci. Adv.* 6:eaba8245.

Schneider, C., Langer, R., Loveday, D. and Hair, D., 2017. Applications of ethylene vinyl acetate copolymers (EVA) in drug delivery systems. *J. Contr. Release* 262:284–295.

Shi, D., Ran, M., Zhang, L, Huang, H., Li, X., Chen, M. and Akashi, M. 2016. Fabrication of biobased polyelectrolyte capsules and their application for glucose-triggered insulin delivery. *ACS Appl Mater Interfaces* 8:13688–13697.

Singh, S.K., Kulkarni, P.P. and Dash, D., 2013. Biomedical applications of nanomaterials: An overview. In Debasis Bagchi, Manashi Bagchi, Hiroyoshi Moriyama, Fereidoon Shahidi (Eds.), *Bio-Nanotechnology: A Revolution in Food. Biomedical and Health* Sciences (pp. 1–32), Wiley-Blackwell, Chichester, UK.

Singh, T.G. and Sharma, N., 2016. Nanobiomaterials in cosmetics: Current status and future prospects. In Alexandru Mihai Grumezescu (ed.), *Nanobiomaterials in Galenic Formulations and Cosmetics* (pp. 149–174), William Andrew Publishing (Elsevier imprint), New York, USA.

Stoicea, N., Fiorda-Diaz, J., Joseph, N., Shabsigh, M., Arias-Morales, C., Gonzalez-Zacarias, A.A., Mavarez-Martinez, A., Marjoribanks, S. and Bergese, S.D. 2017. Advanced analgesic drug delivery and nanobiotechnology. *Drugs* 77(10):1069–1076.

Sua, H., Wanga, Y., Gua, Y., Bowmanb, L., Zhaoa, J. and Ding, M. 2018. Potential applications and human biosafety of nanomaterials used in nanomedicine. *J. Appl. Toxicol.* 38:3–18.

Thapa, A., Miller, D.C., Webster, T.J. and Haberstroh, K.M. 2003. Nano-structured polymers enhance bladder smooth muscle cell function. *Biomaterials* 24:2915–2926.

Toumey C. 2013. Nanobots today. *Nat. Nanotechnol.* 8:475–476.

Tran, P. A., Sarin, L., Hurt, R.H. and Webster, T.J. 2010. Titanium surfaces with adherent selenium nanoclusters as a novel anticancer orthopedic material. *J. Biomed. Mater. Res. A* 93:1417–1528.

Traverso, G. and Langer, R., 2015. Engineering precision. *Sci. Transl. Med.* 7(289):289ed6.

Velu, R., Calais, T., Jayakumar, A. and Raspall, F., 2019. A comprehensive review on bio-nanomaterials for medical implants and feasibility studies on fabrication of such implants by additive manufacturing technique. *Materials* 13(1):92–125.

Wang, X., Gu, X., Wang, H., Yang, J. and Mao, S. 2018. Enhanced delivery of doxorubicin to the liver through self-assembled nanoparticles formed via conjugation of glycyrrhetinic acid to the hydroxyl group of hyaluronic acid. *Carbohydr. Polym.* 195:170–179

Yang, L., Sheldon, B.W. and Webster, T.J. 2009. Orthopedic nano diamond coatings: Control of surface properties and their impact on osteoblast adhesion and proliferation. *J. Biomed. Mater. Res. A* 91:548–556.
Yang, L., Zhang, L. and Webster, T.J. 2011. Nanobiomaterials state of the art and future trends. *Adv. Eng. Mater.* 13(6):B197–B217.
Yu, M., Jambhrunkar, S., Thorn, P., Chen, J., Gu, W. and Yu, C. 2013. Hyaluronic acid modified mesoporous silica nanoparticles for targeted drug delivery to CD44-overexpressing cancer cells. *Nanoscale* 5:178–183.
Zaman, M., Good, M.F. and Toth, I. 2013. Nanovaccines and their mode of action. *Methods* 60:226–231.
Zhang, L., Chun, Y.W. and Webster, T.J. 2010. Decreased lung carcinoma cell density on select polymer nanometer surface features for lung replacement therapies. *Int. J. Nanomed.* 5:269–275.
Zhao, J.X., Xu, L.J., Zhang, T., Ren, G.G. and Yang, Z. 2009. Influences of nanoparticle zinc oxide on acutely isolated rat hippocampal CA3 pyramidal neurons. *Neurotoxicology* 30:220–230.

2 Nanoparticles for Tissue Engineering and Regenerative Medicines

Mohsina Afrooz
MEMS, Microfluidics and Nanoelectronics Laboratory (MMNE Lab), BITS-Pilani, Hyderabad, India

2.1 INTRODUCTION: BACKGROUND AND DRIVING FORCES

It has been a dream for mankind to fully repair or regenerate damaged tissues and restore their functions effectively. The alternative approach to transplantation is to restore or make an organ functional which has been lost due to age, damage, disease, or congenital defects; a global challenge to explore innovative solutions by scientists was started when they clubbed tissue engineering and regenerative medicine (TERM). TERM has been proving itself as one of the promising and evolved steps towards the future needs of humankind. Tissue engineering has quite evolved in the last decade by regenerating almost every tissue from stem cells. The enormous applaudable discoveries were the artificial skin for the people with burns, cartilage for knee replacement, artificial blood vessels generated using tissue engineering, urinary bladder replacement, cellular therapy, etc. Tissue engineering is gaining popularity due to its application of technologies in nanomedicine such as computer-aided design (CAD) and 3D bioprinting tools. Due to never-ending demand for artificial organs at present, tissue engineering is emerging to be the single point-of-care solution for mankind.[1] Tissue engineering follows some general methods such as cell substitution into organism with or without scaffold, implantation of isolated cells, and tissue-inducing biologics. Scaffold is a 3D structure made up of nanofibres, biodegradable materials which provide support, adhesion, nutrition to the tissues along with proper structure to the organ to be regenerated.[2] This porous 3D biomaterial allows gas exchange, cell proliferation, cell differentiation, and promotes cell-biomaterial interactions (Figure 2.1).

Regenerative medicine is the process of curing the wounded organ either by replacing or by regenerating tissues or organs to restore the normal functioning of the body. This process stimulates the body's natural capability to revert to its normalcy. Regenerative medicine involves stem cells to provide clinical therapies. These therapies can be performed either by injecting stem cells called cell therapy or by administrating biologically active molecules called immunomodulation therapy.[3] Out of these approaches, tissue engineering has captured the attention due to its multiple successful attempts in regenerative medicine. Today, these two terms are together referred as "Tissue Engineering and Regenerative Medicine" or in short "TERM" (Figure 2.2).

TERM aims to create a three-dimensional scaffold made up of biomaterials which will help in growing tissues/organs in laboratories from stem cells to regenerate failed organs/tissues. The scaffold needs to be biocompatible to provide cell-biomaterial interaction, which is biodegradable to easily provide the shape and remove itself from the organ after transplantation and non-toxic to avoid any reactions with the physiological systems of the body. It should also be porous, able to provide nutrition, gas exchange, cell differentiation, and cell growth in the given shape.[4]

Nanoparticles (NPs) are the bridge between micromolecules and macromolecules varying in size between 1 and 100 nm in every dimension. The unique size of NPs makes it attractive due to its high

 DOI: 10.1201/9781003473015-2

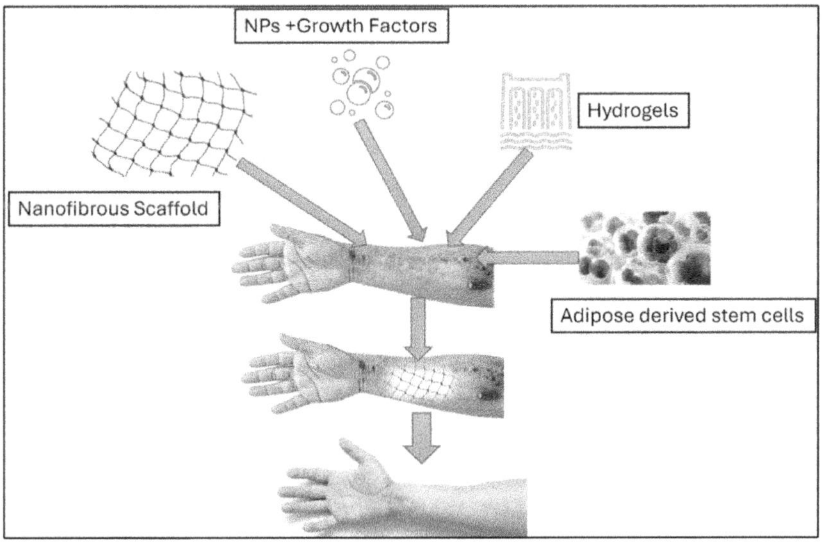

FIGURE 2.1 Process of tissue engineering in regenerative medicine.

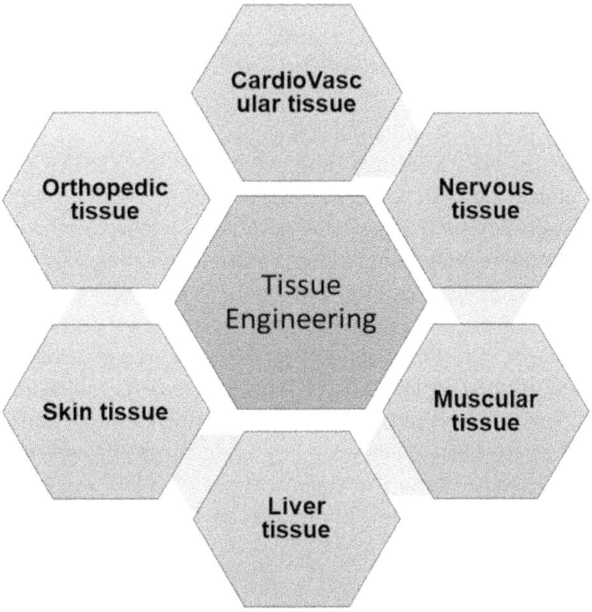

FIGURE 2.2 TERM in various applications.

surface-to-volume ratio. These NPs possess quantum effect which allows extreme control over surface energy of NPs which can regulate cellular interaction and are differentiated based on its vast range of compositions from soft to hard materials. NPs can have zero-dimensional (0D) to three-dimensional (3D) structures based on their shape. Based on their composition, NPs are divided into different types such as semiconductor-based, ceramic-based, polymeric-based, and metal-based. Top-down and bottom-up are the two main approaches of synthesizing NPs, furthermore dividing into chemical, biological, and mechanical synthesis processes. Chemical synthesis can be performed by precipitation method, emulsion method, sol-gel method, chemical vapour deposition, etc. Mechanical method

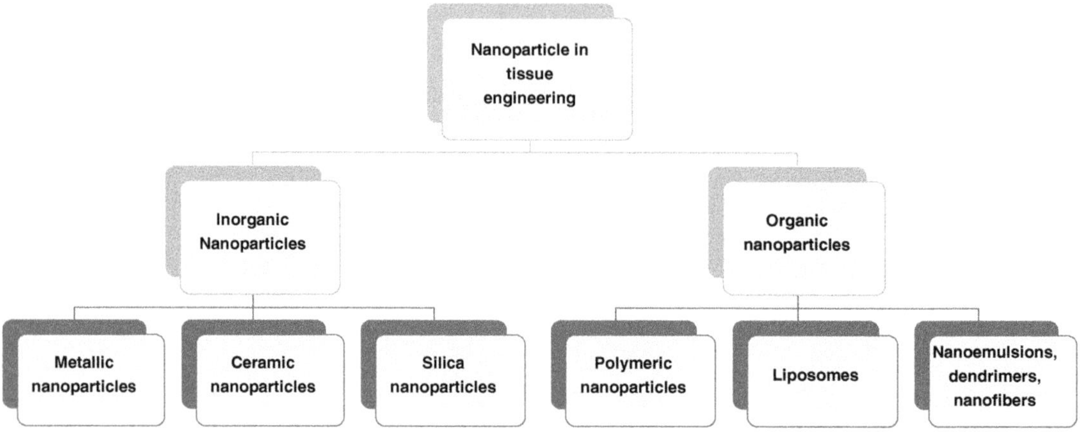

FIGURE 2.3 Various nanoparticles used in TERM.

of synthesis can be achieved by mechanical grinding method, ball and reactive milling method, mechanical milling method, etc. Similarly, biological synthesis can be achieved by bio-polymerization, green synthesis, biomineralization, etc.[5] After synthesis, nanomaterials are characterized based on its composition and types using various analytical equipment such as polarized optical microscope (POM), X-ray diffraction (XRD), scanning electron microscope (SEM), atomic force microscopy (AFM), transmission electron microscopy (TEM), Fourier transform infrared (FT-IR) spectroscopy, and ultraviolet spectroscopy.[6] The synthesized particles are used in fields such as nanoelectronics, biomedical sciences, optics, and environmental sciences.

The amusing properties of NPs have a significant impact on TERM, especially because of the demand of control over nanoscale systems. NPs have helped in overcoming the restrictions faced by TERM with its diverse properties such as targeted stimuli response, controllable size, precise control over behaviour when subjected to magnetic field or external stimulus, low toxicity, tailorable characteristics, and contrasting agent properties. To exert control over engineered tissue, some factors that play major roles are contrast agents in a controlled manner and local delivery of bioactive agents such as chemokines, growth factors, cytokines, and genes.[7] High degree of control over spatial, biological, and temporal events is required to replace a functional tissue or organ. Along with the control over spatial and temporal properties of NPs, control over real-time monitoring is very important for the delivery of growth factors or contrast agents for imaging and controlling scaffold properties.

In this chapter, we will discuss about the various types of NPs used in TERM for the treatment of different organs either by replacement or by healing or transplanting (Figure 2.3).

2.2 TYPES OF NPS USED IN TERM

Types of NPs used in TERM are inorganic and organic NPs.

2.2.1 Inorganic NPs

Inorganic NPs used in TERM are composed of metallic NPs, ceramic NPs, silica NPs (SiNPs), etc. Gold nanoparticles (AuNPs), SiNPs, and hydroxyapatite (HA) NPs are widely used inorganic formulations for TERM.

2.2.1.1 Gold NPs

These NPs are famous for their excellent biocompatibility. They are easy to functionalize. These NPs are primarily used in osteogenesis for bone cell therapy and angiogenesis for blood vessel applications. In tissue engineering, AuNPs are used as growth factors, or for supporting cell proliferation and promoting tissue regrowth. Some of the major roles of AuNPs in tissue engineering are promotion of cell adhesion and cell proliferation where AuNPs are added with the polymer matrices of the scaffolds to enhance biocompatibility of the cell with the scaffold, which leads to increased cellular interactions. AuNPs are also used for osteogenic differentiation in bone tissue engineering where AuNPs help stem cells differentiate into osteoblasts, i.e., bone regeneration. AuNPs are also used in neural tissue and cardiac tissue engineering where they promote the electrical conductivity of scaffolds by supporting signal transmission in electroactive tissues. AuNPs are functionalized and embedded in scaffolds for specific and controlled delivery of growth factors to aid tissue regeneration.

From a rehabilitation engineering point of view, AuNPs are vital for regenerative therapies such as neuroregeneration where AuNPs enhance the neurite outgrowth to repair the damaged nerve tissues by neural stem cell differentiation. AuNPs also work as anti-inflammatory agents for tissue recovery after injury or surgery. Theranostic applications of AuNPs include localized photothermal therapy for treating fibrosis and the cells used in photoacoustic imaging such as computed tomography or magnetic resonance imaging (MRI). AuNPs can be incorporated into biomaterials to support healing muscle injuries by promoting muscle regeneration through inflammatory response angiogenesis. Some examples of AuNPs are AuNP-functionalized hydrogels for cardiovascular applications, AuNP-loaded nanofibres for peripheral nerve repair, and muscle tissue rehabilitation through AuNP-assisted electrical stimulation.[8]

2.2.1.2 Silica NPs

These NPs offer greater surface areas and porosity. These properties make them ideal for applications such as drug delivery and biomolecule activation. SiNPs show biodegradability, biocompatibility, and stability. These NPs can mimic the scaffolds, thereby promoting cell proliferation and release of bioactive agents. SiNPs play important roles in bone tissue engineering by enhancing bioactivity through mimicking bone mineral structures, thereby promoting HA formation. SiNPs also facilitate stem cell differentiation via osteogenic differentiation of mesenchymal stem cells (MSCs). SiNPs also promote scaffold reinforcement by improving strength and porosity of the polymeric scaffolds such as polylactic acid (PLA) or polycaprolactone (PCL). Mesoporous SiNPs also actively take part in the delivery of growth factors such as bone morphogenetic proteins (BMPs), vascular endothelial growth factor (VEGF), antibiotics, and anti-inflammatory agents due to their high surface-to-volume ratio.[9] SiNPs are vastly used for coating of implants or scaffolds, for increasing cell adhesion to the scaffold, and for tissue integration and antibacterial resistance.

From a rehabilitation point of view, SiNPs can deliver neural growth factors called neurotrophic factors for neural regeneration via axon regrowth, or they can be used in conjunction with hydrogels or conductive polymers for peripheral nerve repair or spinal cord repair. SiNPs can be loaded with anti-inflammatory agents such as insulin-like growth factor (IGF)-1 embedded in hydrogels and injected to injured muscle tissue for tissue regeneration. For theranostic applications, SiNPs can be used for delivering therapeutic agents and also as imaging agents as MRI contrast to monitor the rehabilitation progress.

2.2.1.3 Ceramics

Calcium phosphate-based materials are important for bone and teeth in TERM. HA-calcium-phosphate-based scaffolds are optimum for cell proliferation and osteogenic differentiation.[10] A great potential has been seen in calcium silicate materials for bone regeneration and cartilage regeneration. Bioactive glass contains ions such as Si, Ca, and P and has the stimulating effect of bone metabolism and osteogenesis. Mesoporous bioactive glass scaffolds can even promote the process of biomineralization (Figure 2.4).[11]

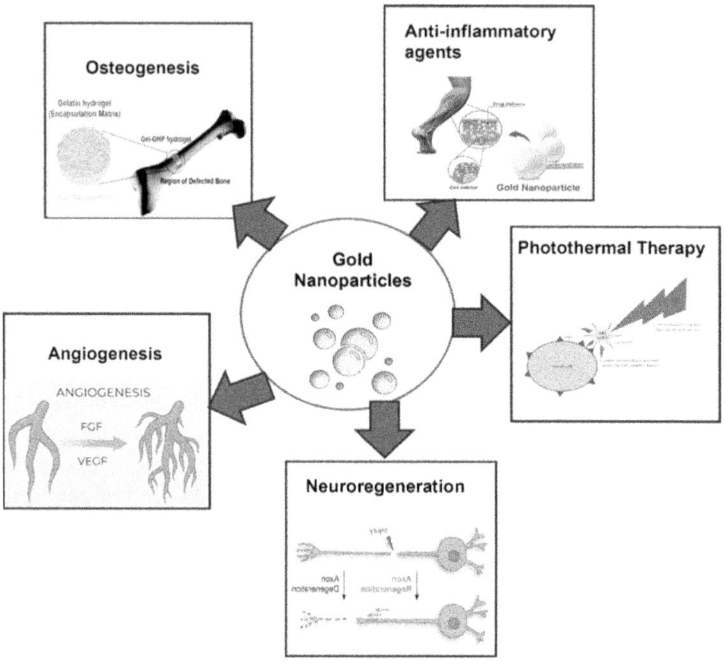

FIGURE 2.4 Application of gold nanoparticles in TERM.

2.2.2 Organic NPs

Organic NPs used in TERM are mainly categorized into polymeric NPs, liposomes, and various nanoemulsions.[12]

2.2.2.1 Polymeric NPs

Polymeric NPs have attracted an increased interest in osteogenic applications due to their biodegradability, tuneable properties, and high biocompatibility with loaded drugs. Specifically, the growth factors can be loaded with various polymers to deliver to the MSCs. For example, growth factors such as BMP-2 and BMP-7 can be loaded to polymers such as chitosan and poly(lactic-co-glycolic acid) (PLGA) to improve the cell differentiation profile.[13] Chitosan can also be used for delivering dexamethasone for gene expression and calcium deposition to MSCs, which results in bone-healing effect.[14]

2.2.2.2 Liposomes

Liposome formulations have found increased applications in osteogenesis for bone regeneration, an important part for TERM. Liposomes are used for preventing the metastasis of bone cancer by delivering cytotoxic elements to the tumour cells such as doxorubicin or peptide.[15] Liposomes also deliver phytoconstituents that are hydrophobic in nature such as icariin or coumaric acid or curcuminoid to prevent osteoporosis, thereby providing early protection from bone fracture.[16] Osteoporosis can be prevented by inhibiting osteoclast formation and osteoblast differentiation enhancement. Liposomes also enhance bone regeneration and prevent infections at bone injury site.[17] Coated liposome delivers BMP-2, inhibits bacterial biofilms, and provides osteogenic differentiation.[18]

2.2.2.3 Composites

Collagen and HA are the two most common organic–inorganic compounds found in bone. Composite hydrogels are made for bone healing by biomimetic process. These composites are used for bone tissue engineering.[19] Combination of organic–inorganic materials can improve mechanical properties and bioactivity. For example, incorporating Zn oxide NPs into chitosan–collagen porous scaffold enhances biocompatibility and mechanical property.[20] Similarly, incorporating titanium dioxide with chitosan–collagen scaffold increases antimicrobial property and resistance to degradation.

2.3 TECHNOLOGY INCORPORATED WITH TERM

2.3.1 3D Printing

Bioprinting is a method of fabricating engineered tissue through biomolecules or biomaterials. Bioprinting greatly impacted skin tissue engineering. 3D-ECM (extracellular matrix) could be prepared through 3D bioprinting which can promote cell differentiation or even possess the ability to regenerate functional skin.[21] By printing polyethylene glycol diacrylate using ink-jet printer and use of chondrocytes as source cells, engineered human cartilages can be constructed. Alginate, gelatine, and fibrin materials are used for construction of liver, adipose tissue, and nerve tissues.[22] Bioprinting is also widely used in ear reconstruction and functional vascular reconstruction. After cardiac transplantation, for rapid vascularization and cardiac repair, 3D-ECM could be used specially prepared with stem cell patch and bioink. 3D liver micro-organ produced using micropatterning technique could be used as in vitro liver model for drug metabolism.[23]

2.3.2 Genome Editing

The method of making changes to human DNA by either editing, removing, or altering the genome to avoid passing the inherited defective gene or disease-carrying gene from one generation to another is called genome editing. In genome editing, safety of the technology is the primary concern while editing the genome sequence because of highly sensitive DNA strand. The system needs to be very much precise to avoid mutation which may cause cancer or damage organs or even cause death to the patient. CRISPR/Cas is the technology used for genome editing.[24] CRISPR/Cas9 variant incorporated with polyethylene glycolysed NP could be used in genome editing with a higher efficiency. Cas9 variant shows a switched ON–OFF system which can be safely used in "off-switch" state to avoid unwanted mutations while genome editing, and it is accepted as a safe technology so far for genome editing in cells/tissues.[25]

2.3.3 Microfluidics and Organ-on-a-Chip Technology

Microfluidics is a technique to encapsulate various cells in microfibres and microbeads.[26] Microfluidics technology is flexible, and it allows preparation of multi-structured fibres, grooves, and helical and other complex structures. Using capillary array microfluidic technology, cell micro carrier can be constructed using controllable pores and heterogenous structures. Microdroplets using *Escherichia coli* may be used for biotransformation, biosensing, and bioremediation.[27] These microfibres produced using microfluidics technique can mimic human blood vessels and act as nutrition and oxygen carriers in tissues grown in vitro. Microfluidics offers a great advantage in developing organ/tissues in vitro. Here, on a chip, stem cells and other pluripotent cells are put on a scaffold to grow organ/tissue like human organs. These cells are nourished with the help of microfluidic fibres which act like capillaries and carriers providing nutrition and oxygen into the intercellular spaces. This laboratory-grown organ-on-a-chip can be used to analyse human organs more closely and systematically.[28] Body-on-a-chip technology will slowly revolutionize the study of whole body on a singular link and control (Figure 2.5).

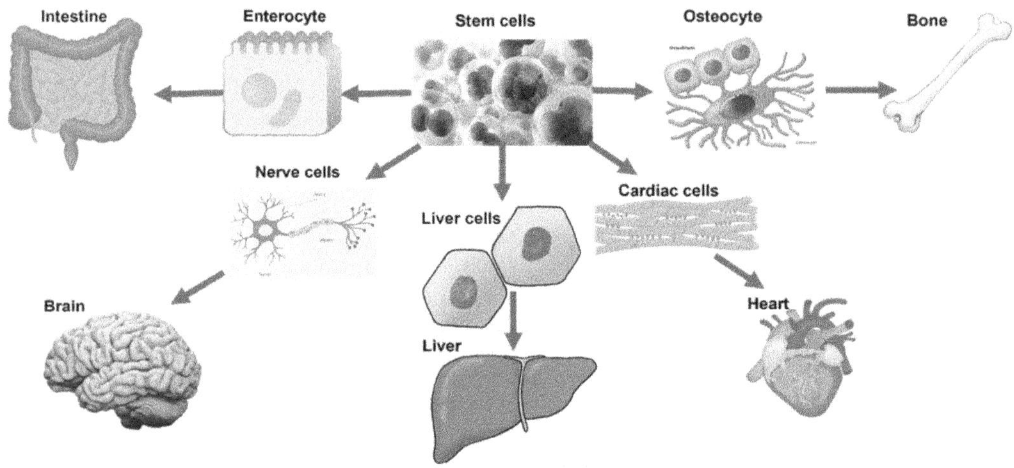

FIGURE 2.5 Use of stem cells on various organs for TERM.

2.4 APPLICATION OF TERM IN DIFFERENT TISSUES

2.4.1 Cartilage

Repair and regeneration of cartilages of ears and joints are achieved to an extent to treat cartilaginous damages. Engineered cartilages can be constructed using suitable cell source with scaffolds to replace damaged or injured tissue. This is a new way to mimic the structure and functioning of natural ears for application in TERM.[29] Cartilages are constructed using various methods by directly differentiating mesenchymal cells or chondrocytes into the required shaped scaffold which could be implanted in mice for growth observation. Other ways of regenerating ear cartilage tissue are by using 3D printing technology where the scaffold is designed using 3D scanner of ear and filled with medical-grade silicon.[30] Cartilage design of weight-bearing zone remains a major challenge due to its mechanical load. Various biomaterials have been used in cartilage tissue engineering such as collagen composite hydrogel or carboxymethylated chondroitin sulphate hydrogel.[31] Chitosan microspheres could also be used to construct cartilage-like composite, and collagen incorporated with carbon dot NPs is extensively used in tissue engineering for better stiffness and mechanical support. Silicate-based bioceramic and acellular matrix microsphere can be used as scaffold in tissue engineering, and porcine cartilage-derived ECM can be used for the fabrication of scaffold to provide suitable environment for chondrocyte to grow.[32]

2.4.2 Skin

Skin wounds caused by burn, radiation, or surgical procedure can be replaced by TERM to promote skin repair and wound healing. Various skin substitutes such as polymer scaffold consisting of collagen, hyaluronic acid, and various cell sources such as melanocytes, keratinocyte, mesenchymal cells, and fibroblasts are used for skin repair.[33] Dermal fibroblast–conditioned medium, together with plasma-derived fibrin, has been reported to promote wound repair. Scaffold systems incorporating nanofibers, hydrogels, bio-scaffolds, and bio-adhesives are used for skin repair. Silver NPs, polyaniline, and polyvinyl alcohol are used in diabetic foot wound dressings; glucan-based hydrogels are used for skin regeneration.[34] Hollow mesoporous silica doped with zinc enhances skin regeneration and wound healing. Bioactive hydrogel in collaboration with 3D printed polymer can be used for treating skin defects.[35]

2.4.3 Bone

Bone tissue engineering aims to develop bone replacements with substantial support and similar cell behaviour. Various scaffolds are designed to mimic the natural bone ECM by developing nano-hyaluronic acid or nano-collagen or porous scaffolds or adding collagen into PMMA (polymethylmethacrylate).[36] Synthetic scaffolds are also prepared with tenable size to provide mechanical support for bone repair along with addition of calcium carbonate with plaster of Paris, which increases mechanical strength and biodegradability of regenerated bone tissue.[37] Osteoporosis can be prevented by the targeted delivery of phyto molecules, and growth factors such as VEGF are injected to promote bone repair.[38] For orofacial tissue regeneration, PLGA/PCL scaffolds are modified using collagen coating or silver coating for providing antimicrobial and osteogenic properties. Biomaterials such as Mg and calcium Mg silicate bioceramic scaffolds regenerate bone and promote angiogenesis.[39] Magnesium alloy or 3D-printed magnesium plays an important role in repairing bone defect.[40]

2.4.4 Cornea

Application of TERM in cornea has helped many in restoring eyesight by corneal repair and regeneration. AuNPs loaded with microRNA in collagen membrane can rapidly repair cornea and prevent scar formation.[41] In an effort to make scaffolds which can mimic the optical and mechanical properties of cornea, scientists discovered nanofibrous scaffolds that show similar traits as cornea and can be used to form biofunctionalized film for corneal regeneration.[42] Corneal stroma cells are responsible for functioning of cornea. Hence, using corneal stroma cell sheets and keratocytes in polyglycolic acid (PGA) scaffold can repair cornea. Using genetically modified embryonic stroma cells with corneal stroma cells promotes wound healing in cornea and helps in the regeneration of cornea.[43]

2.4.5 Nerve

Regeneration of injured, traumatic central nervous system (CNS) and peripheral nervous system (PNS) is still a pressing issue where adult CNS is difficult to regenerate by itself and PNS has limited regeneration capacity. TERM has contributed to nerve regeneration by developing chitosan-based scaffold with neurotrophin-3 (NT-3) which promotes functional axon regeneration and enhances neurogenesis and vascularization, which helps to recover sensory and motor behaviours.[44] To regenerate nerve fibres, Schwann cells could be incorporated with gelatine scaffold which can induce neurite elongation. Acellular nerve allograft can also be a method of nerve regeneration.[45]

2.4.6 Cardiovascular Tissue

Cardiovascular tissue regeneration comes into force due to significant death of cardiac patients. Hence, TERM constructed substitutes of heart valves, arteries, myocardium, etc. Cardiovascular tissues are constructed using scaffolds incorporated with HA hydrogel; alginate hydrogel is used for myocardial infarction.[46] A type of stent called Xinsorb has been used for coronary angioplasty. Xinsorb is a bioabsorbable sirolimus-loaded poly (L-lactic acid) (PLLA) stent.[47] Vascular graft with fusion protein can be used for vascular regeneration. 3D printing associated with HA and hydrogel can mimic vascular structure for tissue regeneration. Collagen hydrogel, decellularized matrix, microRNA can be used for heart regeneration.

2.5 CONCLUSION

TERM has proved as an effective application in biology, engineering, and clinical science for the repair or regeneration of damaged tissues and organs. Advancement in TERM is the result of cumulative efforts through stem cell technology, growth factors, NPs, biomaterials, and 3D bioprinting navigating through challenges such as biocompatibility, biodegradability, non-toxicity, and vascularization. From a patient perspective, factors such as reduced reliance on organ transplantation, faster healing, and more effective clinical therapies are important considerations in tissue engineering and regenerative medicine (TERM). Overall, TERM has taken into consideration both technical and patient-oriented aspects for the betterment of healthcare to provide more personalized treatment to patients.

NOTES

1 Sahai, Nitin, Manashjit Gogoi, and Ravi P. Tewari. 2021. "3D Printed Chitosan Composite Scaffold for Chondrocytes Differentiation." *Current Medical Imaging* 17 (7): 832–42. https://doi.org/10.2174/1573405616666201217112939.

2 Lee, Se-Hwan, Kang-Gon Lee, Jong-Hyun Hwang, et al. 2019b. "Evaluation of Mechanical Strength and Bone Regeneration Ability of 3D Printed Kagome-Structure Scaffold Using Rabbit Calvarial Defect Model." *Materials Science and Engineering: C* 98 (May): 949–59. https://doi.org/10.1016/j.msec.2019.01.050.

3 Chaudhury, Koel, Vishu Kumar, Jayaprakash Kandasamy, and Sourav RoyChoudhury. 2014. "Regenerative Nanomedicine: Current Perspectives and Future Directions." *International Journal of Nanomedicine* 9 (1): 4153–67. https://doi.org/10.2147/IJN.S45332.

4 Chaudhury, Koel, Vishu Kumar, Jayaprakash Kandasamy, and Sourav RoyChoudhury. 2014. "Regenerative Nanomedicine: Current Perspectives and Future Directions." *International Journal of Nanomedicine* 9 (December): 4153–67. doi:10.2147/IJN.S45332.

5 Chaudhury, Koel, Vishu Kumar, Jayaprakash Kandasamy, and Sourav RoyChoudhury. 2014. "Regenerative Nanomedicine: Current Perspectives and Future Directions." *International Journal of Nanomedicine* 9 (1): 4153–67. https://doi.org/10.2147/IJN.S45332.

6 Chaudhury et al.

7 Chaudhury et al.

8 Sahai, Nitin, Nabeel Ahmad, and Manashjit Gogoi. 2018a. "Nanoparticles Based Drug Delivery for Tissue Regeneration Using Biodegradable Scaffolds: A Review." *Current Pathobiology Reports* 6 (4): 219–24. https://doi.org/10.1007/s40139-018-0184-8.

9 Sahai, Nitin, Nabeel Ahmad, and Manashjit Gogoi. 2018a. "Nanoparticles Based Drug Delivery for Tissue Regeneration Using Biodegradable Scaffolds: A Review." *Current Pathobiology Reports* 6 (4): 219–24. https://doi.org/10.1007/s40139-018-0184-8.

10 Zhao, Ningbo, Yanen Wang, Lei Qin, Zhengze Guo, and Dehua Li. 2017. "Effect of Composition and Macropore Percentage on Mechanical and in Vitro Cell Proliferation and Differentiation Properties of 3D Printed HA/β-TCP Scaffolds." *RSC Advances* 7 (68): 43186–96. https://doi.org/10.1039/C7RA07204J.

11 Zhou, Yinghong, Mengchao Shi, Julian R. Jones, et al. 2017. "Strategies to Direct Vascularisation Using Mesoporous Bioactive Glass-Based Biomaterials for Bone Regeneration." *International Materials Reviews* 62 (7): 392–414. https://doi.org/10.1080/09506608.2016.1266744.

12 Gupta, Archita, and Sneha Singh. 2022. "Multimodal Potentials of Gold Nanoparticles for Bone Tissue Engineering and Regenerative Medicine: Avenues and Prospects." *Small* 18 (29): 2201462. https://doi.org/10.1002/smll.202201462.

13 Cao, Lingyan, Jerome A. Werkmeister, Jing Wang, Veronica Glattauer, Keith M. McLean, and Changsheng Liu. 2014. "Bone Regeneration Using Photocrosslinked Hydrogel Incorporating rhBMP-2 Loaded *2-N, 6-O*-Sulfated Chitosan Nanoparticles." *Biomaterials* 35 (9): 2730–42. https://doi.org/10.1016/j.biomaterials.2013.12.028.

14 Oliveira, Joaquim M., Rui A. Sousa, Noriko Kotobuki, Mika Tadokoro, Motohiro Hirose, João F. Mano, Rui L. Reis, and Hajime Ohgushi. 2009. "The Osteogenic Differentiation of Rat Bone Marrow Stromal Cells Cultured with Dexamethasone-loaded Carboxymethylchitosan/Poly(amidoamine) Dendrimer Nanoparticles." *Biomaterials* 30 (5): 804–13, ISSN 0142-9612. https://doi.org/10.1016/j.biomaterials.2008.10.024.

15 Feng, Shuaishuai, Zi-Xin Wu, Ziyan Zhao, et al. 2019. "Engineering of Bone- and CD44-Dual-Targeting Redox-Sensitive Liposomes for the Treatment of Orthotopic Osteosarcoma." *ACS Applied Materials & Interfaces* 11 (7): 7357–68. https://doi.org/10.1021/acsami.8b18820.

16 Chang, Shun-Fu, Chih-Chang Yeh, Pin-Jyun Chen, et al. 2018a. "The Impact of Lipid Types and Liposomal Formulations on Osteoblast Adiposity and Mineralization." *Molecules* 23 (1). https://doi.org/10.3390/molecules23010095.
17 Chang, Shun-Fu, Chih-Chang Yeh, Pin-Jyun Chen, et al. 2018a. "The Impact of Lipid Types and Liposomal Formulations on Osteoblast Adiposity and Mineralization." *Molecules* 23 (1). https://doi.org/10.3390/molecules23010095.
18 Zhou, Tian-Hua, Min Su, Bei-Cheng Shang, et al. 2012. "Nano-Hydroxyapatite/β-Tricalcium Phosphate Ceramics Scaffolds Loaded with Cationic Liposomal Ceftazidime: Preparation, Release Characteristics in Vitro and Inhibition to Staphylococcus Aureus Biofilms." *Drug Development and Industrial Pharmacy* 38 (11): 1298–304. https://doi.org/10.3109/03639045.2011.648196.
19 Ma, Xin, Zhiwei He, Fengxuan Han, Zhiyuan Zhong, Liang Chen, and Bin Li. 2016. "Preparation of Collagen/Hydroxyapatite/Alendronate Hybrid Hydrogels as Potential Scaffolds for Bone Regeneration." *Colloids and Surfaces B: Biointerfaces* 143 (July): 81–87. https://doi.org/10.1016/j.colsurfb.2016.03.025.
20 Sahai, Nitin, Manashjit Gogoi, and Ravi P. Tewari. 2021. "3D Printed Chitosan Composite Scaffold for Chondrocytes Differentiation." *Current Medical Imaging* 17 (7): 832–42. https://doi.org/10.2174/1573405616666201217112939.
21 Huang, Sha, Bin Yao, Jiangfan Xie, and Xiaobing Fu. 2016. "3D Bioprinted Extracellular Matrix Mimics Facilitate Directed Differentiation of Epithelial Progenitors for Sweat Gland Regeneration." *Acta Biomaterialia* 32 (March): 170–77. https://doi.org/10.1016/j.actbio.2015.12.039.
22 Mishra, Sundeep. 2016. "Application of 3D Printing in Medicine." *Indian Heart Journal* 68 (1): 108–9. https://doi.org/10.1016/j.ihj.2016.01.009.
23 Sahai, N. I. T. I. N., and M. Gogoi. 2019. "Techniques and Software Used in 3D Printing for Nanomedicine Applications." *3D Printing Technology in Nanomedicine* (2019): 23–41.
24 Komor, Alexis C., Ahmed H. Badran, and David R. Liu. 2017. "CRISPR-Based Technologies for the Manipulation of Eukaryotic Genomes." *Cell* 168 (1): 20–36. https://doi.org/10.1016/j.cell.2016.10.044.
25 Wang, Hong-Xia, Ziyuan Song, Yeh-Hsing Lao, et al. 2018. "Nonviral Gene Editing via CRISPR/Cas9 Delivery by Membrane-Disruptive and Endosomolytic Helical Polypeptide." *Proceedings of the National Academy of Sciences* 115 (19): 4903–8. https://doi.org/10.1073/pnas.1712963115.
26 Alkayyali, Talal, Thomas Cameron, Blake Haltli, Russell G Kerr, and Ali Ahmadi. 2019. "Microfluidic and Cross-Linking Methods for Encapsulation of Living Cells and Bacteria - A Review." *Analytica Chimica Acta* 1053 (April): 1–21. https://doi.org/10.1016/j.aca.2018.12.056.
27 Jia, Luanluan, Fengxuan Han, Huili Yang, et al. 2019. "Microfluidic Fabrication of Biomimetic Helical Hydrogel Microfibers for Blood-Vessel-on-a-Chip Applications." *Advanced Healthcare Materials* 8 (13): 1900435. https://doi.org/10.1002/adhm.201900435.
28 Mobini, Sahba, Young Hye Song, Michaela W. McCrary, and Christine E. Schmidt. 2019. "Advances in Ex Vivo Models and Lab-on-a-Chip Devices for Neural Tissue Engineering." *Biomaterials*, Organoids and Ex Vivo Tissue On-Chip Technologies, vol. 198 (April): 146–66. https://doi.org/10.1016/j.biomaterials.2018.05.012.
29 Zhang, Lu, Aijuan He, Zongqi Yin, et al. 2014. "Regeneration of Human-Ear-Shaped Cartilage by Co-Culturing Human Microtia Chondrocytes with BMSCs." *Biomaterials* 35 (18): 4878–87. https://doi.org/10.1016/j.biomaterials.2014.02.043.
30 He, Yong, Guang-huai Xue, and Jian-zhong Fu. 2014. "Fabrication of Low Cost Soft Tissue Prostheses with the Desktop 3D Printer." *Scientific Reports* 4 (1): 6973. https://doi.org/10.1038/srep06973.
31 Zheng, Rui, Huichuan Duan, Jixin Xue, et al. 2014. "The Influence of Gelatin/PCL Ratio and 3-D Construct Shape of Electrospun Membranes on Cartilage Regeneration." *Biomaterials* 35 (1): 152–64. https://doi.org/10.1016/j.biomaterials.2013.09.082.
32 Bunpetch, Varitsara, Xiaoan Zhang, Tian Li, et al. 2019. "Silicate-Based Bioceramic Scaffolds for Dual-Lineage Regeneration of Osteochondral Defect." *Biomaterials* 192 (February): 323–33. https://doi.org/10.1016/j.biomaterials.2018.11.025.
33 Liu, Shiyu, Lan Jiang, Haijian Li, et al. 2014. "Mesenchymal Stem Cells Prevent Hypertrophic Scar Formation via Inflammatory Regulation When Undergoing Apoptosis." *Journal of Investigative Dermatology* 134 (10): 2648–57. https://doi.org/10.1038/jid.2014.169.
34 Tang, Xin, Hua Qin, Xiaosong Gu, and Xiaobing Fu. 2017. "China's Landscape in Regenerative Medicine." *Biomaterials* 124 (April): 78–94. https://doi.org/10.1016/j.biomaterials.2017.01.044.
35 Im, Heejung, Su Hee Kim, Soo Hyun Kim, and Youngmee Jung. 2018. "Skin Regeneration with a Scaffold of Predefined Shape and Bioactive Peptide Hydrogels." *Tissue Engineering Part A*, ahead of print, October 4. Sage CA: Los Angeles, CA. https://doi.org/10.1089/ten.tea.2017.0489.

36 Li, Tao, Xisheng Weng, Yanyan Bian, Lei Zhou, Fuzhai Cui, and Zhiye Qiu. 2015. "Influence of Nano-HA Coated Bone Collagen to Acrylic (Polymethylmethacrylate) Bone Cement on Mechanical Properties and Bioactivity." *PLOS ONE* 10 (6): e0129018. https://doi.org/10.1371/journal.pone.0129018.
37 Lee, Se-Hwan, Kang-Gon Lee, Jong-Hyun Hwang, et al. 2019a. "Evaluation of Mechanical Strength and Bone Regeneration Ability of 3D Printed Kagome-Structure Scaffold Using Rabbit Calvarial Defect Model." *Materials Science and Engineering: C* 98 (May): 949–59. https://doi.org/10.1016/j.msec.2019.01.050.
38 Qu, Xiangyang, Yujiang Cao, Cong Chen, Xiaohong Die, and Quan Kang. 2015. "A Poly(Lactide-Co-Glycolide) Film Loaded with Abundant Bone Morphogenetic Protein-2: A Substrate-Promoting Osteoblast Attachment, Proliferation, and Differentiation in Bone Tissue Engineering." *Journal of Biomedical Materials Research Part A* 103 (8): 2786–96. https://doi.org/10.1002/jbm.a.35379.
39 Zhai, Wanyin, Hongxu Lu, Lei Chen, et al. 2012. "Silicate Bioceramics Induce Angiogenesis during Bone Regeneration." *Acta Biomaterialia* 8 (1): 341–49. https://doi.org/10.1016/j.actbio.2011.09.008.
40 Lai, Yuxiao, Ye Li, Huijuan Cao, et al. 2019. "Osteogenic Magnesium Incorporated into PLGA/TCP Porous Scaffold by 3D Printing for Repairing Challenging Bone Defect." *Biomaterials* 197 (March): 207–19. https://doi.org/10.1016/j.biomaterials.2019.01.013.
41 Kobayashi, Takeshi, Atsushi Shiraishi, Yuko Hara, et al. 2015. "Stromal–Epithelial Interaction Study: The Effect of Corneal Epithelial Cells on Growth Factor Expression in Stromal Cells Using Organotypic Culture Model." *Experimental Eye Research* 135 (June): 109–17. https://doi.org/10.1016/j.exer.2015.02.009.
42 Zheng, Canbin, Qingtang Zhu, Xiaolin Liu, et al. 2014. "Improved Peripheral Nerve Regeneration Using Acellular Nerve Allografts Loaded with Platelet-Rich Plasma." *Tissue Engineering Part A* 20 (23–24): 3228–40. https://doi.org/10.1089/ten.tea.2013.0729.
43 Sahai, Nitin, Manashjit Gogoi, and Ravi P. Tewari. 2021. "3D Printed Chitosan Composite Scaffold for Chondrocytes Differentiation." *Current Medical Imaging* 17 (7): 832–42. https://doi.org/10.2174/1573405616666201217112939.
44 Yang, Zhaoyang, Aifeng Zhang, Hongmei Duan, et al. 2015. "NT3-Chitosan Elicits Robust Endogenous Neurogenesis to Enable Functional Recovery after Spinal Cord Injury." *Proceedings of the National Academy of Sciences* 112 (43): 13354–59. World. https://doi.org/10.1073/pnas.1510194112.
45 Zheng, Canbin, Qingtang Zhu, Xiaolin Liu, et al. 2014. "Improved Peripheral Nerve Regeneration Using Acellular Nerve Allografts Loaded with Platelet-Rich Plasma." *Tissue Engineering Part A* 20 (23–24): 3228–40. https://doi.org/10.1089/ten.tea.2013.0729.
46 Han, Fengxuan, Jiayuan Wang, Luguang Ding, et al. 2020. "Tissue Engineering and Regenerative Medicine: Achievements, Future, and Sustainability in Asia." *Frontiers in Bioengineering and Biotechnology* 8 (March). https://doi.org/10.3389/fbioe.2020.00083.
47 Wu, Yizhe, Jiasheng Yin, Jiahui Chen, et al. 2020. "Final Report of the 5-Year Clinical Outcomes of the XINSORB Bioresorbable Sirolimus-Eluting Scaffold in the Treatment of Single de Novo Coronary Lesions in a First-in-Human Study." *Annals of Translational Medicine* 8 (18): 1162–1162. https://doi.org/10.21037/atm-20-5668.

3 Nanomaterials in Biomedical Implants

Shrimanta Sundar Ramchiary[1], *Bethuel Daurai*[1], *Manashjit Gogoi*[1], *and Gautam Saha*[2]
[1]Department of Biomedical Engineering, North-Eastern Hill University, Shillong, India
[2]Department of Information Technology, North-Eastern Hill University, Shillong, India

3.1 INTRODUCTION

A biomedical implant is a device that is intended to replace, strengthen, or improve a biological structure that is missing or has been damaged. The implant's surface is determined by the placement of an implant component, viz. titanium (Ti), silicone (Si), or apatite [$Ca_5(PO_4)_3(F,Cl,OH)$], that will come into touch with living tissues in the body (Wong et al. 2013). Cochlear implants and artificial pacemakers are two examples of implants that contain electronics. Bioactive implants include subcutaneous drug delivery systems (implantable tablets) and drug-eluting stents.

In general, biomedical implants can be divided into groups based on the conditions for which they are used (Arsiwala et al. 2014).

An orthopaedic prosthesis is one of the most often-used implants relating to the body's bones and joints (Thomas and Singh 2017). Orthotic implants include fins, fusion devices, bone grafts, and bone plates. Interference screws may be used as additional orthopaedic fixation devices in regions of the ankle, knee, and hand. To fix fractures, pins and rods are also utilized as implants. Craniomaxillofacial repair has been known to use screws and plates. The only orthopaedic implants that respond to magnetic fields under 1.0 Tesla magnetic resonance imaging (MRI) scanners are external fixator clamps, according to a 2005 study (Kumar et al. 2006). But at the 7.0 Tesla MRI scan, several orthopaedic implants, including fibular and heel implants, would interact significantly with the MRI magnetic fields (Feng et al. 2015).

Dental implants and bone-preserving scaffolds created through tissue engineering fall under the category of orthopaedic implants. Some of the most recent prospective metallic biomaterials used in biodegradable medical implants include metallic glasses based on magnesium (Mg) with zinc (Zn) and calcium (Ca) addition (Nowosielski et al. 2016; Ibrahim et al. 2017).

Heart valves, defibrillators, vascular grafts, stents, pacemakers, and other implantable biomedical devices are used to treat cardiovascular problems (McLatchie et al. 2013; Wong et al. 2013). Angina pectoris, atherosclerosis, cardiac arrhythmia, heart failure, valvular heart disease, and ventricular tachycardia are the main cardiovascular symptoms that could require implants.

There are some neural devices used as implants and prostheses for the cochlear and retinal applications, central nervous system (CNS), and peripheral nervous system (PNS). Patients with rheumatoid arthritis can benefit from neck-implanted electrical implants that send electrical signals to vagus nerve electrodes (Peeples 2019). Implants are used to treat various illnesses, including erectile dysfunction, gastroparesis, gastro-oesophageal reflux disease (GERD), respiratory failure, and sleep apnoea. Examples of such devices include penile implant, implantable stomach stimulator, LINX, diaphragmatic/phrenic nerve stimulator, neurostimulator, surgical mesh, and artificial urinary sphincter (Simmons and Montague 2008; Hjort et al. 2012; McLatchie et al. 2013).

DOI: 10.1201/9781003473015-3

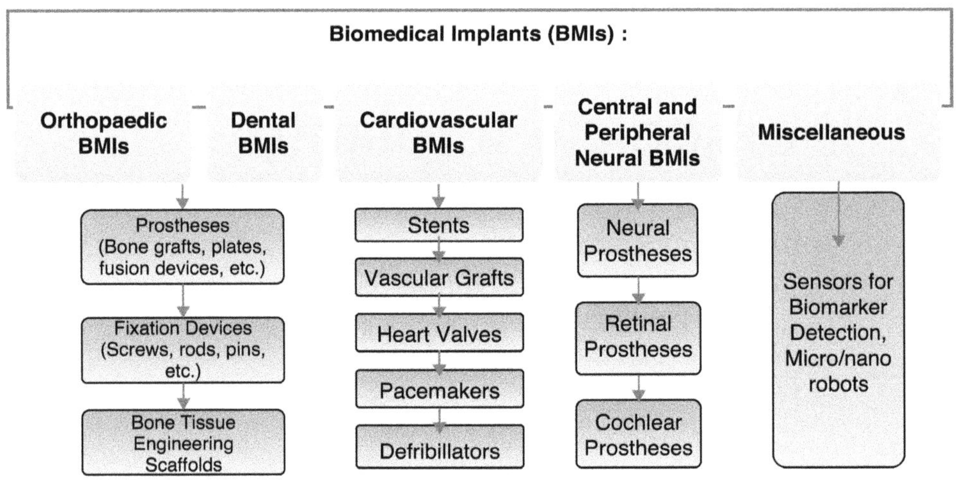

FIGURE 3.1 Biomedical implants (BMIs). (Arsiwala et al. 2014.)

The primary goals of contraceptive implants, including copper and other hormone-based intrauterine devices, are to prevent unwanted pregnancies and treat illnesses, including non-pathological types of menorrhagia (Falcone and Hurd 2007; McLatchie et al. 2013). Breast implants, nasal prostheses, ocular prostheses, and injectable fillers are cosmetic implants attempting to bring the body back up to acceptable aesthetic standards. After a mastectomy for breast cancer, they are used to treat various types of deformities and change physical body characteristics (like augmentation of the buttock and chin) (McLatchie et al. 2013; Wong et al. 2013) (Figure 3.1).

As can be seen from the categories above, technologies at the micro and nano levels have enabled to affect cellular processes starting at sub-micron scales positively. Medical bionic implants are a term that is beginning to be used to refer to biomedical implanted devices as a whole. Bionics is the study of biological systems for creating artificial systems that perform biological systems' functions. From 2012 to 2017, this market expanded at a cumulative annual growth rate (CAGR) of 7.1%, reaching $17.82 billion. The many principles of the aforementioned related subjects are being combined in this field, which is experiencing a surge in the research effort. After the COVID-19 epidemic, the market for medical devices is seeing an increase in demand for biomedical implants. Implant technology may undergo a revolution thanks to micro/nano interventions' ability to design and modulate its features precisely. Nanostructuring makes it possible to duplicate the nanostructures found in the body, giving micro/nanoscale implants unique ability to beneficially influence cellular biomolecular events.

3.2 COMPOSITION OF CONVENTIONAL BIOMEDICAL IMPLANTS

3.2.1 Metallic Implants

Historically, titanium (Ti), Ti alloys, and particular stainless steel grades have been used to make metallic implants for use in medical procedures (Brunette et al. 2001; Geetha et al. 2009; Niinomi et al. 2012; Chen and Thouas 2015; Wang et al. 2016). Due to incredible strength together with outstanding plastic properties, high chemical stability, and biocompatibility, Ti and its alloys were utilized to make load-bearing implants (Brunette et al. 2001).

Additional research is being done to create novel Ti alloys having low Young's moduli, super elasticity, and shape memory behaviour. Also, several surface treatment methods affecting wear resistance and osteointegration were being developed (Chissov et al. 2008; Hench 2015). Therefore, porous metal implant could be modified to match host bone mechanically and encourage its growth into its porous structure generating a permanent synthetic substitute with good Young's modulus of bone (Chen and Thouas 2015). Porous networks formed by nitinol or titanium nickelide (NiTi) are essential for different applications (e.g., reconstructive surgery after breast cancer operations and laryngeal replacement post-radiation therapy). It possesses outstanding strength, flexibility, and a shape memory effect (Chen and Thouas 2015; Muhamedov et al. 2015). The process is repeated as the connective tissue eventually fills the NiTi structure's pores. High biological compatibility between the substance and bodily tissues was evident. 10% of NiTi complications are surgical and not connected to the material (Berthet et al. 2011). Thin elastic NiTi nets are promising for reconstructing complicated abnormalities, including soft tissues, but their small thread diameters make them difficult to see using X-ray technologies, and therefore we need to make them more contrasting (Cheng et al. 2006; Chen and Thouas 2015; Zaworonkow et al. 2018).

Additionally, under development are stainless steel (nickel-free), cobalt-chromium (Co-Cr) alloys, newly created zirconium (Zr)-based alloys, tantalum (Ta), niobium (Nb) and Nb alloys, magnesium (Mg)-based biomaterials, and iron (Fe)-based biomaterials (Chen and Thouas 2015). The main drawback found with their application in the physiological environment is gradual leaching of metal ions, which could result in the development of toxic or allergic reactions, despite alloys' corrosion resistance or formation of protective oxide film as in NiTi and other Ti-containing alloys (Brunette et al. 2001; Kurtz and Devine 2007; Geetha et al. 2009; Berthet et al. 2011; Chen and Thouas 2015; Muhamedov et al. 2015; Wang et al. 2016). Increasing the biointegration capacity and biocompatibility of metal implants is a crucial field of research for preventing the emergence of infections and rejection reactions at body-implant interface (Linkevicius and Apse 2009, 2013, 2009; Geetha et al. 2009).

3.2.2 Ceramic Implants

Ceramic implants are made of materials obtained by sintering clays and their mixtures with mineral additives, metal oxides, and inorganic compounds. Interestingly, the late 1960s marked the beginning of using metal-free ceramics for biomedical applications to increase biocompatibility (Conrad et al. 2007; Andreiotelli et al. 2009; Dorozhkin 2010; Kirilova et al. 2013; Hench 2015). Bioceramic materials can be classified into the following categories depending on how the body reacts to the implant: bioinert bioceramics (ZrO_2, Al_2O_3) and bioactive bioceramics, which can be further divided into low-reactivity bioceramics glass, based on Na_2O-CaF_2-P_2O_5-SiO_2, medium-reactivity bioceramics glass, based on Na_2O-$CaOP_2O_5$-SiO_2, and fully digestible bioceramics, e.g., hydroxyapatite [$Ca_{10}(PO_4)_6(OH)_2$] (HA) and tricalcium phosphate [$Ca_3(PO_4)_2$] (TCP) (Doremus 1992; Vallet-Regí 2001; Best et al. 2008; Chissov et al. 2008; Bayazit et al. 2010; Barinov 2010).

According to a study, bioactive ceramics can osseointegrate by degrading and releasing ions resulting in chemical linkage between implant and bone mineral component (Andreiotelli et al. 2009). Therefore, by adjusting the composition of bioactive ceramics, it is possible to alter the bioactivity and resorbability of implants. The surface alteration after implantation is a characteristic of bioglass materials like bioactive glasses that include specific quantities of silicon dioxide (SiO_2), calcium oxide (CaO), and phosphorous pentoxide (P_2O_5), which are frequently utilized to fill up bone deformities. This bio-porosity glass helps in bioactivity and resorption (Doremus 1992).

Because they essentially do not undergo chemical changes under physiological conditions of living creature, bioinert ceramics maintain their physical and mechanical qualities (Best et al. 2008). Corundum ceramics based on zirconium dioxide (ZrO_2) and ceramics based on aluminium oxide (Al_2O_3) are examples of high-density ceramics having good mechanical properties like high strength and wear resistance and are used to make dental and trauma-orthopaedic implants and prostheses. They are produced utilizing various techniques, including the conventional way of sintering, the hot-pressing method, the plasma-chemical technique, the cold pressing with subsequent sintering technique, and the process of casting from thermoplastic slips (Kirilova et al. 2013).

Researchers are working to make ceramic implants survive longer and be more dependable for creating newer-generation nanocomposites of Al and Zr, highly resistant to crack propagation (de Aza et al. 2005). Developing composite materials with novel features has been suggested as an alternative and creative method to transform ceramics. For instance, laser ablation technology can functionalize ZrO_2 surfaces with gold (Au) nanoparticles (NPs) or silver (Ag) microparticles. According to findings in the most recent studies, friction testing demonstrated that functionalized surface's integrity was not compromised during implant implantation and that ZrO_2's surface has uniformly distributed particles. Hence, the direction of this research development was regarded as the development of antibacterial surface integrating functionalization at nano- and micro-levels, leading to production of biomedical ceramic materials class with superior qualities (Hak et al. 2014).

3.2.3 Polymers and Their Composites

3.2.3.1 Polymeric Implants

In biomedical applications, a wide range of inert or absorbable polymeric biomaterials are commonly used such as ultrahigh molecular weight polyethylene (UHMWPE), polyethylene (PE), polyurethane (PU), polytetrafluoroethylene (PTFE), polyacetal (PA), polymethylmethacrylate (PMMA), polyethylene terephthalate (PET), silicone rubber (SR), polyetheretherketone (PEEK), poly(lactic acid) (PLA), and polysulphone (PS) (Patel and Gohil 2012). Polymers are poorly interchangeable but highly specialized with their unique properties of flexibility, resistance to biochemical effects, good biocompatibility, and lightness. Besides, polymer products can be manufactured of desired shape by varying their composition to change their physical and mechanical properties. Macromolecular chains' composition, structure, and molecular weight determine polymer mechanical properties. For example, polyaryletherketones (PAEKs) are high-temperature thermoplastic polymers having a molecular chain of aromatic backbone connected by functional groups of ketone and ether (May 2008). They are increasingly used after confirming their biocompatibility (Williams et al. 1987) as biomaterials for orthopaedic, trauma, and spinal implants. Two widely used PAEK polymers are PEEK, a semi-crystalline polymer consisting of benzene, ketone, and simple ether groups, and poly(aryl-ether-ketone-ether ketone ketone) (PEKEKK), having high wear resistance and relative inertia inside human body. Polyaromatic ketones are stable at high temperatures (up to 350°C), resistant to radiation and chemical attacks, compatible with stimulating modifiers (viz., glass and carbon fibres), and have high strength (May 2008).

3.2.3.2 Polymer-Based Composites

The ever-growing demand for developing PEEK composite materials is based on biocompatible polymers and carbon fibres (Scholz et al. 2011; Hak et al. 2014; Li et al. 2014, 2016; Zaworonkow et al. 2018). Carbon fibre is high-strength and high-modulus bending filaments with micron-level diameter (Doremus 1992; Vallet-Regí 2001), while graphite has a structure with anisotropic crystal covalent bonds, but with weak van der Waals interactions between the layers (Doremus 1992; Vallet-Regí 2001; Best et al. 2008). It has a density of 1.6–2.2 g/cm^3 (Doremus 1992; Vallet-Regí 2001; Best et al. 2008), close to a compact bone density of 2.0 g/cm^3 (Park and Lakes 1992). In polymer composite implants, carbon fibres act as reinforcing agents in developing high-strength composite materials. Besides their structural and mechanical characteristics (Kurtz and Devine 2007; Ohtsuki et al. 2009), carbon fibres possess biocompatible properties which were clinically proven (de Aza et al.; Barinov 2010; Beljakov et al. 2010; Kenar et al. 2013) both in animal trials (Petersen 2011; Price et al. 2011; Guitchounts et al. 2013) and in laboratory experiments (May 2008; Khonsari et al. 2014). For example, composite rod, reinforced with bisphenol, carbon fibre, and epoxy resin, was compared with a Ti-6–4 alloy (Petersen and Phillips 2016). It was seen that carbon-reinforced composite had significantly improved stimulated osteointegration. Carbon fibre-reinforced polyetheretherketone (CFR-PEEK) plate is a highly effective bioactive composite used in orthopaedics and traumatology. CFR-PEEK is a promising and suitable material for orthopaedic implants due to its biocompatibility and mechanical strength (Li et al. 2014). Several advantages of CFR-PEEK implants can be seen over traditional metal ones. Their lower modulus of elasticity matches that of bone, and fatigue strength is greater than most metal implants (Hak et al. 2014). The data of the studies showed that CFR-PEEK plates have promising short-term results and could be an excellent alternative to stainless steel plates in fixing distal femoral fractures (Mitchell et al. 2018). Similar studies were carried out where biomechanical comparisons of stainless steel, Ti, and CFR-PEEK plates were conducted (Hak et al. 2017; Mugnai et al. 2018). CFR-PEEK plates provide an optimal alternative for metal plates for distal radius fractures treatment too due to their biomechanical properties. However, the modification of the PEEK surface is required because of biological inertia for improving its biocompatibility. Covalently bounded coating of phosphorylated gelatine loaded with bone morphogenetic protein 2 (BMP-2) was used on hydroxylated microporous PEEK films for PEEK surface modification. This novel biological modification technique changed their biological inertia expanding medical application of PEEK nanomaterials in orthopaedic implants (Wu et al. 2018). CFR-PEEK implants showed benefits for radiation therapy with lesser impact by radiation than standard metal systems (Khonsari et al. 2014; Muhamedov et al. 2015; Nevelsky et al. 2017; Liu et al. 2020). But the main disadvantages of CFR-PEEK plates were low resistance to plastic deformation and low fracture load. However, more clinical trials are needed for accurate clinical results on their safety to determine the prospects of using such materials in other areas of orthopaedics, including oncosurgery (Berthet et al. 2011; Khonsari et al. 2014; Li et al. 2014). They also have X-ray transparency feature, which prevents direct visualization by X-ray methods and requires labelling (Hak et al. 2014). Polymer composite materials are characterized by threat of peri-implant infections and insufficient osteoconductivity due to their bioinertness requiring surface modification (Sargeant and Goswami 2006; Berthet et al. 2011) (Figure 3.2).

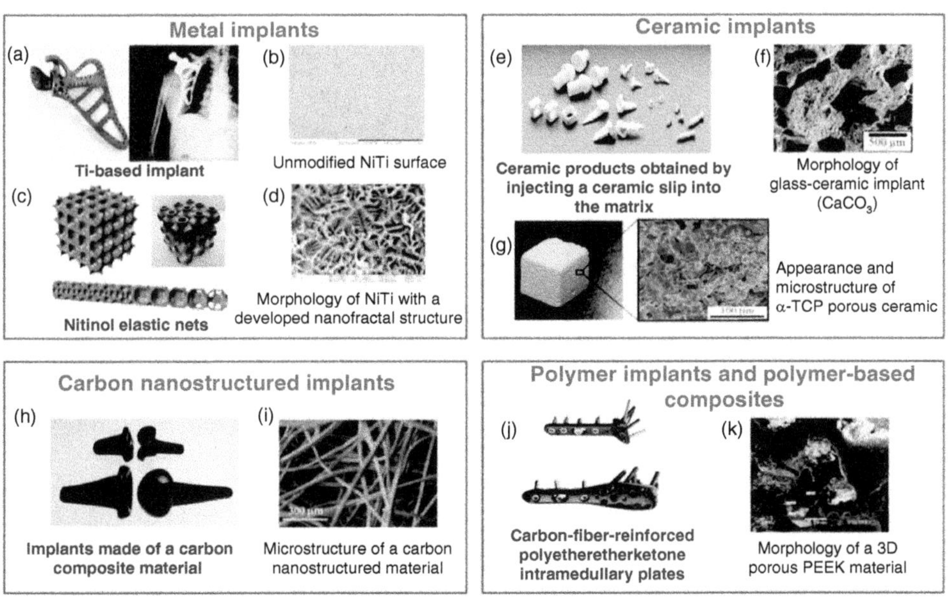

FIGURE 3.2 Biomedical products and their surface morphology: (a) A Ti-based implant (Image courtesy of Ltd. LOGO, Novosibirsk, Russia); (b) unmodified NiTi surface; (c) example of the approaches for scaffold design: representative blocks and unit cells; (d) morphology of a NiTi implant fabricated by selective laser sintering; (e) ceramic products made by injecting ceramic slip into matrix; (f) morphology of a glass-ceramic implant; (g) α-TCP porous ceramic microstructure; (h) example of carbon composite material implants; (i) a CNI microstructure; (j) CFR-PEEK intramedullary plates; and (k) morphology of a 3D porous PEEK material.

3.2.4 Drawbacks of Existing Implants

The current trend in implant development is focused on choosing effective biomaterials and techniques for changing the implant surface since the existing modern implants still have a number of drawbacks, such as infectious problems and cytotoxicity. Implant infection and inflammation continue to be among the most serious side effects of bone surgery. These issues frequently necessitate revision surgery, which adds to the patients' suffering and costs. Ag NPs and coatings have historically been applied as antibacterial agents to enhance the qualities of noble metal biomaterials. The metal gold (Au) was also considered as a possible alternative. Currently, the prospects for using combinations of noble metals (bimetallic NPs and nano-objects made of one metal on top of another) are shown. Such composite materials have osteointegration characteristics in addition to having dramatically improved antibacterial activity.

The problem of metal corrosion seen in metallic implants when they come into contact with biological systems and continuous electrochemical processes is the production of metal ions that can activate the immune system by building complexes with endogenous proteins. Contrarily, dermatitis, urticaria, and vasculitis are linked to implant degradation products. However, there isn't yet a widely acknowledged test for identifying metal allergy clinically. Nanomaterials can be used to create multifunctional biocompatible coatings that can interact with surrounding bone tissue and efficiently enhance the surface properties of bulk biomaterials.

Despite the apparent advantages of bioceramic materials in terms of biochemical compatibility with the body when compared to metals and polymers currently used for the reconstruction of the musculoskeletal system, a number of factors limit the use of bioactive or bioinert ceramics in bone prosthetics. Due to the shielding of mechanical loads that cause the resorption of bone tissue surrounding the implant and the loss of the latter, such ceramics have a severe problem of low durability. Recently, failures in the implantation of Zr prostheses have been reported due to the rapid growth of cracks on the implants.

According to their toxicological and sanitary-chemical indicators, carbon nanostructured implants (CNIs) are compliant with the standards for materials in contact with the internal environment and tissues of the human body. However, it should be noted that when assessing the potential uses of carbon products, all studies that were known up until recently were not carried out in a systematic manner. A severe factor hindering the use of carbon implants in clinical practice was the lack of industrial mass production. The literature lacks pertinent information on the many ways used to modify the surface of CNIs.

Therefore, creating bioactive coatings that can enhance implants' biointegrative qualities (i.e., encourage osteo- and histogenesis) and also have a sustained bactericidal impact is a crucial first step in enhancing the efficacy of contemporary permanent implants (Albrektsson et al. 2009; Michelle Grandin et al. 2012). Traditional approaches to creating such coatings include silver, antibiotics, or bioactive ceramics (Albrektsson et al. 2009; Michelle Grandin et al. 2012). Talk of a comprehensive solution to this issue is, however, undermined by the tolerance to drugs, particularly to antibiotics, associated with their active use and the risk of toxic reactions, such as argyrosis.

The use of biodegradable polymeric bionanomaterials is gaining momentum with the implants with clinical data to be verified and tested for biomedical use with enhanced efficacies and properties due to their usage. As a result of the high demand for entirely bioresorbable stents (BRS), there is delay in bringing nanocoated/nanostructured stents to the market. The next-generation stents, BRS, are now being developed by larger stent manufacturers. Even then, microporous stents have established themselves on the market; nonetheless, there aren't many nano-stents available in the still-developing market. The re-popularization of bare metallic stents is a result of opposing market trends that call for polymer-free methods. On the other hand, the most recent product on the market is the popular trend of entirely biodegradable polymeric stents.

3.3 NANOMATERIALS USED IN IMPLANTS

3.3.1 Metal and Metal Oxide Nanomaterials

Varying research has been performed to test the antimicrobial capacity of metallic and metallic oxide NPs. A few of them have been discussed in the following.

3.3.1.1 Silver (Ag) and Silver Oxide (Ag_2O) NPs

Because of their strong biocidal properties, Ag NPs have been used in multiple areas, such as coating and tissue regeneration. New research and development have been conducted to better understand their inherent anti-inflammatory, antibacterial, antiviral, antifungal, and anti-yeast activities and their potential toxicity as well.

Xiu et al. (2012), in their study, found that Ag ions affect bacteria but not Ag NPs. However, Prabhu and Poulose (2012) found that Ag NPs attach themselves to bacterial cell and then penetrate it, damaging cell membranes and causing cell death. Reactive oxygen species (ROS) generated by Ag NPs is also a reason for their antimicrobial ability. Ag NPs can suppress inflammation nearby, making Ag NPs a suitable adjunct for bone healing treatment. Sarraf et al. applied Ag_2O NPs to thin film of tantalum oxide (Ta_2O_5) nanotubes and then coated them with titanium (Ti) alloy for increasing osseointegration and antibacterial activity (Sarraf et al. 2018; Ranga et al. 2019). In another study, creative collagen scaffold was created for encapsulating Ag NPs and BMP-2 (Sun et al. 2015). The hybrid structure of Ag NPs, BMP-2, and collagen together built up antimicrobial ability, and the surface roughness of scaffold increased cell adhesion and proliferation.

Nandi et al. (2018) determined that Ag NPs deposited in bone implants could be exercised for treatment of osteomyelitis *in vivo*. Ag_2O NPs, when embedded in a titanium oxide nanotube, it was found that the novel structure had superior cytocompatibility and better osteoblast proliferation and differentiation than titanium oxide nanotube (Gao et al. 2014). Ag NPs also promote *in vitro* and *in vivo* osteogenic differentiation and proliferation of human mesenchymal stem cells (hMSCs) (Zhang et al. 2015). Ag NPs may enter hMSCs and trigger expression of the gene hypoxia-inducible factor (HIF)-1, which protects the cell from stressful situations, including hypoxia, ROS production, etc. Qureshi et al. (2013, 2015) functionalized Ag NPs with photoactivated microRNA (miR-148b), improving the differentiation of human adipose stromal/stem cells (hASCs). It also helped with closure of mouse calvarial defects. However, further investigation of Ag NPs is necessary to ensure its safety in bone-related applications.

3.3.1.2 Copper (Cu) and Copper Oxide (CuO) NPs

Copper is an essential mineral for many proteins and enzymes in humans. Cu NPs are toxic to bacteria and are of low cost and therefore have been the subject of increased interest. Their antibacterial ability is high, even at low dosages. Several reports suggested that Cu NPs could be used to develop materials for infection prevention and treating bone defects due to their excellent bioactivity and antimicrobial ability. Sahmani et al. (2019) used CuO NPs to improve mechanical properties, cell viability, and electrical conductivity of HA scaffold. In a different study, chitosan and Cu NPs were mixed to form antimicrobial coating; the most potent antimicrobial effects against gram (+)ve and gram (−)ve bacteria were obtained with 1.25 wt% of Cu NPs (Tabesh et al. 2019).

van Hengel et al. (2020) biofunctionalized a Ti-6Al-4V bone implant with Ag and Cu NPs ranging from 0% to 100%. It boosted the antimicrobial and osteoconductive abilities of the implant. When exposed to air, Cu NPs will rapidly form CuO NPs that are toxic to human cells and organs. Wang et al. (2012) investigated how CuO NPs could affect human lung epithelial (A549) cells and found that the CuO NPs were engulfed by A549 cells mainly through endocytosis. CuO NPs inside cells, especially in mitochondria or nucleus, can cause ROS generation and lead to cell apoptosis and necrosis. These results indicate that exposure to Cu and CuO NPs carries risks, such as gene alteration and homeostasis disturbance.

3.3.1.3 Gold (Au) NPs

Au NPs have remarkable chemical properties, excellent physical properties, superior biocompatibility, antimicrobial ability, ease of synthesis, controlled geometrical and optical properties, and versatility in surface modification resulting in their extensive use in many biomedical applications, e.g., orthopaedic implants, bioimaging, and drug delivery. Au NPs also have positive effects on bone formation.

Lee et al. (2018a) used an injectable hydrogel system containing functionalized Au NPs to promote bone differentiation in human adipose-derived stromal/stem cells (hADSCs). Poly(lactic-co-glycolic acid) (PLGA) scaffolds were coated with Au particles as osteoinductive agents for enhancing osteogenesis and osteogenic differentiation of hADSCs. Similar results were seen when Au NPs were coated with polycaprolactone (PCL) scaffolds (Lee et al. 2018b). In another study, Au NPs were embedded in Ti implants for treatment of osteopenia and osteoporosis, and *in vitro* results indicated that Au NPs significantly improved osteointegration (Ko et al. 2020).

Furthermore, because of biocompatibility, mild toxicity, and high X-ray attenuation of Au NPs, Russo et al. (2017) determined that loading PMMA-based bone cement with Au NPs within a specific range enhances its mechanical and antimicrobial abilities.

Zhang et al. (2010) employed them as an X-ray contrast agent to detect damaged bone tissue. Au NPs can enhance X-ray attenuation without affecting the physicochemical properties of the scaffolds.

Celikkin et al. (2019) 3D printed scaffold with Au NPs embedded to ensure suitable biological properties and imaging function. Multiple experiments showed that Au NPs could carry drugs, peptides, proteins, DNA, RNA, etc. Therefore, Au NPs provide possible solution for real-time tracking of cells and may lead to new advancements in molecular diagnostics and nano-therapeutic fields in bone-related research.

3.3.1.4 Zinc (Zn) and Zinc Oxide (ZnO) NPs

Zn is a mineral found in all biological tissues. It stimulates bone mineralization, maintains cell membrane structure, and helps with pathological calcification. Zn also plays an essential role, for instance, through DNA synthesis, enzyme activity, and apoptosis control at the cellular level. About 30% of Zn is stored in bone, making it the main Zn reservoir. Research has shown that Zn can improve cytocompatibility. For example, Bageshlooyafshar et al. (2019) applied zinc silicate mineral NPs via coating to nanofibrous scaffold surface, which helped to enhance proliferation and osteogenic differentiation of stem cells. Begam et al. (2017) cultured MG63 osteoblasts on pure and Zn-doped HA and found improved cell viability and adhesion rate on the Zn-doped HA compared with the pure HA. ZnO NPs also possess antimicrobial ability. ZnO/HA coating has shown excellent bacterial killing efficacy against gram (+)ve and gram (−)ve bacteria. In addition, Wu et al. (2012) reported that Zn-incorporated Ti coating also has antimicrobial ability and could build up adhesion, proliferation, and differentiation of rat bone marrow stem cells (rBMSCs) (Hu et al. 2012). However, the exact mechanism driving antibacterial ability of ZnO NPs has not been entirely determined. As with strontium (Sr), Zn NPs are often applied conjugated with other biomaterials to achieve multiple qualities, such as antimicrobial ability, cytocompatibility, and corrosion resistance. On the other hand, an excess of Zn may cause cell apoptosis or necrosis, and ZnO NPs can alter cell morphology, damage DNA, and cause other harmful effects. Moreover, Kononenko et al. (2017) confirmed that ZnO NPs could induce genotoxic effects and damage cellular defence system.

3.3.1.5 Aluminium (Al) and Alumina (Al_2O_3) NPs

Aluminium is an essential element of life. However, compared with Al, Al_2O_3 NPs have more applications for orthopaedic implants and scaffolds because of their superior biomechanical properties and excellent biocompatibility. Al_2O_3 NPs possess antimicrobial ability as they can easily attach themselves to the bacterial cell wall and deform it, resulting in apoptosis. For instance, researchers have found that Al_2O_3 NPs can act against gram (+)ve and gram (−)ve bacteria. However, Al_2O_3

NPs showed only mild toxicity towards certain other strains of bacteria, such as *Escherichia coli*. According to Sadiq et al. (2009), Al_2O_3 NPs have been used to enhance various bone scaffolds' mechanical and biological properties.

Aghajani Derazkola and Simchi (2018) employed Al_2O_3 NPs to reinforce PMMA nanocomposites. With increase in the volume of Al_2O_3 NPs, the results showed that the hardness, flexural strength, and tensile strength of the PMMA nanocomposites were all improved. Hesaraki explored β-TCP scaffolds with Al_2O_3 NPs incorporated into them (Hesaraki 2016). The mechanical strength of the enhanced scaffolds was greater because of the more compacted microstructure that was created.

Zafar et al. (2020) created a silk fibroin scaffold embedded with Al_2O_3 NPs to boost the osteogenic differentiation of rabbit adipose-derived stem cells (rADSCs). The Al_2O_3 NPs considerably improved the compressive strength and mineralization of the scaffold, and the scaffold showed the least possible toxic effect on cell proliferation *in vitro*.

Hence Al_2O_3 NPs could be used to enhance scaffolds to improve their physicochemical, mechanical, and biological properties. Both cytotoxicity and genotoxicity have been observed in connection with Al_2O_3 NPs. Al_2O_3 NPs can be engulfed by the cells, forming vesicles and generating ROS and radicals through the interaction with the cell, inducing damage to DNA. Zhang et al. (2017) found that Al_2O_3 NPs (13 and 50 nm) could enter the cells and trigger ROS generation, DNA damage, micronucleus in bone marrow cells, and other potential issues. However, Al_2O_3 NPs (10 µm) did not show severe cytotoxicity and genotoxicity in the cells. Further research is required to study the detailed mechanism of the toxicity of Al_2O_3 NPs (Figure 3.3).

3.3.1.6 Magnesium (Mg) and Magnesium Oxide (MgO) NPs

Magnesium is a necessary component of human body. Mg deficiency can decrease bone-related cell activities, cause osteopenia and bone fragility, and inhibit bone growth. Mg has many unique properties, such as bone-forming stimulation, biocompatibility, biodegradability, and low Young's modulus compared with other metals. These rare features make MgO NPs extremely valuable in orthopaedic implants and scaffolds. MgO NPs possess antimicrobial ability, which, with their low cost and environmental friendliness, makes them extremely useful. MgO NPs have been applied in bone substitutes and HA for their antimicrobial ability to prevent dental and orthopaedic infections.

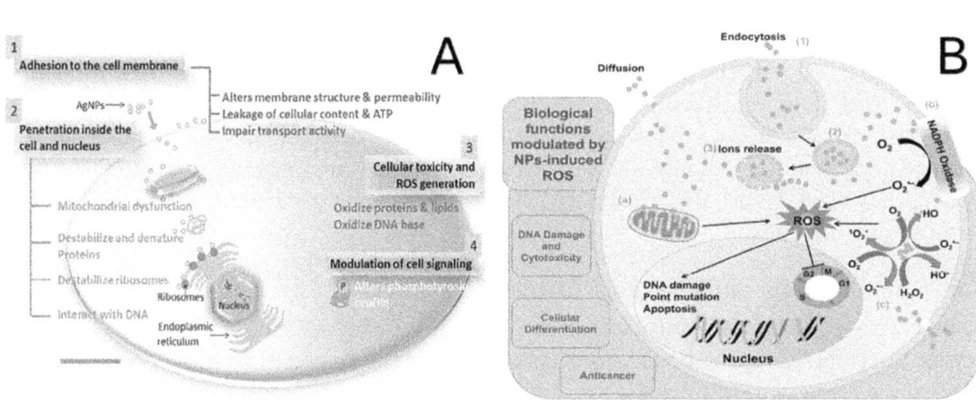

FIGURE 3.3 A pictorial diagram of antimicrobial action of Ag NPs. (a) Four antimicrobial action routes of Ag NPs. (b) NP-induced ROS production mechanisms. NPs internalized into cell via (1) endocytosis, (2) endocytotic vesicle formation, and (3) particle ions released from vesicles into cell. NP ROS generation factors include (a) interaction with mitochondria, (b) interaction with NADPH oxidase, and (c) factors related to physicochemical properties (size, shape, photoreactive properties, and surface chemistry). These factors result in ROS generation leading to consequences, including DNA damage, cell cycle arrest, apoptosis alterations, and cell membrane damage.

Researchers have tried varied methods using Mg NPs to improve shortcomings of existing scaffolds. For instance, Nasri-Nasrabadi et al. (2018) fabricated a porous sodium alginate scaffold with MgO NPs embedded to magnify its mechanical strength and antimicrobial ability. Dittler et al. (2019) embedded Mg NPs in a bioactive glass-based scaffold to give it better biological behaviour and antibacterial ability. Lih et al. (2018) used modified magnesium hydroxide NPs loaded on PLGA biodegradable scaffold to obtain reduced *in vivo* inflammatory effects, strong mechanical strength, and biocompatibility. MgO NPs have low toxicity but can still cause DNA damage directly or by inducing ROS and inflammatory responses in cells which can cause cell apoptosis or necrosis. They can also induce cell apoptosis, DNA damage, and intracellular ROS at different concentrations (Ghobadian et al. 2015). Mg NPs can also harm osteoblastic SaOS-2 sarcoma cells in a dosage- and time-dependent manner. Nevertheless, research into Mg and MgO NPs toxicity has not been pervasive and needs further study to gain more comprehensive knowledge of their exact mechanism of toxicity.

3.3.1.7 Titanium (Ti) and Titania (TiO_2) NPs

Titanium, titania, and alloys are extensively used in orthopaedic implants because of their outstanding mechanical properties and biocompatibility. However, debris or particles can be generated from load-bearing orthopaedic implants' daily wear and tear. The wear and tear effect may be main reasons for aspect loosening that leads to implant failure. Ti and TiO_2 NPs can damage DNA and induce genotoxicity. TiO_2 NPs may also bind with specific proteins that generate hypersensitivity reactions in implant area. Liu et al. (2010) addressed that TiO_2 NPs could induce cytotoxicity in brain neuron cells (PC12) and generate ROS in a specific dosage and length of time.

TiO_2 NPs also have toxic effects on many organs. However, it is well-established that reinforcing wear resistance of Ti and its alloys is essential. Therefore, more novel coatings and structures are necessary to obtain functional, long-lived Ti-based orthopaedic implants. Like many other metallic NPs, TiO_2 NPs possess antibacterial ability against bacteria and fungi.

TiO_2 NPs can induce ROS on bacterial surface, damage cell membrane integrity of bacteria, and finally, cause excretion of bacterial components. Kim et al. (2014) used silk fibroin and TiO_2 NPs to produce scaffolds with highly porous architecture; TiO_2 NPs helped to maintain shape, reduced swelling ratio of scaffold, and amplified scaffold's mechanical strength, which was a positive result in the context of using silk as bone-implant material. Ikono et al. (2019) hybridized chitosan with TiO_2 NPs to make a sponge for bone healing. The TiO_2 NPs improved sponge tenacity, biomineralization, and bone healing capability. Johari et al. (2018) created a novel scaffold with silk fibroin and fluoridated TiO_2 NPs; the NPs improved their mechanical behaviour, cell attachment, and viability. Furthermore, PEEK upgraded with TiO_2 NPs was tested *in vitro* and *in vivo* by Wu et al. (2012), who confirmed that no or little cytotoxicity and genotoxicity were detected and found that bond between implant and bone was significantly fortified during *in vivo* testing. In conclusion, as Ti is one of the most commonly used metals, it is critical for safe and permanent incorporation of Ti NPs and alloys into orthopaedic implants.

3.3.1.8 Tantalum (Ta) and Tantalum Oxide (Ta_2O_5) NPs

Compared with Ti-based implants, tantalum implants can induce more significant proliferation, osteogenic differentiation, and better bioactivity. The bioactivity and biological bond to bone makes Ta promising material for orthopaedic implants and scaffolds, and Ta naturally forms an outer layer of Ta_2O_5 with anti-corrosion ability. Many inorganic NPs have been tested in medical imaging. Ta_2O_5 NPs are chemically inert, biocompatible, and have excellent radiopacity, making them suitable for X-ray and computed tomography (CT) contrast agents. Freedman et al. (2014) used Ta_2O_5 NPs as a CT contrast agent to successfully image human articular cartilage. Chen et al. (2017) loaded chemotherapeutics like doxorubicin on Ta_2O_5 NPs to treat cancers and found that these NPs could offer an intrinsic radio sensitization effect to induce DNA damage in cancer cells during radiotherapy. Ta_2O_5-poly (acrylic acid) (Ta_2O_5-PAA) nanocomposites were combined by Bogusz et al. (2019), who loaded methotrexate on Ta_2O_5-PAA nanocomposites to treat cancer. The team observed the release of the drug in media with different pH levels and found that the media with lower pH levels could release the drug in a more controlled and sustained manner, which was suitable for long-term cancer treatment. Ta NPs can also improve the mechanical properties of bone scaffolds. Kang et al. (2017) performed a series of tests using Ta NPs deposited on Ta implants with MC3T3-E1 mouse osteoblasts. Ta NPs promoted the proliferation of the MC3T3-E1 osteoblasts and showed strong biocompatibility and osteogenic properties. Moreover, other studies have reported that Ta NPs can induce autophagy in osteoblasts, improving the proliferation and differentiation of the osteoblasts and protecting them from ROS damage and apoptosis.

3.3.1.9 Zirconium (Zr) and Zirconia (ZrO_2) NPs

Zirconium, zirconia, and alloys have outstanding biocompatibility and antimicrobial ability, excellent corrosion resistance, and enhanced mechanical properties. Zr and ZrO_2 are primarily employed in alloy or coating forms rather than NPs and have various bio-applications, such as orthopaedic implants, dentistry, and biosensors. Wang et al. (2017) used Zn to dope ZrO_2/TiO_2 coatings and found that ZrO_2 was stable. There was no release of Zr ions but only Zn ions. ZrO_2/TiO_2 layers doped with Zn killed much more bacteria than Zr; combining Zn and Zr produced more remarkable antimicrobial ability.

Zr NPs could help strengthen scaffolds' mechanical properties, cytocompatibility, and corrosion resistance. Yu et al. (2015) used Zr NPs in HA bone cement to substantially improve its mechanical strength. The inertness of Zr and ZrO_2 may affect its application. Gillani et al. (2010) prepared functionalized ZrO_2 NPs as bone cement additives and reported refined osteoconductivity and improved mechanical properties. Bashir et al. (2018) created organic, additive-based ZrO_2 NPs as bone substitutes to minimize the inertness of the ZrO_2. Because of their low cost, the team used glucose and fructose as organic additives. However, ZrO_2 NPs have also been reported to have mild toxic effects. Ye and Shi (2018) determined that ZrO_2 and TiO_2 NPs could induce apoptosis and morphology changes in osteoblast MC3T3-E1 cells. It was found that ZrO_2 and TiO_2 NPs could affect osteogenesis and hinder osteoblast differentiation at higher dosages and that ZrO_2 NPs were more toxic than TiO_2 NPs. Overall, further analysis and research on ZrO_2 NPs are necessary, as they have enormous potential for bone-related applications.

3.3.2 Magnetic Nanomaterials

In general, magnetic nanoparticles (MNPs) can be pure metallic NPs, metallic oxide NPs, or magnetic nanocomposites. MNPs have been extensively analysed for their biomedical applications, such as drug delivery, diagnostic imaging, biosensors, cancer therapy, and bone tissue engineering. Iron oxide NPs (usually Fe_3O_4 or Fe_2O_3) are the most promising material derived from MNPs, because of their feasible cost and low-toxicity profile. MNPs can be implemented in complex tissue repair, like bone regeneration and healing, or even dental applications. Kharaziha and Fathi (2009) synthesized forsterite NPs with superb bioactivity and biocompatibility, which could be used as bioactive bone grafting materials. MNPs and other metallic NPs can be coated to alter their surface chemistry and reduce their toxicity. Different coating methods, such as *in situ* coatings (carried out during synthesis) and post-synthesis coating, have been implemented to form the core-shell MNPs. Other polymeric coatings, such as polyethylene glycol (PEG), PLGA, and chitosan, have also been studied. Silica coatings can also prevent MNPs from developing toxicity. As reported by Mahmoudi et al. (2009), although superparamagnetic iron oxide nanoparticles (SPIONs) exhibited toxicity, SPIONs coated with polyvinyl alcohol (PVA) showed minimal toxic effects even at a very high concentration.

Furthermore, different organic and inorganic materials, such as polymeric NPs, metallic NPs, and liposomes, have been studied as drug delivery carriers. Therapeutic agents like drugs, genes, growth factors (GFs), and enzymes can be loaded on MNPs, especially SPIONs. MNPs are one of the most suitable carriers for delivering bioactive molecules because of their unique advantages, especially the ease with which they can be monitored and visualized through MRI with guidance from an external magnetic field. Multiple SPIONs, SPION liposomes, SPION nanospheres, and SPION encapsulated hydrogels have been tested for drug delivery. These SPIONs, with various modifications, increase the delivery efficiency of external magnetic fields and enable multiple therapeutic agents simultaneously.

3.3.3 Metal Nanocomposites

Many metallic and metallic oxide NPs can be toxic to humans or animals in the long term. Incorporation of the second bioactive compound, or even more than two, is a promising solution to mitigate the toxicity of NPs while maintaining their desired ability. For instance, Geng et al. (2016) incorporated Ag and Sr NPs into HA coatings. Sr was deployed as secondary dopant to ease potential toxicity of the Ag NPs while allowing them to bring their antimicrobial ability to orthopaedic implants. Similarly, Ti bone implants dual-loaded with Zn and Ag demonstrated excellent osteogenic and antibacterial activity. Tao et al. (2016) prepared coatings composed of HA, containing 10% Zn, Mg, and Sr ions, which built up implant osseointegration and improved the microstructure of bone implant.

Osteomyelitis is a progressive infection that is often caused by *Staphylococcus aureus*, a gram (+)ve bacteria, and can sometimes lead to limb amputation or even death. Ag and Cu NPs can be used to treat it instead of antibiotics. The antimicrobial ability of Ag and Cu combined is better than that of Ag or Cu alone, but that antimicrobial ability rapidly decreases as Cu oxidizes. Qadri et al. (2017) designed and synthesized silver-copper-boron (AgCuB) NPs by introducing boron to maintain an extended period of antimicrobial ability. AgCuB NPs could act as an alternative to antibiotics to treat osteomyelitis. Other promising research with sundry combinations has been carried out to improve bioactivity and corrosion resistance, escalate the osteoblast proliferation and differentiation rate, and reinforce antibacterial function. The combinations include Cu and Ag NPs, Zn and Ag NPs, Zn and Ti NPs, Sr and Ag NPs, and many others.

In many cases, metallic/ceramic/polymeric NPs can be mixed as nanocomposites to upgrade their mechanical properties and adjust their biological ones. The most well-established metallic and metallic oxide NPs have been discussed above, emphasizing their excellent mechanical and biological abilities and different applications in orthopaedic implants and scaffolds. Nanocomposite materials that mimic the bone structure with appropriately tailored mechanical and biological properties are possibly the best candidates for generating functional bone tissues compared with monolithic materials and micro-composites. Although considerable bone-related research and applications already exist for nanocomposites, more still needs to be done to understand the long-term *in vitro* and *in vivo* effects of nanocomposites (Niinomi et al. 2012; Arsiwala et al. 2014).

3.3.4 Carbon Nanostructured Implants

Resorption phenomena often occur due to significant differences between elastic modulus of metals and biological tissues (Petersen and Phillips 2016). The bone implants, therefore, should have biomechanical characteristics as close as possible to bones. In this regard, we can see the usage of CNI having high biological compatibility, possessing good strength characteristics, non-toxicity, lack of sensitizing effects and rejection reactions (Govindaraj et al. 1999; Baker et al. 2004; Beljakov et al. 2010; Vandrovcová and Bačáková 2011; Kenar et al. 2013; Petersen and Phillips 2016). Joint implants made of carbon nanomaterials are less susceptible to destruction, with an estimated 20–25 years of service life, while metal endoprostheses usually have an estimated 5–7 years of service life. CNIs, unlike metal plates, screws, and rods, do not require rapid removal after bone fusion. Carbon has been widely used as an artificial material in the manufacture of implants (Nevelsky et al. 2017; Wu et al. 2018). Researchers were looking into the possibilities of using carbon nanomaterials in orthopaedics, traumatology, neurosurgery, and maxillofacial surgery at the beginning of the 21st century

(Muhamedov et al. 2015). However, due to its mechanical properties, ordinary carbon material can't be allowed under mechanical load (Baker et al. 2004). The surface structure, porosity, possibility of modelling mechanical properties of CNIs, according to bone tissue parameters and its invasion into CNI by forming a strong bone-carbon block, allow us to consider bone-implant biomechanical system ensuring its survival duration (Nandi et al. 2010; Kirilova et al. 2012; Campoccia et al. 2013). CNIs, made of strong porous composite of carbon fibres, bonded by nanostructured carbon matrix and characterized by high structural and biomechanical compatibility, can withstand large compression and bending load, while difference between strength of implants and bone is not too large compared to high-strength ceramic and Ti implants.

3.3.5 Bionanomaterials for Drug Delivery

Bionanomaterials are critical in developing innovative targeted drug delivery systems and diagnosis and therapies for various life-threatening disorders. The production of bionanomaterials utilizing biological processes is quick, safe, and ecologically beneficial. Different metallic NPs are widely used in drug delivery applications (Singh and Lillard 2009). This nano-drug's significant advantage is reducing the cytotoxic drug loading during systemic distribution, requiring a small dose, i.e., more efficient with site-specific targeting (Onoue et al. 2014). NPs capped with biocompatible molecules using a linker also increase the circulatory half-life time (Lee et al. 2010). The nature of the NPs can be multimodal starting with enhancing their drug delivery efficiency, transport and targeting inside the cells, and also controlled drug release (Cho et al. 2008; Torchilin 2014). This drug delivery technique is currently being used for treating certain types of cancer comparatively different from what is seen either in chemotherapy or radiotherapy (Cherukuri et al. 2010). Conventional treatments have harmful side effects and attack both normal/healthy cells and the infected ones. While nanomaterial-based drug delivery is used for treating several types of cancer, this therapy helps reduce the drug's toxic effects, does not affect healthy cells, and targets only damaged (cancer) cells (Rai et al. 2011). These drug/carrier complexes are systemically administered to the patients through the bloodstream, usually in the form of a biocompatible liquefied drug (Daum et al. 2012).

In case of targeted therapy using MNPs, a cytotoxic drug is attached to an NP carrier, enters into blood, and is targeted by magnetic fields to reach a specific site within the body (Bhaumik et al. 2015). After reaching the site, the drug is released either by enzymatic activity or by altering physiological conditions (pH, osmolality, temperature, and uptake by the tumour cells) (Rai et al. 2011). The availability of metallic NPs has created new opportunities for medical technologies. Nanomaterials' distinctive properties make them valuable in a number of industries, including electronics, antimicrobials, biosensors, medication delivery, and catalysis. Pharmaceutical sciences are actively using metal NPs as a cutting-edge drug delivery technology. Nanomaterials used in medication delivery could serve both therapeutic and diagnostic purposes. Life-threatening disorders can now be treated in novel ways thanks to nanomedicines. There are some restrictions, such as the extremely restricted number of functionalized pharmaceuticals that individual NPs can carry and the difficulty in quantifying them. To create a targeted medication delivery system, NPs must be conjugated with either an antibody or a ligand. However, toxic effects of metallic NPs must be considered before using them for therapeutic applications (Sahai et al. 2018).

3.3.6 Bionanomaterials for GF Delivery

These are a few examples of bionanomaterials used for GF delivery:

- Synthetic polymer NPs, e.g., biocompatible synthetic NPs made of copolymers PLA, polyglycolide, and PLGA;
- Protein-based NPs for delivery of GFs, e.g., albumin NPs, polysaccharide-coated bovine serum albumin (BSA) NPs, and BMP-2-encapsulated NPs;

- Polysaccharide-based NPs, e.g., epidermal growth factor (EGF)- and fibroblast growth factor (FGF)-incorporated chitosan/tripolyphosphate (TPP) NPs, *N*-succinyl-chitosan/TPP NPs, vascular endothelial growth factor (VEGF)-loaded low-molecular-weight heparin–*N*-trimethyl chitosan (LMWH-TMC) NPs, heparin-immobilized chitosan (EHC)/poly(γ-glutamic acid) (γ-PGA) NPs;
- Lipid-based nanocarriers for controlled release of GFs, e.g., liposomes, solid lipid particles (SLN), and nanostructured lipid carriers (NLC);
- Mesoporous silica NPs as GF carriers, e.g., BMP2-functionalized nanoporous silicon NPs (NPSNPs), NPSNPs;
- Polymer nanocapsules for controlled GF release, e.g., VEGF-loaded protein nanocapsules, BMP-2-loaded degradable protein nanocapsules, VEGF-loaded magnetic PLGA nanocapsules;
- Other GF nanocarriers like EGF-incorporated dextran-coated superparamagnetic iron oxide NPs (EGF-SPION^{Dex}), calcium phosphate (CaP) NPs, HA NPs and silk fibroin, polydopamine NPs, poly(*N*-isopropyl acrylamide) (PNIPAM) and PLGA nanocarriers.

Due to nanostructures' high surface area and careful control of various proteins that are essential for controlling cellular adhesion, proliferation, differentiation, and the production of extracellular matrix, NP-based GF delivery systems have demonstrated a number of benefits (Sahai et al. 2018). Nanotoxicology and related toxicity issues like cytotoxicity, ecotoxicity, and genotoxicity are crucial to improving their future usage in clinical trials. Additionally, these nanocarriers can be joined with microporous scaffolds employing sophisticated nanotechnology techniques in order to mediate GF release kinetics in a predesigned manner to enhance tissue healing and regeneration. Successful GF delivery in the clinic is significantly hampered by the requirement for huge amounts of biomolecules during tissue regeneration.

GF delivery from various bionanomaterials has produced positive results in bone fractures and fibular deformities, improvements in Alzheimer's disease and periprosthetic fractures, and advancements in peripheral nerve regeneration, cutaneous healing, and skeletal muscle regeneration. Thus, a lot of smart nanomaterials responsive to physiological or environmental stimuli have been employed to deliver GFs at the right time and place. In fact, the creation of novel materials—many of which are based on biomaterials that resemble the ECM—promises to present a viable future option for the more controlled distribution of a number of GFs.

3.4 TOXICITY ASSESSMENT

We can see that burden may come along with micro-/nanotechnology. According to what has been said thus far and what is clear from the aforementioned sections, as the field of biomedical implants undergoes a revolution thanks to the development of micro- and nanointerventions that improve sustainability, performance, and efficacy, it is crucial to pay close attention to how these innovations will affect cellular sites over the course of prolonged use. These nanocarriers' ability to replicate biomolecular and cellular structures may have special toxicities due to their small size, necessitating a thorough assessment. Addressing the problems with the host immune response brought on by the foreign nature of these biomedical implants is the other issue at hand. Even though there are numerous methods, such as hydrophilic polymer coatings and functionalized surfaces, for creating biocompatible implant-tissue interface, a thorough examination of their cellular interactions is still needed. The widespread use of carbon nanostructures, for which there is currently conflicting information regarding their safety, is one such key cause for concern. Despite numerous findings indicating the safety and biocompatibility of carbon nanostructures *in vivo* and *in vitro*, a distinct thought process based on experimental evidence raises the possibility of toxicity, mostly as a result of functional variation, dose, contact duration, agglomeration, etc.

As a result, acute and chronic toxicity studies are required since accumulation of these carbon nanostructures at focal areas may result in delayed damage. The other category of nanocomposite that has found widespread use in orthopaedics and dental implants is nanoTiO_2. Recent data suggest that these NPs can cause cardiac toxicity, especially in people who already have cardiac conditions. Therefore, before employing these, one must also take into account the patient's entire pathophysiological state. In conclusion, given the increased use of inorganic, carbon-based, and nonbiodegradable microparticles and NPs in the field of bionics, it is important to remember the battery of toxicological tests determining their safety when used over an extended period of time to support their successful entry into the market (Das et al. 2021).

3.5 CHALLENGES AND FUTURE PERSPECTIVES

Over the years, we've come a long way from surgically introducing foreign objects into the human body to hide their foreignness and make the body more aesthetically pleasing. Medical implants have developed from straightforward support devices to cutting-edge healing techniques. There are certain aspects of challenges that are seen when dealing with biomedical implants.

One of the commonest complications of biomedical implants is infection. This is due to the fact that the implant is an artificial device in the body and can be a breeding ground for bacteria. It is a major challenge with biomedical implants, as any foreign material introduced into the body carries the risk of infection. Due to the foreign substance that is inserted into the body, they can raise the risk of infection.

Another challenge is potential for the body to reject the implant, either because of the material it is made from or due to antibodies that attack the foreign object. The body's immune system can reject biomedical implants, as it does with organ transplants. The body may reject the implant, leading to pain and inflammation.

Biomedical implants can fail due to mechanical issues such as wear and tear, corrosion, or other mechanical problems leading to the need for replacement or repair. For example, implants, such as joint replacements, can wear out over time due to natural wear and tear.

Biomedical implants may interfere with other medical devices, such as pacemakers and defibrillators. External electrical fields, such as those from MRI machines, can interfere with the functioning of certain biomedical implants if they are not properly shielded. Also, electrical interference from the environment or from other electronic devices can disrupt the function of a biomedical implant.

As with any device, biomedical implants can experience device failure and malfunction due to a variety of reasons, such as faulty components or incorrect programming. This can range from poor design to manufacturing issues to everyday wear and tear. The process of inserting a medical implant can also lead to potential complications from the surgical procedure, including bleeding and infection.

Certain medications used to treat medical implants can lead to adverse reactions, including allergic reactions and other side effects. Allergic reactions to the materials involved in the implant can occur. The cost associated with the implants and their maintenance can be expensive, and they may not be covered by insurance. Biomedical implants may have limited lifespans, requiring replacement or repair. There is shortage of long-term data regarding safety and effectiveness of biomedical implants, as most studies only focus on short-term outcomes.

Biomedical implants are devices that are designed to replace, support, or enhance a biological system in some way. The future of biomedical implants is promising, with existing technology being improved and new technologies being developed. They are expected to become increasingly sophisticated and effective over the next few decades. Advances in materials science, biosensor technology, computing power, and artificial intelligence will allow implants to become smaller, more complex, and more interactive with the body in more effective ways. Implants will be able to monitor and respond to changes in the body, provide feedback to the patient in real time, and even offer personalized treatments. For instance, implants may soon be able to monitor and adjust levels of neurotransmitters in the brain or detect and respond to changes in blood sugar levels. Implants may also be designed to deliver drugs or hormones directly to the body, as well as provide novel stem cell therapies. The field of nanotechnology is one of the most promising for the future development of biomedical implants. Implants might possibly get so minuscule with the advancement of nanotechnology that they can be inserted right into the bloodstream. Nanotechnology has the potential to create devices that are smaller, more efficient, and more precise than current devices. This could allow for the creation of implants that are more closely integrated into the body and capable of detecting and responding to a wider range of biological signals.

Implants may also be further enhanced through the use of "smart" technology. For instance, implants could be programmable and able to detect and respond to changes in the body's internal environment. They could also be developed to respond to external stimuli, such as voice commands or changes in the environment. In addition, advances in biotechnology, including gene editing and tissue engineering, could allow for the creation of implants that are better able to replicate or replace biological functions. For example, gene editing could be used to create implants that are able to detect and respond to a wider range of biological signals. Also, advances in biotechnology, including gene editing and tissue engineering, could allow for the creation of implants that are better able to replicate or replace biological functions. For example, gene editing could be used to create implants that are able to detect and respond to a wider range of biological signals.

Finally, advances in 3D printing and tissue engineering are expected to make implants more lifelike and durable. For instance, using 3D printing can create personalized implants that properly match the body. Tissue engineering could also be used to generate living cells or tissues that could be used to create more robust and more durable implants. Also, advances in artificial intelligence, machine learning, and robotics could lead to development of implants which are able to interact with the body in increasingly sophisticated ways. This could include the development of implants that are able to learn and adapt to their environment, in addition to being able to detect and respond to biological signals. Overall, the future of biomedical implants is very promising. With existing technology being improved and new technologies being developed, biomedical implants could be used to replace, support, or enhance biological systems in increasingly sophisticated ways. They have the potential to revolutionize medical care and offer unprecedented levels of personalization for healthcare applications.

3.6 CONCLUSIONS

Medical implants were the first products to use nanomaterials a few decades ago. However, compatibility with advanced additive manufacturing (AM) techniques like 3D printing poses a challenge, especially for niche medical applications. Researchers from a variety of disciplines, including bioengineering and mechanical engineering, can now better understand how to choose the right materials for 3D printing based on the application. AM technology for medical implant applications can quickly become economically feasible if the physics of material selection, process optimization, and design architecture requirements are thoroughly studied.

Using microfluidic chips, created over the past few decades, might be an alternative strategy. Microfabrication and 3D printing both allow for the production of organ-on-chips. As one sort of organ-on-ships, bone-on-chips are a multidisciplinary approach based on micro-/nanofluidic chips specifically created for advanced management of the 3D biological microenvironment to imitate a tissue- or organ-level function of the human body. Bone-on-chips will create a real-time system replicating the intricate human bone structure. This system will show how bone cells interact with one another in real time when exposed to stressors like medications or NPs. Bone-on-chips may be able to save animals since they offer a more moral method with more specific toxicity and efficacy as well as cost and time savings because fewer ingredients are needed. As stem cells from specific individuals can be used to further customize medications and implants, bone-on-chips can also aid patients. Complete human-on-chips can be created by combining bone-on-chips with other organs-on-chips for more complicated stimulations. Bone-on-chips must prove their effectiveness and safety in preclinical therapy before moving on to human clinical trials.

NPs are linked to enormous advantages and potential in bone-related research that vastly outweigh their drawbacks. It is challenging to create orthopaedic implants and scaffolds that can adhere to existing bone structures and restore all complex activities in a living environment because of the constantly coordinated interaction of bone cells. Therefore, the development of nanotechnology concerning orthopaedic implants is essential. The development of NP use in orthopaedic implants, scaffolds, and other biomedical fields depends on further research into various forms of NPs.

REFERENCES

Aghajani Derazkola H, Simchi A (2018) Effects of alumina nanoparticles on the microstructure, strength and wear resistance of poly(methyl methacrylate)-based nanocomposites prepared by friction stir processing. *J Mech Behav Biomed Mater* 79:246–253. https://doi.org/10.1016/J.JMBBM.2018.01.007

Albrektsson T, Brånemark PI, Hansson HA, Lindström J (2009) Osseointegrated titanium implants: Requirements for ensuring a long-lasting, direct bone-to-implant anchorage in man. *Acta Orthop* 52:155–170. https://doi.org/10.3109/17453678108991776

Andreiotelli M, Wenz HJ, Kohal RJ (2009) Are ceramic implants a viable alternative to titanium implants? A systematic literature review. *Clin Oral Implants Res* 20:32–47. https://doi.org/10.1111/J.1600-0501.2009.01785.X

Arsiwala A, Desai P, Patravale V (2014) Recent advances in micro/nanoscale biomedical implants. *J Contr Release* 189:25–45. https://doi.org/10.1016/J.JCONREL.2014.06.021

Bageshlooyafshar B, Vakilian S, Kehtari M, et al. (2019) Zinc silicate mineral-coated scaffold improved in vitro osteogenic differentiation of equine adipose-derived mesenchymal stem cells. *Res Vet Sci* 124:444–451. https://doi.org/10.1016/J.RVSC.2017.09.015

Baker D, Kadambande SS, Alderman PM (2004) Carbon fibre plates in the treatment of femoral periprosthetic fractures. *Injury* 35:596–598. https://doi.org/10.1016/J.INJURY.2003.10.014

Barinov SM (2010) Calcium phosphate-based ceramic and composite materials for medicine. *Russ Chem Rev* 79:13–29. https://doi.org/10.1070/RC2010V079N01ABEH004098

Bashir M, Riaz S, Kayani ZN, Naseem S (2018) Synthesis of bone implant substitutes using organic additive based zirconia nanoparticles and their biodegradation study. *J Mech Behav Biomed Mater* 88:48–57. https://doi.org/10.1016/J.JMBBM.2018.07.035

Bayazit V, Bayazit M, Bayazit E (2010) Evaluation of bioceramic materials in biology and medicine. *Dig J Nanomater Biostruct* 5:267–278

Begam H, Kundu B, Chanda A, Nandi SK (2017) MG63 osteoblast cell response on Zn doped hydroxyapatite (HAp) with various surface features. *Ceram Int* 4:3752–3760. https://doi.org/10.1016/J.CERAMINT.2016.12.010

Beljakov MV, Guseva VN, Mushkin AY et al. (2010) Multifunction carbon implants in surgical treatment of inflammatory spinal diseases. *Hirurgiâ pozvonočnika (Spine Surgery)* 1:057–061. https://doi.org/10.14531/SS2010.1.57-61

Berthet JP, Canaud L, D'Annoville T, et al. (2011) Titanium plates and dualmesh: A modern combination for reconstructing very large chest wall defects. *Ann Thorac Surg* 91:1709–1716. https://doi.org/10.1016/J.ATHORACSUR.2011.02.014

Best SM, Porter AE, Thian ES, Huang J (2008) Bioceramics: Past, present and for the future. *J Eur Ceram Soc* 28:1319–1327. https://doi.org/10.1016/J.JEURCERAMSOC.2007.12.001

Bhaumik J, Mittal AK, Banerjee A, et al. (2015) Applications of phototheranostic nanoagents in photodynamic therapy. *Nano Res* 8:1373–1394.

Bogusz K, Zuchora M, Sencadas V, et al. (2019) Synthesis of methotrexate-loaded tantalum pentoxide–poly(acrylic acid) nanoparticles for controlled drug release applications. *J Colloid Interface Sci* 538:286–296. https://doi.org/10.1016/J.JCIS.2018.11.097

Brunette DM, Tengvall P, Textor M, Thomsen P (2001) *Titanium in Medicine*. https://doi.org/10.1007/978-3-642-56486-4

Campoccia D, Montanaro L, Arciola CR (2006) The significance of infection related to orthopedic devices and issues of antibiotic resistance. *Biomaterials* 27:2331–2339. https://doi.org/10.1016/J.BIOMATERIALS.2005.11.044

Campoccia D, Montanaro L, Arciola CR (2013) A review of the biomaterials technologies for infection-resistant surfaces. *Biomaterials* 34:8533–8554. https://doi.org/10.1016/J.BIOMATERIALS.2013.07.089

Celikkin N, Mastrogiacomo S, Frank Walboomers X, Swieszkowski W (2019) Enhancing X-ray attenuation of 3D printed gelatin methacrylate (GelMA) hydrogels utilizing gold nanoparticles for bone tissue engineering applications. *Polymers* 11. https://doi.org/10.3390/POLYM11020367

Chen Q, Thouas GA (2015) Metallic implant biomaterials. *Mater Sci Eng R Rep* 87:1–57. https://doi.org/10.1016/J.MSER.2014.10.001

Chen Y, Song G, Dong Z, et al. (2017) Drug-loaded mesoporous tantalum oxide nanoparticles for enhanced synergetic chemoradiotherapy with reduced systemic toxicity. *Small* 13:1602869. https://doi.org/10.1002/SMLL.201602869

Cheng Y, Cai W, Li HT, Zheng YF (2006) Surface modification of NiTi alloy with tantalum to improve its biocompatibility and radiopacity. *J Mater Sci* 41:4961–4964. https://doi.org/10.1007/S10853-006-0096-6

Cherukuri P, Glazer ES, Curley SA (2010) Targeted hyperthermia using metal nanoparticles. *Adv Drug Deliv Rev* 62:339–345. https://doi.org/10.1016/J.ADDR.2009.11.006

Chissov VI, Sviridova IK, Sergeeva NS, et al. (2008) In vitro study of matrix surface properties of porous granulated calcium phosphate ceramic materials made in Russia. *Bull Exp Biol Med* 145:499–503. https://doi.org/10.1007/S10517-008-0128-0

Cho K, Wang X, Nie S, et al. (2008) Therapeutic nanoparticles for drug delivery in cancer. *Clin Cancer Res* 14:1310–1316. https://doi.org/10.1158/1078-0432.CCR-07-1441

Conrad HJ, Seong WJ, Pesun IJ (2007) Current ceramic materials and systems with clinical recommendations: A systematic review. *J Prosthet Dent* 98:389–404. https://doi.org/10.1016/S0022-3913(07)60124-3

Das B, Chabukdhara M, Patra S, Gogoi M (2021) Current knowledge on toxicity of nanomaterials: Toxicity assessment and impact. *Nanotoxicology* 339–375. https://doi.org/10.1201/9780429299742-14

Daum N, Tscheka C, Neumeyer A, Schneider M (2012) Novel approaches for drug delivery systems in nanomedicine: Effects of particle design and shape. *Wiley Interdiscip Rev Nanomed Nanobiotechnol* 4:52–65. https://doi.org/10.1002/WNAN.165

De Aza, P. N., De Aza, A. H., & De Aza, S. (2005). Crystalline bioceramic materials. *Bol. Soc. Esp. Ceram*, *44*(3), 135-145.doi: 10.1002/chin.200629272

Dittler ML, Unalan I, Grünewald A, et al. (2019) Bioactive glass (45S5)-based 3D scaffolds coated with magnesium and zinc-loaded hydroxyapatite nanoparticles for tissue engineering applications. *Colloids Surf B Biointerfaces* 182:110346. https://doi.org/10.1016/J.COLSURFB.2019.110346

Doremus RH (1992) Bioceramics. *J Mater Sci* 27:285–297. https://doi.org/10.1007/BF00543915

Dorozhkin SV (2010) Bioceramics of calcium orthophosphates. *Biomaterials* 31:1465–1485. https://doi.org/10.1016/J.BIOMATERIALS.2009.11.050

Falcone, Tommaso, and William W. Hurd. "Clinical reproductive medicine and surgery." 2007,*Springer Cham.* doi: 10.1007/978-3-319-52210-4

Feng DX, McCauley JP, Morgan-Curtis FK, et al. (2015) Evaluation of 39 medical implants at 7.0T. *Br J Radiol* 88. https://doi.org/10.1259/BJR.20150633

Freedman JD, Lusic H, Snyder BD, Grinstaff MW (2014) Tantalum oxide nanoparticles for the imaging of articular cartilage using X-ray computed tomography: Visualization of ex vivo/in vivo murine tibia and ex vivo human index finger cartilage. *Angew Chem Int Ed* 53:8406–8410. https://doi.org/10.1002/ANIE.201404519

Gao A, Hang R, Huang X, et al. (2014) The effects of titania nanotubes with embedded silver oxide nanoparticles on bacteria and osteoblasts. *Biomaterials* 35:4223–4235. https://doi.org/10.1016/J.BIOMATERIALS.2014.01.058

Geetha M, Singh AK, Asokamani R, Gogia AK (2009) Ti based biomaterials, the ultimate choice for orthopaedic implants – A review. *Prog Mater Sci* 54:397–425. https://doi.org/10.1016/J.PMATSCI.2008.06.004

Geng Z, Cui Z, Li Z, et al. (2016) Strontium incorporation to optimize the antibacterial and biological characteristics of silver-substituted hydroxyapatite coating. *Mater Sci Eng* C 58:467–477. https://doi.org/10.1016/J.MSEC.2015.08.061

Ghobadian M, Nabiuni M, Parivar K, et al. (2015) Toxic effects of magnesium oxide nanoparticles on early developmental and larval stages of zebrafish (Danio rerio). *Ecotoxicol Environ Saf* 122:260–267. https://doi.org/10.1016/J.ECOENV.2015.08.009

Gillani R, Ercan B, Qiao A, Webster TJ (2010) Nanofunctionalized zirconia and barium sulfate particles as bone cement additives. *Int J Nanomedicine* 5:1. https://doi.org/10.2147/ijn.s7603

Govindaraj S, Costantino PD, Friedman CD (1999) Current use of bone substitutes in maxillofacial surgery. *Facial Plast Surg* 15:73–81. https://doi.org/10.1055/S-2008-1064302/BIB

Guitchounts G, Markowitz JE, Liberti WA, Gardner TJ (2013) A carbon-fiber electrode array for long-term neural recording. *J Neural Eng* 10:046016. https://doi.org/10.1088/1741-2560/10/4/046016
Hak DJ, Fader R, Baldini T, Chadayammuri VBS (2017) Locking screw-plate interface stability in carbon-fibre reinforced polyetheretherketone proximal humerus plates. *Int Orthop* 41:1735–1739. https://doi.org/10.1007/S00264-017-3562-7
Hak DJ, Mauffrey C, Seligson D, Lindeque B (2014) Use of carbon-fiber-reinforced composite implants in orthopedic surgery. *Orthopedics* 37:825–830. https://doi.org/10.3928/01477447-20141124-05
Hench LL (2015) The future of bioactive ceramics. *J Mater Sci Mater Med* 26:1–4. https://doi.org/10.1007/S10856-015-5425-3
Hesaraki S (2016) Feasibility of alumina and alumina-silica nanoparticles to fabricate strengthened betatricalcium phosphate scaffold with improved biological responses. *Ceram Int* 42:7593–7604. https://doi.org/10.1016/J.CERAMINT.2016.01.167
Hjort H, Mathisen T, Alves A, et al. (2012) Three-year results from a preclinical implantation study of a long-term resorbable surgical mesh with time-dependent mechanical characteristics. *Hernia* 16:191. https://doi.org/10.1007/S10029-011-0885-Y
Hu H, Zhang W, Qiao Y, et al. (2012) Antibacterial activity and increased bone marrow stem cell functions of Zn-incorporated TiO_2 coatings on titanium. *Acta Biomater* 8:904–915. https://doi.org/10.1016/J.ACTBIO.2011.09.031
Ibrahim H, Esfahani SN, Poorganji B, et al. (2017) Resorbable bone fixation alloys, forming, and post-fabrication treatments. *Mater Sci Eng C* 70:870–888. https://doi.org/10.1016/J.MSEC.2016.09.069
Ikono R, Li N, Pratama NH, et al. (2019) Enhanced bone regeneration capability of chitosan sponge coated with TiO_2 nanoparticles. *Biotechnol Rep* 24:e00350. https://doi.org/10.1016/J.BTRE.2019.E00350
Johari N, Madaah Hosseini HR, Samadikuchaksaraei A (2018) Novel fluoridated silk fibroin/TiO_2 nanocomposite scaffolds for bone tissue engineering. *Mater Sci Eng* C 82:265–276. https://doi.org/10.1016/J.MSEC.2017.09.001
Kang C, Wei L, Song B, et al. (2017) Involvement of autophagy in tantalum nanoparticle-induced osteoblast proliferation. *Int J Nanomedicine* 12:4323. https://doi.org/10.2147/IJN.S136281
Kenar H, Akman E, Kacar E, et al. (2013) Femtosecond laser treatment of 316L improves its surface nanoroughness and carbon content and promotes osseointegration: An in vitro evaluation. *Colloids Surf B Biointerfaces* 108:305–312. https://doi.org/10.1016/J.COLSURFB.2013.02.039
Kharaziha M, Fathi MH (2009) Synthesis and characterization of bioactive forsterite nanopowder. *Ceram Int* 35:2449–2454. https://doi.org/10.1016/J.CERAMINT.2009.02.001
Khonsari RH, Berthier P, Rouillon T, et al. (2014) Severe infectious complications after PEEK-derived implant placement: Report of three cases. *J Oral Maxillofac Surg Med Pathol* 26:477–482. https://doi.org/10.1016/J.AJOMS.2013.04.006
Kim JH, Sheikh FA, Ju HW, et al. (2014) 3D silk fibroin scaffold incorporating titanium dioxide (TiO_2) nanoparticle (NPs) for tissue engineering. *Int J Biol Macromol* 68:158–168. https://doi.org/10.1016/J.IJBIOMAC.2014.04.045
Kirilova IA, Sadovoy M, Podorozhnaya VT (2012) Comparative characteristics of materials for bone grafting: Composition and properties. *Hirurgiâ pozvonočnika (Spine Surgery)* 72–83. https://doi.org/10.14531/SS2012.3.72-83
Kirilova IA, Sadovoy MA, Podorozhnaya VT, et al. (2013) Ceramic and osteoceramic implants: Upcoming trends. *Hirurgiâ pozvonočnika (Spine Surgery)* 052–062. https://doi.org/10.14531/SS2013.4.52-62
Ko WK, Kim SJ, Heo DN, et al. (2020) Double layers of gold nanoparticles immobilized titanium implants improve the osseointegration in rabbit models. *Nanomedicine* 24:102129. https://doi.org/10.1016/J.NANO.2019.102129
Kononenko V, Repar N, Marušič N, et al. (2017) Comparative *in vitro* genotoxicity study of ZnO nanoparticles, ZnO macroparticles and $ZnCl_2$ to MDCK kidney cells: Size matters. *Toxicol In Vitro* 40:256–263. https://doi.org/10.1016/J.TIV.2017.01.015
Kumar R, Lerski RA, Gandy S, et al. (2006) Safety of orthopedic implants in magnetic resonance imaging: An experimental verification. *J Orthop Res* 24:1799–1802. https://doi.org/10.1002/JOR.20213
Kurtz SM, Devine JN (2007) PEEK biomaterials in trauma, orthopedic, and spinal implants. *Biomaterials* 28:4845–4869. https://doi.org/10.1016/J.BIOMATERIALS.2007.07.013
Lee D, Heo DN, Nah HR, et al. (2018a) Injectable hydrogel composite containing modified gold nanoparticles: Implication in bone tissue regeneration. *Int J Nanomedicine* 13:7019. https://doi.org/10.2147/IJN.S185715
Lee MJE, Veiseh O, Bhattarai N, et al. (2010) Rapid pharmacokinetic and biodistribution studies using cholorotoxin-conjugated iron oxide nanoparticles: A novel non-radioactive Method. *PLoS One* 5:e9536. https://doi.org/10.1371/JOURNAL.PONE.0009536

Lee SJ, Lee HJ, Kim SY, et al. (2018b) In situ gold nanoparticle growth on polydopamine-coated 3D-printed scaffolds improves osteogenic differentiation for bone tissue engineering applications: In vitro and in vivo studies. *Nanoscale* 10:15447–15453. https://doi.org/10.1039/C8NR04037K

Li CS, Vannabouathong C, Sprague S, Bhandari M (2014) The use of carbon-fiber-reinforced (CFR) peek material in orthopedic implants: A systematic review. *Clin Med Insights Arthritis Musculoskelet Disord* 8:33–45. https://doi.org/10.4137/cmamd.s20354

Li H, Cong Y, Zheng Y, Cui L (2016) In vitro investigation of NiTiW shape memory alloy as potential biomaterial with enhanced radiopacity. *Mater Sci Eng* C 60:554–559. https://doi.org/10.1016/J.MSEC.2015.12.006

Lih E, Kum CH, Park W, et al. (2018) Modified magnesium hydroxide nanoparticles inhibit the inflammatory response to biodegradable poly(lactide- *co*-glycolide) implants. *ACS Nano* 12:6917–6925. https://doi.org/10.1021/ACSNANO.8B02365

Linkevicius T, Apse P (2009) Influence of abutment material on stability of peri-implant tissues: A systematic review. *J Prosthet Dent* 101:143. https://doi.org/10.1016/s0022-3913(09)60012-3

Liu S, Xu L, Zhang T, et al. (2010) Oxidative stress and apoptosis induced by nanosized titanium dioxide in PC12 cells. *Toxicology* 267:172–177. https://doi.org/10.1016/J.TOX.2009.11.012

Liu Y, Rath B, Tingart M, Eschweiler J (2020) Role of implants surface modification in osseointegration: A systematic review. *J Biomed Mater Res A* 108:470–484. https://doi.org/10.1002/JBM.A.36829

Mahmoudi M, Simchi A, Milani AS, Stroeve P (2009) Cell toxicity of superparamagnetic iron oxide nanoparticles. *J Colloid Interface Sci* 336:510–518. https://doi.org/10.1016/J.JCIS.2009.04.046

May R (2008) Polyetheretherketones. In *Encyclopedia of Polymer Science and Technology*. https://doi.org/10.1002/0471440264.PST266

McLatchie GR, Borley NR, Joanna, C (2013) *Oxford Handbook of Clinical Surgery*. Oxford University Press (OUP), Oxford, UK.

Michelle Grandin H, Berner S, Dard M (2012) A review of titanium zirconium (TiZr) alloys for use in endosseous dental implants. *Materials* 5:1348–1360. https://doi.org/10.3390/MA5081348

Mitchell PM, Lee AK, Collinge CA, et al. (2018) Early comparative outcomes of carbon fiber-reinforced polymer plate in the fixation of distal femur fractures. *J Orthop Trauma* 32:386–390. https://doi.org/10.1097/BOT.0000000000001223

Mugnai R, Tarallo L, Capra F, Catani F (2018) Biomechanical comparison between stainless steel, titanium and carbon-fiber reinforced polyetheretherketone volar locking plates for distal radius fractures. *Orthop Traumatol Surg Res* 104:877–882. https://doi.org/10.1016/J.OTSR.2018.05.002

Muhamedov M, Kulbakin D, Gunther V, et al. (2015) Sparing surgery with the use of tini-based endografts in larynx cancer patients. *J Surg Oncol* 111:231–236. https://doi.org/10.1002/JSO.23779

Nandi SK, Roy S, Mukherjee P, et al. (2010) Orthopaedic applications of bone graft & graft substitutes: A review. *Indian J Med Res* 132:15–30

Nandi SK, Shivaram A, Bose S, Bandyopadhyay A (2018) Silver nanoparticle deposited implants to treat osteomyelitis. *J Biomed Mater Res B Appl Biomater* 106:1073. https://doi.org/10.1002/JBM.B.33910

Nasri-Nasrabadi B, Kaynak A, Heidarian P, et al. (2018) Sodium alginate/magnesium oxide nanocomposite scaffolds for bone tissue engineering. *Polym Adv Technol* 29:2553–2559. https://doi.org/10.1002/PAT.4367

Nevelsky A, Borzov E, Daniel S, Bar-Deroma R (2017) Perturbation effects of the carbon fiber-PEEK screws on radiotherapy dose distribution. *J Appl Clin Med Phys* 18:62–68. https://doi.org/10.1002/ACM2.12046

Niinomi M, Nakai M, Hieda J (2012) Development of new metallic alloys for biomedical applications. *Acta Biomater* 8:3888–3903. https://doi.org/10.1016/J.ACTBIO.2012.06.037

Nowosielski R, Cesarz-Andraczke K, Sakiewicz P, et al. (2016) Corrosion of biocompatible $Mg_{66+X}Zn_{30-X}Ca_4$ (x=0.2) bulk metallic glasses. *Arch Metall Mater* 61:807–810. https://doi.org/10.1515/AMM-2016-0136

Ohtsuki C, Kamitakahara M, Miyazaki T (2009) Bioactive ceramic-based materials with designed reactivity for bone tissue regeneration. *J R Soc Interface* 6. https://doi.org/10.1098/RSIF.2008.0419.FOCUS

Onoue S, Yamada S, Chan HK (2014) Nanodrugs: Pharmacokinetics and safety. *Int J Nanomedicine* 9:1025–1037. https://doi.org/10.2147/IJN.S38378

Park JB, Lakes RS (1992) Hard tissue replacement II: Joints and teeth. *Biomaterials* 317–354. https://doi.org/10.1007/978-1-4757-2156-0_14

Patel NR, Gohil PP (2012) A review on biomaterials: Scope, applications & human anatomy significance. *Int J Emerg Technol Adv Eng* 2:91–101.

Peeples L (2019) Core concept: The rise of bioelectric medicine sparks interest among researchers, patients, and industry. *Proc Natl Acad Sci USA* 116:24379. https://doi.org/10.1073/PNAS.1919040116

Petersen R, Phillips J (2016) Carbon fiber biocompatibility for implants. *Fibers* 4:1. https://doi.org/10.3390/FIB4010001

Petersen RC (2011) Bisphenyl-polymer/carbon-fiber-reinforced composite compared to titanium alloy bone implant. *Int J Polym Sci*. https://doi.org/10.1155/2011/168924

Prabhu S, Poulose EK (2012) Silver nanoparticles: Mechanism of antimicrobial action, synthesis, medical applications, and toxicity effects. *Int Nano Lett* 2:1–10. https://doi.org/10.1186/2228-5326-2-32

Price RL, Elias KL, Haberstroh KM, Webster TJ (2011) Small diameter, high surface energy carbon nanofiber formulations that selectively increase osteoblast function. *MRS Online Proc Libr* 711:1–4. https://doi.org/10.1557/PROC-711-HH3.11.1

Qadri S, Haik Y, Mensah-Brown E, et al. (2017) Metallic nanoparticles to eradicate bacterial bone infection. *Nanomedicine* 13:2241–2250. https://doi.org/10.1016/J.NANO.2017.05.013

Qureshi AT, Doyle A, Chen C, et al. (2015) Photoactivated miR-148b-nanoparticle conjugates improve closure of critical size mouse calvarial defects. *Acta Biomater* 12:166–173. https://doi.org/10.1016/J.ACTBIO.2014.10.010

Qureshi AT, Monroe WT, Dasa V, et al. (2013) miR-148b-nanoparticle conjugates for light mediated osteogenesis of human adipose stromal/stem cells. *Biomaterials* 34:7799–7810. https://doi.org/10.1016/J.BIOMATERIALS.2013.07.004

Rai M, Duran N, De DO, Wirtschaft S (2011) Metal Nanoparticles in Microbiology Zu Inhaltsverzeichnis schnell und portofrei erhältlich bei An Insight into the Bacterial Biogenesis of Silver Nanoparticles, Industrial Production and Scale-up. Metal Nanoparticles in Microbiology. https://doi.org/10.1007/978-3-642-18312-6

Ranga N, Poonia E, Jakhar S, et al. (2019) Enhanced antimicrobial properties of bioactive glass using strontium and silver oxide nanocomposites. 7:75–81. https://doi.org/10.1080/21870764.2018.1564477

Russo T, Gloria A, de Santis R, et al. (2017) Preliminary focus on the mechanical and antibacterial activity of a PMMA-based bone cement loaded with gold nanoparticles. *Bioact Mater* 2:156–161. https://doi.org/10.1016/J.BIOACTMAT.2017.05.002

Sadiq IM, Chowdhury B, Chandrasekaran N, Mukherjee A (2009) Antimicrobial sensitivity of *Escherichia coli* to alumina nanoparticles. *Nanomedicine* 5:282–286. https://doi.org/10.1016/J.NANO.2009.01.002

Sahai N, Ahmad N, Gogoi M (2018) Nanoparticles based drug delivery for tissue regeneration using biodegradable scaffolds: A review. *Curr Pathobiol Rep* 6:219–224.

Sahmani S, Shahali M, Ghadiri Nejad M, et al. (2019) Effect of copper oxide nanoparticles on electrical conductivity and cell viability of calcium phosphate scaffolds with improved mechanical strength for bone tissue engineering. *Eur Phys J Plus* 134. https://doi.org/10.1140/EPJP/I2019-12375-X

Sargeant A, Goswami T (2006) Hip implants: Paper V. Physiological effects. *Mater Des* 27:287–307. https://doi.org/10.1016/J.MATDES.2004.10.028

Sarraf M, Dabbagh A, Abdul Razak B, et al. (2018) Silver oxide nanoparticles-decorated tantala nanotubes for enhanced antibacterial activity and osseointegration of Ti6Al4V. *Mater Des* 154:28–40. https://doi.org/10.1016/J.MATDES.2018.05.025

Scholz MS, Blanchfield JP, Bloom LD, et al. (2011) The use of composite materials in modern orthopaedic medicine and prosthetic devices: A review. *Compos Sci Technol* 71:1791–1803. https://doi.org/10.1016/J.COMPSCITECH.2011.08.017

Simmons M, Montague DK (2008) Penile prosthesis implantation: Past, present and future. *Int J Impot Res* 20(5):437–444. https://doi.org/10.1038/ijir.2008.11

Singh R, Lillard JW (2009) Nanoparticle-based targeted drug delivery. *Exp Mol Pathol* 86:215–223. https://doi.org/10.1016/J.YEXMP.2008.12.004

Sun CY, Che YJ, Lu SJ (2015) Preparation and application of collagen scaffold-encapsulated silver nanoparticles and bone morphogenetic protein 2 for enhancing the repair of infected bone. *Biotechnol Lett* 37:467–473. https://doi.org/10.1007/S10529-014-1698-8

Tabesh E, Salimijazi HR, Kharaziha M, et al. (2019) Development of an in-situ chitosan-copper nanoparticle coating by electrophoretic deposition. *Surf Coat Technol* 364:239–247. https://doi.org/10.1016/J.SURFCOAT.2019.02.040

Tao ZS, Zhou WS, He XW, et al. (2016) A comparative study of zinc, magnesium, strontium-incorporated hydroxyapatite-coated titanium implants for osseointegration of osteopenic rats. *Mater Sci Eng* C 62:226–232. https://doi.org/10.1016/J.MSEC.2016.01.034

Thomas D, Singh D (2017) 3D printing in surgery – The evolving paradigm-shift in surgical implants on demand. *Int J Surg* 42:58–59. https://doi.org/10.1016/J.IJSU.2017.04.027

Torchilin VP (2014) Multifunctional, stimuli-sensitive nanoparticulate systems for drug delivery. *Nat Rev Drug Discov* 13(11):813–827. https://doi.org/10.1038/nrd4333

Vallet-Regí M (2001) Ceramics for medical applications. *J Chem Soc Dalton Trans* 97–108. https://doi.org/10.1039/B007852M

van Hengel IAJ, Tierolf MWAM, Valerio VPM, et al. (2020) Self-defending additively manufactured bone implants bearing silver and copper nanoparticles. *J Mater Chem B* 8:1589–1602. https://doi.org/10.1039/C9TB02434D

Vandrovcová M, Bačáková L (2011) Adhesion, growth and differentiation of osteoblasts on surface-modified materials developed for bone implants. *Physiol Res* 60:403–417

Wang R, He X, Gao Y, et al. (2017) Antimicrobial property, cytocompatibility and corrosion resistance of Zn-doped ZrO_2/TiO_2 coatings on Ti6Al4V implants. *Mater Sci Eng* C 75:7–15. https://doi.org/10.1016/J.MSEC.2017.02.036

Wang X, Xu S, Zhou S, et al. (2016) Topological design and additive manufacturing of porous metals for bone scaffolds and orthopaedic implants: A review. *Biomaterials* 83:127–141. https://doi.org/10.1016/J.BIOMATERIALS.2016.01.012

Wang Z, Li N, Zhao J, et al. (2012) CuO nanoparticle interaction with human epithelial cells: Cellular uptake, location, export, and genotoxicity. *Chem Res Toxicol* 25:1512–1521. https://doi.org/10.1021/TX3002093/SUPPL_FILE/TX3002093_SI_001.PDF

Williams DF, McNamara A, Turner RM (1987) Potential of polyetheretherketone (PEEK) and carbon-fibre-reinforced PEEK in medical applications. *J Mater Sci Lett* 1987 6:2 6:188–190. https://doi.org/10.1007/BF01728981

Wong, Joyce Y., Joseph D. Bronzino, and Donald R. Peterson, eds. *Biomaterials: principles and practices.* CRC Press, 2013..

Wu J, Li L, Fu C, et al. (2018) Micro-porous polyetheretherketone implants decorated with BMP-2 via phosphorylated gelatin coating for enhancing cell adhesion and osteogenic differentiation. *Colloids Surf B Biointerfaces* 169:233–241. https://doi.org/10.1016/J.COLSURFB.2018.05.027

Wu X, Liu X, Wei J, et al. (2012) Nano-TiO2/PEEK bioactive composite as a bone substitute material: In vitro and in vivo studies. *Int J Nanomedicine* 7:1215. https://doi.org/10.2147/IJN.S28101

Xiu ZM, Zhang QB, Puppala HL, et al. (2012) Negligible particle-specific antibacterial activity of silver nanoparticles. *Nano Lett* 12:4271–4275. https://doi.org/10.1021/NL301934W/SUPPL_FILE/NL301934W_SI_001.PDF

Ye M, Shi B (2018) Zirconia nanoparticles-induced toxic effects in osteoblast-like 3T3-E1 cells. *Nanoscale Res Lett* 13:1–12. https://doi.org/10.1186/S11671-018-2747-3/FIGURES/8

Yu W, Wang X, Zhao J, et al. (2015) Preparation and mechanical properties of reinforced hydroxyapatite bone cement with nano-ZrO_2. *Ceram Int* 41:10600–10606. https://doi.org/10.1016/J.CERAMINT.2015.04.159

Zafar B, Mottaghitalab F, Shahosseini Z, et al. (2020) Silk fibroin/alumina nanoparticle scaffold using for osteogenic differentiation of rabbit adipose-derived stem cells. *Materialia* 9:100518. https://doi.org/10.1016/J.MTLA.2019.100518

Zaworonkow D, Chekan M, Kusnierz K, et al. (2018) Evaluation of TiNi-based wire mesh implant for abdominal wall defect management. *Biomed Phys Eng Express* 4:027010. https://doi.org/10.1088/2057-1976/AAA0B0

Zhang Q, Wang H, Ge C, et al. (2017) Alumina at 50 and 13 nm nanoparticle sizes have potential genotoxicity. *J Appl Toxicol* 37:1053–1064. https://doi.org/10.1002/JAT.3456

Zhang R, Lee P, Lui VCH, et al. (2015) Silver nanoparticles promote osteogenesis of mesenchymal stem cells and improve bone fracture healing in osteogenesis mechanism mouse model. *Nanomedicine* 11: 1949–1959. https://doi.org/10.1016/J.NANO.2015.07.016

Zhang Z, Ross RD, Roeder RK (2010) Preparation of functionalized gold nanoparticles as a targeted X-ray contrast agent for damaged bone tissue. *Nanoscale* 2:582–586. https://doi.org/10.1039/B9NR00317G

4 Organic–Inorganic Hybrid Nanomedicine for Drug Delivery

Himanshu Sekhar Panda and Megha Vaddatti
Defence Institute of Advance Technology

4.1 INTRODUCTION

The discoveries in the present drug delivery system (DDS) need to have persistent progress in increased drug efficiency, minimized toxicity, improved macromolecular specificity, and more economical and diverse biological and chemical properties (Patra et al. 2018). All these factors have therefore contributed to the evolution of novel drug delivery methods that are more convenient and controlled, with elevated levels of pharmacological activities and pharmacokinetic properties (Ezike et al. 2023). Recently, in the last few decades, nanoparticles (ultrafine particles that have a measurement of between 1 and 100 nm) have been used as the carriers of drugs in various forms like liposomes, dendrimers, nanowires, nanoshells, micelles, quantum dots and carbon nanotubes (Altammar 2023; Yadav, Ghune, and Kumar Jain 2011). Nanomedicine is the application of nanotechnology to the medical field, which helps us to invigilate, mend, and manage the biological activities of humans using engineered devices and structures of a nanoscale range and treat diseases accurately and efficiently (Yadav, Ghune, and Kumar Jain 2011). Due to their extremely small size, which is much less than the cells present in our body, nanoparticles can pass through our circulatory system with much ease and penetrate numerous organs and provide us with the required specific information(Olariu, Yiu, and Bouffier 2012).

Recently, hybrid nanomaterials—which comprise both organic and inorganic components—have been investigated as potentially beneficial platforms for drug delivery applications. This unique class of nanomaterials can combine functional components in a way that allows it to methodically alter the hybrid material's characteristics while retaining the advantageous aspects of the constituents, both organic and inorganic (Taylor-Pashow et al. 2010). Between the inorganic and organic carrier types, the inorganic types are recognized for offering superior mechanical, optical, and electrical qualities, smaller particle size, and targeting capability (Madni et al. 2017). However, it is well known that organic drug carriers tend to be more biocompatible and versatile when it involves delivering the two types of hydrophilic and hydrophobic medications. But organic DDSs, like liposomes, have difficulties with their chemical and thermal stability and are immediately identified by the body's defences (Corma et al. 2009). The primary disadvantage of nanoparticles made of inorganic materials is the surface functionalization, which is required to improve both stability and dispersibility. To achieve this, the addition of organic molecules to the surface of inorganic nanoparticles is done to improve their biocompatibility and biodegradability (Sarkar et al. 2018). Furthermore, these organic coverings are necessary to initiate site-specific drug transport and release while minimizing the adverse effects of chemotherapy medications without harming healthy tissues (Le et al. 2018).

Because of their advantageous physicochemical characteristics, organic and inorganic nanohybrids, which combine both organic and inorganic components into a single system, have drawn interest over time and have become a great success in recent years (Oshiro et al. 2016). Because of their combined effect, these combinations not only display their features, but they also create new

DOI: 10.1201/9781003473015-4

ones (Manatunga et al. 2020). By using these medication techniques with unique qualities, drug delivery may be improved through a variety of channels, such as enhanced site-specific targeting, improved drug permeability through advanced barriers, altered drug pharmacokinetics, and reduced toxicity, but sometimes the outcomes of investigations of these hybrid nanomedicine particles used for drug delivery frequently fall short of our expectations (Öchsner and Da Silva n.d.).

The scope of this chapter is to know the history and evolution of nanomaterials in drug delivery and their classification, synthesis methods, characterization, and applications. This chapter will ultimately be completed by discussing about the future perspective of utilizing this inorganic and organic hybrid nanomedicine in medication administration.

4.2 HISTORY AND EVOLUTION OF NANOMEDICINE

The field of nanomedicine is a new area of research. Potential applications of nanotechnology in medical technology, medicine, and pharmacology date back only to the 1990s (Krukemeyer et al. 2015). The field of nanoscience originated in the 5th century B.C., during the time of Democritus and the Greeks. They wondered if the matter was made up of atoms, which are tiny, unbreakable, and indivisible particles, or if it continued without restriction, which would further be divisible into smaller pieces (Bayda et al. 2020). The field of nanotechnology has only been around for the past few decades (Figure 4.1).

In the year 1997, Elghanian et al. published an article regarding an instrument for colorimetric polynucleotide detection using hybridized nucleotide nanoparticles of gold, which was the first hybrid nanosystem mentioned in the biomedical sector (Elghanian et al. 1997). In 1998, Caruso et al. announced the development of silica-polymer hybrid spheres at the nanoscale, which signalled the start of actual hybrid nanosystems with structural elements that are both organic and inorganic (Caruso, Caruso, and Möhwald 1998). The revelation of high-resolution microscopy in the 20th century gave rise to new fields like biochemistry, microelectronics, and molecular biology. Understanding nanobiotechnology, which deals with the study of the composition and operation of cells and also intra- and intercellular mechanisms and cell communication, is crucial in the realm of nanomedicine and scientific study, which was first opened at the start of the 20th century

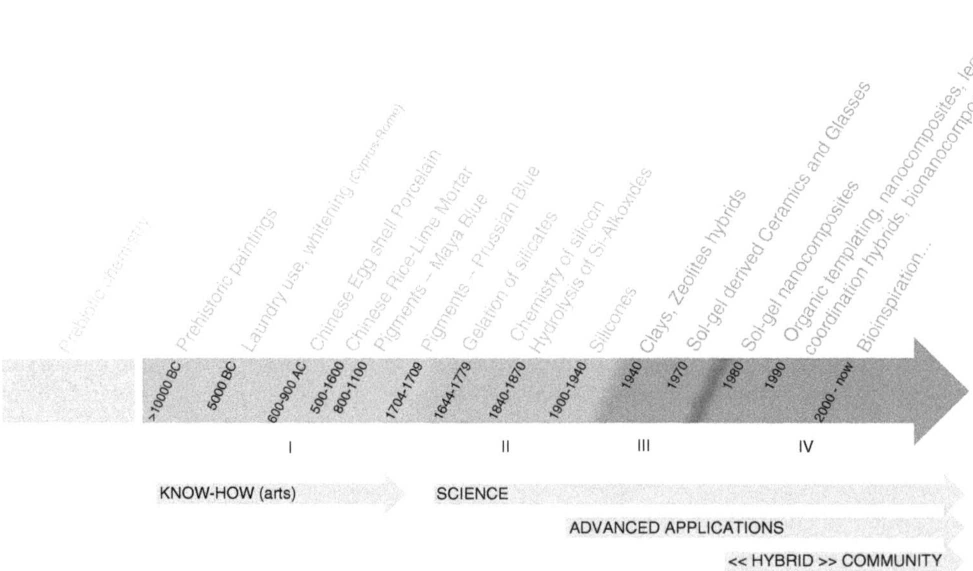

FIGURE 4.1 Timeline of the development and multidisciplinary evolution of the organic–inorganic hybrid materials. (Reproduced from Faustini et al. (2018) with permission.)

with the development of advanced microscopes (Krukemeyer et al. 2015). Along with this, the creation of hybrid nanosystems saw a significant expansion at the beginning of the 21st century with the introduction of metallic nanoparticles functionalized with polymers and the formation of hybrids of silica with polymers, micelles, and liposomes. Review articles on these systems began to surface in 2003 as interest in them developed significantly. Over the previous two decades, there has been a steady rise in the quantity of results returned by the National Library of Medicine's "hybrid nanoparticle" search. In 2003, there were just 42 results returned, but there were about 2,000 matches around 2021 (Mukherjee et al. 2021).

The last decade has seen enormous developments in the advancement of hybrid nanomedicine for the purpose of drug delivery, like targeted drug delivery with nanoparticles, stimuli-responsive DDSs, and theragnostic nanomedicine. Ligand-conjugated and stimuli-responsive nanoparticles are used for targeted drug delivery. Theragnostic nanomedicine and multifunctional nanoparticles are used as combinational therapies for drug delivery.

In ligand-conjugated nanoparticles drug delivery, the therapeutic agent (ligand) that can identify specific receptors or diseased cells is attached to the nanoparticles. This allows for precise delivery of drugs, minimizing side effects on healthy tissues. Stimuli-responsive nanoparticles-based drug delivery of the nanoparticles that react to biological or physical stimuli, such as alterations in enzyme levels, redox potential, or pH due to the presence of specific enzymes found in diseased areas, is used to treat diseases (Singh and Lillard 2009). Theragnostic nanomedicine is a new and rapidly emerging field that uses nanoparticles to combine treatment and diagnostics on a single platform. Nanoparticles can deliver drugs while simultaneously allowing for disease imaging, enabling real-time monitoring of treatment effectiveness (Esposti, Tampieri, and Iafisco 2017). Multifunctional nanoparticles can incorporate contrast agents and deliver one or more therapeutic drugs. They can also provide biomolecular targeting via attached antibodies or different recognizing agents, hence amplifying imaging signals (Vasile 2018). Other novel carriers like polymeric micelles, dendrimers, and microfluidics techniques that enable exact control over the dimensions, morphology, and surface characteristics of nanoparticles, leading to more uniform and efficient DDSs, have also been developed (Gimondi et al. 2023).

These advancements highlight the growing sophistication of nanomedicine for drug delivery. Researchers are constantly pushing boundaries to develop even more targeted, effective, and safe therapeutic strategies.

4.3 HYBRID NANOMEDICINE

4.3.1 Different Types of Organic–Inorganic Nanoparticles

Depending upon the binding force causing how both organic and inorganic elements interact, there are two types of hybrid materials consisting of organic and inorganic components. They are Class I and Class II.

The organic and inorganic constituents of Class I hybrid compounds interact weakly via hydrogen bonding, van der Waals, or electrostatic forces. Class II hybrid compounds, on the other hand, are bound together via strong interactions such as ionic-covalent or covalent bonds (Figure 4.2). There has been an advancement in the development of Class II hybrid compounds with strong and stable binding in recent years (Park et al. 2020).

4.3.2 Constituents of Hybrid Nanomedicine

Hybrid nanomedicine consists of both organic and inorganic nanoparticle constituents (Figure 4.3). These hybrid nanomaterials are made up of inorganic nanoparticles, such as gold, magnetic, and silica materials, which are encased in organic nano compartments, like poly(lactic-co-glycolic acid), dendrimers, liposomes, or micelles (Yanar, Carugo, and Zhang 2023).

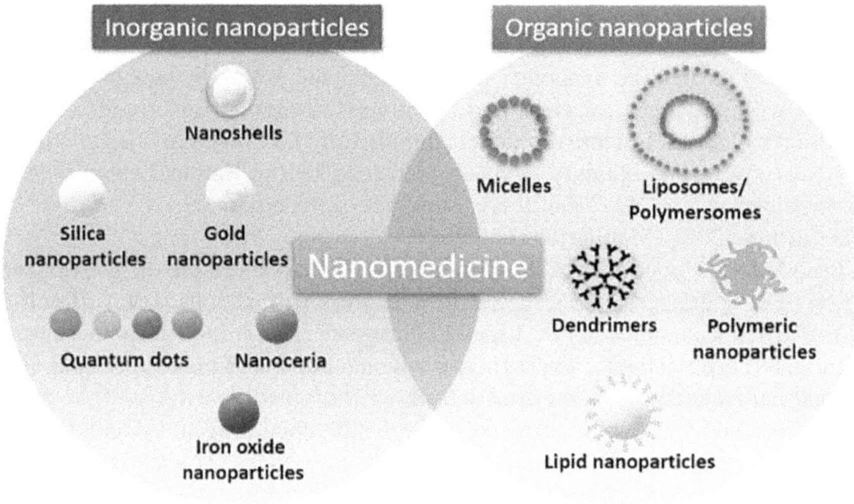

FIGURE 4.2 Types of organic–inorganic hybrid materials. (Reproduced from Faustini et al. (2018) with permission.)

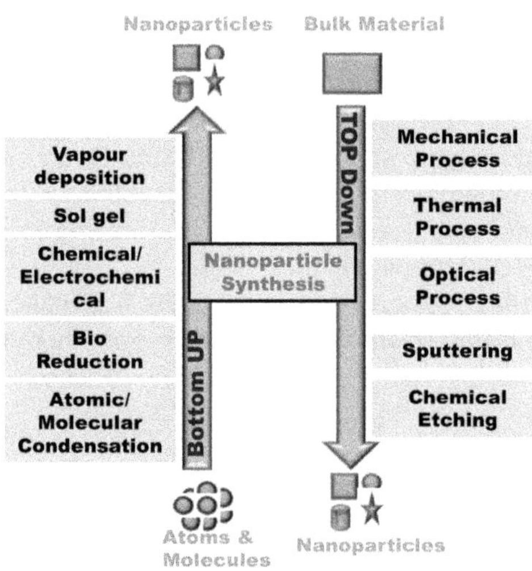

FIGURE 4.3 Organic and inorganic hybrid nanomedicine. (Reproduced from Martinelli, Pucci, and Ciofani (2019) with permission.)

4.3.3 Factors to Be Considered While Designing Nanohybrid Materials for Medicine

For an efficient DDS, the design of nanomedicine needs to be such that it has maximum saturation solubility rise, so the therapeutic nanoparticles used for this purpose should be amorphous and should have a size of 20–50 nm. It is also important to remember that the blood type is to be determined while taking a certain medication. Often, a very rapid dissolution of the drug is not recommended. In many cases, drug nanocrystals must be used in conjunction with conventional controlled-release technology (such as coated pellets) to achieve sustained blood levels and prevent rapid breakdown. In summary, the ideal drug nanocrystal form and crystalline/amorphous state will be determined by: the administrative path of the drug, blood purity requirements, and the ability of the product's amorphous condition to remain stable over its shelf life (Junghanns and Müller 2008).

Furthermore, many additional properties like the microstructure, charge, and composition of particular tissues/cartilages/organs of the body are to be considered while designing a nanohybrid medicine to ensure that the drug is delivered to the appropriate place. All these factors determine the depth to which nanohybrid medicine can penetrate (Zhou et al. 2024). Also, other facts like being secure and efficient, biocompatible, having a long half-life, being metabolically stable, being nontoxic, and having few to no adverse effects need to be distributed selectively to the intended tissues; high potency and efficiency, better distribution and metabolism should also be considered (Baldi 2010).

4.3.4 Mechanism of Interaction between Organic and Inorganic Nanomaterials

The bonding between the inorganic and organic nanomaterials is a vital element for constructing hybrid systems with specialized features for use in electronics, catalytic activity, sensors, medicine, and other fields. This interaction method depends upon the distinctive properties of both the inorganic and organic elements, like their chemical integrity, physical features, and surface functioning (Vallet-Regí, Colilla, and González 2011).

Organic and inorganic hybrid nanomaterials can be prepared by various types of interactions, like covalent bonds (Imai et al. 2000; Imai, Naka, and Chmot 1998), hydrogen bonds, ionic interactions (Ogoshi and Chujo 2005), π–π interactions (Tamaki, Samura, and Chujo n.d.), metal–ligand coordination (Ogoshi et al. 2002, 2003), host-guest interactions (Ogoshi and Chujo 2003), and many others. In situ polymerization is also helpful for producing hybrid materials (Tamaki, Naka, and Chujo 1997).

Covalent Bond Interactions: These bonds are one of the strongest linkages between materials. It is feasible to create stimuli-responsive hybrid materials by employing versatile procedures that form covalent bonds. The Diels–Alder reaction between maleimide and furan was used to create polymer hybrids, which are an IPN (interpenetrating polymer network) comprising organic polymer and silica gel (Imai et al. 2000).

Ionic Bond Interactions: The ionic interactions between cations and anions are also used to produce hybrid materials. For example, the ionic interactions between the amino groups of 3-aminopropyltrimethoxysilane (APTMOS) and the sulphonic groups of the organic polymer were used to produce homogeneous polystyrene and silica gel polymer (Tamaki and Chujo 1999).

π-π Interactions: π-π interactions between the organic and inorganic components are helpful to produce hybrid materials. For example, phenyltrimethoxysilane sol-gel reaction has been used for producing homogeneous polystyrene and silica gel polymer hybrids. The π-π interactions between the silica gel and the organic polymer's phenyl groups were crucial to the uniformity (Tamaki, Samura, and Chujo n.d.).

The interactions between organic and inorganic phases in hybrid nanomaterials are diverse and application-dependent. By tailoring these interactions—through covalent modifications, optimization of non-covalent forces, or employing hybrid bonding techniques—researchers can design materials with customized properties. Future developments in this field will likely focus on enhancing the precision and scalability of these bonding techniques for advanced applications in electronics, energy, and medicine.

4.3.5 Advantages of Organic and Inorganic Hybrid Nanomaterials

The formation of hybrid materials is significantly impacted by the combined presence of organic and inorganic components. There are different forms and compositions of hybrid nanomaterials, such as nanorods, nanotubes, nanoparticles, and nanospheres (Singh and Singh 2023). By altering their composition and shape, hybrid nanomaterials' features can be adjusted to produce materials with improved performance characteristics such as increased thermal stability, electron conductivity, mechanical strength, and light emission (Hayami et al. 2017). Due to their accessible features and multifunctionality, these hybrid materials are becoming platforms for applications across a wide range of sectors like health and diagnostics, solar and fuel cells, smart coatings, optics, microelectronics, catalysis, and sensing (Meroni and Ardizzone 2018).

There have been many reports of biomedical and medicinal applications of inorganic-organic hybrid systems and their therapeutic uses in biological environments. Encasing inorganic nanoparticles in organic component vesicles (such as liposomes or polymers) improves bioavailability, reduces possible toxicity while functionality is maintained, and improves stability in biological systems, making them suitable for drug administration and theragnostics (Sanchez et al. 2005; Yanar, Carugo, and Zhang 2023). Microwindow-equipped hollow nanospheres offered a flexible framework for using organic and inorganic hybrid materials in drug delivery and encapsulation (Sonia and Sharma 2014a). The potential for gold nanoparticles, nanoshells, nanorods, and nanowires to be an essential part of our imaging equipment and helpful in the battle against cancer is enormous. Biocompatible quantum dot conjugates are used for tumour targeting, metastatic cell tracking, tumour angiogenesis imaging, and sentinel lymph node mapping (Sekhon and Kamboj 2010a). Dendrimers are used as contrast agents, medication or gene carriers, and metal ion sensors (Sekhon and Kamboj 2010b). Due to their small size, lipid nanoparticles improve mucosal adhesion, shield the loaded insulin from enzymatic and chemical degradation, and release insulin from their lipid matrix gradually into the bloodstream, all of which contribute to better therapeutic action (Sonia and Sharma 2014a).

Organic and inorganic hybrid nanomaterials have many advantages as they have combinational properties of both the organic and inorganic constituents; they also come with certain limitations and challenges that can affect their practical applications, like complexity in synthesis, stability concerns, and transitioning from lab-scale synthesis to industrial-scale production due to the complexity of the process (Yanar, Carugo, and Zhang 2023). The modern age of hybrid organic–inorganic hybrid systems has recently begun. The profound structural insights and mechanics comprehension reached in recent years will direct a new trend in the atomic and molecular design of hybrid materials (Ananikov 2019).

4.4 SYNTHESIS METHOD

Numerous nanomaterials have been employed in nanomedicine applications. Based upon their constitution, they can be broadly classified into three types (McDonald et al. 2015):

1. Solid drug nanoparticles (SDNs)
2. Polymer therapeutics
3. Nanocarriers.

4.4.1 Solid Drug Nanoparticles

SDNs are created using various techniques, each with its advantages and considerations, but the most prominent techniques among them are "top-down" and "bottom-up" (McDonald et al. 2015).

The **top-down method** involves the process in which the massive material is disintegrated into small constituents or structures in the nanoscale range. This technique is less complex by nature and depends on either reducing the size of bulk production processes or splitting or eliminating bulk material to create the intended structure with the appropriate qualities. The primary issue with the top-down approach is flawed surface structure (Figure 4.4).

The **bottom-up method** involves the technique in which a substance is assembled starting at the base or bottom via molecule per molecule, atom per atom, or cluster per cluster (Figure 4.4). There

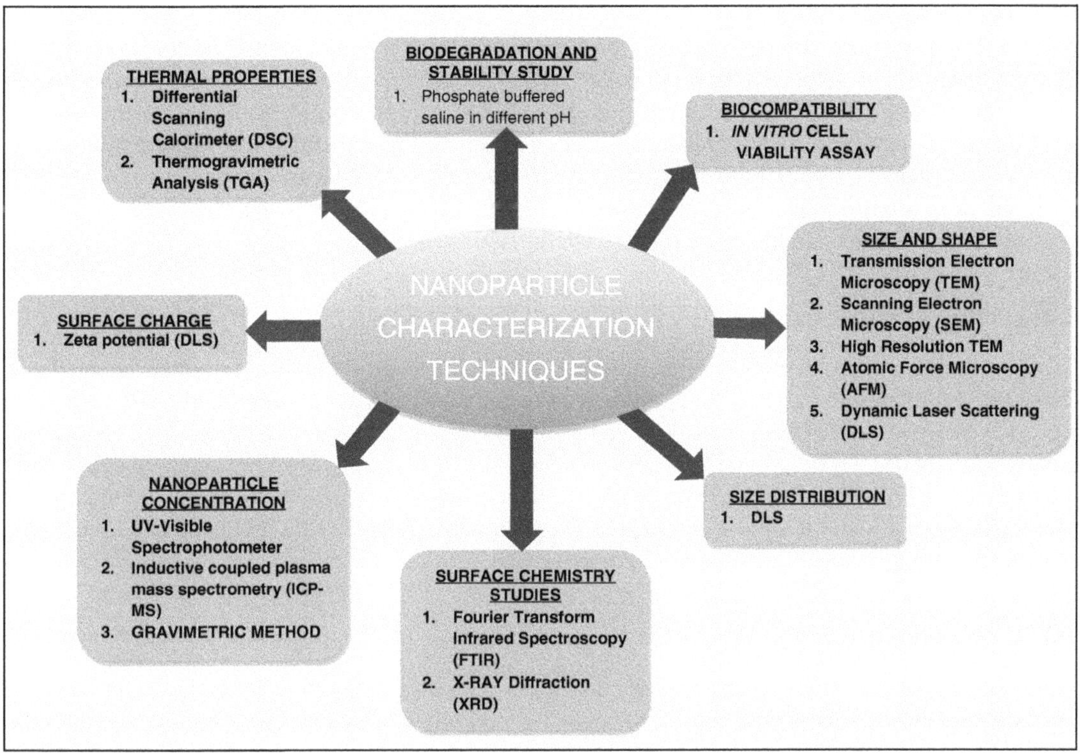

FIGURE 4.4 Different methods of nanoparticle synthesis. (Reproduced from Bayda et al. (2020) with permission.)

have been reports of several renowned bottom-up methods for producing nanoparticles, including the reverse-micelle route, electrodeposition, hydrothermal synthesis, sol-gel synthesis, organometallic chemical route, and colloidal precipitation (Beer Pal Singh n.d.).

The methods that are generally employed for the formulation of hybrid nanomedicine are as follows:

1. *Milling Method*:

   The process of milling is used to create SDN-based nanomedicines, which is the most effective technique. It is also referred to as bead or pearl milling. In a grinding mill, media milling occurs in either a liquid or solid state. An abrasive substance is used in a grinding mill to provide stress to the particle, causing it to break down into small particles (Buse and El-Aneed 2010). Nanosuspensions are made in pearl mills or high-shear media mills. The three components of the media mill are the recirculation chamber, the milling shaft, and the milling chamber (Nagpal et al. 2012). The required drug is then fed into the mill, which has tiny pearl-like grinding balls submerged in an aqueous solution, and then the temperature is properly regulated. These balls further go through the interior of the grinding jar, striking the specimen material against the wall across from them. They revolve at an extremely elevated shear rate. The joined actions of both the attrition and impact may cause a substantial decrease in particle size. Materials like highly cross-linked polystyrene resin with exceptional resistance to abrasion, aluminium oxide, or zirconium oxide sintered in ceramic are used to create balls or milling media. The planetary ball mill is a component of machinery that can produce particles smaller than 0.1 μm (Aldeeb et al. 2024). Numerous nano-therapies that are currently available on the market were created using this technique (Möschwitzer 2013).

2. *Homogenization Method*:

   High-pressure homogenization, or HPH, has become a practical method for producing inorganic/hybrid-type nanoparticles. Initially, the extruder barrel could be filled with raw materials at a temperature higher than the lipids' melting point. Furthermore, the solid lipid nanoparticles (SLNs) may be reduced in size by using an insulated connector to fasten a homogenizer by applying intense pressure to the hot melt extruder barrel's rear. The previously described strategy produced SLNs with better-reduced size and process parameters as compared to the usual method (Setia et al. 2024).

4.4.2 Polymer Therapeutics

Usually, polymer therapeutics are created by slightly altering standard polymer chemistries. Different techniques can be used to conjugate an active pharmaceutical ingredient (API) to a polymer; polyethylene glycol (PEG)-based polymer therapies, such as conjugating PEG directly to a protein, frequently use the functionality that is present at the PEG chain's termination point connecting the two halves. By reacting with the protein's lysine or cysteine residues, the functionalized polymer can be conjugated to the protein by adding functional groups such as maleimide and aldehyde to the chain end of the polymer (Larson and Ghandehari 2012).

4.4.3 Nanocarriers

Nanocarriers are described as the vehicles that are utilized to deliver the medicine to the desired location, and these nanocarriers control the distribution and pharmacokinetics of the delivery of the drug. The use of nanocarriers has the benefit of protecting active drugs from degradation, enabling higher and more effective amounts in the tissue being targeted, and minimizing the intensity of unfavourable toxic side effects (Esfahani et al. 2018). There is a wide range of nanocarriers like SLNs, polymer nanoparticles, metal nanoparticles, nanoemulsions, dendrimers, and virosomes (McDonald et al. 2015).

SLNs are used for specialized and controlled administration of drugs. These are present in the range of 50–1,000 nm (submicron) in size and are composed of biodegradable and biocompatible materials that can incorporate both hydrophilic and lipophilic drugs. Water, emulsifiers, and lipids (matrix materials) are commonly used in SLN formulations.

The most often used platforms for polymeric nanoparticles are liposomes, micelles, dendrimers, nanoshells, conjugates of polymer and protein, conjugates of polymer and drug, polymersomes, polyplexes, and many more (Vasile 2018).

Metal nanoparticles are being used for various purposes, such as magnetic separation, target analyte preconcentration, targeted gene and drug administration, and diagnostic imaging. Among them, gold and silver are the most often employed types of nanoparticles for delivering drugs because of their antifungal and antimicrobial properties and are efficiently functionalized using a range of target ligands (Almeida et al. 2020). Other metal nanoparticles include platinum nanoparticles, palladium nanoparticles, copper nanoparticles, zinc-oxide nanoparticles, titanium dioxide nanoparticles, and metal sulphide nanoparticles (Chandrakala, Aruna, and Angajala 2022).

The two primary approaches utilized in the synthesis of metal nanoparticles are the top-down technique (dispersion method) and the bottom-up approach (condensation method). Considering these approaches, numerous researchers have documented a variety of chemical and physical processes for creating metal nanoparticles (Chandrakala, Aruna, and Angajala 2022).

4.4.3.1 Lithography

Lithography involves a printing method where images are formed by dipping a substrate covered with a stamp into ink. There are hydrophobic and hydrophilic areas on the stamp; the hydrophobic area absorbs ink while the hydrophilic area does not. Lithography typically reproduces (Vasile 2018) a pattern that is similar to the substrate patterning. Photolithography, e-beam lithography, scanning probe lithography, ultraviolet (UV) lithography, nanolithography, and soft lithography are the various types of lithography used for the delivery of drugs (Paramasivam et al. 2021).

4.4.3.2 Sol-Gel Method

The manufacture of carriers of drugs using the **sol-gel method** is an inexpensive, easy procedure that yields particles characterized by a significant degree of uniformity and purity. The process of hydrolysis, polymerization, or condensation of the employed monomers, particle development, and gel formation are involved in the sol-gel method. Owing to all the advantages this process has, it is extensively employed in composing the drug carrier (Nasr Azadani et al. 2021).

4.4.3.3 Chemical Vapour Deposition

Chemical vapour deposition, or CVD, is comparatively economical to other processes. It involves exposing a volatile precursor to a substrate that is kept at a high temperature. The reactant separates into a number of products that disperse over the surface, undergo a chemical process, develop into nuclei, and then mature into the required material. This hybrid method can be used to cover both organic and inorganic materials. There are numerous CVD methods that are accessible, such as plasma-accelerated CVD, vapour phase epitaxy, molecular beam epitaxy, and metallocene organic CVD (Yu et al. 2015; Pirtarighat, Ghannadnia, and Baghshahi 2019).

4.4.3.4 Laser Ablation

In this process, the concentrated laser energy creates pores or microchannels by damaging the skin's outermost layers. Lasers like erbium-doped yttrium aluminium garnet (Er: YAG) are used. By acting as channels, these microchannels greatly improve the absorption and therapeutic effectiveness of nanomedicines. The noncontact nature of the laser ablation technique reduces the possibility of contamination. Furthermore, it enables exact regulation of the extent of ablation, guaranteeing that only the specified skin layers are impacted and protecting the healthy tissue around them, and therefore they are involved in the production of nanomedicine, which encapsulates drugs that are involved in targeted drug delivery (Hsiao et al. 2019).

4.4.3.5 Hydrothermal Synthesis/Solvothermal Synthesis

The hydrothermal technique uses water as a solvent at high temperatures and pressures to synthesize nanomaterials. These chemical reactions are carried out in autoclaves, which are sealed vessels that heat water to temperatures close to its critical point (374°C) while applying high pressures (up to 22.1 MPa), which involve two important steps of crystal nucleation and crystal growth (Li, Wu, and Wu 2015).

Solvothermal procedures use organic solvents in place of water, just like hydrothermal processes do. This makes it possible to synthesize a greater range of materials, such as transitional metals and metal-organic frameworks (MOFs) (Li, Wu, and Wu 2015).

4.4.3.6 Sputtering Deposition

This process is usually involved in the creation of thin films for various processes. Using energetic ions, usually from a plasma, material is ejected from the target's (source) surface and deposited onto a substrate, which is used in the production of hybrid nanomaterials used for various processes (Seshan 2002).

Many other techniques like plasma electrolytic oxidation (PEO), electrospinning, polymerization-induced self-assembly (PISA), block co-polymerization, and many others are used for the production of organic and inorganic hybrid nanomedicine (Lee et al. 2023; Macchione, Biglione, and Strumia 2018; Niu et al. 2022; Alshammari et al. 2023).

The fabrication of hybrid organic–inorganic nanomedicine has improved considerably due to creative fabrication methods designed to satisfy the requirements of present-day biomedical applications. These nanomedicine synergies between organic and inorganic constituents provide advances in targeted therapeutics, implantable devices, and theragnostics. Despite the enormous potential of these methods, issues including cost, reproducibility, and scalability still prevail. Future developments might concentrate on combining real-time monitoring during synthesis, ecologically friendly fabrication techniques, and machine learning for reliable synthesis (Patra et al. 2018; Serov and Vinogradov 2022).

4.5 CHARACTERIZATION TECHNIQUES

Nanomaterials used for drug delivery have different attributes depending on their size; thus, it's important to characterize their optical, structural, and physical characteristics (Figure 4.5). The following discusses the various characterization procedures of the nanomaterials, which are majorly of two categories: chemical characterization and structural characterization (Sharma et al. 2020).

4.5.1 Chemical Characterization

Chemical characterization of nanomaterials is the process of determining the elemental and chemical composition of a nanomaterial.

4.5.1.1 Fourier-Transform Infrared Spectroscopy

Fourier-transform infrared spectroscopy (FTIR) is a kind of vibratory spectroscopy that relies on how infrared light interacts with an atom's inherent vibrations that form the material's chemical bonds. In infrared spectroscopy, a source of infrared light is used to irradiate the sample, and the variations in the radiation that the sample absorbs are monitored. It depends upon the molecular vibrations (stretching and bending) of the sample. FTIR is employed to determine the types of chemical bonds and functional groups that exist in a substance (Sampath Kumar 2013).

4.5.1.2 Energy-Dispersive X-Ray Spectroscopy

Energy-dispersive X-ray spectroscopy (EDS) is employed in the characterization of chemicals, micrometre dimension measurement, and elemental analysis of the sample. Depending on the sample being analysed, scanning electron microscopy (SEM) or transmission electron microscopy (TEM) is typically attached to the EDS instrument. EDS also provides sample image analysis in addition to elemental mapping. Using EDS has numerous advantages, including quicker contamination and identification of sources, greater yields, more control over outside influences, and the ability to identify the source of the problem (Senthil Kumar, Grace Pavithra, and Naushad 2019).

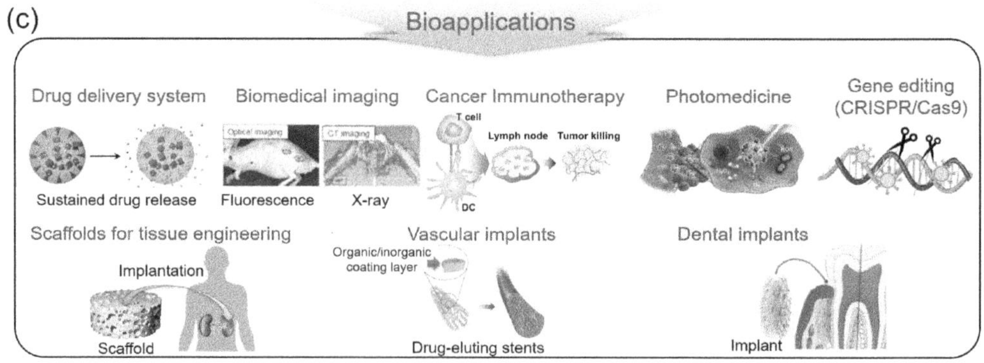

FIGURE 4.5 Characterization of nanoparticles. (Reproduced from Dhilip Kumar and Abrahamse (2020) with permission.)

4.5.1.3 UV-Visible Spectroscopy

The range of wavelengths during which absorption happens and the intensity at each wavelength are recorded using a UV-visible (Vis) spectrometer. The application of UV-Vis spectroscopy allows for evaluating the effects of various signals on the optical characteristics of metal nanoparticles. The kinetics of a process can be evaluated using the UV-Vis spectroscopy time course, polymeric network, and development of particles (Heera and Shanmugam 2015).

4.5.1.4 Nuclear Magnetic Resonance Spectroscopy

Nuclear magnetic resonance (NMR) uses a strong magnetic field to estimate the interaction of nuclear spins to determine a material's molecular structure. Additionally, it permits the assessment of molecular structural mobility to various generated pulse sequences. It has been utilized to identify conformational changes taking place within the molecule as well as physical characteristics like structure, functionality, and purity of dendrimers, polymers, and other physicochemical parameters (Lin et al. 2014).

4.5.1.5 Brunauer-Emmett-Teller Surface Area Analysis Method

The Brunauer-Emmett-Teller (BET) technique is helpful for using the gas sorption process to analyse the properties of nanomaterials, including area of the surface, size of the pore, form, and also the amount of adsorbent that is on the surface. This method involves exposing a solid sample to a controlled atmosphere of gas, typically nitrogen gas, to obtain the isotherms for adsorption and desorption at a very low temperature. An increasing number of gas molecules adhere to the solid's surface as the gas pressure rises. The amount of gas needed to produce a single layer on the solid surface is then calculated by using the BET equation to the isotherm of adsorption data. Then the total area of the surface of the solid sample can be determined by using this value combined with the specified area represented by an individual gas molecule (Sinha et al. 2019).

4.5.2 Structural Characterization

Structural characterization is used to determine the nanomaterials' size, shape, lattice, and crystallinity.

4.5.2.1 X-ray Diffraction Technique

X-ray diffraction (XRD) technique is employed to evaluate properties like strain, crystallite size, and structure of the sample (Akbari, Pirhadi Tavandashti, and Zandrahimi 2011). The samples of XRD are analysed in the powder form, and a "reflection" is created when the constructive interference Bragg criteria are met. Usually, the quantity of grains in a favoured orientation is directly correlated with the relative peak height. The Scherrer equation is used to determine the average crystallite size from the diffraction peaks (Akbari, Pirhadi Tavandashti, and Zandrahimi 2011).

4.5.2.2 Electron Microscopy

4.5.2.2.1 Scanning Electron Microscope

SEM is a surface scanning technique where the incident electron beam moves across the specimen's surface and reacts with it to produce signals that show the topography and atomic constitution of the specimen surface (Hall et al. 2007). Electrons on a sample's surface or near-surface substance emit elastic scattering (also known as backscattered electrons), inelastic scattering (also known as low-energy secondary electrons), and characteristic X-ray light (also known as cathodoluminescence) as a result of the incident electrons, and later these scattering patterns are converted to a signal which helps surface imaging (Lin et al. 2014).

4.5.2.2.2 Transmission Electron Microscopy

TEM is a precise technique for electronic spectroscopic imaging that provides superior resolution compared to SEM. Typically, conventional TEM operates at around 100 keV, while for high-resolution imaging, the energy level is increased to 1 MeV (Misof, Roschger, and Fratzl 2011). It utilizes an electron beam to engage with a specimen, resulting in the formation of an image captured either on a specific camera or photographic plate. It is a quantitative approach for examining the particle's form, size, and dispersion. TEM has two major advantages in comparison to SEM: they have greater spatial resolution and more analytical measurements (Sonia and Sharma 2014b).

4.5.2.2.3 Atomic Force Microscopy

AFM, or atomic force microscopy, offers analytical and visualizing capabilities of the samples in three dimensions (Rao et al. 2007). It can produce images at an atomic resolution, providing height information accurate to the Angstrom scale, all with minimal sample preparation requirements. It scans the sample's surface using a cantilever that has a pointed tip. AFM scanning can be done in three different ways: tapping, noncontact, and contact. It is used for examining the nanomaterials' surface texture (Rao et al. 2007).

4.5.2.2.4 Magnetic Force Microscopy

Magnetic force microscopy (MFM) is a technique that is derived from AFM, employing an AFM tip coated with a magnetic material to examine local magnetic fields. This technique provides spatial resolution akin to standard AFM, enabling the capture of images that depict the nanoscale magnetic characteristics of samples (Passeri et al. 2014). MFM can be used to analyse a wide range of magnetic interactions, such as the magnetic dipole-dipole interaction. It is also used for identifying different biological components (Nasrollahzadeh et al. 2019).

4.5.2.3 Differential Scanning Calorimetry

The measurement of heat evolution or absorption during chemical reactions, transitions in phase, and other physical changes is known as calorimetry (Mansfield and Banash). Differential scanning calorimetry (DSC) is a technique in thermal analysis utilized for evaluating the quantity of energy absorbed or released by a sample for temperature changes. Specific heat, enthalpy, entropy, glass transition temperature (Tg), and phase diagram can all be measured with DSC equipment (Koshy, Subramanian, and Thomas 2017). This seems like a quick, easy, and economical way to be used in laboratories. Due to all these features, DSC is the most applicable method for research and the process of drug development (Demetzos 2008).

4.5.2.4 Dynamic Light Scattering

Dynamic light scattering (DLS) enables in the precise measurement of the submicron range particle size distribution profiles (Mukherjee and Sasikala 2013). It is a specific, harmless, and effective analytical tool that is frequently used to characterize colloids and macromolecules in solution. It is also utilized for evaluating a nanoparticle's size and size dispersion profile (Nimesh 2013). The DLS approach has several benefits, including automated operation, quick measurement times, sensitivity to aggregates, non-invasiveness for colloids, lack of calibration, and no need for a particular kind of sample preparation. Thus, this method is being employed extensively in many areas of science to characterize nanoparticles used for drug delivery (Krzyzowska et al. 2017).

4.6 PROGRESS, CHALLENGES, AND FUTURE OF ORGANIC AND INORGANIC HYBRID NANOMEDICINE

In recent years, hybrid nanomedicine has emerged as a hopeful strategy in both preclinical and clinical research for the timely detection of illnesses (Rajana et al. 2022). Because of their small size (10–100 nm), high surface area, and flexible surface functionalization, nanomedicine frequently shows higher therapeutic efficacy than traditional small-molecule medicines (Zhang et al. 2021).

The field of hybrid nanomedicine encompasses a wide range of applications, such as high-throughput screening platforms, wearable devices, antibacterial agents, vaccine development, medication delivery, and diagnostic (in vivo and in vitro) and imaging instruments utilizing materials that are biological, biomimetic, nonbiological, or hybrid (Figure 4.6) (Pelaz et al. 2017). These hybrid nanomedicines are used to treat a wide range of diseases such as cancer (oncology), neurological disorders related to central nervous system, diseases of the bones and joints (orthopaedics), cardiovascular disorders (cardiology), and diseases of the eyes (ophthalmology) (Jain 2008). Nanomedicine is also used in the development of personalized diseases and to treat autoimmune diseases like rheumatoid arthritis, systemic lupus erythematosus, type I diabetes, multiple sclerosis, inflammatory bowel diseases, and Parkinson's diseases (Yuan, Thiele, and Wang 2011; Shankar, Geetha, and Wilson 2021).

Compared to conventional treatment approaches, they offer several benefits, including enhanced drug solubility, preferred drug accumulation in the tumour site, prolonged drug release, increased bioavailability, improved pharmacokinetics, and enhanced biocompatibility (Niveditha 2019). Yet, every opportunity has its own set of obstacles. Since hybrid systems are made of numerous materials and involve a variety of technologies, their complexity could be a significant barrier. The intricacy of the particles adds to the difficulties in achieving large-scale manufacturing, consistency, the hybrid systems' affordability, and homogeneity, necessitating significant focus and effort. The characteristics of hybrid nanoparticles, including excretion and biodegradation, are extremely concerning from a safety standpoint for in vivo applications, particularly for the inorganic constituents in the hybrid systems (Chen et al. 2021). Even many toxicity considerations of nanomedicine are to be examined before using them to treat any kind of disease (Li et al. 2012).

Nanomedicine is a swiftly advancing domain that involves the utilization of nanoparticles for diagnosing and treating various illnesses, alongside applications in regenerative medicine. In the future, we need to put efforts into developing potential strategies to prevent toxicity or to develop techniques for examining biodistribution to produce nanomaterials that can be applied for clinical applications. Internationally, efforts are underway to realize the clinical implementation of diverse nanomaterials, yet there exists a pervasive doubt regarding the practicality of employing nanomaterials within living organisms (Chang et al. 2015).

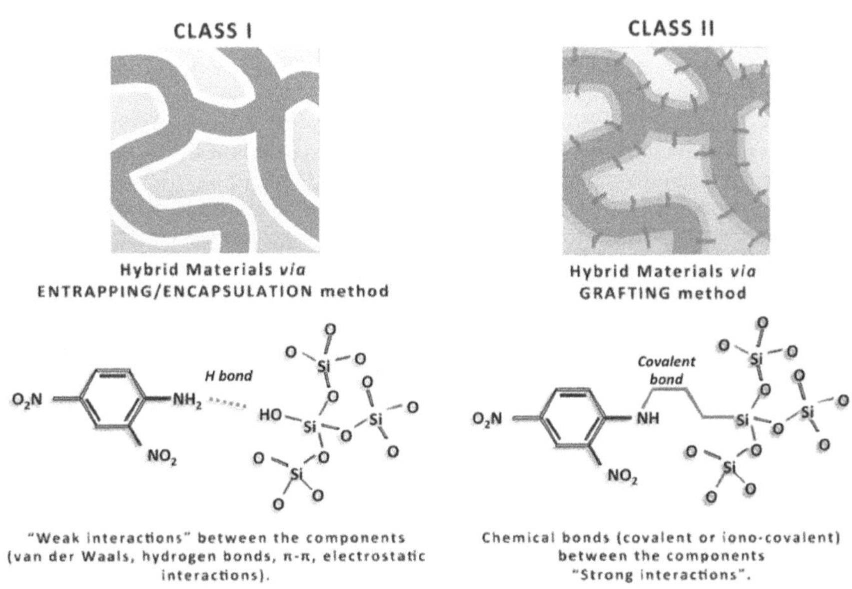

FIGURE 4.6 Application of organic–inorganic hybrid nanoparticles in the medical field. (Reproduced from Park et al. (2020) with permission.)

4.7 CONCLUSION

Many different synthetic approaches have been used for developing inorganic-organic hybrid nanomaterials. The presence of both the organic and inorganic constituents in the hybrid nanomedicine allows them to be altered for a wide range of diverse biological applications. Comprehensive research in the field of nanomedicine will undoubtedly result in the development of safe, extremely effective, and extremely sensitive medications for intravenous and oral use, as well as early-stage cancer monitoring and detection systems in the future. We conclude by saying that in the future there shall definitely be the development of hybrid nanomedicine overcoming all the present drawbacks and new designs, and formulations of the drugs that might help to treat the disease more efficiently than at present with minimal side effects and pave way for new avenues of research in the respective field.

REFERENCES

Akbari, Behzad; Pirhadi Tavandashti, Mohammad; and Zandrahimi, Morteza. 2011. *Particle Size Characterization of Nanoparticles – A Practical Approach.*

Aldeeb, Mohamed Mahmud E., Gofarana Wilar, Cecep Suhandi, Khaled M. Elamin, and Nasrul Wathoni. 2024. "Nanosuspension-Based Drug Delivery Systems for Topical Applications." *International Journal of Nanomedicine*. doi:10.2147/IJN.S447429.

Almeida, Mafalda R., Márcia C. Neves, Sergio Morales-Torres, Mara G. Freire, Joaquim L. Faria, Valéria C. Santos-Ebinuma, Cláudia G. Silva, and Ana P.M. Tavares. 2020. "Biomedical-Related Applications of Functionalized Nanomaterials." In *Handbook of Functionalized Nanomaterials for Industrial Applications*, 205–230. doi:10.1016/B978-0-12-816787-8.00009-0.

Alshammari, Basmah H., Maha M.A. Lashin, Muhammad Adil Mahmood, Fahad S. Al-Mubaddel, Nasir Ilyas, Nasir Rahman, Mohammad Sohail, Aurangzeb Khan, Sherzod Shukhratovich Abdullaev, and Rajwali Khan. 2023. "Organic and Inorganic Nanomaterials: Fabrication, Properties and Applications." *RSC Advances*. doi:10.1039/d3ra01421e.

Altammar, Khadijah A. 2023. "A Review on Nanoparticles: Characteristics, Synthesis, Applications, and Challenges." *Frontiers in Microbiology*. doi:10.3389/fmicb.2023.1155622.

Ananikov, Valentine P. 2019. "Organic-Inorganic Hybrid Nanomaterials." *Nanomaterials*. doi:10.3390/nano9091197.

Baldi, A. 2010. "Computational Approaches for Drug Design and Discovery: An Overview." *Systematic Reviews in Pharmacy*. doi:10.4103/0975-8453.59519.

Bayda, Samer, Muhammad Adeel, Tiziano Tuccinardi, Marco Cordani, and Flavio Rizzolio. 2020. "The History of Nanoscience and Nanotechnology: From Chemical-Physical Applications to Nanomedicine." *Molecules*. doi:10.3390/molecules25010112.

Beer Pal Singh. *Top-Down and Bottom-Up Approaches for Synthesis of Nanomaterials.* [SCRIBD website] https://www.scribd.com/document/483386153/Nano-material-Synthesis-Techniques-Top-down-and-bottom-up-nanofabrication-Synthesis-of

Buse, Joshua, and Anas El-Aneed. 2010. "Properties, Engineering and Applications of Lipid-Based Nanoparticle Drug-Delivery Systems: Current Research and Advances." *Nanomedicine*. doi:10.2217/nnm.10.107.

Caruso, Frank, Rachel A. Caruso, and Helmuth Möhwald. 1998. "Nanoengineering of Inorganic and Hybrid Hollow Spheres by Colloidal Templating." *Science* 282 (5391): 1111–1114. doi:10.1126/science.282.5391.1111.

Chandrakala, Vinayagasundaram, Valmiki Aruna, and Gangadhara Angajala. 2022. "Review on Metal Nanoparticles as Nanocarriers: Current Challenges and Perspectives in Drug Delivery Systems." *Emergent Materials*. doi:10.1007/s42247-021-00335-x.

Chang, Esther H., Joe B. Harford, Michael A.W. Eaton, Patrick M. Boisseau, Admire Dube, Rose Hayeshi, Hulda Swai, and Dong Soo Lee. 2015. "Nanomedicine: Past, Present and Future - A Global Perspective." *Biochemical and Biophysical Research Communications*. doi:10.1016/j.bbrc.2015.10.136.

Chen, Gang, Yuna Qian, Hang Zhang, Aftab Ullah, Xiaojun He, Zaigang Zhou, Hicham Fenniri, and Jianliang Shen. 2021. "Advances in Cancer Theranostics Using Organic-Inorganic Hybrid Nanotechnology." *Applied Materials Today*. doi:10.1016/j.apmt.2021.101003.

Corma, Avelino, Urbano Díaz, María Arrica, Eduardo Fernández, and Ílida Ortega. 2009. "Organic-Inorganic Nanospheres with Responsive Molecular Gates for Drug Storage and Release." *Angewandte Chemie - International Edition* 48 (34): 6247–6250. doi:10.1002/anie.200902208.

Demetzos, Costas. 2008. "Differential Scanning Calorimetry (DSC): A Tool to Study the Thermal Behavior of Lipid Bilayers and Liposomal Stability." *Journal of Liposome Research* 18 (3): 159–173. doi:10.1080/08982100802310261.

Dhilip Kumar, Sathish Sundar, and Heidi Abrahamse. 2020. "Advancement of Nanobiomaterials to Deliver Natural Compounds for Tissue Engineering Applications." *International Journal of Molecular Sciences*. doi:10.3390/ijms21186752.

Elghanian, Robert, James J. Storhoff, Robert C. Mucic, Robert L. Letsinger, and Chad A. Mirkin. 1997. "Selective Colorimetric Detection of Polynucleotides Based on the Distance-Dependent Optical Properties of Gold Nanoparticles." *Science* 277 (5329): 1078–1081. doi:10.1126/science.277.5329.1078.

Esfahani, Darian R., Kevin M. Tangen, Morteza Sadeh, Akop Seksenyan, Brandon L. Neisewander, Ankit I. Mehta, and Andreas A. Linninger. 2018. "Systems Engineers' Role in Biomedical Research. Convection-Enhanced Drug Delivery." In *Computer Aided Chemical Engineering*, vol. 42, pp. 271–302. doi:10.1016/B978-0-444-63964-6.00009-X.

Esposti, Lorenzo Degli, Anna Tampieri, and Michele Iafisco. 2017. "Targeted and Theranostic Applications for Nanotechnologies in Medicine: Nanostructured Calcium Phosphates for Theranostic Nanomedicine." In *Nanotechnologies in Preventive and Regenerative Medicine: An Emerging Big Picture*, pp. 465–487. doi:10.1016/B978-0-323-48063-5.00006-X.

Ezike, Tobechukwu Christian, Ugochukwu Solomon Okpala, Ufedo Lovet Onoja, Chinenye Princess Nwike, Emmanuel Chimeh Ezeako, Osinachi Juliet Okpara, Charles Chinkwere Okoroafor, et al. 2023. "Advances in Drug Delivery Systems, Challenges and Future Directions." *Heliyon*. doi:10.1016/j.heliyon.2023.e17488.

Faustini, Marco, Lionel Nicole, Eduardo Ruiz-Hitzky, and Clément Sanchez. 2018. "History of Organic–Inorganic Hybrid Materials: Prehistory, Art, Science, and Advanced Applications." *Advanced Functional Materials*. doi:10.1002/adfm.201704158.

Gimondi, Sara, Helena Ferreira, Rui L. Reis, and Nuno M. Neves. 2023. "Microfluidic Devices: A Tool for Nanoparticle Synthesis and Performance Evaluation." *ACS Nano*. doi:10.1021/acsnano.3c01117.

Hall, Jennifer B., Marina A. Dobrovolskaia, Anil K. Patri, and Scott E. McNeil. 2007. "Characterization of Nanoparticles for Therapeutics." *Nanomedicine*. doi:10.2217/17435889.2.6.789.

Hayami, Ryohei, Keisuke Wada, Izumi Nishikawa, Takuya Sagawa, Kazuki Yamamoto, Satoru Tsukada, and Takahiro Gunji. 2017. "Preparation and Properties of Organic-Inorganic Hybrid Materials Using Titanium Phosphonate Cluster." *Polymer Journal* 49 (9): 665–669. doi:10.1038/pj.2017.34.

Heera, P, and S Shanmugam. 2015. Review Article Nanoparticle Characterization and Application: An Overview. *International Journal of Current Microbiology and Applied Sciences* 4. https://www.ijcmas.com.

Hsiao, Chien Yu, Shih Chun Yang, Ahmed Alalaiwe, and Jia You Fang. 2019. "Laser Ablation and Topical Drug Delivery: A Review of Recent Advances." *Expert Opinion on Drug Delivery*. doi:10.1080/17425247.2019.1649655.

Imai, Yusuke, Hideaki Itoh, Kensuke Naka, and Yoshiki Chujo. 2000a. "Thermally Reversible IPN Organic–Inorganic Polymer Hybrids Utilizing the Diels-Alder Reaction." *Macromolecules* 33 (12): 4343–4346. doi:10.1021/ma991899b.

Imai, Yusuke, Kensuke Naka, and Yoshiki Chmot. 1998. "Reversible Formation of Interpenetrating Polymer Network Structure in Organic-Inorganic Polymer Hybrids." *Polymer Journal* 30.

Jain, K. K. 2008. "Nanomedicine: Application of Nanobiotechnology in Medical Practice." *Medical Principles and Practice*. doi:10.1159/000112961.

Junghanns, Jens-Uwe AH, and Rainer H. Müller. 2008. "Nanocrystal Technology, Drug Delivery and Clinical Applications." *International Journal of Nanomedicine* 3, 295–309.

Koshy, Obey, Lakshmanan Subramanian, and Sabu Thomas. 2017. "Differential Scanning Calorimetry in Nanoscience and Nanotechnology." In *Thermal and Rheological Measurement Techniques for Nanomaterials Characterization*, vol. 3, pp. 109–122. doi:10.1016/B978-0-323-46139-9.00005-0.

Krukemeyer, M. G., V. Krenn, F. Huebner, W. Wagner, and R. Resch. 2015. "History and Possible Uses of Nanomedicine Based on Nanoparticles and Nanotechnological Progress." *Journal of Nanomedicine & Nanotechnology* 6 (6). doi:10.4172/2157-7439.1000336.

Krzyzowska, Malgorzata, Emilia Tomaszewska, Katarzyna Ranoszek-Soliwoda, Karolina Bien, Piotr Orlowski, Grzegorz Celichowski, and Jaroslaw Grobelny. 2017. "Tannic Acid Modification of Metal Nanoparticles: Possibility for New Antiviral Applications." *Nanostructures for Oral Medicine*, 335–363. doi:10.1016/B978-0-323-47720-8.00013-4.

Larson, Nate, and Hamidreza Ghandehari. 2012. "Polymeric Conjugates for Drug Delivery." *Chemistry of Materials*. doi:10.1021/cm2031569.

Le, Thi Thu Huong, Thuc Quang Bui, Thi Minh Thi Ha, Mai Huong Le, Hong Nam Pham, and Phuong Thu Ha. 2018. "Optimizing the Alginate Coating Layer of Doxorubicin-Loaded Iron Oxide Nanoparticles for Cancer Hyperthermia and Chemotherapy." *Journal of Materials Science* 53 (19): 13826–13842. doi:10.1007/s10853-018-2574-z.

Lee, Donghyun, Jeongsu Shin, Hangyu Son, Seo Young Cheon, Yeeun Lee, Joonhyuck Park, and Heebeom Koo. 2023. "Organic and Inorganic Nanomedicine for Combination Cancer Therapies." *Nanoscale Advances*. doi:10.1039/d3na00043e.

Li, Jianlin, Qingliu Wu, and Ji Wu. 2015. "Synthesis of Nanoparticles via Solvothermal and Hydrothermal Methods." In *Handbook of Nanoparticles*, pp. 295–328. Springer International Publishing. doi:10.1007/978-3-319-15338-4_17.

Li, Xiaoming, Lu Wang, Yubo Fan, Qingling Feng, and Fu Zhai Cui. 2012. "Biocompatibility and Toxicity of Nanoparticles and Nanotubes." *Journal of Nanomaterials*. doi:10.1155/2012/548389.

Lin, Ping Chang, Stephen Lin, Paul C. Wang, and Rajagopalan Sridhar. 2014. "Techniques for Physicochemical Characterization of Nanomaterials." *Biotechnology Advances*. doi:10.1016/j.biotechadv.2013.11.006.

Macchione, Micaela A., Catalina Biglione, and Miriam Strumia. 2018. "Design, Synthesis and Architectures of Hybrid Nanomaterials for Therapy and Diagnosis Applications." *Polymers*. doi:10.3390/polym10050527.

Madni, Asadullah, Nayab Tahir, Mubashar Rehman, Ahmed Raza, Muhammad Ahmad Mahmood, Muhammad Imran Khan, and Prince Muhammad Kashif. 2017. "Hybrid Nano-Carriers for Potential Drug Delivery." In *Advanced Technology for Delivering Therapeutics*. doi:10.5772/66466.

Manatunga, Danushika C., V. Umayangana Godakanda, Rohini M. de Silva, and K. M. Nalin de Silva. 2020. "Recent Developments in the Use of Organic–Inorganic Nanohybrids for Drug Delivery." *Wiley Interdisciplinary Reviews: Nanomedicine and Nanobiotechnology*. doi:10.1002/wnan.1605.

Mansfield, Elisabeth, and Mark Banash. *Thermal Analysis of Nanoparticles: Methods, Kinetics, and Recent Advances*. www.nanodb.dk.

Martinelli, Chiara, Carlotta Pucci, and Gianni Ciofani. 2019. "Nanostructured Carriers as Innovative Tools for Cancer Diagnosis and Therapy." *APL Bioengineering*. doi:10.1063/1.5079943.

McDonald, Tom O., Marco Siccardi, Darren Moss, Neill Liptrott, Marco Giardiello, Steve Rannard, and Andrew Owen. 2015. "The Application of Nanotechnology to Drug Delivery in Medicine." In *Nanoengineering: Global Approaches to Health and Safety Issues*, pp. 173–223. doi:10.1016/B978-0-444-62747-6.00007-5.

Meroni, Daniela, and Silvia Ardizzone. 2018. "Preparation and Application of Hybrid Nanomaterials." *Nanomaterials*. doi:10.3390/nano8110891.

Misof, B., P. Roschger, and P. Fratzl. 2011. "Imaging Mineralized Tissues in Vertebrates." *Comprehensive Biomaterials* 3 (January): 407–426. doi:10.1016/B978-0-08–055294-1.00112-4.

Möschwitzer, Jan P. 2013. "Drug Nanocrystals in the Commercial Pharmaceutical Development Process." *International Journal of Pharmaceutics*. doi:10.1016/j.ijpharm.2012.09.034.

Mukherjee, Arnab, and Wilbee D. Sasikala. 2013. "Drug-DNA Intercalation: From Discovery to the Molecular Mechanism." *Advances in Protein Chemistry and Structural Biology* 92 (January): 1–62. doi:10.1016/B978-0-12–411636-8.00001-8.

Mukherjee, Priyabrata, Ali Khademhosseini, Joshua Seaberg, Hossein Montazerian, Md Nazir Hossen, and Resham Bhattacharya. 2021. "Hybrid Nanosystems for Biomedical Applications." *ACS Nano*. doi:10.1021/acsnano.0c09382.

Nagpal, Manju, Meetali Mudgil, Nidhi Gupta, and Pravin Pawar. 2012. *Nanotechnology: A New Approach for Ocular Drug Delivery System. Article in International Journal of Pharmacy and Pharmaceutical Sciences*. https://www.researchgate.net/publication/272495532.

Nasr Azadani, Reyhaneh, Milad Sabbagh, Haniye Salehi, Amir Cheshmi, Ali Raza Beena Kumari, and Gisou Erabi. 2021. "Sol-Gel: Uncomplicated, Routine and Affordable Synthesis Procedure for Utilization of Composites in Drug Delivery: Review." *Journal of Composites and Compounds* 2 (5): 57–70. doi:10.52547/jcc.3.1.6.

Nasrollahzadeh, Mahmoud, Monireh Atarod, Mohaddeseh Sajjadi, S. Mohammad Sajadi, and Zahra Issaabadi. 2019. "Plant-Mediated Green Synthesis of Nanostructures: Mechanisms, Characterization, and Applications." *Interface Science and Technology* 28 (January): 199–322. doi:10.1016/B978-0-12-813586-0.00006–7.

Nimesh, Surendra. 2013. "Tools and Techniques for Physico-Chemical Characterization of Nanoparticles." In *Gene Therapy*, pp. 43–63. Elsevier. doi:10.1533/9781908818645.43.

Niu, Bing, Ying Chen, Li Zhang, and Jianbo Tan. 2022. "Organic-Inorganic Hybrid Nanomaterials Prepared via Polymerization-Induced Self-Assembly: Recent Developments and Future Opportunities." *Polymer Chemistry*. doi:10.1039/d2py00180b.

Niveditha, T. M. A. 2019. "Applications of Nanomedicine-Overview." *International Journal of Advance Research*. doi:10.2967/jnumed.

Öchsner, Andreas, and Lucas F M Da Silva. n.d. *Advanced Structured Materials Volume* 104 *Series Editors*. https://www.springer.com/series/8611.

Ogoshi, Tomoki, and Yoshiki Chujo. 2003. "Synthesis of Organic-Inorganic Polymer Hybrids by Means of Host-Guest Interaction Utilizing Cyclodextrin." *Macromolecules* 36 (3): 654–660. doi:10.1021/ma0213089.

Ogoshi, Tomoki, and Yoshiki Chujo. 2005. "Synthesis of Amorphous and Nanostructured Cationic Polyacetylene/Silica Hybrids by Using Ionic Interactions." *Macromolecules* 38 (22): 9110–9116. doi:10.1021/ma050296z.

Ogoshi, Tomoki, Hideaki Itoh, Kyung Min Kim, and Yoshiki Chujo. 2002. "Synthesis of Organic-Inorganic Polymer Hybrids Having Interpenetrating Polymer Network Structure by Formation of Ruthenium-Bipyridyl Complex." *Macromolecules* 35 (2): 334–338. doi:10.1021/ma010819c.

Ogoshi, Tomoki, Hideaki Itoh, Kyung-Min Kim, and Yoshiki Chujo. 2003. "Thermal and Solvent-Resistant Properties of Organic-Inorganic Polymer Hybrids Having Interpenetrating Polymer Network Structure by Formation of Metal-Bipyridyl Complex." *Polymer Journal* 35.

Olariu, Cristina I., Humphrey H.P. Yiu, and Laurent Bouffier. 2012. "Inorganic–Organic Hybrid Nanoparticles for Medical Applications." In *Advanced Structured Materials* 4: 85–133. doi:10.1007/8611_2010_30.

Oshiro, João Augusto, Marina Paiva Abuçafy, Eloísa Berbel Manaia, Bruna Lallo Da Silva, Bruna Galdorfini Chiari-Andréo, and Leila Aparecida Chiavacci. 2016. "Drug Delivery Systems Obtained from Silica Based Organic-Inorganic Hybrids." *Polymers*. doi:10.3390/polym8040091.

Paramasivam, Gokul, Vishnu Vardhan Palem, Thanigaivel Sundaram, Vickram Sundaram, Somasundaram Chandra Kishore, and Stefano Bellucci. 2021. "Nanomaterials: Synthesis and Applications in Theranostics." *Nanomaterials*. doi:10.3390/nano11123228.

Park, Wooram, Heejun Shin, Bogyu Choi, Won Kyu Rhim, Kun Na, and Dong Keun Han. 2020. "Advanced Hybrid Nanomaterials for Biomedical Applications." *Progress in Materials Science*. doi:10.1016/j.pmatsci.2020.100686.

Passeri, Daniele, Chunhua Dong, Melania Reggente, Livia Angeloni, Mario Barteri, Francesca A. Scaramuzzo, Francesca de Angelis, et al. 2014. "Magnetic Force Microscopy: Quantitative Issues in Biomaterials." *BioMatter* 4 (6). doi:10.4161/biom.29507.

Patra, Jayanta Kumar, Gitishree Das, Leonardo Fernandes Fraceto, Estefania Vangelie Ramos Campos, Maria Del Pilar Rodriguez-Torres, Laura Susana Acosta-Torres, Luis Armando Diaz-Torres, et al. 2018a. "Nano Based Drug Delivery Systems: Recent Developments and Future Prospects." *Journal of Nanobiotechnology*. doi:10.1186/s12951-018-0392-8.

Pelaz, Beatriz, Christoph Alexiou, Ramon A. Alvarez-Puebla, Frauke Alves, Anne M. Andrews, Sumaira Ashraf, Lajos P. Balogh, et al. 2017. "Diverse Applications of Nanomedicine." *ACS Nano* 11 (3): 2313–2381. doi:10.1021/acsnano.6b06040.

Pirtarighat, Saba, Maryam Ghannadnia, and Saeid Baghshahi. 2019. "Green Synthesis of Silver Nanoparticles Using the Plant Extract of Salvia Spinosa Grown in Vitro and Their Antibacterial Activity Assessment." *Journal of Nanostructure in Chemistry* 9 (1): 1–9. doi:10.1007/s40097-018-0291-4.

Rajana, Naveen, Aare Mounika, Padakanti Sandeep Chary, Valamla Bhavana, Anuradha Urati, Dharmendra Khatri, Shashi Bala Singh, and Neelesh Kumar Mehra. 2022. "Multifunctional Hybrid Nanoparticles in Diagnosis and Therapy of Breast Cancer." *Journal of Controlled Release* 352 (December): 1024–1047. doi:10.1016/J.JCONREL.2022.11.009.

Rao, A., M. Schoenenberger, E. Gnecco, Th Glatzel, E. Meyer, D. Brändlin, and L. Scandella. 2007. "Characterization of Nanoparticles Using Atomic Force Microscopy." *Journal of Physics: Conference Series* 61 (1): 971–976. doi:10.1088/1742-6596/61/1/192.

Sampath Kumar, T. S. 2013. "Physical and Chemical Characterization of Biomaterials." In *Characterization of Biomaterials*, pp. 11–47. doi:10.1016/B978-0-12-415800-9.00002-4.

Sanchez, Clément, Beatriz Julián, Philippe Belleville, and Michael Popall. 2005. "Applications of Hybrid Organic–Inorganic Nanocomposites." *Journal of Materials Chemistry* 15 (35–36): 3559–3592. doi:10.1039/b509097k.

Sarkar, Chandrani, Angshuman Ray Chowdhuri, Amit Kumar, Dipranjan Laha, Subhadra Garai, Jui Chakraborty, and Sumanta Kumar Sahu. 2018. "One Pot Synthesis of Carbon Dots Decorated Carboxymethyl Cellulose- Hydroxyapatite Nanocomposite for Drug Delivery, Tissue Engineering and Fe3+ Ion Sensing." *Carbohydrate Polymers* 181 (February): 710–718. doi:10.1016/j.carbpol.2017.11.091.

Sekhon, Bhupinder S., and Seema R. Kamboj. 2010a. "Inorganic Nanomedicine-Part 1." *Nanomedicine: Nanotechnology, Biology, and Medicine*. doi:10.1016/j.nano.2010.04.004.

Sekhon, Bhupinder S., and Seema R. Kamboj. 2010b. "Inorganic Nanomedicine-Part 2." *Nanomedicine: Nanotechnology, Biology, and Medicine*. doi:10.1016/j.nano.2010.04.003.

Senthil Kumar, P., K. Grace Pavithra, and Mu Naushad. 2019. "Characterization Techniques for Nanomaterials." In *Nanomaterials for Solar Cell Applications*, pp. 97–124. doi:10.1016/B978-0-12–813337-8.00004–7.

Serov, Nikita, and Vladimir Vinogradov. 2022. "Artificial Intelligence to Bring Nanomedicine to Life." *Advanced Drug Delivery Reviews* 184 (May): 114194. doi:10.1016/J.ADDR.2022.114194.

Seshan, Krishna. 2002. *Handbook of Thin-Film Deposition Processes and Techniques : Principles, Methods, Equipment and Applications*. Noyes Publications/William Andrew Pub, Norwich, New York.

Setia, Aseem, Bhaskar Vallamkonda, Randheer Reddy Challa, Abhishesh Kumar Mehata, Paresh Badgujar, and Madaswamy S. Muthu. 2024. "Herbal Theranostics: Controlled, Targeted Delivery and Imaging of Herbal Molecules." *Nanotheranostics*. doi:10.7150/ntno.94987.

Shankar, Jyotsna, K.M. Geetha, and Barnabas Wilson. 2021. "Potential Applications of Nanomedicine for Treating Parkinson's Disease." *Journal of Drug Delivery Science and Technology*. doi:10.1016/j.jddst.2021.102793.

Sharma, Manu, Pandey Easha, Gupta Tapasvi, and Rawat Reetika. 2020. "Nanomaterials in Biomedical Diagnosis." In *Nanomaterials in Diagnostic Tools and Devices*, pp. 57–83. doi:10.1016/B978-0-12–817923-9.00002-X.

Singh, Nitu, and S. P Singh. 2023. "Advanced Hybrid Nanomaterials for Various Application: A Comprehensive Overview." *Journal of Science and Technological Researches* 5 (3): 33–37. doi:10.51514/jstr.5.3.2023.33–37.

Singh, Rajesh, and James W. Lillard. 2009. "Nanoparticle-Based Targeted Drug Delivery." *Experimental and Molecular Pathology*. doi:10.1016/j.yexmp.2008.12.004.

Sinha, Priya, Archit Datar, Chungsik Jeong, Xuepeng Deng, Yongchul G. Chung, and Li Chiang Lin. 2019. "Surface Area Determination of Porous Materials Using the Brunauer-Emmett-Teller (BET) Method: Limitations and Improvements." *Journal of Physical Chemistry C* 123 (33): 20195–20209. doi:10.1021/acs.jpcc.9b02116.

Sonia, Thundiparambil Azeez, and Chandra P. Sharma. 2014a. "Lipids and Inorganic Nanoparticles in Oral Insulin Delivery." In *Oral Delivery of Insulin*, pp. 219–256. doi:10.1533/9781908818683.219.

Sonia, Thundiparambil Azeez, and Chandra P. Sharma. 2014b. "Experimental Techniques Involved in the Development of Oral Insulin Carriers." In *Oral Delivery of Insulin*, pp. 169–217. doi:10.1533/9781908818683.169.

Tamaki, Ryo, and Yoshiki Chujo. 1999. "Synthesis of Polystyrene and Silica Gel Polymer Hybrids Utilizing Ionic Interactions." *Chemistry of Materials* 11 (7): 1719–1726. doi:10.1021/cm9810741.

Tamaki, Ryo, Ken Samura, and Yoshiki Chujo. 1998. Synthesis of Polystyrene and Silica Gel Polymer Hybrids via Π–Π Interactions. *Chemical Communications*, 1131–1132.

Tamaki, Ryo, Kensuke Naka, and Yoshiki Chujo. 1997. Synthesis of Polystyrene/Silica Gel Polymer Hybrids by in-Situ Polymerization Method. *Polymer Bulletin* 39, 1131–1132.

Taylor-Pashow, Kathryn M. L., Joseph Della Rocca, Rachel C. Huxford, and Wenbin Lin. 2010. "Hybrid Nanomaterials for Biomedical Applications." *Chemical Communications*. doi:10.1039/c002073g.

Vallet-Regí, María, Montserrat Colilla, and Blanca González. 2011. "Medical Applications of Organic–Inorganic Hybrid Materials within the Field of Silica-Based Bioceramics." *Chemical Society Reviews* 40 (2): 596–607. doi:10.1039/c0cs00025f.

Vasile, Cornelia. 2018. "Polymeric Nanomaterials: Recent Developments, Properties and Medical Applications." In *Polymeric Nanomaterials in Nanotherapeutics*, pp. 1–66. doi:10.1016/B978-0-12-813932-5.00001-7.

Yadav, Akash, Meenal Ghune, and Dinesh Kumar Jain. 2011. "Nano-Medicine Based Drug Delivery System." *Journal of Advanced Pharmacy Education & Research* 1 (4): 201–213.

Yanar, Fatih, Dario Carugo, and Xunli Zhang. 2023. "Hybrid Nanoplatforms Comprising Organic Nanocompartments Encapsulating Inorganic Nanoparticles for Enhanced Drug Delivery and Bioimaging Applications." *Molecules*. doi:10.3390/molecules28155694.

Yu, Jingxue, Jie Li, Wenfeng Zhang, and Haixin Chang. 2015. "Synthesis of High Quality Two-Dimensional Materials via Chemical Vapor Deposition." *Chemical Science* 6 (12): 6705–6716. doi:10.1039/c5sc01941a.

Yuan, Fang, Geoffrey M. Thiele, and Dong Wang. 2011. "Nanomedicine Development for Autoimmune Diseases." *Drug Development Research*. doi:10.1002/ddr.20479.

Zhang, Chenyang, Xin Wang, Jiangfeng Du, Zhanjun Gu, and Yuliang Zhao. 2021. "Reactive Oxygen Species-Regulating Strategies Based on Nanomaterials for Disease Treatment." *Advanced Science*. doi:10.1002/advs.202002797.

Zhou, Huiqun, Zhen Zhang, Yulei Mu, Hang Yao, Yi Zhang, and Dong-An Wang. 2024. "Harnessing Nanomedicine for Cartilage Repair: Design Considerations and Recent Advances in Biomaterials." *ACS Nano*. doi:10.1021/acsnano.4c00780.

5 Nanoparticles in Nuclear Medicines

Biji Balakrishnan[1] *and Madhava B. Mallia*[2,3]
[1]Somaiya Centre for Integrated Science Education and Research, Somaiya Vidyavihar University, Mumbai, India
[2]Radiopharmaceuticals Division, BARC, Mumbai, India
[3]Homi Bhabha National Institute, Mumbai, India

5.1 INTRODUCTION

Nuclear medicine market had reached a value of US$4.9 billion in 2021, and is projected to grow at a compound annual growth rate (CAGR) of 11.3% to reach a value of US$9.4 billion by 2028 [URL: https://www.marketsandmarkets.com/Market-Reports/radiopharmaceuticals-market-417.html#]. Development of advanced technology for radioisotope production and the increasing occurrence of cancer and cardiovascular diseases contribute majorly to the growth of nuclear medicine. Since the majority of cancer and cardiovascular disease cases can be prevented by quick detection and treatment, nuclear medicine plays a major role in its diagnostics and therapy. Nuclear medicine has shown applications in other areas also such as nephro-urology, orthopedics, rheumatology, and neuropsychiatry. This chapter will provide an overview of nuclear medicine, classification, properties, and production of radioisotopes and how radioisotope-tagged nanoparticles (NPs) has been explored as radiopharmaceuticals for therapy and diagnostics.

5.2 NUCLEAR MEDICINE

For a common man, the word 'nuclear' is often associated with atom bomb and the dreaded consequences of its use on humanity in a nuclear war. When probed further, this word may be associated with 'nuclear power' (electricity) which lies under the domain of peaceful applications of nuclear energy. The potential of nuclear energy in applications such as nuclear agriculture (Gautam & Tripathi, 2016) and, most importantly, human healthcare (Vaz et al., 2020) is often less obvious. In present-day healthcare, man-made radioisotopes find immense applications in the diagnosis of a variety of diseases such as cardiovascular diseases, kidney, thyroid and liver dysfunctions, Alzheimer's and Parkinson's disease, and cancer (Lever, 2002). Apart from diagnostic applications, radioisotopes can also be used for effective clinical management of various types of cancers at an affordable cost. The application of radioisotopes for organ function evaluation, diagnosis, or therapy can be broadly considered under the umbrella of 'nuclear medicine' (Vaz et al., 2020). As of today, this is the only technique which can provide functional information of organs, for example, kidney, heart, and liver, with such sensitivities not obtainable with any other technique.

The essential difference between nuclear medicine and medicines that we use in our daily life is that the former contains a radioisotope. Another significant difference is the amount required for a given application. While nuclear medicines are used in very small amounts as injections (micrograms to nanograms or even less), conventional medicines are used in milligram quantities mostly through oral route. Again, while conventional medicines have a relatively long shelf-life, nuclear medicines are not off-the-shelf products owing to the peculiar nature of the radioisotopes that disintegrate with time. Therefore, nuclear medicines are produced on-demand.

DOI: 10.1201/9781003473015-5

It is important to note that radioisotopes are rarely used directly for nuclear medicine applications. Instead, radioisotopes are chemically bonded to suitable molecules to obtain a 'radiopharmaceutical'. Radiopharmaceuticals can be broadly defined as a radioactive drug safe to administer in human body to obtain diagnostic information or to deliver therapy in a noninvasive manner. Before going into the details of radiopharmaceuticals, it is essential to understand about radioisotopes which form the essential component of a radiopharmaceutical (Lever, 2002).

5.3 RADIOISOTOPES

Isotopes of elements with unstable nuclei are called radioisotopes. In an attempt to attain stability, they undergo spontaneous transformation into another nucleus with concomitant emission of energy in the form of particulate or electromagnetic radiation such alpha, beta, Auger electrons, or gamma photons. Alpha particles are mono-energetic helium nuclei whereas beta particles are electrons which can have a positive or negative charge. While electrons with unit negative charge are well known, electrons with positive charge are called positrons. While the energy spectrum of beta particles emitted from the nucleus is continuous, the Auger electrons are mono-energetic and they originate from atomic orbital rather than the nucleus. Gamma radiations are electromagnetic radiation of fixed energy with very high penetrating properties. Positron-emitting radioisotopes also fall under the category of diagnostic radioisotopes. The positrons undergo an interesting phenomenon called 'annihilation'. In this process, the positron emitted from the nucleus of the radioisotope after losing its energy to near zero value, by continuous interaction with the matter through which it passes, combines with an electron from the surroundings to produce two 511 keV gamma photons. The reason for instability of some nuclei leading to the display of radioactivity is beyond the scope of this chapter. However, it is strongly associated with the neutron-to-proton (N/P) ratio in the nucleus. The phenomenon of radioactivity is actually the process of 'adjusting' the N/P ratio of the unstable nucleus to attain a stable N/P ratio.

The conventional unit of radioactivity is Curie (Ci), which is defined as the quantity of any radioactive substance which undergoes 3.7×10^{10} disintegrations per second. The SI unit of radioactivity is Becquerel (Bq). One Becquerel is one disintegration per second. Every radioisotope has its characteristic half-life, which is defined as the time taken to reduce the radioactivity to half the initial value. It is interesting to note that half-lives of radioisotopes vary over a wide range. Nonetheless, they find application in almost every field of science.

5.4 PRODUCTION OF RADIOISOTOPES

It is very important to recognize that radioisotopes used for nuclear medicine applications are all man-made and not from natural sources. Though several radioisotopes, such as tritium (^{3}H), carbon-14 (^{14}C), and potassium-40 (^{40}K), are available in nature, they are less abundant and their isolation is challenging. More importantly, the choice of radioisotope for a given application depends on several factors including the half-life of the radioisotope, energy and type of emitted radiation, ease of availability, and most importantly, the chemistry of the element. These factors necessitate the production of artificial radioisotopes with nuclear characteristics appropriate for the intended application. The production of radioisotopes is a vast subject in itself. Therefore, only a brief description covering the basic concepts of radioisotope production is intended here.

Of few thousand isotopes known, only about 251 isotopes are stable. The stability of an isotope can be traced back to the N/P ratio in its nucleus. An N/P ratio different from that required for nuclear stability will make that nucleus unstable and, therefore, radioactive. Altering the N/P ratio of stable nucleus forms the basis of radioisotope production. The N/P ratio can be altered by adding a neutron or a proton to the nucleus of an atom. The former process is carried out in a nuclear reactor and the latter is carried out in a device called cyclotron. Tables 5.1 and 5.2 list some of the most important radioisotopes used in nuclear medicine for diagnosis and therapy (AC07607271, A, 2009; International Atomic Energy Agency, n.d.).

TABLE 5.1
Nuclear Characteristics and Production Route of Some Medically Important Radioisotopes

Radioisotopes for diagnosis (AC07607271, A, 2009; International Atomic Energy Agency, n.d.)

Radionuclide	Half-Life	Mode of Decay	E_γ, keV (%)	Production Method/Route(s)
^{99m}Tc	6.0 hours	IT[a]	140.5 (88.9)	Generator (^{99}Mo/^{99m}Tc)
^{123}I	13.3 hours	EC[$]	159.0 (82.8)	Cyclotron, ^{124}Te (p,2n) ^{123}I
^{111}In	2.8 days	EC[$]	245.4 (94.2)	Cyclotron, ^{111}Cd (p,n) ^{111}In
^{201}Tl	72.9 hours	EC[$]	167.4 (10.0)	Cyclotron, ^{203}Tl (p,3n) ^{201}Pb → ^{201}Tl
^{67}Ga	3.3 days	EC[$]	93.3 (38.3)	Cyclotron, ^{66}Zn (d,n) ^{67}Ga, ^{68}Zn (p, 2n) ^{67}Ga
^{18}F	109.8 minutes	β^+	0.635 (97)	Cyclotron, ^{18}O (p, n) ^{18}F
^{11}C	20.4 minutes	β^+	0.960 (99.8)	Cyclotron, ^{14}N (p, α)^{11}C
^{13}N	9.9 minutes	β^+	1.199 (100)	Cyclotron, ^{16}O (p, α) ^{13}N
^{15}O	122.2 seconds	β^+	1.732 (100)	Cyclotron, ^{15}N (p, n) ^{15}O
^{82}Rb	1.2 minutes	β^+, EC	3.150 (95)	Generator, ^{82}Sr/^{82}Rb
^{68}Ga	68.3 minutes	β^+, EC	1.897 (89.3)	Generator, ^{68}Ge/^{68}Ga
^{64}Cu	12.7 hours	β^+, β^-, EC	0.656 (17.4)	Cyclotron, ^{64}Ni (p, n) ^{64}Cu
^{89}Zr	78.1 hours	β^+, EC	0.900 (22.7)	Cyclotron, ^{89}Y (p, n) ^{89}Zr

IT, Isomeric transition; EC, Electron capture.

TABLE 5.2
Physical Characteristics of Therapeutic Radionuclides (International Atomic Energy Agency, n.d.)

Radionuclide	Half-Life	E_{max}, MeV (%)	Max Tissue Penetration Range (mm)	Production
^{90}Y	64.1 hours	β 2.2 (100)	12	**Generator** ^{90}Sr/^{90}Y
^{188}Re	16.9 hours	β 2.12 (100); γ 0.155 (15)	11	**Nuclear reactor** ^{187}Re (n,γ)^{188}Re **Generator** ^{188}W/^{188}Re
^{131}I	8.0 days	β 0.606 (89); γ 0.364 (81)	2.1	**Nuclear reactor** ^{130}Te (n, γ)^{131}Te → ^{131}I
^{177}Lu	6.7 days	β 0.497 (78.6), 0.384 (9.1), 0.176 (12.2); γ 0.208 (11.1), 0.113 (6.6)	2.2	**Nuclear reactor** ^{176}Yb (n,γ)^{177}Yb (β^-) ^{177}Lu; ^{176}Lu (n,γ)^{177}Lu
^{153}Sm	46.3 hours	β 0.81 (20), 0.71 (30), 0.64 (50); γ 0.103 (28)	3.1	**Nuclear reactor** ^{152}Sm (n,γ)^{153}Sm
^{166}Ho	26.8 hours	β 1.774 (48.8), 1.854 (49.9); γ 0.080 (6.7)	8.7	**Nuclear reactor** ^{165}Ho (n,γ) ^{166}Ho

5.5 CLASSIFICATION OF RADIOISOTOPES

Radioisotopes can be broadly classified into two categories based on their clinical application, viz. diagnostic radioisotopes and therapeutic radioisotopes. Diagnostic radioisotopes emit tissue-penetrating gamma radiations of energy, preferably 100–200 keV, suitable for efficient detection with thallium-activated sodium iodide [NaI (TL)] detectors generally employed in gamma camera or SPECT (single-photon emission computed tomography) camera. Positron-emitting radioisotopes are also used for diagnostic purposes since the annihilation of positron leads to the formation of two gamma photons of 511 keV. These two gamma photons of equal energy moving in opposite directions can be used for obtaining high-resolution diagnostic images using PET (positron emission tomography) camera. It is desirable that a diagnostic radioisotope is a pure gamma emitter since concomitant particulate emissions, if present, do not contribute to any diagnostic information, but give unnecessary radiation dose to the patient. On the other hand, it is preferable that a therapeutic radioisotope emits a gamma radiation, which will permit real-time monitoring of the radiotracer when used in patients.

5.6 RADIOPHARMACEUTICALS FOR THERAPY AND DIAGNOSTICS

It is to be noted that a radioisotope is rarely used directly for diagnostic or therapeutic applications. Instead, the radioisotopes are tagged to molecules that impart an ability to target certain organs, tissues, disease sites, or even certain biological pathways when injected into the human body. Therefore, a radiopharmaceutical can be defined as a radiolabeled drug/pharmaceutical, safe to administer in human body, that has the ability to accumulate in the target organ/tissue or trace certain biological process, and can be used to obtain diagnostic information or to deliver therapy. The radioisotope is tagged to a biomolecule either through a covalent bond or through a coordinate bond. In cases where the biomolecule cannot be directly tagged to a radioisotope, the biomolecule is modified to introduce a chelator which can then be used to tag the radioisotope. This approach is called bifunctional chelator approach. A typical design of a radiopharmaceutical using bifunctional chelator is shown in Figure 5.1. It is highly desirable that the procedure for the preparation of radiopharmaceuticals should be simple, reproducible, and adoptable in a nuclear radiopharmacy setup.

Like radioisotopes, radiopharmaceuticals can also be broadly classified into diagnostic and therapeutic radiopharmaceuticals (Lindsley et al., 2022). Classification in either category is based on the type of radionuclide incorporated into the radiopharmaceutical. A good radiopharmaceutical should accumulate in the organ or tissue of interest with high specificity and at the same time clear rapidly from non-target organs or tissues, resulting in high target-to-non-target ratio.

Gamma or positron-emitting radioisotopes are used for the preparation of diagnostic radioisotopes. Typical diagnostic procedure involves intravenous administration of appropriate amount of activity in a patient. After permitting sufficient time for the radiopharmaceutical to distribute and accumulate in target organ/tissue of interest and clear from the non-target organs, the patient is

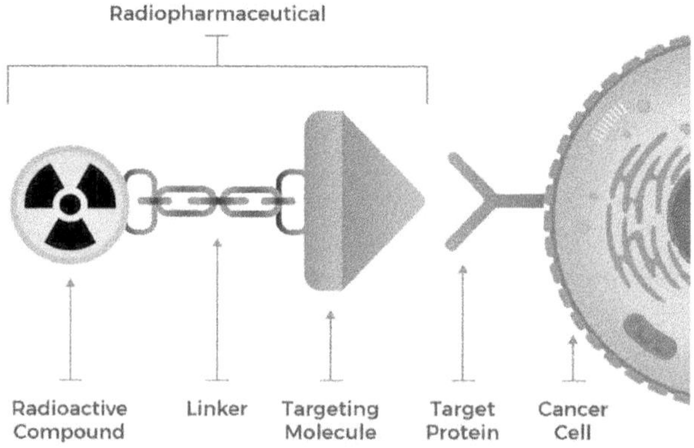

FIGURE 5.1 Radiopharmaceuticals consist of a radioactive molecule, a targeting molecule, and a linker that joins the two. (Credit: National Cancer Institute, https://www.cancer.gov/news-events/cancer-currents-blog/2020/radiopharmaceuticals-cancer-radiation-therapy.)

scanned in a device called gamma camera. There are two types of gamma camera depending on the type of radioisotope used. For a gamma-emitting radioisotope like technetium-99m or iodine-131, SPECT machine is used. For positron-emitting radiopharmaceuticals, PET machine is used. The gamma camera records the gamma emission from the body of the patient which is a representation of the distribution of the radiopharmaceutical. From the scan, a nuclear medicine physician can understand the clinical condition of the patient for further management.

A therapeutic procedure roughly is similar to the diagnostic procedure. The main difference is that a therapeutic radiopharmaceutical containing a beta- or alpha-emitting radioisotope capable of depositing therapeutic dose of radiation in tissue is used. Once the therapeutic radiopharmaceutical accumulates in cancer cells, the particulate radiations can directly interact with the macromolecules in the cells and damage them (direct effect), eventually leading to cell death. Alternately, the particulate radiations can interact with the majority component in cells, which is water, and can generate reactive radicals through the process of radiolysis. These radicals can undergo secondary interaction with macromolecules inside the cells (indirect effect), including DNA, leading to cell death. The dose of therapeutic radiopharmaceutical to be administered in a patient depends on the extent of the disease as well as the pharmacokinetics of the radiopharmaceutical. These parameters are determined through different phases of clinical trials. There is a long list of radiopharmaceuticals, diagnostic as well as therapeutic, that are in clinical use today. Some of the important diagnostic and therapeutic radiopharmaceuticals are listed in Tables 5.3 and 5.4.

To complete the brief discussion on radiopharmaceuticals, it is worth mentioning some of the radioisotopes that can be directly used for diagnosis or therapy. Iodine-131 is an excellent example in this category. Iodine-131 in the form of sodium iodide [$Na^{131}I$] is used for the diagnosis of thyroid dysfunction and also for therapy of thyroid cancer (Souza & McCabe, 2021). This is possible only because of the inherent ability of the thyroid gland to absorb iodine from our diet and use it for biosynthesis of hormones such as T3 (triiodothyronine) and T4 (thyroxin). Iodine-131 (as sodium iodide [$Na^{131}I$]) also has a rare distinction that it can be given orally, while most of the other radiopharmaceuticals are administered through intravenous route to bypass possible metabolism in stomach. Other radioisotopes in this category are phosphorus-32 (Silberstein et al., 1992) (as orthophosphate or polyphosphate) and strontium-89 (Zhang et al., 2013) (as strontium chloride) for bone pain palliation, fluorine-18 (Jadvar et al., 2015) (as sodium fluoride) for skeletal imaging, radium-223 (Gupta et al., 2017) (as radium chloride, also commercially known as Alpharadin®) for the treatment of skeletal metastasis secondary to prostate cancer, etc.

TABLE 5.3
List of Few Diagnostic Radiopharmaceuticals Used in Nuclear Medicine (Pimlott & Sutherland, 2011; Schwochau, 1994)

Radiopharmaceutical	Application
^{99m}Tc-ECD, ^{99m}Tc-TRODAT, ^{99m}Tc-HMPAO	Brain imaging
^{99m}Tc-Sestamibi, ^{99m}Tc-Tetrofosmin, ^{201}TlCl	Cardiac imaging
^{99m}Tc-Sulfur colloid	Liver imaging
^{99m}Tc-Mebrofenin	Hepatobiliary function
^{99m}Tc-MAA, ^{68}Ga-MAA	Lung imaging
^{99m}Tc-MDP, ^{68}Ga-BPAMD, $Na^{18}F$	Bone imaging
^{99m}Tc-GHA, ^{99m}Tc(III)-DMSA, ^{99m}Tc-DTPA, ^{99m}Tc-EC, ^{99m}Tc-MAG_3	Kidney imaging
^{99m}Tc-Leukocytes, ^{99m}Tc-Ciprofloxacin, ^{99m}Tc-UBI	Infection/Inflammation imaging
^{18}F-FDG	Cancer diagnosis
^{99m}Tc-HYNIC-TOC/TATE, ^{68}Ga-DOTA-TOC/TATE	Diagnosis of NETs
^{68}Ga-PSMA	Diagnosis of prostate cancer

TABLE 5.4
Commonly Used Radiopharmaceuticals for Radionuclide Therapy (Chung & Cheon, 2014; Das & Banerjee, 2017; Gulenchyn et al., 2012; Sgouros et al., 2020; Volkert & Hoffman, 1999)

Radiopharmaceutical	Application
$^{89}SrCl_2$, $^{223}RaCl_2$, ^{153}Sm-EDTMP, ^{177}Lu-EDTMP, ^{188}Re-HEDP	Bone pain palliation
^{90}Y-yttrium silicate/citrate colloid, ^{186}Re-rhenium sulfur colloid, ^{169}Er-erbium citrate	Radiosynoviorthesis (RSV)
^{90}Y-loaded glass microspheres (TheraSphere), ^{90}Y-loaded resin microspheres (SIR-Sphere)	Selective internal radiation therapy (SIRT) of liver cancer/hepatocellular carcinoma
^{131}I-MIBG	Treatment of neuroblastoma, pheochromocytoma, carcinoid, paraganglioma, medullary thyroid carcinoma
^{177}Lu-DOTA-TATE	Therapy of neuroendocrine tumors
^{177}Lu-PSMA-617	Therapy of prostate cancer

5.7 NPS IN NUCLEAR MEDICINE

Early nuclear medicine started with simple molecules which could form kinetically stable complexes with a variety of metallic radioisotopes such as technetium-99m (Internationale Atomenergie-Organisation, 2009). Molecular structures of many of the early radio-complexes were not known; nevertheless, they had properties that permitted their use in patients to extract important clinical information in a noninvasive manner. These radiopharmaceuticals are called first-generation radiopharmaceuticals. Most of the 'second generation' ^{99m}Tc-radiopharmaceuticals had well-defined structure and their application was based on their physicochemical properties such as charge, hydrophilicity, and size based on their structure. Few examples are: myocardial perfusion agents ^{99m}Tc-MIBI (sestamibi, Cardiolite®) **and** ^{99m}Tc-tetrofosmin (Myoview®)**, the brain imaging agents** ^{99m}Tc-HMPAO and ^{99m}Tc-ECD (bicisate, Neurolite®)**, renal imaging agent** ^{99m}Tc-MAG3 (Mertiatide), and hepatobiliary agent such as ^{99m}Tc-mebrofenin (Internationale Atomenergie-Organisation, 2009). The 'third generation' of technetium radiopharmaceuticals consisted of a targeting molecule having an affinity toward certain biological targets, such as receptors, apart from its well-defined molecular structure. Herein, the ^{99m}Tc complex in the radiopharmaceutical is kept at a position where the biological activity is not compromised. Third-generation radiotracers extensively use bifunctional chelating agents (BFCAs) such as HYNIC, 1,4,7,10-tetraazacy clododecane-1,4,7,10-tetraacetic acid (DOTA), and NOTA, or novel radiometal chemistries for the preparation of radiopharmaceuticals (Holik et al., 2022).

Recently, there is considerable interest in utilizing nanomaterials for nuclear medicine applications. Nanomaterials in general can be defined as materials with individual units having at least one dimension less than 100 nm. These materials are made of elements or combination of elements, which can be broadly grouped into organic (made of carbon), inorganic (non-carbon based), and hybrid (combination of carbon and other elements) materials. Their small size results in unique physical properties, which has resulted in significant research interest to understand, prepare, and tune the nanomaterials for a specific application. Nanomaterials are already being used in commercial products, such as in high-end displays, automobile components, electronic device, sunscreens, military applications, photovoltaic cells, paints, and catalysts. Nanomaterials are also being investigated for use in solar panels. Most importantly, nanomaterials find wide applications in healthcare, which will be the central point of discussion here. Nanotechnology finds immense applications in medicine as targeted medicinal products, pharmaceutical products, biomedical implants, tissue engineering, and drug delivery vehicles. Nanomaterials when used for drug delivery applications can significantly reduce the toxicity of drug without compromising the efficacy.

In nuclear medicine, nanoplatforms find applications as vehicles to carry radioisotopes, to the intended target in vivo, for diagnostic or therapeutic applications. While the targeting vectors, bifunctional chelators, radioisotopes, etc. remain the same, the research is directed toward enhancing the efficacy of treatment taking advantage of the enhanced permeation retention (EPR) effects of NPs combined with the utilization of the large surface area to load chemotherapeutic drugs as well as radioisotopes to deliver 'chemo-radiotherapy' for cancer management. Large surface area offered by the nanoplatforms also permits decorating with targeting vectors to achieve targeted 'chemo-radiotherapy'. Thus, nanomaterials present immense possibilities in nuclear medicine applications.

Broad class of nanomaterials explored for diagnostic and therapeutic purposes are gold nanoparticles (GNPs) (Gao et al., 2021; Guo et al., 2017), quantum dots (QDs), organic QDs (Dhas et al., 2022; Tripathi et al., 2015), magnetic NPs (Gobbo et al., 2015; Li et al., 2021), upconversion NPs (Li et al., 2019; Chen et al., 2014), nanoemulsions (Curry et al., 2014; Fernandes et al., 2021; Gorain et al., 2020), nanogels (Wang et al. 2022; Soni et al., 2016), micro/nano-bubbles (Jangjou et al., 2021; Martin & Dayton, 2013; Zahiri et al., 2021), carbon NPs (Saleem et al., 2018; Tang et al., 2022), polymeric NPs (Indoria et al., 2020; Luk et al., 2012), liposomes (Fernandes, 2023), and micelles (Varela-Moreira et al., 2017; Zhou et al., 2018).

5.7.1 Gold Nanoparticles

GNPs are widely explored as radiosensitizers in nuclear medicine. Confining numerous hundreds or thousands of high-Z atoms in a single unit provides advantage over molecules having only one high-Z element per unit. Moreover, size, shape, and surface functionalization of GNPs can be easily controlled. Due to its biocompatibility and ease of cellular internalization, it has been used as brachytherapy agent either in nonradioactive or radioactive form. Brachytherapy involves insertion of radioactive material inside the body to treat certain categories of cancers and other conditions. GNP, being a high-Z (atomic number) element, can interact with therapeutic photons (X- and γ-rays) emitted by the radiotherapeutic source (external beam, brachytherapy, or tagged radioisotopes) leading to the generation of secondary products (e.g., Auger electrons, characteristic X-rays, and photoelectrons) to enhance overall local deposition dose (Figure 5.2) (Rosa et al., 2017). The photoelectric effect, the Compton effect, pair production, and Rayleigh scattering are the four major attenuation effects that occur upon collision between photons and materials. The secondary products produced during attenuation ionize the atoms present in the surrounding tissues to cause direct

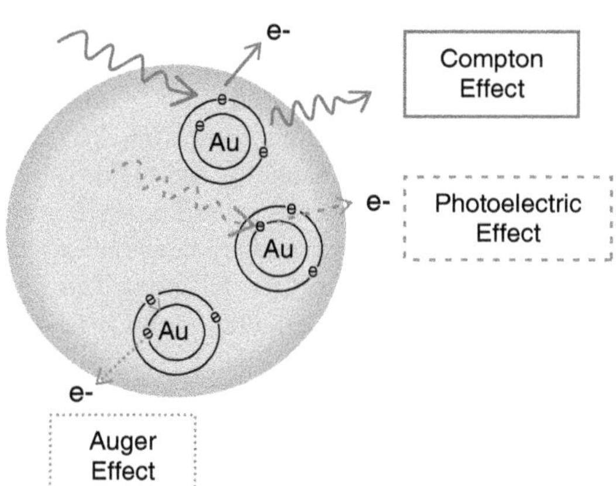

FIGURE 5.2 Schematic illustration of the photoelectric, Compton, and Auger effects. The Compton effect is represented in solid line, the photoelectric effect in dashed line, and the Auger effect in dotted line. (Rosa et al., 2017.)

damage to molecules such as proteins, lipids, and nucleic acids and generate reactive oxygen species (ROS). ROS causes indirect damage to the cells and creates a cascade effect leading to enhanced cellular damage and stress (Laprise-Pelletier et al., 2018).

The performance of GNPs as radiosensitizers is shown to be enhanced at photon energies lower than the k-edge of Au (80.7 keV). It is reported that probability of interaction is significantly high at 20 keV, where the predominant interaction mechanism is the photoelectric effect. Single injection of 1.6–1.7 mCi of radioactive Pd-coated GNPs (^{103}Pd:Pd@Au-polyethylene glycol (PEG) and ^{103}Pd:Pd@198 Au:Au-PEG NPs) demonstrated significant reduction in PC3 tumor growth rate. This is attributed to the effect of a large quantity of Auger and delta electrons produced upon interaction of GNPs with low-energy photons produced by ^{103}Pd (Laprise-Pelletier et al., 2017).

GNPs when intravenously injected into murine xenograft tumors (breast) and irradiated with a 250 kVp X-ray beam at a dose close to its lethal dose (LD50 ≈ 5 g Au/kg), tumor growth inhibition was clearly observed with long-term (1 year) survival rates of 50% (1.35 g Au/kg) and 86% (2.7 g Au/kg) as compared to a survival rate of only 20% for those groups that received radiation alone (Hainfeld et al., 2004). In order to enhance the effect of Auger electrons that can travel only across a short range (up to ≈2 μm), it is necessary to increase the tumor accumulation of GNPs. Small (2.5–3 nm) tiopronin-coated GNPs demonstrated a 94 times higher accumulation in the HCT116 tumor when it was intratumorally administered as compared to intravenous injection and enabled a significant tumor response upon low-energy X-ray irradiation (Shi et al., 2016). Radiosensitization effect is also influenced by particle size, concentration, position, self-absorption, as well as extent of secondary electrons and free radicals' production. GNPs smaller than 50 nm, especially those with size in the range of 2–3 nm, demonstrated enhanced dose deposition (Lechtman et al., 2011). However, small-sized GNPs are prone to rapid removal from the tissues, which would restrict their timeframe of use as radiosensitization agents. GNPs with a hydrodynamic diameter higher than 6 nm surpass the renal filtration threshold, and hinder its excretion by the urinary tract.

To achieve optimal tumor accumulation, GNPs will have to be surface functionalized (Lechtman et al., 2011). The size and shape of GNPs effect their intracellular uptake, transport, and processing in the radiosensitization environment as reported elsewhere (Chithrani et al., 2010; Jain et al., 2011). Proton and electron beams in combination with GNPs also revealed dose enhancement and cancer cell growth inhibition (Chang et al., 2008; Cunningham et al., 2021). Radiosensitizing effect of GNPs injected near low-dose-rate brachytherapy seeds (e.g., ^{125}I and ^{103}Pd) and high-dose-rate (e.g., ^{192}Ir) sources are also investigated. ^{125}I brachytherapy treatment technique for high-risk prostate cancer patients was found to get synergistic effect of enhanced localized energy deposition and radiation shielding of organs at risk (urethra and rectum) via injection of AuNP directly into the prostate (Brivio et al., 2017).

Radioactive and radiolabeled GNPs were also investigated as brachytherapy agents. Radioactive gold-doped GNPs used for treatment were of size ranging from 1 to 90 nm. Heterogeneous distribution of radioactive gold within the tumor was one of the major disadvantages (Wheeler et al., 1955). Radioactive ^{198}Au led to high-energy β emission, and hence is suitable only for large tumors (Knapp & Dash, 2016). Therefore, attempts were made to develop radioactive palladium–gold NPs as an alternative to ^{198}Au-based GNPs as radioactive Pd is used in low-dose-rate brachytherapy (Djoumessi et al., 2015). Radiolabeled GNPs tagged with antibody have been explored for radioimmune therapy. Radiolabeling was achieved by using chelators or radioiodination methods. Further, GNPs coated with suitable polymers having hanging functional groups offer several conjugation opportunities (Chen et al., 2013; Curry et al., 2014; Iram et al., 2020). Tagging of GNPS with radionuclides can be done using bifunctional molecules that can stabilize the NPs and bind the radioisotopes. Direct conjugation of molecules on the surface of AuNPs, especially those having amino and thio functional groups, can be achieved via a ligand exchange or by chemical modification of capping molecules on GNPs. Radioisotopes such as ^{131}I and ^{64}Cu, adsorbed to the surface of GNPs, are few examples (Silva et al., 2020).

For clinical translation, if used either along with external beam radiation or as brachytherapy agent, dose thresholds and their related limits of GNPs are to be identified. Further there should be provisions to spare the surrounding healthy tissues. Long-term biocompatibility, biodistribution, and clearance data must be systematically investigated for each case independently.

5.7.2 Magnetic NPs

Magnetic nanoparticle (MNP)-based strategies have received great attention in diagnostic as well as therapeutics. Since MNPs such as superparamagnetic iron oxide nanoparticles (SPIONs) offer strong image contrast of targeted anatomical sites, it has immense use in magnetic resonance imaging (MRI). Having a magnetic core surrounded by a polymer or metal coating, these NPs offer opportunity to further functionalization.

Since MNPs can be moved under magnetic field, it is possible to guide specifically those particles to the tumor site. MNPs coated with molecules (e.g., antibodies, peptides) can help to specifically target receptors overexpressed in diseased conditions, particularly cancer. PEG-coated Fe_3O_4 NPs coated with a monoclonal antibody implanted in a colon cancer mouse model were effectively directed to targeted localization by MRI (Anbarasu et al., 2015). Magnetic hyperthermia is another application where thermal energy produced via interaction of MNPs with an external alternating (AC) radiofrequency (RF) magnetic field is utilized for inducing apoptosis in cancer cells and tumor thermal ablation.

Hybrid imaging techniques using combination of MNPs and radioisotopes are envisaged to have a more comprehensive and precise assessment of biological processes at molecular and cellular levels. Due to their size-dependent properties, MNPs are considered a potential tool in nuclear imaging techniques in combination with radioisotopes. In order to use MNPs as molecular imaging probes it should have high in vivo chemical, radiochemical, and metabolic stability, target-specific uptake, fast clearance of any unbound imaging agent, and high-sensitive tracking even at low dose with minimal side effects (Kiessling et al., 2014). MRI techniques are based on the interaction of magnetic field with protons of tissues and detection of signal generated during the relaxation. The technique provides good soft tissue contrast even without the contrast agents. SPECT or PET radionuclide could improve signal-to-noise ratios at low uptake region and calculate MRI's contrast uptake (De Rosales, 2014). Moreover, the combination of PET (or SPECT) with MRI that does not produce any ionizing radiation is highly synergistic as compared to PET/SPECT-CT. While using iron oxide NPs for multimodal imaging, selection of radioisotope and mode of incorporation within the NP are important. Radioisotope can either be tagged on the surface of the NP or be incorporated within the core. Whatever method used, tagging with radioisotope can impart change in the surface properties, and zeta potential. However, since mass amount of radioisotope required for nuclear imaging is very less, modifications produce negligible change in macroscopic level (Ai et al., 2016; Pellico et al., 2017). Attempts were also made to investigate the efficacy of such systems as theranostics by incorporating chemotherapeutics. Table 5.5 provides examples on studies on combination of MNPs with radioisotopes for various applications.

5.7.3 Upconversion NPs

The upconversion luminescence is a nonlinear optical process associated with continuous multiphoton absorption and the interionic energy transfer, where low-energy photons are converted into one high-energy (with short wavelength) emission (Haase & Schäfer, 2011). Lanthanide-doped upconversion nanoparticles (UCNPs) are promising bioimaging agents. In the case of lymph node metastasis, inhibition of growth of local as well as sentinel lymph node tumor cells has to be achieved, for which it is essential to identify the regions where tumor cells are located in the lymph nodes. NaGdF4:Yb,Tm@NaLuF4 UCNPs with PEG and anti-human epidermal growth factor receptor (HER)2 monoclonal antibody (trastuzumab, Herceptin) (NP-mAb) were radiolabeled

TABLE 5.5
Magnetic Nanoparticles Investigated for Nuclear Medicine Applications

Radioisotope Used	Nanomaterial	Imaging Technique	Application	Ref.
^{18}F	^{18}F-labeled iron oxide nanoparticles	PET/MRI	Dual-modality imaging	Sun et al. (2016)
^{68}Ga	^{68}Ga-SPION	PET/MRI	Tri-modality agent for diagnostic imaging and potential Cherenkov luminescent-guided resection of sentinel node lymph node	Madru et al. (2013)
^{99m}Tc	^{99m}Tc-labeled and polyethylene glycol-coated IONPs	SPECT/MRI	Dual-mode imaging of sentinel lymph nodes	Madru et al. (2012)
		SPECT/MRI	Multimodal imaging enables visualization of functional and anatomical information	Barrefelt et al. (2013)
	99mTc-PEG-bisphosphonate-ultra small SPION	MRI-SPECT	Multimodal imaging	Sandiford et al. (2013)
	99mTc-labeled and bevacizumab monoclonal antibody (mAb) conjugated ultra small SPION	MRI-SPECT	Targeted imaging of hepatocellular carcinoma	Zhao et al. (2014)
	99mTc-labeled-cRGDfK-Orn3-CGG conjugated iron oxide	Potential thermal therapy delivery vehicle	Molecular imaging of $\alpha\nu\beta3$-mediated tumor expression and hyperthermia treatment	Tsiapa et al. (2014)
^{124}I	^{124}I-labeled serum albumin-coated Mn-doped iron oxide	PET/MR	Lymph nodes imaging with PET and MR	Choi et al. (2008)
$^{44/47}Sc$	$^{44/47}Sc$-labeled PSMA-617 conjugated SPIONs	^{44}Sc for PET diagnosis and ^{47}Sc for therapy and hyperthermia	Diagnosis and therapy even for chemo- and radioresistant tumor cells	Ünak et al. (2023)
^{64}Cu	Dextranated and DTPA-modified iron oxide nanoparticle labeled with Vivotag-680 and 64Cu	PET/MR/optical imaging	Detection of macrophages in atherosclerotic plaques	Nahrendorf et al. (2008)
^{111}In	^{111}In-labeled, trastuzumab-doxorubicin conjugated, and APTES-PEG-coated SPION	SPECT/MRI along with targeted therapy	Imaging along with targeted therapy	Zolata et al. (2015)

with positron-emitting ^{68}Ga and β-emitting ^{177}Lu radionuclides for imaging as well as therapy. Upconversion particles were used for lymphatic cancer cell visualization via near-infrared fluorescence (NIRF), and radionuclides were used for SPECT, PET, and targeted radionuclide therapy (TRT) of HER2-positive breast cancer lymph node metastasis tumor in mice. Results demonstrated a decrease in the incidence and volumes of lymph node metastasis (Zhang et al., 2022).

Combinatorial theranostic agents were prepared using UCNPs in which a fraction of yttrium is substituted by beta-emitting radionuclide yttrium-90 (^{90}Y) and conjugated with fragment of the exotoxin genetically fused with a targeting designed ankyrin repeat protein (DARPin) specific to HER2 receptors. The photoluminescence in the visible and NIR spectral regions originated from UCNPs enables up to 1-cm imaging depth, facilitating the study of pharmacokinetics in animal model xenografts and possibly in millimeter-sized tumor foci (Guryev et al., 2018). Toxicity of upconversion particles needs to be carefully monitored to enhance its efficacy in clinics.

5.7.4 Carbon NPs

Due to remarkable physicochemical properties, carbon-based nanomaterials can function as delivery vehicle for substantial amounts of radionuclides, and can be functionalized with target-specific ligands for targeted therapy. Carbon-based materials include carbon nanotubes (CNTs), graphene, fullerenes, nanodiamonds, or carbon QDs. CNTs are mechanically robust, composed of sp2-bonded carbon atoms, and have highly regular structures of rolled graphene sheets with defined periodicity. Small diameter with high aspect ratios (>200:1 length:width for high-pressure carbon monoxide-produced single-walled tubes), unique pharmacokinetics and cellular interaction, radiolabeling ability, and facility to modify CNT with appropriate chemistries to render them highly biocompatible and dispersible in aqueous media are other advantages (In Het Panhuis, 2003; Kam et al., 2005; Shi Kam et al., 2004).

Many of the carbon-based nanomaterials have strong absorption in the infrared (IR) or NIR regions, and can be used for photothermal therapy (PTT) of cancer. These nanomaterials have fluorescence emission in the visible and IR regions for fluorescence imaging (Tao et al., 2012; Welsher et al., 2009) and are promising agents for photoacoustic imaging that can transform the energy from a laser into acoustic signals (De La Zerda et al., 2008).

Radiolabeled CNTs have demonstrated rapid blood compartment clearance, high specific activity, multimodal imaging capability, renal elimination, and tumor-specific accumulation in vivo (McDevitt et al., 2007) Amino-functionalized CNT(Georgakilas et al., 2002) could be radiolabeled with the short half-life, positron-emitting ^{86}Y ($t_{1/2}$=14.7 hours) or the long half-life, gamma-emitting ^{111}In ($t_{1/2}$=2.81 days) using a DOTA chelator (McDevitt et al., 2007). Actinium-225-labeled single-walled carbon nanotube (SWCNT) conjugated with DOTA and tumor neovascular-targeting antibody E4G10 were investigated for tumor vasculature-targeted anticancer therapy. Same material was labeled with ^{89}Zr for PET radioimmunoimaging of the tumor vessels (McDevitt et al., 2010). Though generally carbon-based nanomaterials are considered to be biocompatible, after modifications the materials should be screened for biocompatibility. ROS generation by CNTs also should be critically followed (Yang et al., 2014).

5.7.5 Quantum Dots

QDs are semiconductor nanocrystals having diameter size in the range from 2 to 10 nm and are based on II-VI or III-V elements in the periodic table. Having unique optical and chemical properties, QDs are found to have beneficial characteristics such as high fluorescence intensity, long lifetime, and photobleaching resistance, suitable for *in vivo* imaging with high signal-to-background ratio (Bentolila et al., 2009). Cadmium-based QDs are commonly prepared and toxicity is a concern if it is used for biomedical applications. Attempts are made to synthesize less toxic QDs based on silica, carbon, zinc, etc. (Juzenas et al., 2008; Sun et al., 2006). High atom and electron density QDs can act as radiosensitizers by absorbing high-energy photons (X-rays and gamma rays), leading to localized and targeted damage to cancer cells. QDs based on CaF (Chen et al., 2007), LaF (Liu et al., 2008), ZnS (Wang et al., 2008), or ZnO (Liu et al., 2008) and carbon dots (Sun et al., 2006) are potential candidates as radiosensitizers (Carter et al., 2007). QDs also have been explored as scintillators for detecting the ionizing radiation for gamma photons (Létant & Wang, 2006a) and alpha particles (Létant & Wang, 2006b), advantage being the size-oriented band gap tunability.

5.7.6 Polymeric NPs

Polymeric NPs have gained much attention in the field of therapy and diagnostics due to their unique advantages which include size and property tunability, ease of surface functionalization and payload incorporation, biocompatibility, biodegradability, option to impart trigger responsiveness, and passive tumor-targeting properties. Commonly used polymeric NPs in nuclear medicine include dendrimer-based, polymersomes, polymer conjugates, micelles, etc.

Due to the ease of synthesis of well-defined monodisperse globular nanovectors, with size and peripheral group tunability, dendrimers are extensively investigated as radiopharmaceuticals. Dendrimers are characterized with a multivalent peripheral shell and an internal core from which the branches grow, and these layers of branches define the generation of dendrimer. The availability of terminal groups increases exponentially with generation number. The controlled architecture of dendrimers opens up various possibilities for the simultaneous attachment of radionuclide chelators and targeting moieties (Patri et al., 2005).

Poly(amidoamine) (PAMAM) dendrimer and its gold composites poly-$^{198}Au^{0}$ have been synthesized from nonradioactive ^{197}Au-PAMAM complexes (size 29 nm) using both gamma radiation and neutron radiation components in a reactor. A slight increase in size of NP was observed due to radiation-induced cross-linking. Biodistribution studies of intratumoral injection of ^{198}Au-PAMAM complexes demonstrated increase in internalization and tumor tissue retention of positively charged particles (Khan et al., 2008). Dendrimers of higher generation provide provision to incorporate considerably higher number of chelating ligands per molecule and thereby binding of a larger number of radiometals. Dendrimers also offer possibility of modification using targeting moieties such as folic acid and chlorotoxin and subsequent radiolabeling with ^{131}I (Zhao et al., 2015).

Polymeric micelles and vesicles are prepared by self-assembly of amphiphilic polymers. In such systems, hydrophobic and hydrophilic payloads are incorporated in the hydrophobic core and inner aqueous cavity regions, respectively, and are potential candidates for drug delivery systems. Other advantages are ease of surface functionalization by appropriately custom-made amphiphilic polymers (Park et al., 2008). Encapsulation of radionuclides in these systems, one of the requisites to be used as radiopharmaceuticals, is achieved by hydrophobizing radionuclides followed by encapsulation into the hydrophobic core region of polymeric micelle (Yamamoto et al., 2013). Other approaches include encapsulation of aqueous radionuclide solution into the inner cavity of vesicular assemblies, and attaching metal radionuclides such as ^{64}Cu and ^{99m}Tc to the NPs using chelates. Radionuclides used for internal radiation therapy include β-ray emitters, such as ^{90}Y and ^{131}I. Radionuclides emitting α-ray (^{211}At, ^{213}Bi) and Auger electron (^{99m}Tc, ^{111}In, and ^{125}I) are also investigated (Makino & Kimura, 2014). Folate-PEG-amine conjugated to the surface of micelle prepared from amphiphilic poly(methyl acrylate)-b-poly(acrylic acid) (PMA164-b-PAA93) has been investigated as a carrier for PET tracer agent after labeling with ^{64}Cu. Biodistribution studies showed high accumulation in liver and spleen, but due to the targeting ability of folate, up to 6% ID/g accumulation was observed in tumor till 24 hours (Rossin et al., 2005). Though PEGylation showed promising results in prolonging residence time in circulation of polymeric systems, it was inferred that molecular weight of the copolymers, structure of polymer, size of the micelle, and characteristics of tumor are controlling factors that determine the intratumor accumulation (Allmeroth et al., 2013).

Polysaccharides such as dextran (Wen et al., 2023), citrus pectin (Balakrishnan et al., 2020), and pullulan (Park et al., 2007)-based NPs also have been radiolabeled for investigation as radiopharmaceuticals. Radioisotope-labeled polymeric nanoparticulate systems have been investigated as therapeutic and/or diagnostic agents in numerous diseases such as ischemia, cardiovascular diseases (Hwang et al., 2014), angiogenesis (Almutairi et al., 2009), atherosclerosis (Stendahl & Sinusas, 2015), sentinel node detection (Subramanian et al., 2013), inflammation (Wu et al., 2020), cancer (Piras et al., 2019), among others. Although a great variety of radioactive polymer-based NPs have reached the preclinical status, none of them has achieved clinical translation. For clinical translation, reliable data pertaining to biodistribution, pharmacokinetic and pharmacodynamic properties are required. With the advent of many technological progresses in the modification of polymers, it is envisaged that many polymeric nano-based radiopharmaceuticals will get regulatory approval in the coming years.

5.7.7 Liposomes

Liposomes are lipid-based spherical vesicles having either unilamellar or multilamellar bilayer where the polar head groups are facing outward and the hydrophobic tails are facing inward, ultimately forming an enclosed amphiphilic system with an aqueous center. Lipids can be glycerophospholipids, sphingomyelins, and cholesterols (Low et al., 2023).

Attempts to use liposomes as vectors to carry radioisotope started in the late 1970s with researches investigating the in vivo behavior of radiolabeled liposomes (Gregoriadis et al., 1977; Richardson et al., 1977). Early studies used liposomes radiolabeled with diagnostic radioisotopes such as indium-111, gallium-67, and technetium-99m (Gabizon et al., 1990; Goto et al., 1989; Harrington et al., 2000a; Hnatowich et al., 1981; Jaggi et al., 1991; Ogihara et al., 1986; Ogihara-Umeda et al., 1992; Presant et al., 1988; Richardson et al., 1979). However, majority of such liposome-based radiotracers showed very high uptake in liver and spleen and very fast clearance from blood, which pose significant limitation to its utility as a carrier vector (Presant et al., 1988; Richardson et al., 1979). One of the successfully implemented methods to improve the circulation time of the liposomes was PEGylation, which involves modifying the liposome surface with pendent PEG chains. Studies indicated significant improvement in circulation time of liposomes in blood after PEGylation (Harrington et al., 1996, 2000b, 2001; Ogihara-Umeda & Kojima, 1988, 1989). The size of the liposome also plays a significant role in its pharmacokinetics. It was observed that liposomes with large size (~200 nm and above) showed poor uptake in tumor, possibly due to fast clearance through the reticuloendothelial system (RES) (Phillips, 1999). A study by Ogihara-Umeda et al. (1996) showing better accumulation of liposomes of smaller size (~80 nm) provided evidence in support of this observation. In addition to size, surface charge of the liposomes was also found to influence its pharmacokinetics, with neutral liposomes faring better in terms of delivering the payload to the tumor site (Bao et al., 2006; Goins et al., 1994; Udayachander et al., 1987). To enhance the target specificity, PEGylated liposomes were further modified with tumor-targeting molecules such as antibodies or peptides and such studies indeed showed significant improvement in tumor accumulation (Dagar et al., 2001; Elbayoumi & Torchilin, 2006; Geng et al., 2004). Apart from single-photon-emitting radioisotopes, liposomes are also radiolabeled with positron-emitting radioisotopes such as fluorine-18. Liposomes radiolabeled with positron-emitting radioisotope, fluorine-18, through the incorporation of F-18 fluorodeoxyglucose (^{18}F-FDG), has shown significant accumulation in tumor (Oku, 1999).

The first report on the preparation of rhenium-186/188-labeled liposome for therapeutic purpose was published by Häfeli et al. Subsequently, Utkhede et al. reported the preparation of yttrium-90-labeled, PEGylated liposome for radiotherapy applications (Häfeli et al., 1991; Utkhede et al., 1994). Subsequently, encouraging dosimetric studies of liposomes radiolabeled with therapeutic radioisotopes in model systems such as avascular tumor spheroids were reported. However, these studies were limited to in vitro evaluations (Emfietzoglou et al., 2001, 2005; Kostarelos & Emfietzoglou, 2000). In vitro studies with liposomes radiolabeled with alpha particle emitters such as radium-223, radium-224, and actinium-225 are also reported. These liposomes incorporating high linear energy transfer (LET) alpha-emitting radioisotopes were found to be stable in serum, which is an important prerequisite for in vivo applications (Henriksen et al., 2004; Sofou et al., 2004). J Tyler French et al. (2010) reported preclinical evaluation of lipid NPs encapsulated with therapeutic, rhenium-186, radionuclide in the form of ^{186}Re-BMEDA complex. They could show significant reduction in tumor volume after intratumoral injection of the radiolabeled lipid NP in nude rats bearing head and neck cancer. Similar approach with nanoliposome and 188Re-BMEDA was also reported and the agent was evaluated in glioma tumor-bearing rats (Huang et al., 2011). In an elaborate study, Anna Helbok et al. (2010) evaluated PEGylated lipid-based NPs with various diagnostic and therapeutic radioisotopes such as indium-111, technetium-99m, gallium-68, and lutetium-177. Diethyl-ethylene-triamene-penta-acetic acid (DTPA) was used as chelator for all radioisotopes. While biodistribution carried out in normal Lewis rats did not reveal any information in particular, the study as a whole indicated the potential of lipid NP systems to carry a variety of radioisotopes (Helbok et al., 2010). Later, they reported evaluation of a tyrosine-3-octreotide-conjugated liposome labeled with indium-111 in murine tumor model wherein moderate uptake was observed (Helbok et al., 2012).

5.8 STRATEGIES FOR RADIOLABELING NPS

Radiolabeling refers to the tagging of suitable radionuclide to the NPs. The radionuclide can be a diagnostic radioisotope or a therapeutic radioisotope depending upon the application for the NP designed. The method adopted for radiolabeling depends on the nature of the NPs as well as the chemical nature of the radioisotope being used. Broadly, the radiolabeling methods can be divided into direct and indirect methods (Bentivoglio et al., 2022, 2023; Varani et al., 2022). In direct method, the radioisotope is tagged to the functional group already present on the nanomaterials' surface. On the contrary, in indirect method, the surface of the NP is further modified with a suitable chelating agent, which is specific to the radioisotope being tagged. Technetium-99m, the most widely used diagnostic radioisotope, can be used for direct radiolabeling of NPs possessing functional groups such as –COOH and –OH (Gupta et al., 2021; Mondal et al., 2019; Psimadas et al., 2013). The radiolabeling procedure involves reduction of technetium-99m in its +7 oxidation state (in sodium pertechnetate [$Na^{99m}TcO_4$]) to a lower oxidation state (generally +5) using reducing agents such as stannous chloride ($SnCl_2$) and sodium borohydride ($NaBH_4$) (Geskovski et al., 2013). Technetium-99m in its lower oxidation state is then stabilized by the surface functional groups present on the surface of the NPs. Major disadvantage in this method is low radiolabeling yield and presence of side products of technetium-99m such as $99mTcO_2$ (reduced/hydrolyzed technetium) and sodium pertechnetate [$Na99mTcO_4$]. Purification of 99mTc-NPs from the impurities is often difficult and using the unpurified 99mTc-NPs is not advisable since the impurities may impact the diagnosis (Deutsch et al., 1983; Vallabhajosula et al., 2010). In some cases, radioiodine (iodine-125/131) was directly conjugated to GNPs taking advantage of the high affinity of gold atoms for iodine (Walsh, 2017; Zhang et al., 2017). Direct radiolabeling of liposomes with iodine-124 was reported to be more efficient than the indirect route (Mougin-Degraef et al., 2006). Fluorine-18 is another important diagnostic PET radioisotope that can be directly radiolabeled with certain types of rare-earth NPs, though this approach has significant limitations for widespread applicability (Liu et al., 2011). Copper-64 is used for direct labeling of electron donor-type NPs that have a high affinity for radiometals such as copper (Shaffer et al., 2015). Indium-111, zirconium-89, lutetium-177, and alpha emitters such as astatine-211, actinium-225, and radium-223 were also radiolabeled with appropriate NPs by direct route (Bentivoglio et al., 2023; Boros et al., 2015).

Most of the radioisotopes discussed herein can also be tagged to the NPs through indirect route. Indirect methods of radiolabeling significantly eliminate the problems posed by direct methods of radiolabeling. In this method, the surface of the NPs is synthetically modified with bifunctional chelators such as hydrazinonicotinamide (HYINIC), N-hydroxysuccinimide derivative of S-acetylmercaptoacetyltriglycine (NHS-MAG3), and DTPA (Kumar et al., 2021; Mushtaq et al., 2021; Peiris et al., 2015; Wang et al., 2007), which are efficiently radiolabeled with technetium-99m. These chelators can efficiently radiolabel with technetium-99m eliminating the need for purification of the 99mTc-NPs post-radiolabeling. For indirect radiolabeling with radioiodine, prosthetic groups suitable for tagging radioiodine are conjugated on the NP surface. For example, to permit nucleophilic exchange of radioiodine, NP surface is modified with tyrosine residues wherein the orthoposition of its phenolic group can be substituted with radioiodine. This requires generation of I+ species from iodide (I-) form of radioactive iodine-124/125/131 using strong oxidizing agent like N-chlorobenzenesulfonamide (Chloramine-T) (Tashtoush et al., 2001). The entire radiolabeling process takes only a few seconds to a minute and then terminated by adding a reducing agent (usually sodium metabisulfite). Iodogen is a less aggressive reducing agent, which can be used for radio-iodination of suitably surface-modified NPs. Indirect radiolabeling with fluorine-18 (Tang et al., 2022) requires specific modification of the NP surface to enable copper-catalyzed azide-alkyne cycloaddition, often termed as 'click chemistry' (Wang et al., 2003).

While chelators such as HYNIC and MAG3 are often used for radiolabeling with technetium-99m, DTPA can also be used for radiolabeling with indium-111, yttrium-90, and lutetium-177 (Pentsova et al., 2021; Wang et al., 2015; Winter et al., 2023). There are other chelators such as 2,2′,2″,2‴-DOTA and 2-[1,4,7,10-tetraazacyclododecane-4,7,10-tetrayl]-pentanedioic acid (DOTAGA), which can be used for radiolabeling with radioisotopes such as indium-111, yttrium-90, zirconium-89, copper-64, gallium-68, and lutetium-177 (Holik et al., 2022). AAZTA-5 (6-amino-6-(5-methoxy-5-oxopentyl)-1,4-diacepine-tetraacetate) is an emerging chelator for radiolabeling with radioisotopes such as gallium-68, scandium-44, and lutetium-177 (Sinnes et al., 2020).

5.9 CONCLUSIONS

Nuclear medicine has gained much attention recently as it provides solution for precise diagnosis, management, and therapy of various diseases. Combination of radioisotopes and NPs that are able to concurrently treat and diagnose diseased conditions can make various advancements in nuclear medicine. While the combination of nanocarrier-based chemotherapeutic drugs, hyperthermia agents, and radiosensitizers with radioisotopes can have synergistic enhanced therapeutic effects, combination of diagnostic agents such as MNPs, upconversion particles, and QDs, with radioisotopes can result in better resolution in diagnostic procedures. Factors that govern the feasibility of clinical translation of a therapeutic and diagnostic NP-based nuclear medicine are its biocompatibility, biodegradability, biodistribution data, pharmacokinetics, ease of scaling up, reproducibility, and cost-effectiveness. Though studies on many nano-based radiopharmaceuticals are reported, only very few based on liposomes and inorganic materials have achieved clinical translation. Increasing number of references related to nano-based radiopharmaceuticals shows that many nano-based systems will reach clinical translation in the near future.

REFERENCES

AC07607271, A. (2009). *Cyclotron Produced Radionuclides: Physical Characteristics and Production Methods*. International Atomic Energy Agency.

Ai, F., Ferreira, C. A., Chen, F., & Cai, W. (2016). Engineering of radiolabeled iron oxide nanoparticles for dual-modality imaging. *WIREs Nanomedicine and Nanobiotechnology*, 8(4), 619–630. https://doi.org/10.1002/wnan.1386

Allmeroth, M., Moderegger, D., Gündel, D., Koynov, K., Buchholz, H.-G., Mohr, K., Rösch, F., Zentel, R., & Thews, O. (2013). HPMA-LMA copolymer drug carriers in oncology: An in vivo PET study to assess the tumor line-specific polymer uptake and body distribution. *Biomacromolecules*, 14(9), 3091–3101. https://doi.org/10.1021/bm400709z

Almutairi, A., Rossin, R., Shokeen, M., Hagooly, A., Ananth, A., Capoccia, B., Guillaudeu, S., Abendschein, D., Anderson, C. J., Welch, M. J., & Fréchet, J. M. J. (2009). Biodegradable dendritic positron-emitting nanoprobes for the noninvasive imaging of angiogenesis. *Proceedings of the National Academy of Sciences*, 106(3), 685–690. https://doi.org/10.1073/pnas.0811757106

Anbarasu, M., Anandan, M., Chinnasamy, E., Gopinath, V., & Balamurugan, K. (2015). Synthesis and characterization of polyethylene glycol (PEG) coated Fe_3O_4 nanoparticles by chemical co-precipitation method for biomedical applications. *Spectrochimica Acta. Part A, Molecular and Biomolecular Spectroscopy*, 135, 536–539. https://doi.org/10.1016/j.saa.2014.07.059

Balakrishnan, B., Subramanian, S., Mallia, M. B., Repaka, K., Kaur, S., Chandan, R., Bhardwaj, P., Dash, A., & Banerjee, R. (2020). Multifunctional core–shell glyconanoparticles for galectin-3-targeted, trigger-responsive combination chemotherapy. *Biomacromolecules*, 21(7), 2645–2660. https://doi.org/10.1021/acs.biomac.0c00358

Bao, A., Phillips, W. T., Goins, B., Zheng, X., Sabour, S., Natarajan, M., Ross Woolley, F., Zavaleta, C., & Otto, R. A. (2006). Potential use of drug carried-liposomes for cancer therapy via direct intratumoral injection. *International Journal of Pharmaceutics*, 316(1–2), 162–169. https://doi.org/10.1016/j.ijpharm.2006.02.039

Barrefelt, Å. A., Brismar, T. B., Egri, G., Aspelin, P., Olsson, A., Oddo, L., Margheritelli, S., Caidahl, K., Paradossi, G., Dähne, L., Axelsson, R., & Hassan, M. (2013). Multimodality imaging using SPECT/CT and MRI and ligand functionalized ^{99m}Tc-labeled magnetic microbubbles. *EJNMMI Research*, 3(1), 12. https://doi.org/10.1186/2191-219X-3-12

Bentivoglio, V., Nayak, P., Varani, M., Lauri, C., & Signore, A. (2023). Methods for radiolabeling nanoparticles (Part 3): Therapeutic use. *Biomolecules*, *13*(8), 1241. https://doi.org/10.3390/biom13081241

Bentivoglio, V., Varani, M., Lauri, C., Ranieri, D., & Signore, A. (2022). Methods for radiolabelling nanoparticles: PET use (Part 2). *Biomolecules*, *12*(10), 1517. https://doi.org/10.3390/biom12101517

Bentolila, L. A., Ebenstein, Y., & Weiss, S. (2009). Quantum dots for in vivo small-animal imaging. *Journal of Nuclear Medicine*, 50(4), 493–496. https://doi.org/10.2967/jnumed.108.053561

Boros, E., Bowen, A. M., Josephson, L., Vasdev, N., & Holland, J. P. (2015). Chelate-free metal ion binding and heat-induced radiolabeling of iron oxide nanoparticles. *Chemical Science*, 6(1), 225–236. https://doi.org/10.1039/C4SC02778G

Brivio, D., Nguyen, P. L., Sajo, E., Ngwa, W., & Zygmanski, P. (2017). A Monte Carlo study of I-125 prostate brachytherapy with gold nanoparticles: Dose enhancement with simultaneous rectal dose sparing via radiation shielding. *Physics in Medicine and Biology*, 62(5), 1935–1948. https://doi.org/10.1088/1361-6560/aa5bc7

Carter, J. D., Cheng, N. N., Qu, Y., Suarez, G. D., & Guo, T. (2007). Nanoscale energy deposition by X-ray absorbing nanostructures. *The Journal of Physical Chemistry* B, 111(40), 11622–11625. https://doi.org/10.1021/jp075253u

Chang, M., Shiau, A., Chen, Y., Chang, C., Chen, H. H., & Wu, C. (2008). Increased apoptotic potential and dose-enhancing effect of gold nanoparticles in combination with single-dose clinical electron beams on tumor-bearing mice. *Cancer Science*, 99(7), 1479–1484. https://doi.org/10.1111/j.1349-7006.2008.00827.x

Chen, G., Qiu, H., Prasad, P. N., & Chen, X. (2014). Upconversion nanoparticles: Design, nanochemistry, and applications in theranostics. *Chemical Reviews*, *114*(10), 5161–5214. Retrieved June 15, 2024, from https://pubs.acs.org/doi/10.1021/cr400425h

Chen, H., Zhang, X., Dai, S., Ma, Y., Cui, S., Achilefus, S., & Gu, Y. (2013). Multifunctional gold nanostar conjugates for tumor imaging and combined photothermal and chemo-therapy. *Theranostics*, 3(9), 633–649. https://doi.org/10.7150/thno.6630

Chen, W., Westcott, S. L., & Zhang, J. (2007). Dose dependence of x-ray luminescence from CaF_2:Eu^{2+}, Mn^{2+} phosphors. *Applied Physics Letters*, 91(21), 211103. https://doi.org/10.1063/1.2816330

Chithrani, D. B., Jelveh, S., Jalali, F., van Prooijen, M., Allen, C., Bristow, R. G., Hill, R. P., & Jaffray, D. A. (2010). Gold nanoparticles as radiation sensitizers in cancer therapy. *Radiation Research*, 173(6), 719–728. https://doi.org/10.1667/RR1984.1

Choi, J., Park, J. C., Nah, H., Woo, S., Oh, J., Kim, K. M., Cheon, G. J., Chang, Y., Yoo, J., & Cheon, J. (2008). A hybrid nanoparticle probe for dual-modality positron emission tomography and magnetic resonance imaging. *Angewandte Chemie International Edition*, 47(33), 6259–6262. https://doi.org/10.1002/anie.200801369

Chung, J.-K., & Cheon, G. J. (2014). Radioiodine therapy in differentiated thyroid cancer: The first targeted therapy in oncology. *Endocrinology and Metabolism*, 29(3), 233. https://doi.org/10.3803/EnM.2014.29.3.233

Cunningham, C., de Kock, M., Engelbrecht, M., Miles, X., Slabbert, J., & Vandevoorde, C. (2021). Radiosensitization effect of gold nanoparticles in proton therapy. *Frontiers in Public Health*, 9, 699822. https://doi.org/10.3389/fpubh.2021.699822

Curry, T., Kopelman, R., Shilo, M., & Popovtzer, R. (2014). Multifunctional theranostic gold nanoparticles for targeted CT imaging and photothermal therapy. *Contrast Media & Molecular Imaging*, 9(1), 53–61. https://doi.org/10.1002/cmmi.1563

Dagar, S., Sekosan, M., Lee, B. S., Rubinstein, I., & Onyüksel, H. (2001). VIP receptors as molecular targets of breast cancer: Implications for targeted imaging and drug delivery. *Journal of Controlled Release: Official Journal of the Controlled Release Society*, 74(1–3), 129–134. https://doi.org/10.1016/s0168-3659(01)00326-1

Das, T., & Banerjee, S. (2017). Radiopharmaceuticals for metastatic bone pain palliation: Available options in the clinical domain and their comparisons. *Clinical & Experimental Metastasis*, 34(1), 1–10. https://doi.org/10.1007/s10585-016-9831-9

De La Zerda, A., Zavaleta, C., Keren, S., Vaithilingam, S., Bodapati, S., Liu, Z., Levi, J., Smith, B. R., Ma, T.-J., Oralkan, O., Cheng, Z., Chen, X., Dai, H., Khuri-Yakub, B. T., & Gambhir, S. S. (2008). Carbon nanotubes as photoacoustic molecular imaging agents in living mice. *Nature Nanotechnology*, 3(9), 557–562. https://doi.org/10.1038/nnano.2008.231

De Rosales, R. T. M. (2014). Potential clinical applications of bimodal PET-MRI or SPECT-MRI agents. *Journal of Labelled Compounds and Radiopharmaceuticals*, 57(4), 298–303. https://doi.org/10.1002/jlcr.3154

Deutsch, E., Libson, K., Jurisson, S., & Lindoy, L. F. (1983). Technetium chemistry and technetium radiopharmaceuticals. In S. J. Lippard (Ed.), *Progress in Inorganic Chemistry* (1st ed., Vol. 30, pp. 75–139). Wiley. https://doi.org/10.1002/9780470166314.ch2

Dhas, N., Pastagia, M., Sharma, A., Khera, A., Kudarha, R., Kulkarni, S., … & Patel, M. (2022). Organic quantum dots: An ultrasmall nanoplatform for cancer theranostics. *Journal of Controlled Release*, *348*, 798–824. Retrieved June 15, 2024, from https://www.sciencedirect.com/science/article/abs/pii/S0168365922003741?via%3Dihub

Djoumessi, D., Laprise-Pelletier, M., Chevallier, P., Lagueux, J., Côté, M. F., & Fortin, M.-A. (2015). Rapid, one-pot procedure to synthesise ^{103}Pd:Pd@Au nanoparticles en route for radiosensitisation and radiotherapeutic applications. *Journal of Materials Chemistry* B, 3(10), 2192–2205. https://doi.org/10.1039/C4TB01663G

Elbayoumi, T. A., & Torchilin, V. P. (2006). Enhanced accumulation of long-circulating liposomes modified with the nucleosome-specific monoclonal antibody 2C5 in various tumours in mice: Gamma-imaging studies. *European Journal of Nuclear Medicine and Molecular Imaging*, 33(10), 1196–1205. https://doi.org/10.1007/s00259-006-0139-x

Emfietzoglou, D., Kostarelos, K., & Sgouros, G. (2001). An analytic dosimetry study for the use of radionuclide-liposome conjugates in internal radiotherapy. *Journal of Nuclear Medicine: Official Publication, Society of Nuclear Medicine*, 42(3), 499–504.

Emfietzoglou, D., Kostarelos, K., Papakostas, A., Yang, W.-H., Ballangrud, A., Song, H., & Sgouros, G. (2005). Liposome-mediated radiotherapeutics within avascular tumor spheroids: Comparative dosimetry study for various radionuclides, liposome systems, and a targeting antibody. *Journal of Nuclear Medicine: Official Publication, Society of Nuclear Medicine*, 46(1), 89–97.

Fernandes, D. A. (2023). Liposomes for cancer theranostics. *Pharmaceutics*, 15(10), 2448. https://doi.org/10.3390/pharmaceutics15102448

Fernandes, D. A., Appak-Baskoy, S., Berndl, E., & Kolios, M. C. (2021). Laser activatable perfluorocarbon bubbles for imaging and therapy through enhanced absorption from coupled silica coated gold nanoparticles. *RSC Advances*, 11(9), 4906–4920. https://doi.org/10.1039/D0RA08009H

French, J. T., Goins, B., Saenz, M., Li, S., Garcia-Rojas, X., Phillips, W. T., Otto, R. A., & Bao, A. (2010). Interventional therapy of head and neck cancer with lipid nanoparticle–carried rhenium 186 radionuclide. *Journal of Vascular and Interventional Radiology*, 21(8), 1271–1279. https://doi.org/10.1016/j.jvir.2010.02.027

Gabizon, A., Price, D. C., Huberty, J., Bresalier, R. S., & Papahadjopoulos, D. (1990). Effect of liposome composition and other factors on the targeting of liposomes to experimental tumors: Biodistribution and imaging studies. *Cancer Research*, 50(19), 6371–6378.

Gao, Q., Zhang, J., Gao, J., Zhang, Z., Zhu, H., & Wang, D. (2021). Gold nanoparticles in cancer theranostics. *Frontiers in Bioengineering and Biotechnology*, 9. https://doi.org/10.3389/fbioe.2021.647905

Gautam, S., & Tripathi, J. (2016). Food processing by irradiation——An effective technology for food safety and security. *Indian Journal of Experimental Biology*, 54(11), 700–707.

Geng, L., Osusky, K., Konjeti, S., Fu, A., & Hallahan, D. (2004). Radiation-guided drug delivery to tumor blood vessels results in improved tumor growth delay. *Journal of Controlled Release: Official Journal of the Controlled Release Society*, 99(3), 369–381. https://doi.org/10.1016/j.jconrel.2004.07.024

Georgakilas, V., Tagmatarchis, N., Pantarotto, D., Bianco, A., Briand, J.-P., & Prato, M. (2002). Amino acid functionalisation of water soluble carbon nanotubes. *Chemical Communications*, 24, 3050–3051. https://doi.org/10.1039/b209843a

Geskovski, N., Kuzmanovska, S., Simonoska Crcarevska, M., Calis, S., Dimchevska, S., Petrusevska, M., Zdravkovski, P., & Goracinova, K. (2013). Comparative biodistribution studies of technetium-99 m radiolabeled amphiphilic nanoparticles using three different reducing agents during the labeling procedure: Technetium-99 m direct labeling of nanoparticles-effects of reductants. *Journal of Labelled Compounds and Radiopharmaceuticals*, 56(14), 689–695. https://doi.org/10.1002/jlcr.3097

Gobbo, O. L., Sjaastad, K., Radomski, M. W., Volkov, Y., & Prina-Mello, A. (2015). Magnetic nanoparticles in cancer theranostics. *Theranostics*, 5(11), 1249–1263. https://doi.org/10.7150/thno.11544

Goins, B., Klipper, R., Rudolph, A. S., & Phillips, W. T. (1994). Use of technetium-99m-liposomes in tumor imaging. *Journal of Nuclear Medicine: Official Publication, Society of Nuclear Medicine*, 35(9), 1491–1498.

Gorain, B., Choudhury, H., Nair, A. B., Dubey, S. K., & Kesharwani, P. (2020). Theranostic application of nanoemulsions in chemotherapy. *Drug Discovery Today*, 25(7), 1174–1188. https://doi.org/10.1016/j.drudis.2020.04.013

Goto, R., Kubo, H., & Okada, S. (1989). Liposomes prepared from synthetic amphiphiles. I. Their technetium labeling and stability. *Chemical & Pharmaceutical Bulletin*, 37(5), 1351–1354. https://doi.org/10.1248/cpb.37.1351

Gregoriadis, G., Neerunjun, D. E., & Hunt, R. (1977). Fate of a liposome-associated agent injected into normal and tumour-bearing rodents. Attempts to improve localization in tumour tissues. *Life Sciences*, 21(3), 357–369. https://doi.org/10.1016/0024-3205(77)90516-1

Gulenchyn, K. Y., Yao, X., Asa, S. L., Singh, S., & Law, C. (2012). Radionuclide therapy in neuroendocrine tumours: A systematic review. *Clinical Oncology*, 24(4), 294–308. https://doi.org/10.1016/j.clon.2011.12.003

Guo, J., Rahme, K., He, Y., Li, L.-L., Holmes, J. D., & O'Driscoll, C. M. (2017). Gold nanoparticles enlighten the future of cancer theranostics. *International Journal of Nanomedicine*, 12, 6131–6152. https://doi.org/10.2147/IJN.S140772

Gupta, A., Mathur, R., Singh, S., Bag, N., Khan, U. A., Ahmad, F. J., Gabr, G. A., Kesharwani, P., & Jain, G. K. (2021). ^{99m}Tc-methionine gold nanoparticles as a promising biomaterial for enhanced tumor imaging. *Journal of Pharmaceutical Sciences*, 110(2), 888–897. https://doi.org/10.1016/j.xphs.2020.11.008

Gupta, N., Devgan, A., Bansal, I., Olsavsky, T. D., Li, S., Abdelbaki, A., & Kumar, Y. (2017). Usefulness of radium-223 in patients with bone metastases. *Proceedings (Baylor University. Medical Center)*, 30(4), 424–426.

Guryev, E. L., Volodina, N. O., Shilyagina, N. Y., Gudkov, S. V., Balalaeva, I. V., Volovetskiy, A. B., Lyubeshkin, A. V., Sen', A. V., Ermilov, S. A., Vodeneev, V. A., Petrov, R. V., Zvyagin, A. V., Alferov, Z. I., & Deyev, S. M. (2018). Radioactive (^{90}Y) upconversion nanoparticles conjugated with recombinant targeted toxin for synergistic nanotheranostics of cancer. *Proceedings of the National Academy of Sciences*, 115(39), 9690–9695. https://doi.org/10.1073/pnas.1809258115

Haase, M., & Schäfer, H. (2011). Upconverting nanoparticles. *Angewandte Chemie*, 50(26), 5808–5829. https://doi.org/10.1002/anie.201005159

Häfeli, U., Tiefenauer, L. X., Schbiger, P. A., & Weder, H. G. (1991). A lipophilic complex with ^{186}Re/^{188}Re incorporated in liposomes suitable for radiotherapy. *International Journal of Radiation Applications and Instrumentation. Part B, Nuclear Medicine and Biology*, 18(5), 449–454. https://doi.org/10.1016/0883-2897(91)90104-s

Hainfeld, J. F., Slatkin, D. N., & Smilowitz, H. M. (2004). The use of gold nanoparticles to enhance radiotherapy in mice. *Physics in Medicine and Biology*, 49(18), N309–315. https://doi.org/10.1088/0031-9155/49/18/n03

Harrington, K. J., Mohammadtaghi, S., Uster, P. S., Glass, D., Peters, A. M., Vile, R. G., & Stewart, J. S. W. (2001). Effective targeting of solid tumors in patients with locally advanced cancers by radiolabeled pegylated liposomes. *Clinical Cancer Research*, 7(2), 243–254.

Harrington, K. J., Peters, A. M., & Mohammadtaghi, S. (1996). Biodistribution and pharmacokinetics of In-111-labeled Stealth{reg_sign} liposomes in patients with solid tumours. *Journal of Nuclear Medicine*, *37*(Suppl.5), Article CONF-960659-. https://www.osti.gov/biblio/447750

Harrington, K. J., Rowlinson-Busza, G., Syrigos, K. N., Uster, P. S., Abra, R. M., & Stewart, J. S. (2000a). Biodistribution and pharmacokinetics of ^{111}In-DTPA-labelled pegylated liposomes in a human tumour xenograft model: Implications for novel targeting strategies. *British Journal of Cancer*, 83(2), 232–238. https://doi.org/10.1054/bjoc.1999.1232

Harrington, K. J., Rowlinson-Busza, G., Syrigos, K. N., Vile, R. G., Uster, P. S., Peters, A. M., & Stewart, J. S. (2000b). Pegylated liposome-encapsulated doxorubicin and cisplatin enhance the effect of radiotherapy in a tumor xenograft model. *Clinical Cancer Research: An Official Journal of the American Association for Cancer Research*, 6(12), 4939–4949.

Helbok, A., Decristoforo, C., Dobrozemsky, G., Rangger, C., Diederen, E., Stark, B., Prassl, R., & Von Guggenberg, E. (2010). Radiolabeling of lipid-based nanoparticles for diagnostics and therapeutic applications: A comparison using different radiometals. *Journal of Liposome Research*, 20(3), 219–227. https://doi.org/10.3109/08982100903311812

Helbok, A., Rangger, C., Von Guggenberg, E., Saba-Lepek, M., Radolf, T., Thurner, G., Andreae, F., Prassl, R., & Decristoforo, C. (2012). Targeting properties of peptide-modified radiolabeled liposomal nanoparticles. *Nanomedicine: Nanotechnology, Biology and Medicine*, 8(1), 112–118. https://doi.org/10.1016/j.nano.2011.04.012

Henriksen, G., Schoultz, B. W., Michaelsen, T. E., Bruland, Ø. S., & Larsen, R. H. (2004). Sterically stabilized liposomes as a carrier for alpha-emitting radium and actinium radionuclides. *Nuclear Medicine and Biology*, 31(4), 441–449. https://doi.org/10.1016/j.nucmedbio.2003.11.004

Hnatowich, D. J., Friedman, B., Clancy, B., & Novak, M. (1981). Labeling of preformed liposomes with Ga-67 and Tc-99m by chelation. *Journal of Nuclear Medicine: Official Publication, Society of Nuclear Medicine*, 22(9), 810–814.

Holik, H. A., Ibrahim, F. M., Elaine, A. A., Putra, B. D., Achmad, A., & Kartamihardja, A. H. S. (2022). The chemical scaffold of theranostic radiopharmaceuticals: Radionuclide, bifunctional chelator, and pharmacokinetics modifying linker. *Molecules*, 27(10), 3062. https://doi.org/10.3390/molecules27103062

Huang, F.-Y. J., Lee, T.-W., Kao, C.-H. K., Chang, C.-H., Zhang, X., Lee, W.-Y., Chen, W.-J., Wang, S.-C., & Lo, J.-M. (2011). Imaging, autoradiography, and biodistribution of ^{188}Re-labeled PEGylated nanoliposome in orthotopic glioma bearing rat model. *Cancer Biotherapy and Radiopharmaceuticals*, 26(6), 717–725. https://doi.org/10.1089/cbr.2011.1052

Hwang, H., Kwon, J., Oh, P.-S., Lee, T.-K., Na, K.-S., Lee, C.-M., Jeong, H.-S., Lim, S. T., Sohn, M.-H., & Jeong, H.-J. (2014). Peptide-loaded nanoparticles and radionuclide imaging for individualized treatment of myocardial ischemia. *Radiology*, 273(1), 160–167. https://doi.org/10.1148/radiol.14132942

In Het Panhuis, M. (2003). Vaccine delivery by carbon nanotubes. *Chemistry & Biology*, 10(10), 897–898. https://doi.org/10.1016/j.chembiol.2003.10.005

Indoria, S., Singh, V., & Hsieh, M.-F. (2020). Recent advances in theranostic polymeric nanoparticles for cancer treatment: A review. *International Journal of Pharmaceutics*, 582, 119314. https://doi.org/10.1016/j.ijpharm.2020.119314

International Atomic Energy Agency. (n.d.). *Manual for Reactor Produced Radioisotopes*. IAEA.

Internationale Atomenergie-Organisation (Ed.). (2009). *Technetium-99m Radiopharmaceuticals: Status and Trends*. IAEA.

Iram, F., Iqbal, M. S., Khan, I. U., Rasheed, R., Khalid, A., Khalid, M., Aftab, S., & Shakoori, A. R. (2020). Synthesis and biodistribution study of biocompatible ^{198}Au nanoparticles by use of arabinoxylan as reducing and stabilizing agent. *Biological Trace Element Research*, 193(1), 282–293. https://doi.org/10.1007/s12011-019-01700-y

Jadvar, H., Desai, B., & Conti, P. S. (2015). Sodium ^{18}F-fluoride PET/CT of bone, joint and other disorders. *Seminars in Nuclear Medicine*, 45(1), 58–65. https://doi.org/10.1053/j.semnuclmed.2014.07.008

Jaggi, M., Khar, R. K., Chauhan, U. P. S., & Gangal, S. V. (1991). Liposomes as carriers of ^{99m}Tc glucoheptonate for liver imaging. *International Journal of Pharmaceutics*, 69(1), 77–79. https://doi.org/10.1016/0378-5173(91)90089-7

Jain, S., Coulter, J. A., Hounsell, A. R., Butterworth, K. T., McMahon, S. J., Hyland, W. B., Muir, M. F., Dickson, G. R., Prise, K. M., Currell, F. J., O'Sullivan, J. M., & Hirst, D. G. (2011). Cell-specific radiosensitization by gold nanoparticles at megavoltage radiation energies. *International Journal of Radiation Oncology, Biology,* Physics, 79(2), 531–539. https://doi.org/10.1016/j.ijrobp.2010.08.044

Jangjou, A., Meisami, A. H., Jamali, K., Niakan, M. H., Abbasi, M., Shafiee, M., Salehi, M., Hosseinzadeh, A., Amani, A. M., & Vaez, A. (2021). The promising shadow of microbubble over medical sciences: From fighting wide scope of prevalence disease to cancer eradication. *Journal of Biomedical Science*, 28(1), 49. https://doi.org/10.1186/s12929-021-00744-4

Juzenas, P., Chen, W., Sun, Y.-P., Coelho, M. A. N., Generalov, R., Generalova, N., & Christensen, I. L. (2008). Quantum dots and nanoparticles for photodynamic and radiation therapies of cancer. *Advanced Drug Delivery Reviews*, 60(15), 1600–1614. https://doi.org/10.1016/j.addr.2008.08.004

Kam, N. W. S., O'Connell, M., Wisdom, J. A., & Dai, H. (2005). Carbon nanotubes as multifunctional biological transporters and near-infrared agents for selective cancer cell destruction. *Proceedings of the National Academy of Sciences*, 102(33), 11600–11605. https://doi.org/10.1073/pnas.0502680102

Khan, M. K., Minc, L. D., Nigavekar, S. S., Kariapper, M. S. T., Nair, B. M., Schipper, M., Cook, A. C., Lesniak, W. G., & Balogh, L. P. (2008). Fabrication of {$^{198}Au^0$} radioactive composite nanodevices and their use for nano-brachytherapy. *Nanomedicine : Nanotechnology, Biology, and Medicine*, 4(1), 57–69. https://doi.org/10.1016/j.nano.2007.11.005

Kiessling, F., Mertens, M. E., Grimm, J., & Lammers, T. (2014). Nanoparticles for imaging: Top or flop? *Radiology*, 273(1), 10–28. https://doi.org/10.1148/radiol.14131520

Knapp, F. F., & Dash, A. (2016). *Radiopharmaceuticals for Therapy*. Springer India. https://doi.org/10.1007/978-81-322-2607-9

Kostarelos, K., & Emfietzoglou, D. (2000). Tissue dosimetry of liposome-radionuclide complexes for internal radiotherapy: Toward liposome-targeted therapeutic radiopharmaceuticals. *Anticancer Research*, 20(5A), 3339–3345.

Kumar, D., Sakhare, N., Das, S., Kale, P., Mathur, A., Mirapurkar, S., Muralidharan, S., Chaudhari, P., Mohanty, B., Ballal, A., & Patro, P. (2021). Development of technetium-99m labeled ultrafine gold nanobioconjugates for targeted imaging of folate receptor positive cancers. *Nuclear Medicine and Biology*, 93, 1–10. https://doi.org/10.1016/j.nucmedbio.2020.11.001

Laprise-Pelletier, M., Lagueux, J., Côté, M.-F., LaGrange, T., & Fortin, M.-A. (2017). Low-dose prostate cancer brachytherapy with radioactive palladium-gold nanoparticles. *Advanced Healthcare Materials*, *6*(4). https://doi.org/10.1002/adhm.201601120

Laprise-Pelletier, M., Simão, T., & Fortin, M.-A. (2018). Gold nanoparticles in radiotherapy and recent progress in nanobrachytherapy. *Advanced Healthcare Materials*, 7(16), e1701460. https://doi.org/10.1002/adhm.201701460

Lechtman, E., Chattopadhyay, N., Cai, Z., Mashouf, S., Reilly, R., & Pignol, J. P. (2011). Implications on clinical scenario of gold nanoparticle radiosensitization in regards to photon energy, nanoparticle size, concentration and location. *Physics in Medicine and Biology*, 56(15), 4631–4647. https://doi.org/10.1088/0031-9155/56/15/001

Létant, S. E., & Wang, T.-F. (2006a). Semiconductor quantum dot scintillation under γ-ray irradiation. *Nano Letters*, 6(12), 2877–2880. https://doi.org/10.1021/nl0620942

Létant, S. E., & Wang, T.-F. (2006b). Study of porous glass doped with quantum dots or laser dyes under alpha irradiation. *Applied Physics Letters*, 88(10), 103110. https://doi.org/10.1063/1.2182072

Lever, S. Z. (2002). Evolution of radiopharmaceuticals for diagnosis and therapy. *Journal of Cellular Biochemistry.* Supplement, 39, 60–64. https://doi.org/10.1002/jcb.10405

Li, K., Hong, E., Wang, B., Wang, Z., Zhang, L., Hu, R., & Wang, B. (2019). Advances in the application of upconversion nanoparticles for detecting and treating cancers. *Photodiagnosis and Photodynamic Therapy*, 25, 177–192. https://doi.org/10.1016/j.pdpdt.2018.12.007

Li, X., Li, W., Wang, M., & Liao, Z. (2021). Magnetic nanoparticles for cancer theranostics: Advances and prospects. *Journal of Controlled Release*, 335, 437–448. https://doi.org/10.1016/j.jconrel.2021.05.042

Lindsley, C. W., Müller, C. E., & Bongarzone, S. (2022). Diagnostic and therapeutic radiopharmaceuticals. *Journal of Medicinal Chemistry*, 65(19), 12497–12499. https://doi.org/10.1021/acs.jmedchem.2c01403

Liu, Q., Sun, Y., Li, C., Zhou, J., Li, C., Yang, T., Zhang, X., Yi, T., Wu, D., & Li, F. (2011). ^{18}F-Labeled magnetic-upconversion nanophosphors *via* rare-Earth cation-assisted ligand assembly. *ACS Nano*, 5(4), 3146–3157. https://doi.org/10.1021/nn200298y

Liu, Y., Chen, W., Wang, S., & Joly, A. G. (2008). Investigation of water-soluble x-ray luminescence nanoparticles for photodynamic activation. *Applied Physics Letters*, *92*(4). Retrieved June 16, 2024, from https://pubs.aip.org/aip/apl/article-abstract/92/4/043901/335671/Investigation-of-water-soluble-x-ray-luminescence?redirectedFrom=fulltext

Liu, Y., Zhang, Y., Wang, S., Pope, C., & Chen, W. (2008). Optical behaviors of ZnO-porphyrin conjugates and their potential applications for cancer treatment. *Applied Physics Letters*, 92(14), 143901. https://doi.org/10.1063/1.2908211

Low, H. Y., Yang, C.-T., Xia, B., He, T., Lam, W. W. C., & Ng, D. C. E. (2023). Radiolabeled liposomes for nuclear imaging probes. *Molecules*, 28(9), 3798. https://doi.org/10.3390/molecules28093798

Luk, B. T., Fang, R. H., & Zhang, L. (2012). Lipid- and polymer-based nanostructures for cancer theranostics. *Theranostics*, 2(12), 1117–1126. https://doi.org/10.7150/thno.4381

Madru, R., Kjellman, P., Olsson, F., Wingårdh, K., Ingvar, C., Ståhlberg, F., Olsrud, J., Lätt, J., Fredriksson, S., Knutsson, L., & Strand, S.-E. (2012). ^{99m}Tc-labeled superparamagnetic iron oxide nanoparticles for multimodality SPECT/MRI of sentinel lymph nodes. *Journal of Nuclear Medicine*, 53(3), 459–463. https://doi.org/10.2967/jnumed.111.092437

Madru, R., Tran, T. A., Axelsson, J., Ingvar, C., Bibic, A., Ståhlberg, F., Knutsson, L., & Strand, S.-E. (2013). ^{68}Ga-labeled superparamagnetic iron oxide nanoparticles (SPIONs) for multi-modality PET/MR/Cherenkov luminescence imaging of sentinel lymph nodes. *American Journal of Nuclear Medicine and Molecular Imaging*, 4(1), 60–69.

Makino, A., & Kimura, S. (2014). Solid tumor-targeting theranostic polymer nanoparticle in nuclear medicinal fields. *The Scientific World Journal*, *2014*, 1–12. https://doi.org/10.1155/2014/424513

Martin, K. H., & Dayton, P. A. (2013). Current status and prospects for microbubbles in ultrasound theranostics. *WIREs Nanomedicine and Nanobiotechnology*, 5(4), 329–345. https://doi.org/10.1002/wnan.1219

McDevitt, M. R., Chattopadhyay, D., Jaggi, J. S., Finn, R. D., Zanzonico, P. B., Villa, C., Rey, D., Mendenhall, J., Batt, C. A., Njardarson, J. T., & Scheinberg, D. A. (2007). PET imaging of soluble yttrium-86-labeled carbon nanotubes in mice. *PLoS One*, *2*(9), e907. https://doi.org/10.1371/journal.pone.0000907

McDevitt, M. R., Chattopadhyay, D., Kappel, B. J., Jaggi, J. S., Schiffman, S. R., Antczak, C., Njardarson, J. T., Brentjens, R., & Scheinberg, D. A. (2007). Tumor targeting with antibody-functionalized, radiolabeled carbon nanotubes. *Journal of Nuclear Medicine*, 48(7), 1180–1189. https://doi.org/10.2967/jnumed.106.039131

McDevitt, M., McDevitt, M., Alessandro Ruggiero, Carlos H. Villa, Jason P. Holland, Shanna R. Sprinkle, Chad May, Lewis, J., & Scheinberg, D. (2010). Imaging and treating tumor vasculature with targeted radiolabeled carbon nanotubes. *International Journal of Nanomedicine*, 783. https://doi.org/10.2147/IJN.S13300

Mondal, L., Mukherjee, B., Das, K., Bhattacharya, S., Dutta, D., Chakraborty, S., Pal, M. M., Gaonkar, R. H., & Debnath, M. C. (2019). CD-340 functionalized doxorubicin-loaded nanoparticle induces apoptosis and reduces tumor volume along with drug-related cardiotoxicity in mice. *International Journal of Nanomedicine*, 14, 8073–8094. https://doi.org/10.2147/IJN.S220740

Mougin-Degraef, M., Jestin, E., Bruel, D., Remaud-Le Saëc, P., Morandeau, L., Faivre-Chauvet, A., & Barbet, J. (2006). High-Activity Radio-Iodine Labeling of Conventional and Stealth Liposomes. *Journal of Liposome Research*, 16(1), 91–102. https://doi.org/10.1080/08982100500528941

Mushtaq, S., Bibi, A., Park, J. E., & Jeon, J. (2021). Recent progress in technetium-99m-labeled nanoparticles for molecular imaging and cancer therapy. *Nanomaterials*, 11(11), 3022. https://doi.org/10.3390/nano11113022

Nahrendorf, M., Zhang, H., Hembrador, S., Panizzi, P., Sosnovik, D. E., Aikawa, E., Libby, P., Swirski, F. K., & Weissleder, R. (2008). Nanoparticle PET-CT imaging of macrophages in inflammatory atherosclerosis. *Circulation*, 117(3), 379–387. https://doi.org/10.1161/CIRCULATIONAHA.107.741181

Ogihara, I., Kojima, S., & Jay, M. (1986). Tumor uptake of 67Ga-carrying liposomes. *European Journal of Nuclear Medicine*, 11(10), 405–411. https://doi.org/10.1007/BF00261406

Ogihara-Umeda, I., & Kojima, S. (1988). Increased delivery of gallium-67 to tumors using serum-stable liposomes. *Journal of Nuclear Medicine: Official Publication, Society of Nuclear Medicine*, 29(4), 516–523.

Ogihara-Umeda, I., & Kojima, S. (1989). Cholesterol enhances the delivery of liposome-encapsulated gallium-67 to tumors. *European Journal of Nuclear Medicine*, 15(9), 612–617. https://doi.org/10.1007/BF00256940

Ogihara-Umeda, I., Sasaki, T., & Nishigori, H. (1992). Development of a liposome-encapsulated radionuclide with preferential tumor accumulation—The choice of radionuclide and chelating ligand. *International Journal of Radiation Applications and Instrumentation. Part B, Nuclear Medicine and Biology*, 19(7), 753–757. https://doi.org/10.1016/0883-2897(92)90136-m

Ogihara-Umeda, I., Sasaki, T., Kojima, S., & Nishigori, H. (1996). Optimal radiolabeled liposomes for tumor imaging. *Journal of Nuclear Medicine: Official Publication, Society of Nuclear Medicine*, 37(2), 326–332.

Oku, N. (1999). Delivery of contrast agents for positron emission tomography imaging by liposomes. *Advanced Drug Delivery Reviews*, 37(1–3), 53–61. https://doi.org/10.1016/s0169-409x(98)00110-0

Park, J. H., Lee, S., Kim, J.-H., Park, K., Kim, K., & Kwon, I. C. (2008). Polymeric nanomedicine for cancer therapy. *Progress in Polymer Science*, 33(1), 113–137. https://doi.org/10.1016/j.progpolymsci.2007.09.003

Park, K.-H., Song, H.-C., Na, K., Bom, H.-S., Lee, K. H., Kim, S., Kang, D., & Lee, D. H. (2007). Ionic strength-sensitive pullulan acetate nanoparticles (PAN) for intratumoral administration of radioisotope: Ionic strength-dependent aggregation behavior and 99mTechnetium retention property. *Colloids and Surfaces B: Biointerfaces*, 59(1), 16–23. https://doi.org/10.1016/j.colsurfb.2007.04.010

Patri, A., Kukowskalatallo, J., & Bakerjr, J. (2005). Targeted drug delivery with dendrimers: Comparison of the release kinetics of covalently conjugated drug and non-covalent drug inclusion complex. *Advanced Drug Delivery Reviews*, 57(15), 2203–2214. https://doi.org/10.1016/j.addr.2005.09.014

Peiris, P. M., Deb, P., Doolittle, E., Doron, G., Goldberg, A., Govender, P., Shah, S., Rao, S., Carbone, S., Cotey, T., Sylvestre, M., Singh, S., Schiemann, W. P., Lee, Z., & Karathanasis, E. (2015). Vascular targeting of a gold nanoparticle to breast cancer metastasis. *Journal of Pharmaceutical Sciences*, 104(8), 2600–2610. https://doi.org/10.1002/jps.24518

Pellico, J., Llop, J., Fernández-Barahona, I., Bhavesh, R., Ruiz-Cabello, J., & Herranz, F. (2017). Iron oxide nanoradiomaterials: Combining nanoscale properties with radioisotopes for enhanced molecular imaging. *Contrast Media & Molecular Imaging*, *2017*, 1–24. https://doi.org/10.1155/2017/1549580

Pentsova, E., Düring, M., Lind, C. L., & Nielsen, J. R. (2021). 397 A phase I/II trial of intracerebroventricular 177Lu DTPA omburtamab radioimmunotherapy for leptomeningeal metastasis from solid tumors. *Regular and Young Investigator Award Abstracts*, A429–A429. https://doi.org/10.1136/jitc-2021-SITC2021.397

Phillips, W. T. (1999). Delivery of gamma-imaging agents by liposomes. *Advanced Drug Delivery Reviews*, 37(1), 13–32. https://doi.org/10.1016/S0169-409X(98)00108-2

Pimlott, S. L., & Sutherland, A. (2011). Molecular tracers for the PET and SPECT imaging of disease. *Chemical Society Reviews*, 40(1), 149–162. https://doi.org/10.1039/B922628C

Piras, A. M., Fabiano, A., Sartini, S., Zambito, Y., Braccini, S., Chiellini, F., … & Erba, P. A. (2019). pH-Responsive carboxymethylcellulose nanoparticles for 68Ga-WBC labeling in PET imaging. *Polymers*, *11*(10), 1615. https://doi.org/10.3390/polym11101615

Presant, C. A., Proffitt, R. T., Turner, A. F., Williams, L. E., Winsor, D., Werner, J. L., Kennedy, P., Wiseman, C., Gala, K., & McKenna, R. J. (1988). Successful imaging of human cancer with indium-111-labeled phospholipid vesicles. *Cancer*, 62(5), 905–911. https://doi.org/10.1002/1097-0142(19880901)62:5<905::aid-cncr2820620509>3.0.co;2-3

Psimadas, D., Bouziotis, P., Georgoulias, P., Valotassiou, V., Tsotakos, T., & Loudos, G. (2013). Radiolabeling approaches of nanoparticles with ^{99m}Tc. *Contrast Media & Molecular Imaging*, 8(4), 333–339. https://doi.org/10.1002/cmmi.1530

Richardson, V. J., Jeyasingh, K., Jewkes, R. F., Ryman, B. E., & Tattersall, M. H. (1977). Properties of [^{99m}Tc] technetium-labelled liposomes in normal and tumour-bearing rats. *Biochemical Society Transactions*, 5(1), 290–291. https://doi.org/10.1042/bst0050290

Richardson, V. J., Ryman, B. E., Jewkes, R. F., Jeyasingh, K., Tattersall, M. N., Newlands, E. S., & Kaye, S. B. (1979). Tissue distribution and tumour localization of 99m-technetium-labelled liposomes in cancer patients. *British Journal of Cancer*, 40(1), 35–43. https://doi.org/10.1038/bjc.1979.138

Rosa, S., Connolly, C., Schettino, G., Butterworth, K. T., & Prise, K. M. (2017). Biological mechanisms of gold nanoparticle radiosensitization. *Cancer Nanotechnology*, 8(1), 2. https://doi.org/10.1186/s12645-017-0026-0

Rossin, R., Pan, D., Qi, K., Turner, J. L., Sun, X., Wooley, K. L., & Welch, M. J. (2005). ^{64}Cu-labeled folate-conjugated shell cross-linked nanoparticles for tumor imaging and radiotherapy: Synthesis, radiolabeling, and biologic evaluation. *Journal of Nuclear Medicine: Official Publication, Society of Nuclear Medicine*, 46(7), 1210–1218.

Saleem, J., Wang, L., & Chen, C. (2018). Carbon-based nanomaterials for cancer therapy via targeting tumor microenvironment. *Advanced Healthcare Materials*. Retrieved June 15, 2024, from https://onlinelibrary.wiley.com/doi/10.1002/adhm.201800525

Sandiford, L., Phinikaridou, A., Protti, A., Meszaros, L. K., Cui, X., Yan, Y., Frodsham, G., Williamson, P. A., Gaddum, N., Botnar, R. M., Blower, P. J., Green, M. A., & De Rosales, R. T. M. (2013). Bisphosphonate-anchored PEGylation and radiolabeling of superparamagnetic iron oxide: Long-circulating nanoparticles for *in vivo* multimodal (T1 MRI-SPECT) imaging. *ACS Nano*, 7(1), 500–512. https://doi.org/10.1021/nn3046055

Schwochau, K. (1994). Technetium radiopharmaceuticals—Fundamentals, synthesis, structure, and development. *Angewandte Chemie International Edition in English*, 33(22), 2258–2267. https://doi.org/10.1002/anie.199422581

Sgouros, G., Bodei, L., McDevitt, M. R., & Nedrow, J. R. (2020). Radiopharmaceutical therapy in cancer: Clinical advances and challenges. *Nature Reviews Drug Discovery*, 19(9), 589–608. https://doi.org/10.1038/s41573-020-0073-9

Shaffer, T. M., Wall, M. A., Harmsen, S., Longo, V. A., Drain, C. M., Kircher, M. F., & Grimm, J. (2015). Silica nanoparticles as substrates for chelator-free labeling of oxophilic radioisotopes. *Nano Letters*, 15(2), 864–868. https://doi.org/10.1021/nl503522y

Shi Kam, N. W., Jessop, T. C., Wender, P. A., & Dai, H. (2004). Nanotube molecular transporters: Internalization of carbon nanotube–protein conjugates into mammalian cells. *Journal of the American Chemical Society*, 126(22), 6850–6851. https://doi.org/10.1021/ja0486059

Shi, M., Paquette, B., Thippayamontri, T., Gendron, L., Guérin, B., & Sanche, L. (2016). Increased radiosensitivity of colorectal tumors with intra-tumoral injection of low dose of gold nanoparticles. *International Journal of Nanomedicine*, 11, 5323–5333. https://doi.org/10.2147/IJN.S97541

Silberstein, E. B., Elgazzar, A. H., & Kapilivsky, A. (1992). Phosphorus-32 radiopharmaceuticals for the treatment of painful osseous metastases. *Seminars in Nuclear Medicine*, 22(1), 17–27. https://doi.org/10.1016/S0001-2998(05)80153-9

Silva, F., Cabral Campello, M. P., & Paulo, A. (2020). Radiolabeled gold nanoparticles for imaging and therapy of cancer. *Materials*, 14(1), 4. https://doi.org/10.3390/ma14010004

Sinnes, J.-P., Bauder-Wüst, U., Schäfer, M., Moon, E. S., Kopka, K., & Rösch, F. (2020). ^{68}Ga, ^{44}Sc and ^{177}Lu-labeled AAZTA^{5}-PSMA-617: Synthesis, radiolabeling, stability and cell binding compared to DOTA-PSMA-617 analogues. *EJNMMI Radiopharmacy and Chemistry*, 5(1), 28. https://doi.org/10.1186/s41181-020-00107-8

Sofou, S., Thomas, J. L., Lin, H., McDevitt, M. R., Scheinberg, D. A., & Sgouros, G. (2004). Engineered liposomes for potential alpha-particle therapy of metastatic cancer. *Journal of Nuclear Medicine: Official Publication, Society of Nuclear Medicine*, 45(2), 253–260.

Soni, K. S., Desale, S. S., & Bronich, T. K. (2016). Nanogels: An overview of properties, biomedical applications and obstacles to clinical translation. *Journal of Controlled Release*, 240, 109–126. https://doi.org/10.1016/j.jconrel.2015.11.009

Souza, P. B. de, & McCabe, C. J. (2021). *Radioiodine Treatment: An Historical and Future Perspective*. https://doi.org/10.1530/ERC-21-0037

Stendahl, J. C., & Sinusas, A. J. (2015). Nanoparticles for cardiovascular imaging and therapeutic delivery, Part 2: Radiolabeled probes. *Journal of Nuclear Medicine*, 56(11), 1637–1641. https://doi.org/10.2967/jnumed.115.164145

Subramanian, S., Pandey, U., Gugulothu, D., Patravale, V., & Samuel, G. (2013). Modification of PLGA nanoparticles for improved properties as a ^{99m}Tc-labeled agent in sentinel lymph node detection. *Cancer Biotherapy and Radiopharmaceuticals*, 28(8), 598–606. https://doi.org/10.1089/cbr.2013.1511

Sun, Y.-P., Zhou, B., Lin, Y., Wang, W., Fernando, K. A. S., Pathak, P., Meziani, M. J., Harruff, B. A., Wang, X., Wang, H., Luo, P. G., Yang, H., Kose, M. E., Chen, B., Veca, L. M., & Xie, S.-Y. (2006). Quantum-sized carbon dots for bright and colorful photoluminescence. *Journal of the American Chemical Society*, 128(24), 7756–7757. https://doi.org/10.1021/ja062677d

Sun, Z., Cheng, K., Wu, F., Liu, H., Ma, X., Su, X., Liu, Y., Xia, L., & Cheng, Z. (2016). Robust surface coating for a fast, facile fluorine-18 labeling of iron oxide nanoparticles for PET/MR dual-modality imaging. *Nanoscale*, 8(47), 19644–19653. https://doi.org/10.1039/C6NR07298D

Tang, L., Li, J., Pan, T., Yin, Y., Mei, Y., Xiao, Q., Wang, R., Yan, Z., & Wang, W. (2022). Versatile carbon nanoplatforms for cancer treatment and diagnosis: Strategies, applications and future perspectives. *Theranostics*, 12(5), 2290–2321. https://doi.org/10.7150/thno.69628

Tao, H., Yang, K., Ma, Z., Wan, J., Zhang, Y., Kang, Z., & Liu, Z. (2012). In vivo NIR fluorescence imaging, biodistribution, and toxicology of photoluminescent carbon dots produced from carbon nanotubes and graphite. *Small*, 8(2), 281–290. https://doi.org/10.1002/smll.201101706

Tashtoush, B. M., Traboulsi, A. A., Dittert, L., & Hussain, A. A. (2001). Chloramine-T in radiolabeling techniques. *Analytical Biochemistry*, 288(1), 16–21. https://doi.org/10.1006/abio.2000.4832

Tripathi, S. K., Kaur, G., Khurana, R. K., Kapoor, S., & Singh, B. (2015). Quantum dots and their potential role in cancer theranostics. *Critical Reviews™ in Therapeutic Drug Carrier Systems*, *32*(6). https://doi.org/10.1615/CritRevTherDrugCarrierSyst.2015012360

Tsiapa, I., Efthimiadou, E. K., Fragogeorgi, E., Loudos, G., Varvarigou, A. D., Bouziotis, P., Kordas, G. C., Mihailidis, D., Nikiforidis, G. C., Xanthopoulos, S., Psimadas, D., Paravatou-Petsotas, M., Palamaris, L., Hazle, J. D., & Kagadis, G. C. (2014). ^{99m}Tc-labeled aminosilane-coated iron oxide nanoparticles for molecular imaging of $\alpha_{\nu}\beta_{3}$-mediated tumor expression and feasibility for hyperthermia treatment. *Journal of Colloid and Interface Science*, 433, 163–175. https://doi.org/10.1016/j.jcis.2014.07.032

Udayachander, M., Meenakshi, A., Muthiah, R., & Sivanandham, M. (1987). Tumor targeting potential of liposomes encapsulating GA-67 and antibody to Dalton's lymphoma associated antigen (anti-DLAA). *International Journal of Radiation Oncology, Biology,* Physics, 13(11), 1713–1719. https://doi.org/10.1016/0360-3016(87)90168-4

Ünak, P., Yasakçı, V., Tutun, E., Karatay, K. B., Walczak, R., Wawrowicz, K., Żelechowska-Matysiak, K., Majkowska-Pilip, A., & Bilewicz, A. (2023). Multimodal radiobioconjugates of magnetic nanoparticles labeled with ^{44}Sc and ^{47}Sc for theranostic application. *Pharmaceutics*, 15(3), 850. https://doi.org/10.3390/pharmaceutics15030850

Utkhede, D., Yeh, V., Szucs, M., & Tilcock, C. (1994). Uptake of yttrium-90 into lipid vesicles. *Journal of Liposome Research.* https://doi.org/10.3109/08982109409018621

Vallabhajosula, S., Killeen, R. P., & Osborne, J. R. (2010). Altered biodistribution of radiopharmaceuticals: Role of radiochemical/pharmaceutical purity, physiological, and pharmacologic factors. *Seminars in Nuclear Medicine*, 40(4), 220–241. https://doi.org/10.1053/j.semnuclmed.2010.02.004

Varani, M., Bentivoglio, V., Lauri, C., Ranieri, D., & Signore, A. (2022). Methods for radiolabelling nanoparticles: SPECT use (Part 1). *Biomolecules*, *12*(10), 1522. https://doi.org/10.3390/biom12101522

Varela-Moreira, A., Shi, Y., Fens, M. H. A. M., Lammers, T., Hennink, W. E., & Schiffelers, R. M. (2017). Clinical application of polymeric micelles for the treatment of cancer. *Materials Chemistry Frontiers*, 1(8), 1485–1501. https://doi.org/10.1039/C6QM00289G

Vaz, S. C., Oliveira, F., Herrmann, K., & Veit-Haibach, P. (2020). Nuclear medicine and molecular imaging advances in the 21st century. *The British Journal of Radiology*, 93(1110), 20200095. https://doi.org/10.1259/bjr.20200095

Volkert, W. A., & Hoffman, T. J. (1999). Therapeutic radiopharmaceuticals. *Chemical Reviews*, 99(9), 2269–2292. https://doi.org/10.1021/cr9804386

Walsh, A. A. (2017). Chemisorption of iodine-125 to gold nanoparticles allows for real-time quantitation and potential use in nanomedicine. *Journal of Nanoparticle Research*, 19(4), 152. https://doi.org/10.1007/s11051-017-3840-8

Wang, H., Kumar, R., Nagesha, D., Duclos, R. I., Sridhar, S., & Gatley, S. J. (2015). Integrity of 111In-radiolabeled superparamagnetic iron oxide nanoparticles in the mouse. *Nuclear Medicine and Biology*, 42(1), 65–70. https://doi.org/10.1016/j.nucmedbio.2014.08.014

Wang, H., Picchio, M. L., & Calderon, M. (2022). One stone, many birds: Recent advances in functional nanogels for cancer nanotheranostics. *Wiley Interdisciplinary Reviews: Nanomedicine and Nanobiotechnology*, *14*(4), e1791. Retrieved June 15, 2024, from https://wires.onlinelibrary.wiley.com/doi/10.1002/wnan.1791

Wang, Q., Chan, T. R., Hilgraf, R., Fokin, V. V., Sharpless, K. B., & Finn, M. G. (2003). Bioconjugation by copper(I)-catalyzed azide-alkyne [3+2] cycloaddition. *Journal of the American Chemical Society*, 125(11), 3192–3193. https://doi.org/10.1021/ja021381e

Wang, Y. H., Chen, Z., & Zhou, X. Q. (2008). Synthesis and photoluminescence of ZnS quantum dots. *Journal of Nanoscience and Nanotechnology*, *8*(3), 1312–1315. Retrieved June 16, 2024, from https://www.ingentaconnect.com/contentone/asp/jnn/2008/00000008/00000003/art00041?crawler=true

Wang, Y., Liu, X., & Hnatowich, D. J. (2007). An improved synthesis of NHS-MAG3 for conjugation and radiolabeling of biomolecules with ^{99m}Tc at room temperature. *Nature Protocols*, 2(4), 972–978. https://doi.org/10.1038/nprot.2007.144

Welsher, K., Liu, Z., Sherlock, S. P., Robinson, J. T., Chen, Z., Daranciang, D., & Dai, H. (2009). A route to brightly fluorescent carbon nanotubes for near-infrared imaging in mice. *Nature Nanotechnology*, 4(11), 773–780. https://doi.org/10.1038/nnano.2009.294

Wen, J., Liu, C., Liu, J., Wang, L., Miao, S., Chen, D., Wang, Q., Huo, M., & Shen, Y. (2023). Dextran 40 hybrid biomimetic bismuth-nanoflower designed for NIR II-triggered hypoxic tumor thermoradiotherapy via macrophage escape. *Carbohydrate Polymers*, 310, 120697. https://doi.org/10.1016/j.carbpol.2023.120697

Wheeler, H. B., Jaques, W. E., & Botsford, T. W. (1955). Experiences with the use of radioactive colloidal gold in the treatment of cancer. *Annals of Surgery*, 141(2), 208–217.

Winter, G., Hamp-Goldstein, C., Fischer, G., Kletting, P., Glatting, G., Solbach, C., Herrmann, H., Sala, E., Feuring, M., Döhner, H., Beer, A. J., Bunjes, D., & Prasad, V. (2023). Optimization of radiolabeling of a [^{90}Y]Y-anti-CD66-antibody for radioimmunotherapy before allogeneic hematopoietic cell transplantation. *Cancers*, 15(14), 3660. https://doi.org/10.3390/cancers15143660

Wu, S., Helal-Neto, E., Matos, A. P. D. S., Jafari, A., Kozempel, J., Silva, Y. J. D. A., Serrano-Larrea, C., Alves Junior, S., Ricci-Junior, E., Alexis, F., & Santos-Oliveira, R. (2020). Radioactive polymeric nanoparticles for biomedical application. *Drug Delivery*, 27(1), 1544–1561. https://doi.org/10.1080/10717544.2020.1837296

Yamamoto, F., Yamahara, R., Makino, A., Kurihara, K., Tsukada, H., Hara, E., Hara, I., Kizaka-Kondoh, S., Ohkubo, Y., Ozeki, E., & Kimura, S. (2013). Radiosynthesis and initial evaluation of ^{18}F labeled nanocarrier composed of poly(L-lactic acid)-*block*-poly(sarcosine) amphiphilic polydepsipeptide. *Nuclear Medicine and Biology*, 40(3), 387–394. https://doi.org/10.1016/j.nucmedbio.2012.12.008

Yang, M., Zhang, M., Tahara, Y., Chechetka, S., Miyako, E., Iijima, S., & Yudasaka, M. (2014). Lysosomal membrane permeabilization: Carbon nanohorn-induced reactive oxygen species generation and toxicity by this neglected mechanism. *Toxicology and Applied Pharmacology*, 280(1), 117–126. https://doi.org/10.1016/j.taap.2014.07.022

Zahiri, M., Taghavi, S., Abnous, K., Taghdisi, S. M., Ramezani, M., & Alibolandi, M. (2021). Theranostic nanobubbles towards smart nanomedicines. *Journal of Controlled Release*, 339, 164–194. https://doi.org/10.1016/j.jconrel.2021.09.032

Zhang, C., Zhang, Y., Liang, M., Shi, X., Jun, Y., Fan, L., Yang, K., Wang, F., Li, W., & Zhu, R. (2022). Near-infrared upconversion multimodal nanoparticles for targeted radionuclide therapy of breast cancer lymphatic metastases. *Frontiers in Immunology*, 13, 1063678. https://doi.org/10.3389/fimmu.2022.1063678

Zhang, W., Zhao, W., Jia, Z., & Deng, H. (2013). Strontium-89 therapy for the treatment of huge osseous metastases in prostate carcinoma: A case report. *Experimental and Therapeutic Medicine*, 5(2), 608. https://doi.org/10.3892/etm.2012.807

Zhang, Y., Zhang, Y., Yin, L., Xia, X., Hu, F., Liu, Q., Qin, C., & Lan, X. (2017). Synthesis and bioevaluation of iodine-131 directly labeled cyclic RGD-PEGylated gold nanorods for tumor-targeted imaging. *Contrast Media & Molecular Imaging*, *2017*, 1–10. https://doi.org/10.1155/2017/6081724

Zhao, L., Zhu, J., Cheng, Y., Xiong, Z., Tang, Y., Guo, L., Shi, X., & Zhao, J. (2015). Chlorotoxin-conjugated multifunctional dendrimers labeled with radionuclide 131I for single photon emission computed tomography imaging and radiotherapy of gliomas. *ACS Applied Materials & Interfaces*, 7(35), 19798–19808. https://doi.org/10.1021/acsami.5b05836

Zhao, Y., Yao, Q., Tan, H., Wu, B., Hu, P., Wu, P., … & Shi, H. (2014). Design and preliminary assessment of ^{99m}Tc-labeled ultrasmall superparamagnetic iron oxide-conjugated bevacizumab for single photon emission computed tomography/magnetic resonance imaging of hepatocellular carcinoma. *Journal of Radioanalytical and Nuclear Chemistry*, *299*(3), 1273–1280. Retrieved June 15, 2024, from https://link.springer.com/article/10.1007/s10967-013-2846-7

Zhou, Q., Zhang, L., Yang, T., & Wu, H. (2018). Stimuli-responsive polymeric micelles for drug delivery and cancer therapy. *International Journal of Nanomedicine*, 13, 2921–2942. https://doi.org/10.2147/IJN.S158696

Zolata, H., Abbasi Davani, F., & Afarideh, H. (2015). Synthesis, characterization and theranostic evaluation of Indium-111 labeled multifunctional superparamagnetic iron oxide nanoparticles. *Nuclear Medicine and Biology*, 42(2), 164–170. https://doi.org/10.1016/j.nucmedbio.2014.09.007

6 Quantum Dots for Biosensing and Bioimaging Applications

Dhaarini Sakharayapatna Yogaraju and Akshath Uchangi Satyaprasad
Division of Nanobiotechnology, Nitte (Deemed to be University), Nitte University Centre for Science Education and Research-NUCSER, Mangalore, India

ABBREVIATIONS

2-ABA	2-aminobenzyl amine
ALP	alkaline phosphatase
AMF	amifostine
AXL	tyrosine kinase receptor
CdSe	cadmium selenide
CdTe	cadmium telluride
CEA	carcinoembryonic antigen
–COOH	carboxyl
CQDs	carbon QDs
CVDs	cardiovascular diseases
DPV	differential pulse voltammetry
EDAC NHS	1-ethyl-3-(3-dimethylaminopropyl)carbodiimide/N-hydroxysuccinimide
ELISA	enzyme-linked immunosorbent assay
FACS	fluorescence-activated cell sorting
FRET	fluorescence resonance energy transfer
GQDs	graphene QDs
H2O2	hydrogen peroxide
HAD	hexadecyl amine
HF	heart failure
HRP	horse radish peroxidase
HSP70	heat shock protein 70
ICP-MS	inductively coupled plasma mass spectrometry
InAs	indium arsenide
LDH	lactose dehydrogenase
MPA	mercapto propionic acid
MT1-MMP	membrane type-1 matrix metalloproteinase
N	nitrogen
NAD+	nicotinamide adenine dinucleotide
–NH2	amines
OH	hydroxyls
PAGD	GQDs functionalized with polyaniline
PANI	polyaniline
PbSe	lead selenide
PCR	polymerase chain reaction

DOI: 10.1201/9781003473015-6

PNA	p-nitroaniline
PNP	p-nitrophenol
QDs	quantum dots
S	sulfur
–SH	thiols
SPCE	screen-printed carbon electrode
SQDs	semiconductor QDs
TCh	thiocholine
TMB	3,3′,5,5′-tetramethylbenzidine
TOP	trioctyl phosphine
TOPO	trioctyl phosphine oxide
ZnS	zinc sulfide
ZnS	zinc sulfide

6.1 INTRODUCTION

The colloidal semiconductor nanocrystals known as quantum dots (QDs), having a size ranging from 1 to 15 nm, have become the limelight of nanoscience because of their remarkable optical and electrical properties. High quantum yield, broad absorption spectra, size-tunable narrow emission, strong resistance to photobleaching, and photostability: these optical properties of QDs make them preferred over traditional fluorophores (Li and Zhu 2013). The size and shape of QDs affect the optoelectronic properties of QDs, where QDs having smaller sizes of 2–3 nm are blue and green, exhibiting shorter wavelengths of light. In contrast to this, longer wavelengths of light have an orange or red color, as shown by larger QDs having sizes ranging from 5 to 6 nm. The size-tunability associated with these optical characteristics is their most notable feature since the quantum confinement effect is caused because of the spatial confinement of charged particles due to the nanometric scale (Efros and Brus 2021). The composition of the QD, which determines the range of wavelengths in which it may emit, is just as significant as its size. Cadmium, a heavy metal element, is the basis for the most researched QD composition, such as CdSe, CdS, and CdTe QDs (Manna 2023). The primary optical property of QDs is also dependent on the QD's core material chemical composition having indium arsenide (InAs), cadmium selenide (CdSe), and lead selenide (PbSe). The shell layer surrounds the core and is composed of different materials like ZnS (zinc sulfide) that enhance the photoluminescence (PL) efficiency and stability of QDs by protecting the core. The core semiconductor material is the only one that can be stimulated or emitted due to its narrow bandgap. Higher bandgap energy shell coatings limit excitation and emission. This design permits electrons to go from ground to excited states while protecting the core from photobleaching and increasing the quantum yield of PL. The PL intensity, photostability, and PL QY all increase to even unity when they are shielded by a second semiconductor material (Van Avermaet et al. 2022). The increased stability and emission intensities of QDs have beneficial applications in long-term imaging and rapid and ultrasensitive detection (Cheng et al. 2021; Walling, Novak, and Shepard 2009). These properties of QDs can be employed as luminescent probes in biological applications such as histopathology, disease diagnosis, *in vitro* and in vivo biological imaging in case of cancer diagnosis. Prolonged usage of these QDs has raised concerns regarding the safety and biocompatibility in biological applications. The major concern of using QDs for biomedical applications is dependent on factors such as ligand coating on the QD surface, mechanical stability, and heavy metal leakage from the QD core (in the case of cadmium containing QDs) (Jin et al. 2011). Biosensing and bioimaging are two biological applications that are greatly impacted by QDs. Because of their wide surface, biomolecules can be immobilized for *in vivo* tumor detection or tailored antigen detection. The ligand shell needs to protect the QD optical characteristics from oxidation or breakdown and offer colloidal stability (Wegner and Hildebrandt 2024). Although near-infrared (NIR) and infrared (IR) emitting QDs are still being developed, visible-emitting QDs are well-established for biosensing and bioimaging (Li et al. 2020). These areas provide improved signal-to-noise ratios, spatial resolution, a greater penetration depth, and less optical absorption (Chen et al. 2022).

The distinct optical properties of QDs make them fluorescent probes in biosensing applications to detect the biomolecules that are used to study enzymatic activity. QDs surface functionalized with biomolecules and ligands make them less toxic and more biocompatible, which is used in in vivo applications in detecting cancer and also imaging specific tissues and cells. Despite a few limitations with respect to heavy metal toxicity, QDs have wide applications in the biological field as a labeling marker and fluorescent probe.

6.2 PROPERTIES OF QDS

The properties of QDs are majorly dependent on optical properties like high quantum yield, broad absorption spectra, size-tunable narrow emission, strong resistance to photobleaching, and photostability that determine their application in the biomedical field.

The ultrafine particle size of the QDs makes it easy for them to be excreted from the body, which comes from the quantum confinement effect, which is the restricted movement of electrons and holes within smaller-sized QDs. Size decreases with the broadening of the band gap due to the quantum confinement effect (Bera et al. 2010). Through a mechanism known as quantum confinement, QDs can act as fluorophores that aid in the imaging of cellular and subcellular structures by producing electromagnetic radiation that is interpreted as fluorescence. The size-dependent band gap of semiconductor QDs (SQDs) is a well-known quantum confinement effect, which is the special confinement of electron–hole pairs in one or more dimensions within a material. Such behavior is not observed in bulk materials. In fact, as particle size increase beyond the magnitude of the characteristic wave function, particles tend to behave freely and form a continuous state. Hence, bulk materials do not have a specific fluorescence size effect (Ramezani, Ghalehsardi, and Noorizadeh 2023). The efficiency of QDs is often described in terms of quantum yield, which is the ratio of photons released to photons absorbed in a fluorophore. QDs having high quantum yield are usually selected for the application purpose. CQDs (carbon quantum dots) fluorescence was enhanced during their synthesis by using chemicals like ethylenediamine and acids like phosphoric acid, nitric acid, and citric acid (Anpalagan et al. 2024). The fluorescence nature of QDs can be better understood in terms of FRET (fluorescence resonance energy transfer), which is used to measure the fluorescence energy transfer between the donor and acceptor molecules separated by a short distance. For a precise FRET to take place, the donor and acceptor molecules should be within the Förster radius of 3–4 nm and also measure the molecular closeness accurately at Angstrom distances (10–100 Å) (Tandale et al. 2021). The spectral properties of QDs allow them to be used as FRET donors and acceptors to study biomolecular interactions. FRET-based applications include structural analysis, enzymatic tests, immunoassays, sensors for small molecules, and fluorescence imaging. QDs are flexible energy donors for organic and inorganic molecules (dyes, fluorescent proteins), polymers, and metal nanoparticles. They can also be acceptors for fluorescent polymers, other QDs, and compounds based on lanthanides like chelates, cryptates, and nanoparticles (Verma et al. 2023).

6.3 SURFACE FUNCTIONALIZATION

The optical properties of QDs have gained much attention in the application of biological research in biosensing and bioimaging. QDs are generally toxic due to heavy metals, but they can be made biocompatible by functionalizing their surface with polymers or biomolecules. Controlled surface functionalization of QDs is essential for achieving a high level of complexity in *in vitro* or in vivo cellular imaging, even though site-selective targeting of QDs is necessary. The surface area of the QD is dependent on the size of the QD. The size and surface area of the QDs are inversely proportional, which attracts more atoms with unmet coordination (or dangling bonds) and raises the total surface energy. Because of this high energy, the spreading and reconstruction of surface

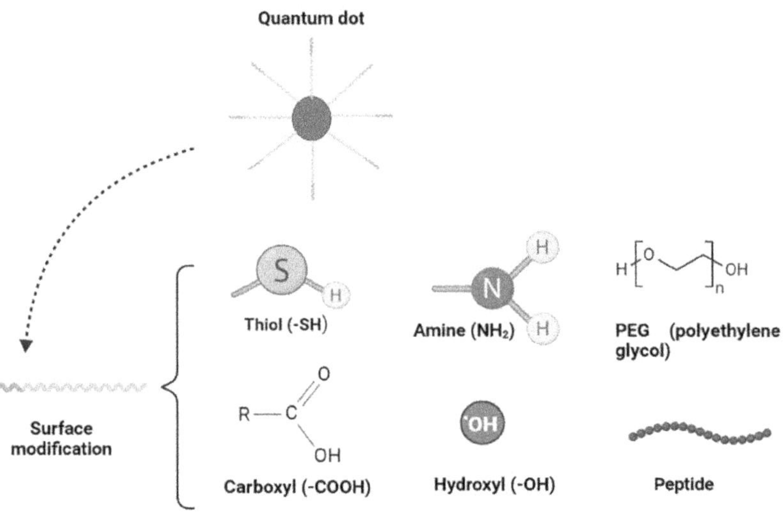

FIGURE 6.1 Surface functionalization of QD with different functional groups.

atoms results in flaws, including vacancies and phase shifts. This defect results in discontinuous fluorescence by trapping the electrons and decreasing the quantum yield. By shielding the core of the QDs against oxidation and chemical reactions, fluorescence application is made possible through surface inactivation/passivation.

The surface of the QDs can be functionalized using aptamers, peptides, and ligands in order to make them biocompatible. Hydrophobic ligands such as TOP (trioctyl phosphine), TOPO (trioctyl phosphine oxide), and HDA (hexadecyl amine) can be used on the surface of QDs. Hydrophilic ligands that have bifunctional groups such as thiols (–SH), carboxyl (–COOH), amines (–NH_2), or hydroxyl (OH) groups bind to the ZnS (zinc sulfide) shell and increase water solubility (Figure 6.1). Polymers like PEG (polyethylene glycol) can also be used (Bilan et al. 2015). Apart from this, silica is also used in surface functionalizing the QD by a process known as silanization.

6.4 APPLICATIONS OF QDS IN BIOSENSING AND BIOIMAGING

The optical properties of QDs make them advantageous in the biomedical field (Figure 6.2). For instance, particle size of QDs allows them to be easily absorbed by the cells when they are incubated with suitable cells. The emission spectra can then be readily observed using fluorescence microscope after stimulation. QDs that have been modified with certain ligands to increase their affinity for the tissue or organ of interest can be used to image various organs and tissues *in vivo*. The popular technique known as FACS (fluorescence-activated cell sorting) is used for various biomedical applications such as cellular absorption of drug delivery systems, isolating cell-specific populations, disease model characterization, cellular marker identification, and immune cell mapping. The high brightness of QDs increases their use with more accuracy in detection purposes compared to traditional organic dyes. Also, QDs stability and cost effectiveness allow them to substitute antibodies for cell surface marker staining by surface functionalizing them with ligands that identify the markers that need to be targeted in case of cancer. (Abdellatif et al. 2022)

6.5 BIOSENSING APPLICATIONS

The ability of NIR/IR QDs to be detected inside or adjacent to biological components is their main benefit in biological applications. The quenching or amplification of the optical probe's PL intensity in the presence of the substance of interest is essential for simple sensing applications. In sensing

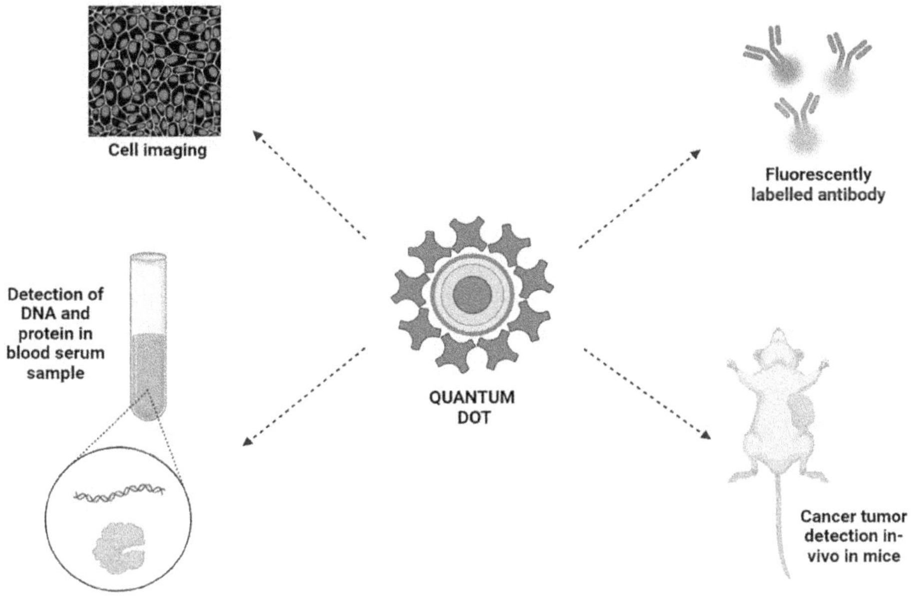

FIGURE 6.2 Different applications of QDs in biosensing and bioimaging.

applications, PL enhancement is preferable as it allows for a higher sensitivity because it is simpler to detect expanding PL signals than declining ones. The quantity of biological interfering chemicals can be comparatively minimal in sensing applications such as typical immunoassays, where the QD is attached to a specific antibody or DNA to identify a target of interest (Wegner and Hildebrandt 2024).

For instance, NIR-II QDs can be used as an activatable probe for observing colon cancer; however, their use is still primarily restricted to either *in vivo* or *ex vivo* biosensing (Jeong et al. 2017). NIR-QDs are ideal for measuring objectives like glucose or tumor cell proliferation in whole blood samples because they eliminate the need for time-consuming separation procedures and blood sample purification (Yu et al. 2017).

6.6 QDS AS ELECTROCHEMICAL BIOSENSORS

An electrochemical biosensor is the one that transforms the presence of biological molecules present on the electrode into an electrical measurable signal through electronic transduction (Akkilic, Geschwindner, and Höök 2020). Graphene, nitrides, black phosphorous, and transition metal oxides are some of the materials that are used in developing QDs that are two-dimensional in nature with simple functionalization, binding sites, and relatively wide surface area. These 2D quantum dots (2D-QDs) are used to identify various biomolecules through electrochemical biosensors (Zhang, Zhang, and Bi 2022). The formation of 2D-QDs happens when the side dimension of 2D materials is decreased below 100 nm. Such smaller versions of 2D-layered nanomaterials provide greater surface-volume ratio, improved solubility, and dispersion while conserving their two-dimensional lattices. Their exceptional electrical qualities, low level of toxicity, and chemical stability allow them to be used in a variety of applications, including optoelectronics, storing energy, and catalysis. GQDs (graphene quantum dots) are used as electrochemical RNA biosensors for the detection of miRNA-155, long non-coding RNA molecules that are used as biomarkers in the diagnosis of cancer. GQDs have more number of carboxyl groups on their surfaces and the HRP (horse radish peroxidase) enzyme immobilized on the QD surface interacts with the single-stranded DNA having an amino group at its end (NH_2-GQDs). A rise in the electrochemical current signal and a color shift from colorless to blue in solution are two signs that the hydrogen peroxide (H_2O_2), an HRP-modified GQD biosensor, can efficiently catalyze the mediated oxidation of 3,3′,5,5′-tetramethylbenzidine (TMB). miRNA was sensitively detected by these GQDs in the concentration range from 1 fM to 100 PM with 0.14 fM as the detection limit; this means that this proposed biosensor has great significance and exceptional compatibility for analyzing other tumor markers (Hu et al. 2016).

Apart from the application in miRNA detection, QDs are more widely used to detect glucose. CQDs, cadmium telluride (CdTe) QDs aerogel, with glucose oxidase (GOx) were used to construct a microfluidic sensor with fluorescence for urinal glucose detection. The sensor, which is integrated onto a microfluidic chip, fluoresces red and green when exposed to ultraviolet light. Green fluorescence intensity is maintained, while H_2O_2 quenches red fluorescence from the glucose/GOx interaction to provide the fluorescence response of the microsensor (Jiang et al. 2017). The color of the sensor varies in response to a slight variation in fluorescence intensities, which indicates the content of glucose. The ideal reaction time was 5 minutes, and the ideal concentration ratio of CdTe QDs to CQDs was 0.5:1. The glucose concentration's limit of detection was 0.223 mM, and its detection range was 0 to 13 mM. With the goal to create a new micro colorimetric sensor, research is being done on miniaturized optical biosensors, which have benefits including minimized sample usage, less pollution, compact size, easy carrying, and protection against hazardous substances. The effectiveness, precision, and sustainability of this glucose sensor are outstanding. The microsensor can be kept in a stable storage environment at –20°C for 30 days. C/CdTe QD-GOx aerogel-based microfluidic assay sensor offers a novel method for the visual and quantifiable measurement of glucose, making it possible for people with diabetes to conveniently monitor their urine glucose levels every day (Hu et al. 2020).

6.7 QDS AS ELECTROCHEMICAL IMMUNOBIOSENSORS

Electrochemical biosensors that use antibody or antigen to detect target based on the electrochemical signal are electrochemical immunological biosensors. Considering its great sensitivity and selectivity, electrochemical immunological sensors are frequently employed in protein analysis, medical research, and environmental monitoring. By enhancing signal amplification, electron transport, and biomolecule immobilization, 2D-QDs improve sensor performance (Zhang, Zhang, and Bi 2022). Identification of depression marker, heat shock protein 70 (HSP70) uses GQDs functionalized with polyaniline (PAGD). HSP70 is detected negatively by the electrochemical immunosensor (HRP-Strept-Biotin-Ab-HSP70/PAGD/GCE) because it interferes with the antibody that is tagged with HRP. Under ideal circumstances, the suggested electrochemical immunosensor (HRP-Strept-Biotin-Ab-HSP70/PAGD/GCE) efficiently detects HSP70 in plasma samples, exhibiting good accuracy stability, and repeatability while achieving broad linearity (0.0976–100 ng/mL) and a narrow detection limit (0.05 ng/mL). In addition to offering a trustworthy and impartial analysis method for the molecular diagnosis of depression, this work offers a new and practical approach for the early clinical screening of depression markers (Sun et al. 2020).

Carcinoembryonic antigen (CEA), whose levels >5 ng/mL in the blood indicate cancer, is one of the main tumor markers. GQDs doped with nitrogen and thiol (N,S-GQDs) and gold nanowire functionalized with polyaniline (PANI) that increases electrochemical activity by enhancing (N,S-GQDs@Au-PANI) are used for the sensitive detection of CEA. By successfully coating 2–9 nm N,S-GQDs onto 30–50 nm Au-PANI nanowires via Au-thiol linkage, they can behave as a bifunctional probe that both anchors anti-CEA and amplifies electrochemical activity. The alteration in impedance of N,S-GQDs/Au-PANI upon CEA injection, which inhibits the transfer of electrons following antibody-antigen conjugation on the N,S-GQDs/Au-PANI surface, served as the basis for the CEA detection principle (Figure 6.3). With a detection limit (LOD) of 0.01 ng/mL, this label-free immunosensor exhibits a broad linear range from 0.5 to 1,000 ng/mL (Ganganboina and Doong 2019).

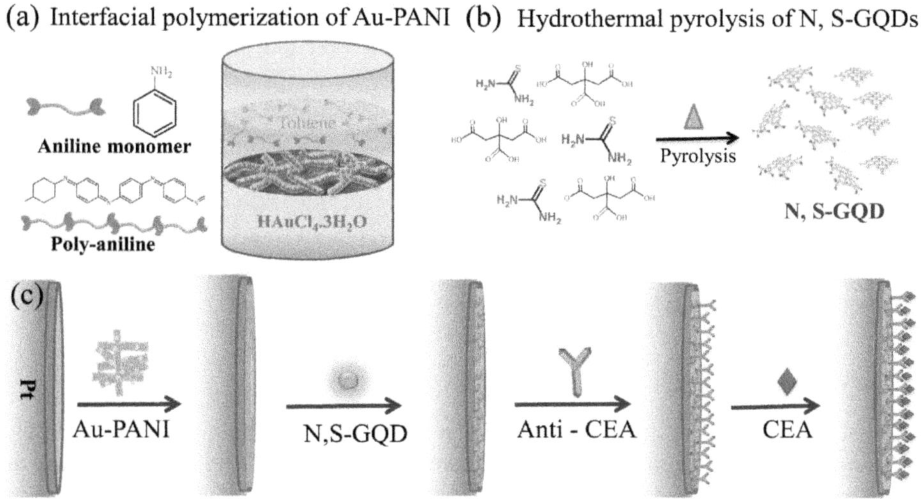

FIGURE 6.3 A label-free electrochemical impedimetric immunosensor for carcinoembryonic antigen (CEA) is constructed step by step. (Ganganboina and Doong 2019, http://creativecommons.org/licenses/by/4.0/ CC BY 4.0.)

Apart from the detection of cancer biomarkers, GQDs are also used in observing cardiovascular diseases (CVDs), which are one of the leading causes of death globally (Mansuriya and Altintas 2019). Extracellular part of the protein (sAXL) is one of the potential bio-marker for the cause of heart failure (HF). (Screen-printed carbon electrode) SPCE/GQDs were functionalized by electropolymerization with 2-aminobenzyl amine (2-ABA) using cyclic voltammetry in a label-free portable electrochemical immunosensor to recognize (tyrosine kinase receptor) AXL (sAXL), which has been purified by proteases. Using functionalized SPCE/GQDs, a label-free electrochemical immunosensor, an anti-AXL antibody, was used to immobilize the electrode after it had been electropolymerized with 2-ABA. By detecting the decrease in the redox probe's DPV (differential pulse voltammetry) response of $Fe(CN)_6^{3-/6-}$, the AXL is detected in human serum by GQDs/SPCE via electropolymerization with 2-ABA (Mollarasouli et al. 2018).

6.8 QDS AS IMMUNOBIOSENSORS

The immunochemical reaction that uses either the antigen or the antibody as recognition elements mounted on a transducer surface that helps in the detection of biological elements like proteins, pathogens, and cancerous conditions with high specificity and sensitivity in a very low concentration range is known as immunosensors (Malhotra and Ali 2018). These immunosensors are used in the detection of proteins, where the chemically modified QDs conjugated with antibody is used. Immunosensing of ferritin in human serum samples is detected using GQDs that are functionalized with amine (afGQDs) based on the fluorescence intensity in the presence of methyl orange as a quencher. For specific immune sensing fluorescence-based detection of ferritin, the anti-ferritin antibody (Ab) is conjugated to afGQDs (Ab@afGQDs) by utilizing the high fluorescence of this material. This fluorescence intensity is diminished by fluorescence quencher methyl orange (MO), which aids in sensing ferritin. Ferritin was spiked in blood serum samples and was determined with a limit of detection of 0.723 ng/mL, an R^2 of 0.994, a linear range of 10–4,000 ng/mL, and a quantum yield of 51% (Garg et al. 2021). Another example is the detection of cancer biomarker (CA15-3 protein) using CdTe QDs. In order to study the interaction via fluorescence between the protein biomarker (CA15-3) and the CA15-3 antibody conjugated on the surface of the QDs, the surface of the CdTe is conjugated with mercapto propionic acid (MPA) so that the molecules binding onto the surface of the QDs interact with free carboxyl groups of MPA and also by EDAC NHS [1-ethyl-3-(3-dimethylaminopropyl) carbodiimide/N-hydroxysuccinimide] chemistry. CA15-3 antibodies bind to CdTe@MPA QDs. The CA15-3, which is being detected here, is the serum biomarker that aids in observing breast cancer, whose normal levels in serum are 30 U/mL but increase in the cancerous condition. Through fluorescence, the interaction between the conjugates and the biomarker is studied in both buffer and commercially available serum samples that is diluted ten times. This method is ultrasensitive, as evidenced by the detection limit of 0.027 U/mL obtained from validation in spiked serum samples, which is 1,000 times less than the clinical range for CA15-3 (25 to 30 U/mL). The proposed method for the detection of the CA15-3 biomarker is a rapid method that gives a response within 10 minutes, a highly sensitive and selective one that is a straightforward and sensitive technique for ultrasensitive surveillance of breast cancer (Sousa et al. 2022).

6.9 QDS AS ENZYMATIC BIOSENSORS

The above discussed biosensors are used in the detection of various biomolecules. One of the most important biomolecules that play a key role in maintaining various cellular functions are enzymes, and their activity is determined using these enzymatic biosensors. Enzymes are vital biocatalysts that accelerate chemical reactions in living things; aberrant activity is associated with a number of disorders. Accurate and sensitive enzyme activity detection is essential, and new techniques, such as fluorescence assays based on QDs/CDs, have enabled high-resolution detection. The effect of enzyme activity based on the interaction of the substrate with QDs/CDs (carbon dots) can be determined based on the fluorescence intensity observed due to QD/CDs. Enzyme activity using QDs can be checked in the following three approaches: The first approach explains that the quenching in the intensity of fluorescence is observed in the case of lactose dehydrogenase (LDH) and alkaline phosphatase (ALP) enzyme activity in the presence of substrates like nicotinamide adenine dinucleotide (NAD^+) for LDH and amifostine (AMF) for ALP enzyme activity. Enzyme activity is determined by "turn on" in the fluorescence intensity upon the addition of an enzyme that converts the substrate to respective products, thereby causing the re-emergence of fluorescence. According to the second approach, the fluorescence of QDs/CDs can be directly quenched by enzymatic products such as p-nitrophenol (PNP) and p-nitroaniline (PNA). Upon the addition of enzymes, a "turn off" in the fluorescence of QDs/CDs aids in the determination of enzyme activity. The fluorescence intensity of QDs/CDs is not altered by the substrates and enzymatic products for some of the enzymes. However, the third approach involves introducing certain chemical interactions with substrates or enzymatic products to form secondary products (such as the Cu^{2+}-thiocholine (TCh) complex), which may impact the fluorescence of QDs/CDs. Enzyme activity is accessed based on the fluorescence observed due to QDs/CDs as sensors, which can be checked via FRET. In the FRET-based method, the two interacting molecules, i.e., donor and acceptor molecules, should be near to each other. In the QDs/CDs FRET-based assay, the donors of energy are QDs/CDs and acceptors are nanomaterials or fluorescent organic molecules. A fluorescent FRET sensor based on QDs immobilizes Cy3 on the QD surface for recognizing MT1-MMP (membrane type-1 matrix metalloproteinase) activity. To increase FRET efficiency, the peptide sequence and QDs form a hairpin loop. Both the QDs' emission and absorption spectra overlap. When MT1-MMP is present, the FRET process is reduced by the active catalytic site (MT1-CAT) on the peptide sequence. The fluorescence proportion between QDs and Cy3 is used to quantify the activity of MT1-MMP (Tong et al. 2020). Another enzyme responsible for the breakdown of proteins in the body and in charge of several biological processes is protease. A caspase-1 nanosensor was engineered by labeling the QD surface with fluorophore-labeled substrates that are exclusive to the protease caspase-1 using polyhistidine linkers. Specifically, FRET between Cy3 tagged onto the QD (emission centered at 538 nm) was used to probe the caspase-1 activity. When the nanosensor was correctly linked up using a substrate peptide, the fluorescence of QD was first quenched by FRET, producing FRET on state. The acceptor fluorophores (Cy3) were released and dispersed into the solution after being recognized and broken by caspase-1. The recovery of QD PL that followed the FRET breakdown then functioned as a sign of the active enzyme activity (Knudsen, Jepsen, and Ho 2013).

6.10 COLORIMETRIC BIOSENSOR

Colorimetric biosensors are a potential diagnostic tool, especially in resource-constrained places, emergency situations, and home care settings wherein no outside resources or chemicals are needed. This tool's benefit is that it can give a visible result to the human eye, overcoming the time, expense, and diagnostic procedure restrictions of the gold standards like (polymerase chain reaction) PCR and (enzyme-linked immunosorbent assay) ELISA methods. The sensitivity of the colorimetric biosensors can be increased using surface-modifiable nanoparticles that enhance signal detection. Detection of SARS-CoV-2 antigens in the initial stages of infection is performed using lateral flow immunoassay (LFIA) using SiO_2@Au/QD (a nanocomposite using gold nanoparticles and QDs on SiO_2), where the sample to be tested can be directly placed onto the apparatus without any pre-treatment. The Spike (S) protein of the virus is observed through the naked eye and fluorescence via SiO_2@Au/QD with an LOD of 33 pg/mL by fluorescence and 1 ng/mL by the naked eye. S protein of the virus was more selectively detected even in the presence of high levels of other interfering viral strains like MERS-CoV (100 ng/mL), influenza H1N1 (5×10^6 copies/mL), SARS-CoV (100 ng/mL). The device's RSD (relative standard deviation) was 3.92%–5.19%, and the recovery assay demonstrated accuracy >92.98%. The novel biosensor's exceptional accuracy and suitability for identifying SARS-CoV-2 in real specimens were validated by this study (Tessaro et al. 2023; Han et al. 2022). It exhibits poor sensitivity in translating the detectable signals to color measurements due to the presence of low sample concentrations and also less accuracy and replicability due to high ionic strength in urine and serum samples, which are some of the limitations of this method (Tessaro et al. 2023).

Carbon source of glucose is used in the synthesis of CQDs, which is doped with heteroatoms like sulfur (S), boron (B), and nitrogen (N). The sensor properties of CQDs are effectively enhanced by doping them with heteroatoms. Doping with heteroatoms had very minor changes in the size of the CQDs based on transmission electron microscopy (TEM) analysis. Still, it had a major effect on their optical properties as there was a shift in the peak, which was characterized through UV-vis and FL (PL) spectrophotometry. Heteroatoms-doped CQDs are used as a colorimetric sensor to detect heavy metals. Different heavy metals like Fe^{3+}, Ag^+, and Ca^{2+} are detected by CQDs and CQDs doped with N, S, and 2B. Fe^{3+} metal ion detection was made possible via CQDs, and the LOD value was determined to be 0.187 μM. Fe^{3+} (LOD: 0.182 μM (B-CQD) and 0.224 μM (S-CQD)) and Ag^+ (LOD: 0.174 μM (B-CQD) and 0.442 μM (S-CQD)) metal ions were detected by B-CQDs and S-CQDs, allowing for the detection of two distinct metals. Ca^{2+} metal ion detection was made possible by N-CQDs, and the LOD value was determined to be 0.391 μM. The findings demonstrate that the introduction of B, N, and S atoms to CQDs contributes to the enhancement and variation of colorimetric sensor characteristics and holds promise for use in sensor applications for heavy metal analysis in fields including the environment and health (Aygun et al. 2024).

Blood glucose levels are an important indicator for clinical diagnosis (Pandya, Sutariya, and Menon 2013). Several techniques, including surface-enhanced Raman scattering, electrochemical analysis, electrochemiluminescence, and chemiluminescence, offer excellent sensitivity but call for specialized equipment. The target concentration can be directly approximated through colorimetry, which is visual and intuitive, and involves monitoring the color with the unaided eye. Due to its benefits, colorimetry and other detection techniques (such as fluorescence and electrochemiluminescence) have been coupled in recent years to create a variety of dual-mode sensors for assessment and identification (Kitte et al. 2017). Between them, colorimetric and fluorescent dual-mode sensors have garnered a lot of interest due to the several benefits that optical techniques may provide, including high sensitivity, straightforward equipment, and ease of use. A luminous dual-mode glucose sensor that is both colorimetric and ratiometric was created using the optical characteristics of o-diaminobenzene oxide (oxODB). oxODB is used as a reporter for the detection of glucose by the colorimetric method as they are able to produce ultraviolet (UV) absorption and also can quench the CQD's fluorescence. Therefore, the ratiometric fluorescence approach for glucose detection can use the intensity of the fluorescence ratio of oxODB to CQDs as the reporter. Hydrogen peroxide oxidizes (o-diaminobenzene oxide) ODB in the presence of HRP, while hydrogen peroxide is produced by oxidizing glucose in the presence of its oxidase. This biological oxidation reaction is another technique for detecting glucose. This means that glucose may be detected in two ways using this method since glucose can determine the creation of oxODB, and oxODB determines the changes in absorbance and fluorescence ratio concurrently. It is also possible to determine the glucose concentration roughly with the naked eye because the color of the glucose detection solution can exhibit a substantial differential change under sunshine and ultraviolet lights (Zhai et al. 2019).

All cells synthesize cholesterol from simpler molecules, and in humans, a total serum cholesterol level below 200 mg/dL is considered desirable. It is vital for the formation of vitamin D, bile acids, steroid hormones, and animal cell membranes. However, uncontrolled production of cholesterol may result in significant medical conditions (Lan Hsia et al. 2000). Thus, it becomes important to detect the cholesterol level by colorimetric means based on the color change using GQDs. For effective cholesterol detection, GQDs are synthesized by mimicking HRP in a straightforward aqueous chemical approach. In the presence of H_2O_2, the catalytic activity of GQDs oxidizes TMB, which is a peroxidase substrate yielding a blue-colored product that is used for the determination of H_2O_2 and cholesterol (Cho). With a detection limit as low as 0.006 mM, the suggested GQD-based detection system enables a broad range of cholesterol sensing (0.02–0.6 mM). Additionally, lower Km (0.01 mM) and higher Vmax (7.3×10^{-6} M/s) demonstrate improved peroxidase-like catalytic activity and a stronger affinity for binding cholesterol oxidase (ChOx) to cholesterol, which leads to good biosensor stability and resilience to environmental interferences (Nirala et al. 2015).

6.11 BIOIMAGING APPLICATION

SQDs are now crucial fluorescent probes for both *in vitro* and *in vivo* bioimaging studies. The primary advantages of QDs over other fluorescence imaging agents are their variable photophysical properties for multiplexed detection, their nanoparticle surfaces for varied bioconjugation, and their higher stability for longer investigation periods.

Significant structural heterogeneity is revealed by detailed electron microscopy (EM), indicating the existence of promising dim and dark populations that lie within a single batch. Issues in the internal structure that reduce PL performance in physiologically realistic cellular contexts must be found and fixed while keeping the lowest size possible if QDs are to become the industry standard fluorescence sensors for 3D samples. By reducing biological components' scattering, absorption, and autofluorescence, NIR optical probes enable deeper light penetration and better spatial and temporal resolution for studying biological processes (Torres et al. 2024).

6.12 *IN VITRO* BIOIMAGING

The distribution of QDs, which are nanoparticles composed of inorganic core components, into cells is the primary obstacle to their use in cellular imaging. For most instances, cellular absorption is facilitated by surface groups containing amines, cationic charges, minuscule sizes, typical cell culture incubation conditions, and body temperatures. The experimental settings must be tailored to the cell type, the subcellular compartment of interest, and the imaging application itself, as no universal approach ensures efficient absorption (Wegner and Hildebrandt 2015). For *in vitro* bioimaging inside the cell, it is crucial to release the entrapped QD–CPP (cell-penetrating peptide) conjugates from the endosomes or lysosomes to allow QDs to be targeted to cell components inside the cytoplasm. One possible way to free QDs is by inducing them with photons that are known to reside at phospholipid membranes, which is done by the amphiphilic photosensitizer, disulfonated aluminum phthalocyanine, which is linked to (transcriptional factor Tat bound to QDs) Tat–QDs. The excitation of the photosensitizer via FRET with the QD as the donor was causing the photo-induced rupture of the endo/lysosomal membrane because of the production of singlet oxygen following the CPP-mediated internalization into the cell. Fluorescence lifetime imaging (FLIM) and steady-state confocal imaging were used to measure the successful release and effective FRET (Kapur et al. 2018). These QD FRET-based sensors are also used in imaging cancerous cells *in vitro*. A DNA-templated hetero-bivalent QD FRET nanosensor that targets and images cancer cells both externally and intracellularly is demonstrated using this probe's dual motifs. In addition to making it easier to target cancer cells, the nucleolin-targeting motif (NTM), the initial component of the DNA-based sensor, also promoted macropinocytosis, which made it possible for the cells to migrate into the cytosol. A Cy5 dye's FRET signal was turned off to demonstrate that the second oligonucleotide component (mRNA-targeting motif, or MTM) inside the cytosol targeted a particular messenger RNA (mRNA). Future imaging applications may employ the technique of evaluating tumor-associated mRNA by combining the cytosolic release of bioactive probes with selective targeting (Martins, LaGrow, and Prior 2022 Wei, He, and Ma 2014). Apart from imaging cancerous tissue, QDs are used in the analysis of proteins that cause cancer based on immunohistofluorometry (IHF) (QD-IHF). IgY, an antibody produced from chicken, exhibited great sensitivity and specificity for the relative quantification of cancer proteins and could be employed for QD-IHF. Western blotting and immunohistochemistry (IHC) on normal and cancer cells revealed that IgY had a higher affinity for antigens than conventional antibodies. A comparison between chromogenic in situ hybridization and tissue microarrays (TMAs) for the measurement of the human epidermal growth factor receptor 2 (HER2) utilizing IgY and QDs revealed favorable agreement. Using Hadamard transform spectrum imaging, a quantitative technique to assess how well QDs stain tissues was studied. In breast cancer tissues labeled with several batches of bioconjugated QDs, they employed proliferating cell nuclear antigens (PCNAs). Using various QD bioconjugation techniques, the study showed consistent bioconjugation efficiency. Additionally, multimodal detection and biomarker quantification by optimizing the labeling technique for QD-IHF probes were shown. The cellular, molecular, and structural diversity of cancer specimens can also be interpreted using spectrally localized fluorescence imaging and multiplexed QD-IHF (Xu et al. 2015; Wegner and Hildebrandt 2015). QDs are also used in the staining of cells other than in the detection of molecules in an *in vitro* condition. One such example is staining and detecting cells undergoing apoptosis (programmed cell death). In order to detect and stain apoptosis, QDs coupled to Annexin V are designed to target apoptotic cells specifically. The 35-kDa protein biotinylated Annexin V, which attaches to phosphatidylserine groups on cell membranes of apoptotic cells, is attached to these probes. Because QDs are not affected by bleaching, this makes them excellent for photographing time-lapses and constant tracking. QD staining has also been used to track individual molecules. For example, QDs have been utilized to stain entire cells upon binding to a particular peptidic signal, or to label organelles specifically (Hu et al. 2021; Le Gac, Vermes, and van den Berg 2006).

The membrane aspartic acid protease, known as β-secretase or β-site amyloid precursor protein (APP) cleaving enzyme (BACE1), is extensively expressed in the brain, particularly in neuronal tissue. Because of its crucial involvement in the pathophysiology of Alzheimer's disease, this enzyme has been the subject of extensive research. In particular, the removal of APP from the senile plaques seen in the postmortem brains of patients indicates that BACE1 is in charge of the hydrolytic production of the β-amyloid peptide (Das and Yan 2017). BACE1 probes require membrane localization and stability at acidic pH in addition to the standard requirements for all biosensors, which include ease of production and usage. The core and shell of QDs are composed of CdSe/CdS/ZnS having a diameter of 4.7 ± 0.4 nm and were checked for colloidal stability at decreased pH with two types of surface functionalization. Based on a bidentate dihydrolipoic acid anchoring group, two distinct surface coatings containing either a sulfonate head (SO_3) or a zwitterionic head (CL_4) were explored. Out of the two types of surface functionalization tested, the CL_4 ligand has demonstrated stability up to the target pH of 4, but if CL_4 turns out to be not feasible, the SO_3 would offer a substitute that might resist lower pH levels (Green et al. 2021; Rogers et al. 2023). So, in order to determine the highest activity of BACE1, QDs (CdSe type) offer easy surface functionalization with peptide substrates because of its increased surface area, improved fluorescence brightness,

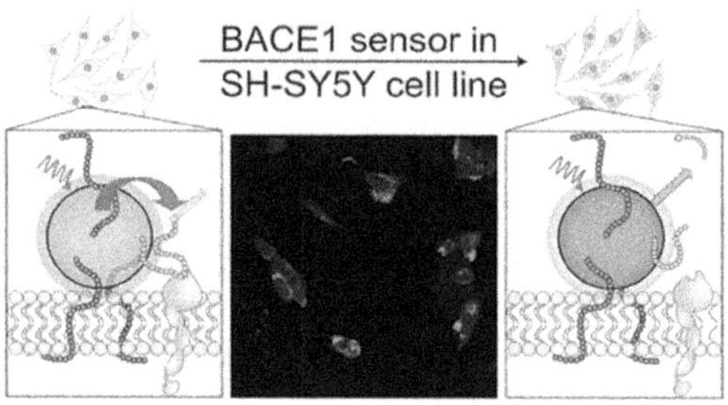

FIGURE 6.4 Illustration showing the sensor's operation. (Tosat-Bitrián et al. 2024, https://creativecommons.org/licenses/by-nc-nd/4.0/ CCBY 4.0.)

and photostability. The study uses CdSe QDs as a sensor to locate the regions of highest BACE1 activity which is achieved using His-tag self-assembly that attach themselves onto the ions of zinc on the surface of the QD (Green et al. 2022). The efficiency of FRET of the QDs modified with two different ligands at various pH levels, from 4 to 7, as well as varied ratios of Cy3B-peptide to QD (1–6:1), was examined in order to choose the most effective sensor. With the exception of PBS, the CL_4-QDs showed centrosymmetric multi-acceptor FRET efficiency dependency (Hildebrandt et al. 2017), whereas the SO_3-QDs showed lower efficiency and FRET curve deviations, which may have been caused by QD surface ligand alteration (Díaz et al. 2017). Testing different BACE1 concentrations against the specified sensor concentration (15 nM) verified the sensor's effectiveness for BACE1 activity. As time proceeded, the emission of fluorescence ratio of the QD over Cy3B rose, suggesting that the peptide was cleaving and moving away from the QD surface, reducing the FRET efficiency. After 60 minutes, the *in vitro* assay's LOD was approximately 10 nM.

The large surface area of QDs allows them to self-assemble a membrane-targeting peptide containing palmitoyl moiety, JB858, which has been demonstrated to stay in the membrane and locate QDs for over 48 hours (Boeneman et al. 2013). Sensor activity is tested in the SH-SY5Y neuroblastoma cell line, which physiologically expresses BACE1 and is a well-used platform for assessing the pharmacological effects of drugs in neurodegeneration (Nopparat et al. 2021; Huang et al. 2020). The ability of membrane-targeted QD to incorporate and be detected, as well as its nontoxicity to cells, were both validated by the study. In time-lapse studies, untreated cells bearing the sensor were compared with cells that had verubecestat added. When BACE1 showed up in SH-SY5Y cells, the fluorescence density was examined and revealed a higher QD emission. There was no variation observed in the fluorescence readings upon introducing an inhibitor of BACE1 activity, verubecestat. This verifies the sensor's performance for use in cellulo BACE1 inhibitor test by clearly differentiating the cellular response whether or not the inhibitor is used (Figure 6.4) (Tosat-Bitrián et al. 2024).

6.13 *IN VIVO* IMAGING

The next goal is to transfer an imaging agent to *in vivo* systems after it has been effectively used *in vitro*. It should be noted that quantum dots (QDs) have so far been used only in animal in vivo applications. This limitation reflects a general restriction of fluorescence imaging, primarily due to the limited penetration depth of light in tissue and the small number of approved imaging agents for humans. Thus, until yet, only endoscopic research, body part imaging, and preliminary studies based on NIR-fluorescence have been carried out. The resolution (spatial and temporal), depth of penetration (in tissues), the energy of stimulation (ionizing vs. non-ionizing), accessibility of biodegradable injectable molecular probes, and identification limits of probes for a particular technology are the five primary characteristics that distinguish the various *in vivo* imaging technologies. Large surfaces and special photophysical and photochemical characteristics of QDs provide numerous *in vivo* imaging benefits that are nearly difficult to achieve with conventional fluorophores. The ability of two-photon absorption to stimulate QDs within the NIR window allows for deeper tissue penetration depths, making it a crucial approach for *in vivo* tissue imaging. The noticeable two-photon absorption traverse section of QDs has been demonstrated in studies using harmless multi-photon imaging of mouse capillaries for evaluating cardiac activity and flow of blood speed. The efficient in vivo efficacy of QDs is also dependent on the surface modifications. Long-chain methoxy-PEG QDs had half-lives of about 70 minutes, while amphiphilic poly(acryl acid), methoxy-PEG, and carboxy-PEG QDs had short half-lives. The investigation additionally looked at how coatings affected *in vivo* spreading and circulation time period (Wegner and Hildebrandt 2015). QDs are also used to target particular cellular receptors. Animal research has employed QDs coupled with folate to identify specific receptors of folate in the lymphoma cells of mice. The findings demonstrated a rise in fluorescence intensity, highlighting the significance of folate toward bio-recognition and homing. Any noticeable rise in folate receptor activity in cancer cells suggests a high level of expression, which may help diagnose cancer. Also, QDs aid in targeting tumor cell receptor integrin. Integrin is bound by a tripeptide-QD conjugate, which offers a cancer diagnostic tool.

Analysis conducted *in vitro* revealed that an integrin antagonist decreased specificity for integrin-positive cells. Large-scale vascular networks were among the effective outcomes of *in vivo* tumor imaging with QDs. This demonstrates how crucial QDs are for imaging applications. To maximize circulation times and offer accuracy for *in vivo* applications, researchers employed antibody-QD conjugates. They used a PEG crosslinking technique to target molecules that bind to cells in the rat retinal vasculature. Spatial resolution lower to individual cells was shown by this noninvasive imaging technique. For noninvasive applications and *in vivo* examination of deep tissue, QDs exhibiting near-IR emission wavelengths were used (Gil et al. 2021). *In vivo* investigations of mouse hearts and femurs were conducted by attaching transferrin to a QD having 750 nm emission wavelength, which enhanced the visibility resolution by up to 800 μm. Along with all these uses of QDs, it becomes necessary to track them *in vivo* as they can be cytotoxic if not surface functionalized with biocompatible polymers. Inductively coupled plasma mass spectrometry (ICP-MS) was used to track the biodistribution of CdSe/CdS, PEG-coated QDs that were injected into the right dorsal flank of mice. ICP-MS sensitivity made it possible to detect traces inside various tissues and organs, such as the kidney, liver, and spleen. The observed presence of the nanoparticles inside organs of the immunological response was verified by quantitative examination. The mice's neck along with upper trunk lymphatic flow was simultaneously observed by injecting five distinct areas with QDs of comparable hydrodynamic dimensions (Zhang et al. 2018). *In vivo* fluorescent pictures were created by conjugating carboxyl groups on QDs, which allowed to examine both individual and composite emptying patterns near basic lymph nodes. This groundbreaking finding has wide-ranging implications regarding anticipating the spread of cancer toward the lymph nodes and will complement noninvasive cancer metastasis route prediction (Matea et al. 2017).

QDs used for targeting, tracking, and imaging organs *in vivo* have to be cleared from the body through excretion. According to the findings of the study of QDs in mice, cadmium was eliminated via urine in 33.3% of cases and by feces in 23.8% of cases. The levels peaked in feces 6–12 hours and urine 24–36 hours after injection. At 120 hours after injection, the kidney displayed the maximum concentration. Urine contained unbound QDs, but feces included QDs bound to proteins. Understanding the toxicity of QDs over the long run requires more investigation into various nanoparticle sizes and coatings (Walling, Novak, and Shepard 2009).

To enhance target sensitivity as well as specificity, the engineering of nanoprobes during *in vivo* tumor imaging has typically focused on improving probe characteristics such as size, surface coating, and signal intensity. Unlike smaller molecules, nanoparticles larger than the renal filtration threshold (~6 nm) circulate longer and aggregate in tumors more effectively. Extended washout times, on the other hand, raise background signals, particularly in the system composed of mononuclear phagocytes (MPS; liver, spleen, etc.). The study uses $Zn_x\ Hg_{1-x}\ Se_y\ S_{1-y}$ QDs (ZHS-QDs) that are widely distributed NIR particles made of zinc (Zn^{2+}), mercury (Hg^{2+}), selenium (Se^{2-}), and sulfur (S^{2-}). As a tracer, Hg^{2+} was doped into the core to examine tissue distribution and clearance rates precisely. PEG was incorporated into the QDs to decrease MPS absorption. The tumor-to-liver ratio (T/Li) of nanoparticles that are not eliminated by the kidneys often declines over time, resulting in diminished image contrast, even if modifying the surface using PEG inhibits nonspecific absorption by liver Kupffer cells (Zelepukin, Shevchenko, and Deyev 2024; Yu and Zheng 2015).

More of the in vivo imaging involves signals from the background fluorescence, which can be overcome by using the QDs that help in imaging the specific tissues/organs. By selectively removing background signals while maintaining tumor signals *in vivo*, photoluminescent QDs are utilized in quenchable nanoprobes to improve tumor selectivity through cation exchange. The capacity of photoluminescent QDs to exchange cations with external metal ions makes them an ideal platform for quenchable nanoprobes (Beberwyck, Surendranath, and Alivisatos 2013). ZHS-QDs injected into mice intravenously exhibited robust signals in the NIR region from the vascular region of the mice (Liu et al. 2017) (Figure 6.5).

A cation donor known as "etchant," which quenches the QDs' PL through cation exchange, is devised. $Zn(OAc)_2$ (zinc acetate dehydrate), by giving extra Zn^{2+} to the QDs, raised the PL, while other compounds having cation-exchange capability quenched the fluorescence of ZHS-QDs. $Ag(S_2O_3)_2^{3-}$ (Ag-TS) was one of the most effective etchants, which is composed of silver ions (Ag^+) fixed with thiosulfate (TS), a type of metal chelator that is used to detoxify heavy metal ions in clinical settings. Zn^{2+} and Hg^{2+} were exchanged for Ag^+ by Ag-TS, which immediately quenched the QD's fluorescence (Figure 6.6) (Liu et al. 2017).

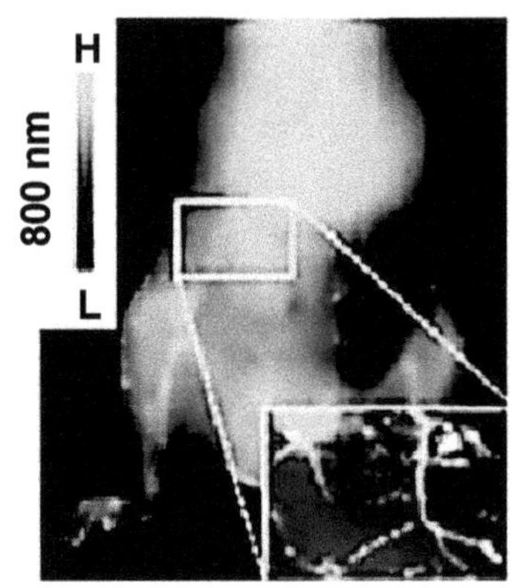

FIGURE 6.5 NIR pictures taken from the ventral side of the mouse that received a ZHS-QD intravenous injection. (Liu et al. 2017, http://creativecommons.org/licenses/by/4.0/ CCBY 4.0.)

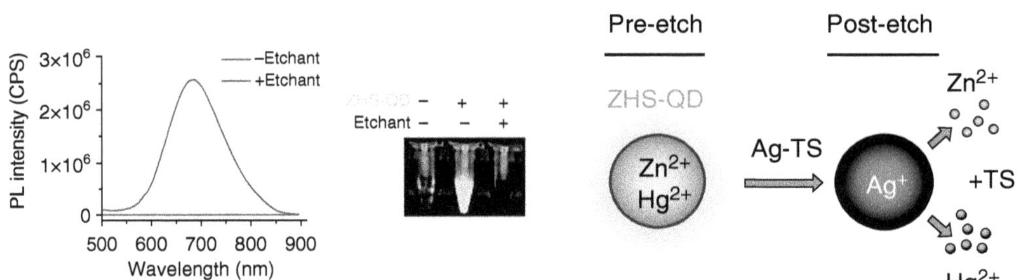

FIGURE 6.6 (a) ZHS-QDs before and after Ag-TS treatment. (b) ZHS-QDs (green) in a NIR picture with and without Ag-TS treatment. (c) ZHS-QD etching diagram. Ag-TS provides Ag^+ in return for Zn^{2+} and Hg^{2+}, quenching ZHS-QDs. (Liu et al. 2017, http://creativecommons.org/licenses/by/4.0/.)

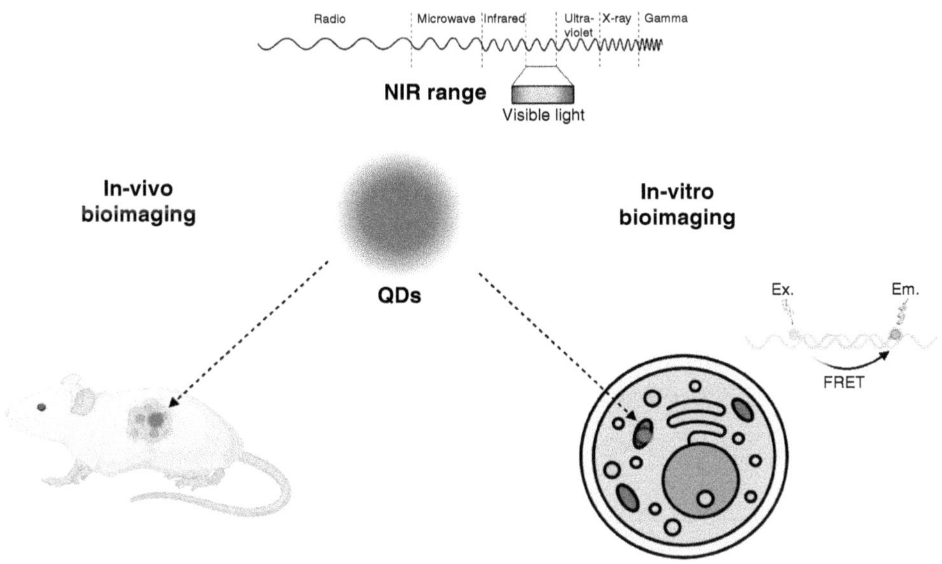

FIGURE 6.7 QDs in *in vitro* and in vivo bioimaging application.

6.14 LIMITATIONS OF QDS

Although usage of QDs has a wide array of applications, there are few safety measures that play a major role with respect to cellular toxicity. Toxicity of QDs is the most important concern as it can be carcinogenic because of the presence of heavy metals like Cd (cadmium) and Pb (lead) in the core structure of QDs. Even after protecting the core of the QDs with shell and functionalizing the surface of QDs with different biocompatible polymers, these strategies do not provide complete protection from the leakage of heavy metals from the core when the shell is damaged. This can be fatal to an organism if treated *in vivo* as some trace amounts of QDs accumulate in some of the organs, like the liver, kidney, and spleen, without being completely excreted from the body through urine (Lin and Chen 2023). Apart from coating the QD surface with peptides and polymers, silica can also be used to surface-functionalized QD via the silanization process. The drawback of this surface functionalization method is that QD size gets larger because of the thick layer of silica coating on the surface. The increased size of QDs will have the emission peak in the blue shift, low QY, and the core's stability is affected (Pham et al. 2021). Another parameter is the synthesis process being followed for the QD synthesis. QDs are synthesized at higher temperatures to maintain chemical stability. Synthesized QDs will be in the organic phase, QDs present in the organic phase are made more biologically applicable /compatible. The procedure of exchanging ligand on the QD surface is one such method of adding biocompatibility, but this method reduces the QY and restricts the fluorescence emission in the NIR region. This limitation can be overcome by synthesizing QDs in one pot with a standardized ligand exchange/phase transfer reaction via efficient hydrothermal routes (Gil et al. 2021). Apart from these limitations, in vivo treatment of QDs will cause aggregation by clumping together that may interfere with the cellular function. Any damage to the structure of QDs like damage caused to the shell or core will decrease the intensity of fluorescence by causing blinking. Aggregation in QDs is also observed when they come in contact with proteins present in the biological samples like blood serum; quenching of fluorescence is also seen as they lose their stability. QDs upon storage for long term by exposing to light may cause photobleaching that diminishes the fluorescence of QDs.

6.15 CONCLUSION

The unique optical properties of QDs, which enhance their efficacy in various biological applications like biosensing and bioimaging, have gained attention recently. Standard fluorescent probes, such as dyes or fluorescent proteins, are still used in many biomolecular detection techniques, such as FRET. While these probes have photophysical limitations, such as fast photobleaching, self-quenching when exposed to elevated concentrations, or instability in biological media, they are extremely versatile and come in nearly every possible color. Instead of substituting dyes or fluorescent proteins, QDs should be considered and used as a substitute for fluorescent nanoprobe that can offer a number of benefits over typical fluorophores.

Although talking about the different applications of QDs as fluorescent probes, as a labeling marker for tissue or cells, and majorly in the detection of cancer, the most important limitation that needs to be addressed is their toxicity with respect to heavy metal leakage.

REFERENCES

Abdellatif, Ahmed A H, Mahmoud A Younis, Mansour Alsharidah, Osamah Al Rugaie, and Hesham M Tawfeek. 2022. "Biomedical Applications of Quantum Dots: Overview, Challenges, and Clinical Potential." *International Journal of Nanomedicine*, 1951–70.

Akkilic, Namik, Stefan Geschwindner, and Fredrik Höök. 2020. "Single-Molecule Biosensors: Recent Advances and Applications." *Biosensors and Bioelectronics* 151: 111944. https://doi.org/https://doi.org/10.1016/j.bios.2019.111944.

Anpalagan, Karthiga, Hong Yin, Ivan Cole, Tian Zhang, and Daniel T H Lai. 2024. "Quantum Yield Enhancement of Carbon Quantum Dots Using Chemical-Free Precursors for Sensing Cr (VI) Ions." *Inorganics* 12 (4). https://doi.org/10.3390/inorganics12040096.

Van Avermaet, Hannes, Pieter Schiettecatte, Sandra Hinz, Luca Giordano, Fabio Ferrari, Céline Nayral, Fabien Delpech, Janina Maultzsch, Holger Lange, and Zeger Hens. 2022. "Full-Spectrum InP-Based Quantum Dots with near-Unity Photoluminescence Quantum Efficiency." *ACS Nano* 16 (6): 9701–12.

Aygun, Aysenur, Ipek Cobas, Rima Nour Elhouda Tiri, and Fatih Sen. 2024. "Hydrothermal Synthesis of B, S, and N-Doped Carbon Quantum Dots for Colorimetric Sensing of Heavy Metal Ions." *RSC Advances* 14 (16): 10814–25.

Beberwyck, Brandon J, Yogesh Surendranath, and A Paul Alivisatos. 2013. "Cation Exchange: A Versatile Tool for Nanomaterials Synthesis." *The Journal of Physical Chemistry C* 117 (39): 19759–70.

Bera, Debasis, Lei Qian, Teng-Kuan Tseng, and Paul H Holloway. 2010. "Quantum Dots and Their Multimodal Applications: A Review." *Materials* 3 (4): 2260–2345. https://doi.org/10.3390/ma3042260.

Bilan, Regina, Fabrice Fleury, Igor Nabiev, and Alyona Sukhanova. 2015. "Quantum Dot Surface Chemistry and Functionalization for Cell Targeting and Imaging." *Bioconjugate Chemistry* 26 (4): 609–24.

Boeneman, Kelly, James B Delehanty, Juan B Blanco-Canosa, Kimihiro Susumu, Michael H Stewart, Eunkeu Oh, Alan L Huston, Glyn Dawson, Sampat Ingale, and Ryan Walters. 2013. "Selecting Improved Peptidyl Motifs for Cytosolic Delivery of Disparate Protein and Nanoparticle Materials." *Acs Nano* 7 (5): 3778–96.

Chen, Lu-Lu, Liang Zhao, Zhi-Gang Wang, Shu-Lin Liu, and Dai-Wen Pang. 2022. "Near-infrared-II Quantum Dots for in Vivo Imaging and Cancer Therapy." *Small* 18 (8): 2104567.

Cheng, Yu, Si Da Ling, Yuhao Geng, Yundong Wang, and Jianhong Xu. 2021. "Microfluidic Synthesis of Quantum Dots and Their Applications in Bio-Sensing and Bio-Imaging." *Nanoscale Advances* 3 (8): 2180–95.

Das, Brati, and Riqiang Yan. 2017. "Role of BACE1 in Alzheimer's Synaptic Function." *Translational Neurodegeneration* 6: 1–8.

Díaz, Sebastián A, Soumyo Sen, Kelly Boeneman Gemmill, Carl W Brown III, Eunkeu Oh, Kimihiro Susumu, Michael H Stewart, Joyce C Breger, Guillermo Lasarte Aragonés, and Lauren D Field. 2017. "Elucidating Surface Ligand-Dependent Kinetic Enhancement of Proteolytic Activity at Surface-Modified Quantum Dots." *ACS Nano* 11 (6): 5884–96.

Efros, Alexander L, and Louis E Brus. 2021. "Nanocrystal Quantum Dots: From Discovery to Modern Development." *ACS Nano* 15 (4): 6192–6210.

Gac, Séverine Le, Istvan Vermes, and Albert van den Berg. 2006. "Quantum Dots Based Probes Conjugated to Annexin V for Photostable Apoptosis Detection and Imaging." *Nano Letters* 6 (9): 1863–69.

Ganganboina, Akhilesh Babu, and Ruey-An Doong. 2019. "Graphene Quantum Dots Decorated Gold-Polyaniline Nanowire for Impedimetric Detection of Carcinoembryonic Antigen." *Scientific Reports* 9 (1): 7214.

Garg, Mayank, Neelam Vishwakarma, Amit L Sharma, and Suman Singh. 2021. "Amine-Functionalized Graphene Quantum Dots for Fluorescence-Based Immunosensing of Ferritin." *ACS Applied Nano Materials* 4 (7): 7416–25.

Gil, Hélio M, Thomas W Price, Kanik Chelani, Jean-Sebastien G Bouillard, Simon D J Calaminus, and Graeme J Stasiuk. 2021. "NIR-Quantum Dots in Biomedical Imaging and Their Future." *IScience* 24 (3): 102189. https://doi.org/https://doi.org/10.1016/j.isci.2021.102189.

Green, Christopher M, David A Hastman, Divita Mathur, Kimihiro Susumu, Eunkeu Oh, Igor L Medintz, and Sebastián A Díaz. 2021. "Direct and Efficient Conjugation of Quantum Dots to DNA Nanostructures with Peptide-PNA." *ACS Nano* 15 (5): 9101–10.

Green, Christopher M, Divita Mathur, Kimihiro Susumu, Eunkeu Oh, Igor L Medintz, and Sebastián A Díaz. 2022. "Polyhistidine-Tag-Enabled Conjugation of Quantum Dots and Enzymes to DNA Nanostructures." In *Bioluminescence: Methods and Protocols,* edited by Sung-Bae Kim *Volume* 2, 61–91. Springer, published in Environmental Management Research Institute, National Institute of Advanced Industrial Science and Technology (AIST), Tsukuba, Ibaraki, Japan.

Han, Han, Chongwen Wang, Xingsheng Yang, Shuai Zheng, Xiaodan Cheng, Zhenzhen Liu, Baohua Zhao, and Rui Xiao. 2022. "Rapid Field Determination of SARS-CoV-2 by a Colorimetric and Fluorescent Dual-Functional Lateral Flow Immunoassay Biosensor." *Sensors and Actuators B: Chemical* 351: 130897.

Hildebrandt, Niko, Christopher M Spillmann, W Russ Algar, Thomas Pons, Michael H Stewart, Eunkeu Oh, Kimihiro Susumu, Sebastian A Diaz, James B Delehanty, and Igor L Medintz. 2017. "Energy Transfer with Semiconductor Quantum Dot Bioconjugates: A Versatile Platform for Biosensing, Energy Harvesting, and Other Developing Applications." *Chemical Reviews* 117 (2): 536–711.

Hu, Tao, Kangkai Xu, Shanhu Qiu, Yu Han, Juan Chen, Jian Xu, Ke Chen, Zilin Sun, Hong Yi, and Zhonghua Ni. 2020. "Colorimetric Detection of Urine Glucose Using a C/CdTe QDs–GOx Aerogel Based on a Microfluidic Assay Sensor." *Journal of Materials Chemistry B* 8 (32): 7160–65.

Hu, Tianxing, Le Zhang, Wei Wen, Xiuhua Zhang, and Shengfu Wang. 2016. "Enzyme Catalytic Amplification of MiRNA-155 Detection with Graphene Quantum Dot-Based Electrochemical Biosensor." *Biosensors and Bioelectronics* 77: 451–56.

Hu, Xi-Min, Zhi-Xin Li, Rui-Han Lin, Jia-Qi Shan, Qing-Wei Yu, Rui-Xuan Wang, Lv-Shuang Liao, Wei-Tao Yan, Zhen Wang, and Lei Shang. 2021. "Guidelines for Regulated Cell Death Assays: A Systematic Summary, a Categorical Comparison, a Prospective." *Frontiers in Cell and Developmental Biology* 9: 634690.

Huang, Pan, Nan Zheng, Hai-bing Zhou, and Jian Huang. 2020. "Curcumin Inhibits BACE1 Expression through the Interaction between ERβ and NFκB Signaling Pathway in SH-SY5Y Cells." *Molecular and Cellular Biochemistry* 463: 161–73.

Jeong, Sanghwa, Jaejung Song, Wonseok Lee, Yeon Mi Ryu, Yebin Jung, Sang-Yeob Kim, Kangwook Kim, Seong Cheol Hong, Seung Jae Myung, and Sungjee Kim. 2017. "Cancer-Microenvironment-Sensitive Activatable Quantum Dot Probe in the Second Near-Infrared Window." *Nano Letters* 17 (3): 1378–86.

Jiang, Chao, Yu Zhang, Haixia Shen, and Chenghui Liu. 2017. "Target-regulated Ce^{3+}/Ce^{4+} Redox Switch for Fluorescence Turn-on Detection of H_2O_2 and Glucose." *ChemistrySelect* 2 (28): 9181–85.

Jin, Shan, Yanxi Hu, Zhanjun Gu, Lei Liu, and Hai-Chen Wu. 2011. "Application of Quantum Dots in Biological Imaging." *Journal of Nanomaterials* 2011 (1): 834139.

Kapur, Anshika, Scott H Medina, Wentao Wang, Goutam Palui, Xin Ji, Joel P Schneider, and Hedi Mattoussi. 2018. "Enhanced Uptake of Luminescent Quantum Dots by Live Cells Mediated by a Membrane-Active Peptide." *ACS Omega* 3 (12): 17164–72.

Kitte, Shimeles Addisu, Wenyue Gao, Yuriy T Zholudov, Liming Qi, Anaclet Nsabimana, Zhongyuan Liu, and Guobao Xu. 2017. "Stainless Steel Electrode for Sensitive Luminol Electrochemiluminescent Detection of H_2O_2, Glucose, and Glucose Oxidase Activity." *Analytical Chemistry* 89 (18): 9864–69.

Knudsen, Birgitta R, Morten Leth Jepsen, and Yi-Ping Ho. 2013. "Quantum Dot-Based Nanosensors for Diagnosis via Enzyme Activity Measurement." *Expert Review of Molecular Diagnostics* 13 (4): 367–75.

Lan Hsia, Sung, Robert Duncan, Alain H Schob, Simon C Chakko, Reinaldo Mulingtapang, Jin Lin He, and Guido O Perez. 2000. "Serum Levels of High-Density Lipoprotein Phospholipids Correlate Inversely with Severity of Angiographically Defined Coronary Artery Disease." *Atherosclerosis* 152 (2): 469–73. https://doi.org/https://doi.org/10.1016/S0021-9150(99)00499-2.

Li, Chunyan, Guangcun Chen, Yejun Zhang, Feng Wu, and Qiangbin Wang. 2020. "Advanced Fluorescence Imaging Technology in the Near-Infrared-II Window for Biomedical Applications." *Journal of the American Chemical Society* 142 (35): 14789–804.

Li, Jingjing, and Jun-Jie Zhu. 2013. "Quantum Dots for Fluorescent Biosensing and Bio-Imaging Applications." *Analyst* 138 (9): 2506–15. https://doi.org/10.1039/C3AN36705C.

Lin, Xiaotan, and Tingting Chen. 2023. "A Review of in Vivo Toxicity of Quantum Dots in Animal Models." *International Journal of Nanomedicine* 18: 8143–68. https://doi.org/10.2147/IJN.S434842.

Liu, Xiangyou, Gary B Braun, Mingde Qin, Erkki Ruoslahti, and Kazuki N Sugahara. 2017. "In Vivo Cation Exchange in Quantum Dots for Tumor-Specific Imaging." *Nature Communications* 8 (1): 343.

Malhotra, Bansi Dhar, and Md Azahar Ali. 2018. "Nanomaterials in Biosensors: Fundamentals and Applications." *Nanomaterials for Biosensors*, 1.

Manna, Liberato. 2023. "The Bright and Enlightening Science of Quantum Dots." *Nano Letters* 23 (21): 9673–76.

Mansuriya, Bhargav D, and Zeynep Altintas. 2019. "Graphene Quantum Dot-Based Electrochemical Immunosensors for Biomedical Applications." *Materials* 13 (1): 96.

Martins, Catarina S M, Alec P LaGrow, and João A V Prior. 2022. "Quantum Dots for Cancer-Related MiRNA Monitoring." *ACS Sensors* 7 (5): 1269–99. https://doi.org/10.1021/acssensors.2c00149.

Matea, Cristian T, Teodora Mocan, Flaviu Tabaran, Teodora Pop, Ofelia Mosteanu, Cosmin Puia, Cornel Iancu, and Lucian Mocan. 2017. "Quantum Dots in Imaging, Drug Delivery and Sensor Applications." *International Journal of Nanomedicine*, 5421–31.

Mollarasouli, Fariba, Verónica Serafín, Susana Campuzano, Paloma Yáñez-Sedeño, José M Pingarrón, and Karim Asadpour-Zeynali. 2018. "Ultrasensitive Determination of Receptor Tyrosine Kinase with a Label-Free Electrochemical Immunosensor Using Graphene Quantum Dots-Modified Screen-Printed Electrodes." *Analytica Chimica Acta* 1011: 28–34.

Nirala, Narsingh R, Shiju Abraham, Vinod Kumar, Anushka Bansal, Anchal Srivastava, and Preeti S Saxena. 2015. "Colorimetric Detection of Cholesterol Based on Highly Efficient Peroxidase Mimetic Activity of Graphene Quantum Dots." *Sensors and Actuators B: Chemical* 218: 42–50. https://doi.org/https://doi.org/10.1016/j.snb.2015.04.091.

Nopparat, Chutikorn, Worawut Chaopae, Parichart Boontem, Pattarawut Sopha, Prapimpun Wongchitrat, and Piyarat Govitrapong. 2021. "Melatonin Attenuates High Glucose-Induced Changes in Beta Amyloid Precursor Protein Processing in Human Neuroblastoma Cells." *Neurochemical Research*, 1–12.

Pandya, Alok, Pinkesh G Sutariya, and Shobhana K Menon. 2013. "A Non Enzymatic Glucose Biosensor Based on an Ultrasensitive Calix [4] Arene Functionalized Boronic Acid Gold Nanoprobe for Sensing in Human Blood Serum." *Analyst* 138 (8): 2483–90.

Pham, Xuan-Hung, Seung-Min Park, Kyeong-Min Ham, San Kyeong, Byung Sung Son, Jaehi Kim, Eunil Hahm, et al. 2021. "Synthesis and Application of Silica-Coated Quantum Dots in Biomedicine." *International Journal of Molecular Sciences* 22 (18). https://doi.org/10.3390/ijms221810116.

Ramezani, Zahra, Fatemeh Kiani Ghalehsardi, and Siamak Noorizadeh. 2023. "Classifications of Quantum Dots and Their Detection Principles in Sensing."

Rogers, Katherine E, Okhil K Nag, Michael H Stewart, Kimihiro Susumu, Eunkeu Oh, and James B Delehanty. 2023. "Multivalent Display of Erythropoietin on Quantum Dots Enhances Aquaporin-4 Expression and Water Transport in Human Astrocytes In Vitro." *Bioconjugate Chemistry* 34 (12): 2205–14.

Sousa, Mariana P, Ana Margarida L Piloto, Ana Cláudia Pereira, Fernando C Schmitt, Ruben Fernandes, and Felismina T C Moreira. 2022. "New Quantum-Dot-Based Fluorescent Immunosensor for Cancer Biomarker Detection." *Chemosensors* 10 (12): 518.

Sun, Bolu, Yanping Wang, Dai Li, Wuyan Li, Xiaodan Gou, Yuqiang Gou, and Fangdi Hu. 2020. "Development of a Sensitive Electrochemical Immunosensor Using Polyaniline Functionalized Graphene Quantum Dots for Detecting a Depression Marker." *Materials Science and Engineering:* C 111: 110797.

Tandale, P, Neeraj Choudhary, Joga Singh, Akanksha Sharma, Ananya Shukla, Pavani Sriram, Udit Soni, Neha Singla, Ravi P Barnwal, and Gurpal Singh. 2021. "Fluorescent Quantum Dots: An Insight on Synthesis and Potential Biological Application as Drug Carrier in Cancer." *Biochemistry and Biophysics Reports* 26: 100962.

Tessaro, Leticia, Adriano Aquino, Pedro Panzenhagen, Nirav Joshi, and Carlos Adam Conte-Junior. 2023. "A Systematic Review of the Advancement on Colorimetric Nanobiosensors for SARS-CoV-2 Detection." *Journal of Pharmaceutical and Biomedical Analysis* 222: 115087.

Tong, Xia, Shuyun Shi, Chaoying Tong, Ali Iftikhar, Ruiqing Long, and Yongfeng Zhu. 2020. "Quantum/Carbon Dots-Based Fluorescent Assays for Enzyme Activity." *TrAC Trends in Analytical Chemistry* 131: 116008.

Torres, Ruben, Lucas B Thal, James R McBride, Bruce E Cohen, and Sandra J Rosenthal. 2024. "Quantum Dot Fluorescent Imaging: Using Atomic Structure Correlation Studies to Improve Photophysical Properties." *The Journal of Physical Chemistry C* 128 (9): 3632–40.

Tosat-Bitrián, Carlota, Jesús Alejandro Bueso de Barrio, Michael H Stewart, Kimihiro Susumu, Igor L Medintz, Sebastián A Díaz, and Valle Palomo. 2024. "Membrane-Targeted Quantum Dot-Based BACE1 Activity Sensors for In Vitro and In Cellulo Assays." *ACS Applied Materials & Interfaces* 16 (46): 63186–94.

Verma, Awadhesh Kumar, Ashab Noumani, Amit K Yadav, and Pratima R Solanki. 2023. "FRET Based Biosensor: Principle Applications Recent Advances and Challenges." *Diagnostics* 13 (8). https://doi.org/10.3390/diagnostics13081375.

Walling, Maureen A, Jennifer A Novak, and Jason R E Shepard. 2009. "Quantum Dots for Live Cell and In Vivo Imaging." *International Journal of Molecular Sciences* 10 (2): 441–91. https://doi.org/10.3390/ijms10020441.

Wegner, K David, and Niko Hildebrandt. 2024. "Near Infrared Quantum Dots for Biosensing and Bioimaging." *TrAC Trends in Analytical Chemistry*, 117922.

Wegner, K David, and Niko Hildebrandt. 2015. "Quantum Dots: Bright and Versatile in Vitro and in Vivo Fluorescence Imaging Biosensors." *Chemical Society Reviews* 44 (14): 4792–4834.

Wei, Wei, Xuewen He, and Nan Ma. 2014. "DNA-templated Assembly of a Heterobivalent Quantum Dot Nanoprobe for Extra-and Intracellular Dual-targeting and Imaging of Live Cancer Cells." *Angewandte Chemie* 126 (22): 5679–83.

Xu, Hao, Chuang Chen, Yue He, Hong-Wu Tang, Zhi-Ling Zhang, Yan Li, and Dai-Wen Pang. 2015. "Analysis of Cancer Marker in Tissues with Hadamard Transform Fluorescence Spectral Microscopic Imaging." *Journal of Fluorescence* 25: 397–402.

Yu, Mengxiao, and Jie Zheng. 2015. "Clearance Pathways and Tumor Targeting of Imaging Nanoparticles." *ACS Nano* 9 (7): 6655–74.

Yu, Mengze, Kunli Zhao, Xiaohua Zhu, Shiyun Tang, Zhou Nie, Yan Huang, Peng Zhao, and Shouzhuo Yao. 2017. "Development of Near-Infrared Ratiometric Fluorescent Probe Based on Cationic Conjugated Polymer and CdTe/CdS QDs for Label-Free Determination of Glucose in Human Body Fluids." *Biosensors and Bioelectronics* 95: 41–47.

Zelepukin, Ivan V, Konstantin G Shevchenko, and Sergey M Deyev. 2024. "Rediscovery of Mononuclear Phagocyte System Blockade for Nanoparticle Drug Delivery." *Nature Communications* 15 (1): 4366.

Zhai, Hong, Yunfeng Bai, Jun Qin, and Feng Feng. 2019. "Colorimetric and Ratiometric Fluorescence Dual-Mode Sensing of Glucose Based on Carbon Quantum Dots and Potential UV/Fluorescence of o-Diaminobenzene." Sensors 19 (3). https://doi.org/10.3390/s19030674.

Zhang, Jian, Xiaoyue Zhang, and Sai Bi. 2022. "Two-Dimensional Quantum Dot-Based Electrochemical Biosensors." *Biosensors* 12 (4): 254.

Zhang, Mingxi, Jingying Yue, Ran Cui, Zhuoran Ma, Hao Wan, Feifei Wang, Shoujun Zhu, et al. 2018. "Bright Quantum Dots Emitting at ~1,600 Nm in the NIR-IIb Window for Deep Tissue Fluorescence Imaging." *Proceedings of the National Academy of Sciences of the United States of America* 115 (26): 6590–95. https://doi.org/10.1073/pnas.1806153115.

7 Gene Therapy Using Polymeric Nanocarriers

Nutan Bhingaradiya[1,2], *Arpita Banerjee*[1], *Nishkal Pisal*[1], *Peixin Shi*[1], *and Nitin Joshi*[1,2]
[1]Center for Nanomedicine and Department of Anesthesiology, Perioperative and Pain Medicine, Brigham and Women's Hospital, Boston, Massachusetts
[2]Harvard Medical School, Boston, Massachusetts

7.1 INTRODUCTION

Gene therapy represents a transformative therapeutic strategy for treating a wide array of diseases by modulating gene expression. This is achieved through the delivery of engineered nucleic acids tailored for specific clinical applications. Key modalities include messenger RNA (mRNA) and plasmid DNA (pDNA) for the expression of therapeutic proteins, antisense oligonucleotides (ASOs), small interfering RNAs (siRNAs), and microRNAs (miRNAs) for targeted gene silencing, and CRISPR-Cas systems for precise genome editing. These platforms hold significant potential for addressing the molecular basis of genetic disorders, greatly expanding therapeutic possibilities. However, several challenges must be addressed to fully realize the potential of nucleic acid-based therapies. A primary challenge is efficient delivery, as nucleic acids face substantial barriers in crossing lipid membranes and are vulnerable to degradation by endogenous nucleases in circulation. Additionally, the immune system can detect and neutralize exogenous genetic material, requiring sophisticated strategies to evade immune detection and minimize inflammatory responses. Overcoming these barriers is crucial to unlocking the full potential of gene-based therapies [1].

To address these physiological challenges, various delivery vehicles have been engineered to navigate the complex biological environment and achieve therapeutic outcomes. Initially, viral vectors were considered highly promising due to their natural infectivity, which facilitated efficient delivery and transfection. Currently, viral vectors represent approximately 70% of clinical gene therapy trials [2], and they have been successfully employed in therapies such as Luxturna for Leber Congenital Amaurosis (LCA) and Retinitis Pigmentosa (RP) [3], Zolgensma for Spinal Muscular Atrophy Type 1 [4], and Zynteglo for Thalassemia [5]. However, concerns regarding immunogenicity and the potential for insertional mutagenesis have raised significant safety issues, limiting the clinical translation of viral vectors. Additionally, the limited cargo capacity and the challenging manufacturing processes have dampened the initial enthusiasm surrounding viral-based delivery systems.

7.2 POLYMERS EXPLORED FOR GENE DELIVERY

Polymeric nanoparticles (PNPs) are highly valued in gene delivery systems due to their straightforward synthesis, tunable functionalization, and high transfection efficiency. Ongoing research on polymeric carriers is focused on optimizing nucleic acid delivery while simultaneously mitigating cytotoxicity. Polymers can be modified in terms of charge, degradability, and molecular weight, all of which influence how they deliver RNA into cells. Various polymers, including polycations, amphiphilic polymers, natural biodegradable polymers (e.g., polysaccharides), and synthetic

 DOI: 10.1201/9781003473015-7

biodegradable polymers (e.g., poly(amino esters), PAEs), have been employed in the fabrication of nanocarriers such as nanogels, micelles, polyplexes, nanoparticles, nanospheres, and polymersomes (Figure 7.1). These nanocarriers have been utilized for the encapsulation and controlled release of nucleic acid-based cargoes, including double-stranded DNA (dsDNA), siRNA, miRNA, and ASOs, with varying base pair lengths and molecular sizes (Figure 7.1) [6].

US Food and Drug Administration (FDA)-approved polymers such as poly(lactic-co-glycolic acid) (PLGA) have been extensively used to make nanoparticles. At neutral pH, PLGA does not have the positive charge required to bind with the anionic RNA phosphodiester backbone. To overcome this limitation, cationic groups, such as chitosan and polyethylenimine (PEI), have been added to PLGA to facilitate the delivery [7]. Polymers containing amine groups, such as PEI and poly(L-lysine) (PLL), can become cationic and form electrostatic interactions with RNA, enabling its delivery into cells. The strong electrostatic attraction between the positively charged groups of the cationic polymer (polycations) and the negatively charged phosphate backbone of nucleic acids leads to the condensation of the genetic material into compact, nanoscale particles, resulting in the formation of polyplexes, which facilitate cellular uptake compared to free nucleic acids [8]. These structures are commonly used in gene delivery systems because they condense and protect the genetic material from degradation by nucleases, while facilitating cellular uptake.

Polycations, typically composed of ionizable amine groups, have been predominantly utilized as the foundational components in the design and fabrication of polymeric nanostructures (Figure 7.2). For instance, PEI has become a benchmark in gene delivery due to its high transfection efficiency [9]. PEI polymers, which come in both linear and branched forms, are versatile in delivering nucleic acids such as pDNA, miRNA, and siRNA [10,11]. Despite their success, PEI's high charge density can cause cellular membrane damage and systemic toxicity, which have been mitigated by blending

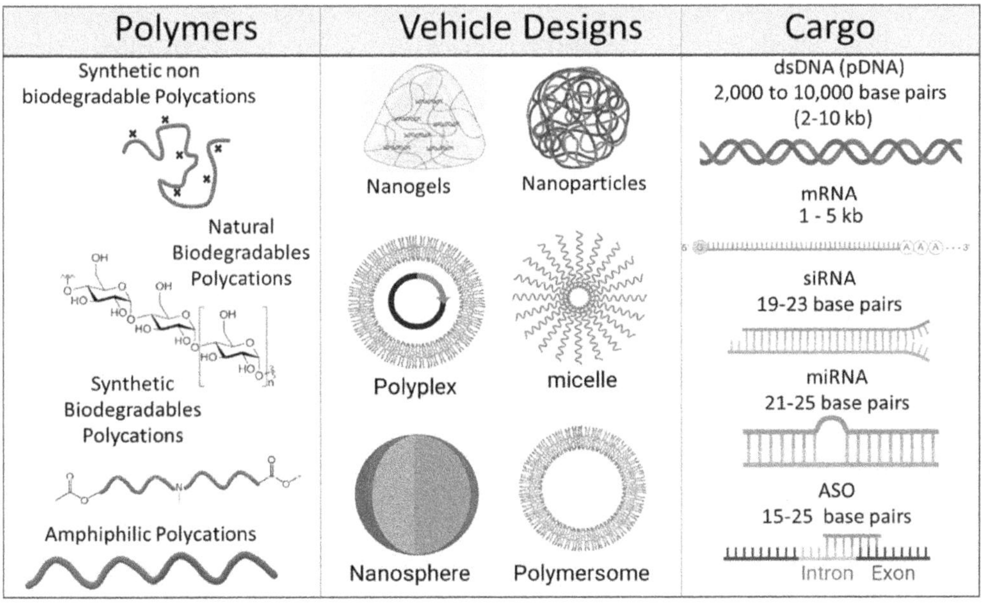

FIGURE 7.1 Overview of polymeric nucleic acid delivery vehicles, including: polyplexes, which are short-lifetime electrostatic complexes utilized for plasmid DNA; micelles, dynamic amphiphilic core-shell complexes designed for small RNA transport; nanoparticles, solid particles with homogeneous nucleic acid loading; nanogels, cross-linked polymer networks that swell in response to environmental stimuli, accommodating various nucleic acids; and polymersomes, self-assembled vesicles formed from block copolymers, prepared using cationic polymers, amphiphilic polymers, natural biodegradable polycations, and synthetic biodegradable polycations used for delivering diverse nucleic acid structures and base pair lengths.

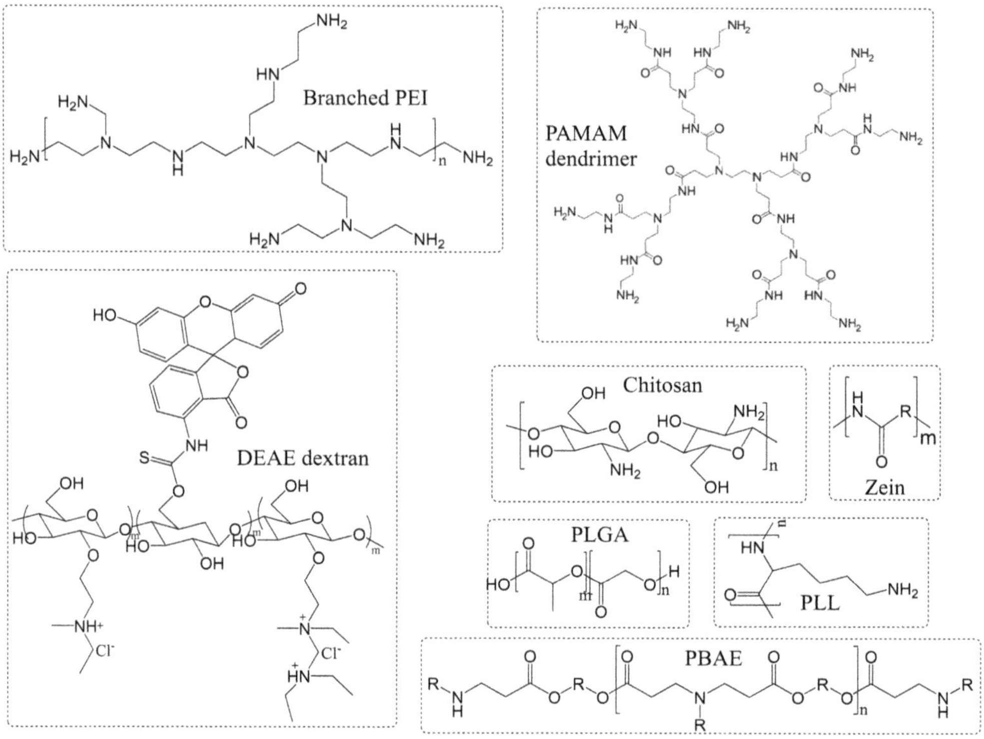

FIGURE 7.2 Polymeric nanoparticles and polymers based on poly(ethylenimine) (PEI), poly(L-lysine) (PLL), modified dextran, zein, chitosan, and poly(beta-amino-ester) (PBAE) utilize cationic amine groups to complex with the anionic phosphodiester backbone of nucleic acid. Polymers like poly(lactic-co-glycolic acid) (PLGA) are often engineered with separate cationic groups. Dendrimers, such as poly(amidoamine) (PAMAM), are polymeric structures with a defined number of molecules branching from a core.

PEI with biocompatible synthetic polymers like PLGA [12]. This combination has been shown to enhance gene transfection while reducing the cytotoxic effects associated with PEI alone. Another class of polymers, dendrimers like polyamidoamine (PAMAM), have demonstrated efficiency in gene delivery, particularly due to their multivalent structure, which offers numerous coupling sites for nucleic acids. PAMAM dendrimers have been used for delivering gene therapies to specific cell types, such as microglia in the brain and tumor cells. To enhance specificity, PAMAM can be conjugated with targeting ligands or with polyethylene glycol (PEG), which improves its biocompatibility and reduces nonspecific uptake [13].

Biodegradable polymers are increasingly being used to enhance the biocompatibility of gene delivery systems. For example, chitosan, a naturally derived polysaccharide, has gained attention for its non-toxic profile and ability to effectively deliver nucleic acids in various therapeutic contexts. Chitosan-based delivery systems have been applied in areas such as bone regeneration and cancer therapy, showing success in the transfection of small and large nucleic acids [14]. Additionally, cyclodextrin (CD), another naturally derived polymer, has been utilized in gene delivery, often in combination with other polymers like PEI or PLGA to form complex polyplexes. These CD-based systems have shown promise in delivering nucleic acids for liver and metastatic tumor therapies. Similarly, biodegradable synthetic polymers like poly(beta-amino) esters (PBAEs) are another group of cationic polymers that combine efficient nucleic acid encapsulation with biodegradability [15]. PBAEs have been successfully used in various applications, such as delivering siRNA to hepatocellular carcinoma cells and targeting pediatric brain cancer cells.

Further innovations in polymer synthesis, such as reversible addition-fragmentation chain transfer (RAFT) polymerization and atom transfer radical polymerization (ATRP), have enabled the creation of sequence-defined synthetic amphiphilic polymers. These methods allow for control of polymer sequence and structure with high precision, facilitating the development of optimized carriers for specific applications [16]. For example, poly(amine-co-esters) (PACEs) have been designed to balance charge density with biocompatibility, making them effective at promoting cellular uptake while minimizing toxicity. PACEs have been successfully formulated into nanoparticles and polyplexes for gene delivery, and their lower charge density compared to polymers like PEI has made them a safer alternative for clinical applications [17]. Figure 7.1 provides an overview of the main categories of polycations commonly used in various polymeric vehicles for the effective loading of genetic material as cargo.

The following section will systematically categorize polycations into first-, second-, and third-generation polymers, providing a concise overview of the key advancements. Notable examples will be discussed, along with the underlying rationale driving their evolutionary development.

7.2.1 First Generation of Polycations

Early efforts centered on using positively charged polymers to enhance viral genome transfection, leading to the discovery of the first-generation polycations [18,19]. These polycations, including diethylaminoethyl-Dextran (DEAE-dextran) and poly (amino acids) like polyornithine, polylysine, and polyarginine, were effective at forming polyplexes for encapsulating DNA and achieving targeted delivery. A significant advancement came with Felgner and Wu's work, which successfully transfected liver cells using DNA encapsulated in polylysine polyplexes and targeted with a complementary ligand (asialo-orosomucoid), whose receptors are expressed exclusively on hepatic cells [20,21]. This breakthrough enabled successful gene delivery both in vitro and in vivo, setting the stage for further innovations in targeted delivery systems, such as the use of transferrin-protamine and polylysine for delivering nucleic acids to cells expressing transferrin receptors, including tumor and hematopoietic cells [22,23].

By the early 1990s, targeted delivery to respiratory cells had been achieved by targeting the immunoglobulin receptor [24]. Despite these successes, researchers recognized the limitations of first-generation polycations in gene transfection. A key breakthrough occurred when Luthman and Magnusson introduced the lysosomotropic drug chloroquine into DEAE-dextran polyplexes [25], significantly enhancing transfection efficiency, a finding also observed with polylysine-based systems upon chloroquine addition [26]. While the mechanisms underlying chloroquine's efficacy were not fully understood during the 1980s, it was hypothesized that chloroquine facilitated DNA escape from lysosomal degradation by causing osmotic swelling, lysis, and subsequent release of polyplexes from endosomes, preventing degradation and improving transfection outcomes [26,27]. This understanding inspired various strategies to mimic viral mechanisms for endolysosomal escape, including the use of viral proteins or inactivated viruses to enhance gene delivery. For example, inactivated adenovirus and rhinovirus were incubated with receptor-targeted polyplex systems to facilitate endolysosomal escape, leveraging viral membrane destabilization domains [27–30]. The attachment of whole inactivated adenoviruses to polyplex systems via biotin-streptavidin linkages marked a significant advancement, leading to highly efficient viral-based transfection [31,32]. This approach proved effective both in vitro and in vivo, even in otherwise difficult-to-transfect primary and tumor cells and culminated in the first clinical trial of polymer-based human gene therapy in 1994. In this trial, autologous melanoma vaccines transfected with interleukin (IL)-2 pDNA were produced for stage 4 melanoma patients [33,34].

Over time, the use of whole viruses was supplanted by viral proteins. For instance, Lee et al. improved pDNA delivery by using a sulfhydryl-activatable listeriolysin O/protamine conjugate [35]. Similar conjugates with viral proteins like perfringolysin O were developed for pDNA delivery, facilitated by biotin-streptavidin conjugation [36]. A significant advancement was the modification of viruses, such as polylysine conjugated with the influenza virus hemagglutinin subunit HA2-derived synthetic fusion peptide and a galactose ligand for targeted delivery to hepatocytes [37,38]. Other innovations included attaching artificial endosomolytic peptides [39–43] and utilizing photochemical internalization for photosensitive release of co-internalized polyplexes [44–46] . Despite these advancements, research continued to develop newer polyplexes with inherent endolysosomal escape capabilities, leading to the development of second-generation polyplexes with built-in endolysosomal escape functionality.

7.2.2 Second Generation of Polycations

Early research by Jean-Paul Behr and his team, who were pioneers in recognizing the need for polycationic polymers with both high transfection efficiency and endosomal buffering capabilities, initiated extensive investigation into polymers that could function effectively as proton sponges [47,48]. First-generation polymers, such as polyhistidine and polyarginine, showed limited success, as they fully protonated at neutral pH despite demonstrating good transfection capabilities. Eventually, PEI was identified as a promising polycationic polymer due to its combination of high transfection efficiency and proton sponge capacity [49–52]. Following the discovery of PEI, research focused on enhancing its performance by exploring modifications, such as the development of branched and linear forms and varying its molecular weight. These modifications were instrumental in tuning specificity, cytotoxicity, and transfection efficiency. Modified PEI derivatives, particularly linear-chain forms, exhibited superior transfection efficiency compared to first-generation polymers like PLL and demonstrated effective endosomal escape [10,52].

Another notable second-generation polymer with endosomal escape properties is PAMAM dendrimers. Endosomal escape in these polymers was assessed using inhibitors or agonists of vesicular proton pumps located on endosomal membranes. For example, the proton pump inhibitor bafilomycin was shown to hinder transfection, while chloroquine, known for its self-protonation ability, enhanced transfection [53]. PAMAM dendrimers, however, demonstrated efficient pDNA transfer without the need for chloroquine, attributed to their pKa value of 6, which promotes protonation and subsequent osmotic pressure buildup within lysosomes, leading to their rupture and content release. Despite these advancements, both PEI and PAMAM were found to have drawbacks. While not inherently cytotoxic, increasing their molecular weight led to heightened cytotoxicity [54,55]. Additionally, these polymers are non-biodegradable, and some in vitro studies indicated activation of the complement system of innate immunity [56].

To address these limitations, amphiphilic cationic polymers were explored for their inherent endosomal escape capabilities. Initial work by Allan Hoffman led to the synthesis of pH-sensitive amphiphilic polymers containing hydrophobic alkyl and hydrophilic acidic carboxyl groups. These facilitated membrane disruption by increasing hydrophobicity due to protonation at acidic pH. Further development involved the polymerization of pyridyl disulfide acrylate (PDSA) with butyl acrylate and methacrylic acid, creating redox-sensitive and pH-dependent polymers that enhanced the cytosolic delivery of functional molecules, such as ASOs. However, these amphiphilic polymers lacked strong DNA-binding capabilities due to the absence of a cationic backbone. To address this, Rozema and colleagues synthesized amphiphilic cationic polyvinyl ethers by introducing amino groups to stabilize DNA complex formation. Alkyl groups containing one to four carbon atoms were added to disrupt cell membranes, with membrane-disruptive activity depending on the length of the carbon chain. Among these, polyvinyl ethers containing butyl groups demonstrated the highest nucleic acid transfection efficiency compared to ethers with shorter alkyl chains [57–60].

Key insights from the first two generations of polymers underscore the significance of charge, pKa, the proton sponge hypothesis, and endosomal escape. These concepts have been critical in advancing gene delivery and identifying factors necessary for stable gene delivery systems. However, challenges such as off-target effects, cytotoxicity, and the need for precision delivery have highlighted the necessity for further research. Ongoing efforts focus on modifying these polymers to achieve enhanced and more efficient gene delivery. As outlined in subsequent sections, the synthesis of biocompatible, biodegradable, and nanoparticle-shielding polymers—ideally derived from natural sources and produced with the highest precision—remains an essential area of research.

7.2.3 Third-Generation Polycations

Given the biocompatibility issues associated with first- and second-generation polycations in gene delivery, there has been a notable transition toward natural-based polymers. These polymers are advantageous due to their biodegradability and enhanced biocompatibility. Initial explorations in this area included chromosomal proteins such as HMG1 [61,62] and histones [63]. More recent advancements have utilized natural polymers like chitosan, protamine, cationic poly(aspartamide)s, and gelatin (a cationic variant of collagen) for gene therapy, particularly in mRNA delivery. Chitosan, derived from chitin through deacetylation, has demonstrated efficacy in forming polyplexes with mRNA, thereby protecting the genetic material and improving cellular uptake [64]. Protamine, an arginine-rich polypeptide, has been employed in RNA delivery since the 1960s, proving effective in RNA payload delivery. Cationic polymers from natural sources, such as poly(aspartamide)s, offer a safer alternative to traditional polycations, balancing biodegradability and endosomal escape with transfection efficiency.

Natural polymers have also been utilized for targeted mRNA delivery. For example, glucose-decorated nanocarriers have shown improved tumor uptake due to the overexpression of glucose transporters on tumor cells. This specificity, combined with natural polymers, enhances the precision and efficacy of gene therapy. Further exploration has included the use of histones and HMG1, either in their native forms or with modifications, as well as cationic forms of gelatin, such as atelocollagen. These have been investigated as gene delivery vectors and have demonstrated the ability to deliver siRNA effectively, particularly in bone metastatic tumors. CDs, carbohydrate-derived polymers, have also been studied for gene transfection. Modifications such as linear cationic β-CD-based polymers with amidine cross-linkages have improved performance [65]. Targeted delivery has been achieved through host-guest interactions between CDs and adamantane. Other modifications, such as tuning the cationic degree of CDs, have led to the synthesis of bio-cleavable polycationic polyrotaxanes, enhancing transfection efficacy. β-CD has also been used to mitigate the toxicity of PEI polyplexes and increasing transfection efficiency. Incorporating adamantane-PEG into PEI polyplexes has facilitated systemic nucleic acid delivery to the liver [66]. New-generation polymers, such as silk from silkworms and arachnids (e.g., *Nephila clavipes* and *Araneus diadematus*), have been explored for gene therapy due to their repetitive amino acid sequences that confer high mechanical strength [67]. For example, ultra-thin silk fibroin (SF) has been utilized for DNA delivery using a layer-by-layer approach on polystyrene templates, resulting in improved transfection efficiency in NIH/3T3 fibroblasts [68]. Zein, a phytoprotein found in maize, has been employed for DNA delivery owing to its hydrophobic nature, which is attributed to its high proline content [69]. Zein nanofibers have been effective in controlled siRNA delivery, achieving gene silencing in skin fibroblast cells for up to 72 hours [70]. Carbohydrates such as glycosides and xylitols have been studied for their ability to modulate membrane permeability through endosomal osmolysis. For instance, cross-linking a small percentage (3.9%) of xylitol diacrylate with PEI improved endosomal escape and cargo release by 50% [71]. Similarly, cross-linking glycerol with low- and high-molecular-weight PEI has shown that the low-molecular-weight variant offers better transfection, while the high-molecular-weight variant provides superior cellular uptake [72,73].

Synthetic polymers continue to be investigated for enhancing gene delivery efficacy through biodegradability. The inverse relationship between molecular weight and biocompatibility in polymers like PEI has led to the development of improved cationic polymers by assembling low-molecular-weight polymers into high-molecular-weight conjugates using bio-reversible linkages. This approach, employing hydrolysable ester bonds and other bio-reversible linkages, has enhanced endosomal escape and transfection efficiency. The trend in polymer design now focuses

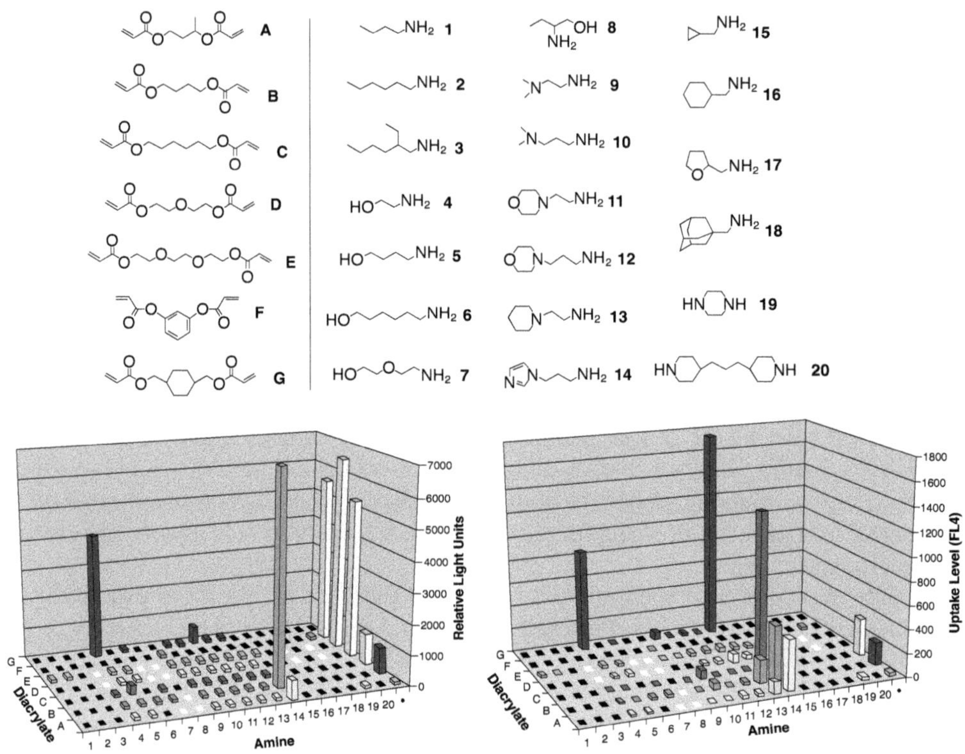

FIGURE 7.3 Transfection and cellular uptake data for the poly(β-amino ester) library synthesized using diacrylate (a–g) and amine (1–20) monomers. (Bottom panel left) Transfection efficiency assessed with pCMV-Luc (600 ng/well, DNA/polymer ratio 1:20). Light units are arbitrary and not normalized to total cell protein. Black squares represent water-insoluble polymers, while white squares indicate water-soluble polymers that did not complex with DNA. Control experiments include no polymer (gray), PEI (black) (DNA/polymer ratio 1:1), and Lipofectamine 2000 (light gray) at 0.1, 0.2, 0.4, and 0.6 μL quantities. (Bottom panel right) Cellular uptake of Cy5-labeled plasmid DNA (DNA/polymer ratio 1:20) was measured by median Cy5 fluorescence of cells (FL4 channel on the flow cytometer. Black squares denote water-insoluble polymers, while white squares represent water-soluble polymers that did not complex with DNA. Control experiments include no polymer (gray), PLL (black) (DNA/polymer ratio 1:1), and PEI (light gray) (DNA/polymer ratio 1:0.75) [77].

on optimizing transfection efficiency through advanced modification strategies. For example, the synthesis of hyperbranched n-PAEs and PBAEs via the Michael addition of amines to acrylate esters has yielded polymers with transfection efficiency comparable to PEI but with improved biocompatibility [74,75] (Figure 7.3). A combinatorial approach involving Michael addition was used by Robert Langer et al. They reacted various primary amines and secondary diamines with different bisacrylates, creating a library of 2,350 biodegradable cationic polymers. Extensive screening for transfection efficiency identified several promising candidates [76–78]. This approach was extended to other polymer libraries.

7.3 POLYMERIC NANOSTRUCTURES FOR GENE DELIVERY

In the realm of advanced materials and nanotechnology, various sophisticated systems have been developed to address diverse scientific and practical challenges. These systems, including micelles, polymersomes, and nanogels, offer unique properties and functionalities that can be tailored for specific applications. Understanding the characteristics and potential applications of each system is crucial for harnessing their full capabilities. The following subsections provide an overview of these advanced materials, exploring their structural attributes, formation processes, and potential uses in research and industry.

7.3.1 Polymeric Micelles

The design of polymeric micelles (PMs) for nucleic acid delivery has advanced significantly, incorporating various strategies to enhance efficacy and specificity. These strategies include selecting suitable polymeric materials, functionalizing PMs for targeted delivery, and optimizing micelle stability and loading capacity.

A key factor in PM design is the choice of polymeric materials. For example, poly(2-(dimethylamino) ethyl methacrylate) (PDMAEMA) forms micelles that facilitate cell internalization and enhance gene expression more effectively than traditional polyplexes [79]. This is due to PDMAEMA's ability to interact with cellular membranes, promoting endocytosis. Additionally, incorporating hydrophobic blocks into the micelle structure can improve stability under physiological conditions, enhancing nucleic acid delivery. Using poly(ε-caprolactone) (PCL) as a core material in PMs has shown effective siRNA delivery with minimal immune response in both in vitro and in vivo studies [80]. Enhancing targeting capabilities through functionalization is another critical strategy. Conjugating targeting ligands, such as folate receptors that are overexpressed in many cancer cells, allows PMs to selectively deliver nucleic acids to tumor tissues, improving specificity and minimizing off-target effects. The use of peptide ligands like angiopep-2, which can cross the blood-brain barrier, demonstrates the versatility of PMs in targeting different tissues, including brain tumors [81].

Ensuring PM stability is crucial for effective nucleic acid delivery. Stability can be enhanced through cross-linking polymer chains and incorporating hydrophobic molecules into the micelle core. These modifications protect nucleic acids from degradation and improve pharmacokinetics, extending circulation time in the bloodstream. The structural plasticity of PMs allows optimization of size, surface charge, and hydrophilicity, all of which are critical for cellular uptake and transfection efficiency. The use of cell membrane coatings is an emerging strategy to enhance the biocompatibility and targeting capabilities of PMs. By mimicking cell membranes, these biomimetic nanosystems evade immune detection and improve cellular uptake, making them promising for targeted drug delivery and gene therapy. Combining different nucleic acids, such as siRNA and mRNA, within a single PM can yield synergistic therapeutic effects. For instance, delivering siRNA targeting apoptosis inhibitory genes along with chemotherapeutic agents has shown enhanced efficacy in cancer treatment by targeting multiple disease pathways.

Charge-neutralized PMs can aggregate and precipitate, but PMs with positive charge ($N/P > 1$) are stable and facilitate cellular uptake through interaction with negatively charged cell membranes [82]. However, excess positive charge also increases nanoparticle toxicity, aggregation, and interactions with serum components, leading to rapid clearance from circulation. To mitigate these issues, conjugating cationic polymers with hydrophilic polymers (such as PEG) can enhance micellar stability, protect nucleic acids from nuclease activity, and reduce undesired interactions with blood components. PEGylation provides solubility and shields the positive charge, but it may also impair cell targeting and uptake due to steric hindrance and charge shielding. Optimal PEGylation is achieved with brush-like PEG topology and a chain length of at least 5 kDa. Studies on micelles composed of methoxy-poly(ethylene glycol)-poly(lactide)-oligoarginine (mPEG-PLA-Rx) reveal that PEG shielding affects charge density, PM stability, RNA loading, and cell uptake [83]. Shorter oligoarginine chains present less effective positive charge, and micelles with lower densities of these chains complex similar amounts of RNA as those with higher densities, indicating reduced surface charge availability. PEG shielding also makes longer cationic chains less resistant to displacement by heparin, highlighting the need for an optimal balance between shielding and functionality. To address PEG shielding limitations, sheddable PEG layers are often introduced. Examples include pH-sensitive systems that expose positive charges under acidic conditions, enhancing endosomal escape and drug release. However, PEGylation can induce immunogenicity, leading to rapid clearance and reduced drug bioavailability in some patients. Alternatives to PEG, such as pluronic, dextran, hyaluronic acid, chitosan, and polyoxazoline, offer potential for improved stability and efficacy without the associated immunogenicity. In the development of poly(2-ethyl-2-oxazoline)-co-poly (ethyleneimine)-poly(ε-caprolactone) (PEtOx-co-PEI-PCL) micelles, the hydrophilic PEtOx block reduces PEI-associated cytotoxicity and improves gene transfection efficiency [84]. PEtOx reduces PEI's cationic charge, and micelles with 60% hydrolyzed PEtOx-co-PEI-PCL showed better transfection efficiency and stability than 30% hydrolyzed ones, due to more free PEI. In MCF7 cells, PEtOx60% had higher transfection at N/P ratios of 20 and 30, while in MDA-MB-468 cells, significant transfection occurred at an N/P ratio of 8. Hydrolysis degree also impacted cell viability, with PEtOx60% having a greater effect. Another approach involved PEGylated micelles composed of fluorinated polypeptides with an amphiphilic triblock structure, such as poly(ethylene glycol)-poly(L-lysine)-poly(L-cysteine) (PEG-PLL-PCys) [85]. In this system, the PEG block reduces serum interactions, PLL condenses nucleic acids, and fluorinated PCys enhance cellular uptake and stability. Fluorine-rich regions promote supramolecular structure formation and improve cell permeability. These fluorinated polypeptides showed low toxicity and superior gene transfection efficiency compared to non-fluorinated micelles, PEI, or Lipofectamine 2000. Cationic polylactides have also been effective for pDNA delivery, outperforming non-PEGylated nanocomplexes with low toxicity and high biodegradability, though the PEG layer can hinder transfection by masking electrostatic interactions. To address this issue, PEG-detachable micelles carrying pDNA were developed. In this system, PEG was attached to cationic poly(aspartamide) copolymers modified with N-(2-aminoethyl)-2-aminoethyl groups through redox-sensitive disulfide linkages, forming micelles of 80–90 nm in size. These pDNA/PEGss-pAsp(DET) micelles showed nearly three times higher transfection efficiency in HeLa cells compared to PEG-pAsp(DET) micelles without disulfide linkages.

Minicircle DNAs (mcDNAs) offer enhanced gene delivery over traditional pDNA by lacking immune-triggering bacterial sequences and providing more efficient, long-lasting gene expression due to their smaller size. Several non-viral methods have been developed to deliver mcDNA effectively to target cells, including mcDNA/polycation nanocomplexes. One such example is micelles made from amphiphilic triblock poly(2-ethyl-2-oxazoline)-PLA-g-PEI (PEOz–PLA-g-PEI), where the PEG units are replaced by poly(2-ethyl-2-oxazoline) (PEOz), a biocompatible polymer [86]. These micelles demonstrated efficient mcDNA delivery, good hemocompatibility, and stability in serum. Furthermore, the potential for co-delivery of mcDNA vectors and chemotherapy was explored. DOX-loaded mcDNA micelles exhibited promising antitumor activity due to the synergistic effects of the chemotherapeutic agent DOX and the therapeutic mcDNA, and reflects the potential of micelles to successfully load and deliver both biologics as well as drugs.

Targeted mRNA delivery to cells using PMs has shown promise, with significant improvements in mRNA stability and expression observed in studies involving tumor models in mice. For instance, anti-angiogenic protein (sFlt-1)-encoding mRNA was loaded into PEG-polyaspartamide (PEG-PAsp) micelles derivatized with cholesterol, enhancing mRNA stability and expression and resulting in significant tumor growth inhibition in pancreatic tumor models [87]. Other approaches to improve RNA stability include pre-hybridizing mRNA with cholesterol-tethered oligonucleotides, which showed enhanced resistance to serum nucleases and improved protein expression while reducing immunogenicity. Furthermore, mRNA-loaded micelles have been explored as potential vaccines, such as for SARS-CoV-2, demonstrating robust immune responses following intramuscular injection. Various micelle-based systems, including those with redox-sensitive properties or pH-responsive functionalities, have been designed for RNA delivery, each tailored to specific therapeutic needs, such as cancer targeting or gene silencing. Overall, the integration of chemical modifications with innovative delivery systems continues to advance the field of nucleic acid therapeutics, though optimizing these systems for clinical applications remains a crucial challenge.

7.3.2 Polymersomes

Polymersomes have gained attention for nucleic acid delivery due to their unique structure, composed of amphiphilic block copolymers that self-assemble into bilayers. Their architecture includes a hydrophilic core for encapsulating nucleic acids and a hydrophobic membrane for protection and controlled release. These vesicles can be tailored to respond to stimuli like temperature, pH, or redox conditions, making them versatile carriers that facilitate cellular entry and release of therapeutic payloads. Their stability and customizable properties make polymersomes a promising option for nucleic acid delivery.

The early designs of polymeric vesicles for DNA delivery were inspired by DNA-polycation polyplexes, with a primary focus on modifying charged poly amino acids and PEI-based polymers to reduce toxicity while enhancing delivery efficiency. One notable example involved polymer vesicles made from poly(amino acid)s, specifically PLL and poly-L-ornithine, which were modified with palmitoyl and methoxy polyethylene glycol (mPEG). These vesicles demonstrated effective gene transfer capabilities to the lungs and liver in vivo, showcasing their potential for systemic delivery. Building on this approach, other researchers utilized galactosamine-targeted poly(ethylene oxide) (PEO) chains to deliver pCMVluc, which significantly increased luciferase expression in HepG2 cells. Similarly, vesicles composed of PEG-*b*-PEI-*b*-PA were developed to mediate GFP transgene expression in the liver following intravenous injection, highlighting the versatility and adaptability of these vesicle systems in targeting specific tissues. Further advancements in vesicle design included the development of cationic diblock copolymer vesicles, such as those made from poly(butadiene-*b*-N-methyl-4-vinylpyridinium) (PBD-*b*-P4VPQ). These vesicles effectively encapsulated and controlled the release of macromolecules, including dsDNA fragments, which facilitated the reverse transfection of plasmids into HeLa cancer cells. Another innovative approach involved polysaccharide-block-polypeptide copolymers like dextran-*b*-poly(γ-benzyl L-glutamate) (DEX-*b*-PBLG), which mimicked the structure of viral capsids and showed significant potential for gene delivery applications.

pH-sensitive diblock copolymer-based vesicles formed from PMPC-*b*-PDPA were designed to physically encapsulate pDNA through pH adjustments [88]. This strategy led to excellent colloidal stability, reduced cytotoxicity, and enhanced GFP expression levels in cells compared to traditional delivery methods. These various designs underscore the evolution of polymeric vesicles as promising carriers for gene delivery, combining innovative materials and functional modifications to improve their safety, stability, and efficiency. To improve cytosolic delivery, researchers developed triblock graft copolymers like lipopolysaccharide-amine (LPSA), which demonstrated high transfection efficiency in mesenchymal stem cells [89]. These triblock copolymers effectively delivered genetic material into cells, making them promising tools for gene therapy. Building on this approach, amphiphilic polyphosphazene-based polymersomes were formulated for systemic pDNA delivery, showcasing notable features such as serum stability, hemocompatibility, and significant tumor suppression in mice [90]. This formulation provided a robust platform for delivering genetic payloads in vivo with minimal toxicity. The exploration of pH-responsive triblock copolymers opened new avenues for targeted nucleic acid delivery. These polymers achieved efficient encapsulation and release of nucleic acids with cell-specific uptake, enhancing therapeutic outcomes. For example, folate-functionalized vesicles were specifically designed to increase uptake in cells overexpressing folate receptors, such as KB cells, thereby improving the precision and effectiveness of the delivery system [91]. Diblock copolymer-based polymersomes were prepared using mPEG-b-PLA, for the simultaneous delivery of multiple therapeutics [92]. These polymersomes co-delivered Bcl-xL siRNA and doxorubicin, a chemotherapy drug, into cancer cells. The combination of gene silencing and chemotherapeutic action resulted in a synergistic effect, significantly enhancing the overall efficacy against cancer cells. This approach highlights the potential of polymersomes as versatile and powerful platforms for multifaceted therapeutic interventions.

A recent innovation in the field of gene delivery involves the development of "dually gated" polymersomes designed specifically for the encapsulation and release of biologics like pDNA under specific environmental conditions. These advanced polymersomes were synthesized using a block copolymer-poly(ethyleneoxide)-block-poly[N-isopropylacrylamide-stat-7-(2methylacryloyloxyethoxy)-4-methylcoumarin-stat-2) (diethylamino)ethyl methacrylate] [PEO-*b*-P(NIPAM-stat-CMA-stat-DEA)] [93]. The hydrophilic PEO chains form the outer corona of the polymersome, while the dual gating is achieved through the temperature and pH-sensitive diblock polymer P(NIPAM-CMA), which creates a heterogeneous membrane. This dual sensitivity allows the encapsulation of pDNA and siRNA at room temperature, with the release of the cargo triggered by the proton sponge effect at acidic pH, facilitating effective intracellular delivery. This design demonstrated higher transfection efficiency of GFP-encoding pDNA compared to systems where pDNA was merely adsorbed rather than encapsulated within the polymersome. This dual-gated setup was also explored for siRNA encapsulation and delivery, representing a novel strategy to address challenges such as surface leakage and low stability in biological fluids, which had previously reduced the efficiency of delivery systems compared to PEGylated liposomes. Further advancing the field, Discher and colleagues pioneered the delivery of siRNA and ASOs using biodegradable block copolymers, including PEG-*b*-PCL, PEG-*b*-PLA, and PEG-*b*-PBD-based polymersomes [94]. These vesicles are capable of transforming into micelles to release their oligonucleotide cargo, effectively knocking down target genes both in vitro and in vivo. Another study utilized biodegradable PEG-*b*-PBD polymersomes for the delivery of ASOs, achieving efficient nuclear uptake and restoring dystrophin expression in mdx-dystrophic mice, highlighting their potential in gene therapy for muscular dystrophies. Amphiphilic α-tocopherol oligochitosan conjugate-based vesicles, termed oligomersomes, were developed to enhance siRNA uptake and target protein knockdown in cancer cells. Peptide-functionalized PBD-b-PEO vesicles achieved moderate siRNA knockdown by releasing their payloads in early endosomes, offering another pathway for targeted gene silencing. Triblock copolymer-based vesicles, such as PEG-b-PCL-b-DEX (PPD) combined with protamine, were shown to efficiently deliver siRNA to liver cells, demonstrating significant gene silencing and preferential liver accumulation in vivo [95].

Polymersomes have also been engineered for the co-delivery of therapeutics, such as the combination of Bcl-xL siRNA and doxorubicin in CPSomes, which showed enhanced efficacy in cancer treatment. pH-sensitive block copolymer vesicles, surface-decorated with targeting molecules, have been effectively used to deliver anticancer drugs and siRNA specifically to cancer stem cells. Additionally, polymeric vesicles based on diblock copolypeptides enabled rapid intracellular release of both chemotherapeutic drugs and siRNA, maximizing therapeutic impact. Recent advancements include the development of "boarding gate" and "debarkation gate" polymersomes, which facilitate controlled loading and release of nucleic acids. These siRNA-based vesicles, referred to as "siRNA-somes," have demonstrated cation-free, controlled payload delivery, showing synergistic therapeutic activity in multidrug-resistant cancer cells. These innovative systems represent a significant leap forward in the targeted and efficient delivery of nucleic acids, paving the way for more effective gene therapies.

7.3.3 Nanogels

Nanogels are hydrophilic, three-dimensional polymer networks that swell in aqueous environments and range from 20 to 200 nm in size, enabling them to penetrate biological barriers and target specific cells. Their stability in biological fluids and tunable physical and chemical properties make them promising carriers for gene therapy. Nanogels can encapsulate genetic materials, protect nucleic acids from degradation, and respond to stimuli like pH or temperature for controlled release. Composed of natural or synthetic polymers, nanogels are being optimized to enhance transfection efficiency and reduce cytotoxicity, though clinical studies remain limited. Nanogels typically have electrostatic interactions between their amine groups and the phosphate groups of nucleic acids. While non-charged nanogels face challenges in cellular uptake and endosomal escape, cationic nanogels, especially those with quaternary or high pKa amines, are favored for their efficient binding, pH-independent charge variation, and effective electrostatic interactions with nucleic acids. The type of amine, its structure, and valency play a critical role in enhancing these electrostatic interactions, which facilitate NA condensation within the nanogels [96]. A notable example is the amines found in spermine and spermidine from sperm whales, which are multivalent and aid in DNA condensation. The specific arrangement of primary and secondary amines within 3:4:3 and 3:4 carbon chains in spermine and spermidine, respectively, makes them ideal candidates for constructing polymeric vehicles [97,98]. The N/P ratio, indicating the balance between charged amine nitrogens in polymers and negatively charged phosphorus in nucleic acids, is crucial for optimizing nanogel encapsulation efficiency. The pKa of the amine group affects this efficiency by influencing amine accessibility under different pH conditions. While adding amines enhances binding, it must be carefully controlled to prevent excessive positive charge, which can hinder cargo release. Aminated nanogels can be synthesized through direct polymerization, cross-linking of aminated biopolymers, or post-synthesis conjugation using methods like activated esters, epoxy groups, or click chemistry [99–101].

In addition to electrostatic interactions, hydrophobic interactions and hydrogen bonding also play important roles in enhancing conjugation [102]. Nucleic acid bases are hydrophobic, and incorporating external hydrophobic moieties, such as surfactants like poly (ethylene glycol) dodecyl ether, can enhance nucleic acid self-assembly and condensation in nanogels. This approach creates varying densities of hydrophobic sites, leading to effective compaction of pDNA. Additionally, fluorescent siRNA nanogels can be synthesized by intercalating aromatic molecules, and hydrogen bonding in PEG-based nanogels can further aid nucleic acid compaction through interactions between PEG moieties and DNA bases [103]. Additionally, introducing phenolic groups can facilitate hydrogen bonding with the phosphate backbone of nucleic acids. This approach has been used in some siRNA-based nanogels, where tannic acid is introduced as a source of phenolic moieties to enhance hydrogen bonding and improve stability [104]. While physical attachments have been explored for loading cargo into nanogels, they often face challenges under physiological conditions, such as charge screening or competition with hydrogen bonding, which can result in leaky cargo release [105]. To ensure more robust and stable loading, chemical bonds are generally preferred. Once optimal loading of nucleic acids is achieved, it is crucial to ensure that the cargo is properly condensed and that the overall system size remains within the 50–500 nm range to enhance cellular uptake [105]. The size of the nanogel pores, as well as the size of the cargo, plays a critical role in determining whether the cargo will pass through the pores of the nanogel or remain restricted to its surface, which can significantly affect delivery efficiency.

DNA-*g*-PCL nanogels cross-linked with siRNA have demonstrated enhanced stability against RNase degradation, even under challenging conditions. Similarly, small oligonucleotides like miRNA show increased stability when encapsulated in nanogels, and proteins such as Cas9 maintain high stability in physiological environments [106]. Embedding nanogels in hydrogel matrices boosts protection and allows targeted, sustained drug delivery. For non-viral gene delivery, cellular uptake occurs via endocytic pathways, and polymeric carriers must escape endosomes before lysosomal degradation. Polycationic nanogels help this process by interacting with negatively charged cell membranes, aiding internalization. Non-viral transfectants can deliver genetic material to the cytoplasm but often cause cytotoxicity, including necrosis, apoptosis, and autophagy. Necrosis leads to inflammatory responses from irreversible damage, while apoptosis is a controlled process that eliminates damaged cells. Polycations can also induce autophagy, where autophagosomes degrade cytoplasmic components [107]. These pathways may be activated early during cellular uptake or later during endosomal escape and intracellular release, with enzymatic dysregulation being the primary cause of polycation transfection cytotoxicity. Before cell internalization, interactions between transporters and membrane phospholipids and proteins can cause structural disruptions, such as membrane thinning, curvature, and pore formation [108]. Polycations can alter membrane permeability by displacing phospholipid molecules, destabilizing the membrane structure. Although reversible destabilization is required for endosome formation during uptake, excessive charges can cause irreversible structural changes. Once internalized within endosomes, polycations need to escape before lysosomal degradation. Lysosomes play a critical role in cellular homeostasis and contain enzymes that can induce apoptosis or necrosis. Polymers with buffering capacities, such as PEI, can escape endosomes via the proton sponge effect, disrupting lysosomal function by altering the lysosomal mass/pH ratio [109,107]. Polycations can also disrupt the stability of essential organelles. For example, branched 25 kDa PEI has been reported to cause mitochondrial dysfunction and reduced ATP levels [110]. This bioenergetic stress results from reduced ATP production due to plasma membrane disruption, decreased mitochondrial membrane potential, and leakage of metabolites. Fluctuations in ATP levels can lead to cell death, and mitochondrial membrane disruption can trigger oxidative stress due to redox homeostasis disturbances. Carrier internalization can trigger simultaneous necrosis and apoptosis. In PEI-mediated cytotoxicity, necrotic changes occur within 30 minutes, followed by mitochondrial-mediated apoptosis after 24 hours [55]. Genetic materials themselves are non-toxic, making gene therapy safer than chemotherapy. Optimizing amine type, polycation architecture, and nanogel structure can reduce polycationic toxicity. Surface modifications, like stealth moieties and targeting ligands, extend circulation time and ensure tissue-specific accumulation [111]. Persistent nanogels may accumulate in organs, but smaller fragments are more easily excreted [112]. To minimize unwanted organ accumulation, nanogels should target specific cells, and encapsulating them within larger hydrogel structures can enhance controlled gene delivery [113,114]. Recently, Wang et al. designed an injectable hydrogel containing nanogels for anti-miRNA delivery as a treatment for intervertebral disc degeneration (IDD) [114]. The mechanical properties, along with ROS, pH, and enzyme responsiveness of peptide-containing dextran-based and chitosan-based hydrogels, ensure sustained delivery within the spine nucleus pulpous over 14 days, limiting cargo leakage and releasing therapeutic oligonucleotides only at the IDD inflammation site.

Aside from organ accumulation, long-term retention in cells after gene delivery can be toxic due to interactions with organelles and functional disruptions. Generally, biodegradable polymers are less toxic than their non-degradable counterparts [115]. Nanogels are designed to minimize cytotoxicity through adjustments to their mechanical properties and surface modifications.

Surface modifications, such as adding peptides or proteins, can improve nanogel uptake and endosome formation. For example, PNIPAM-based nanogels with tumor-specific peptides enhance cancer cell uptake, and R8 peptide-modified heparin nanogels increase transfection efficiency. Functionalizing nanogels with fusogenic peptides can also boost gene silencing. Biodegradable nanogels, made from materials like gelatin, PCL, or heparin, offer sustained release by degrading under physiological conditions, making them effective for gene knockdown. Stimuli-responsive nanogels release cargo in response to environmental changes, such as pH shifts or temperature increases, enhancing delivery efficiency [116]. Disulfide bonds, which cleave in the presence of reducing agents like glutathione, are another common method for controlled release within the reductive environment of cells. These smart nanogels provide precise control over therapeutic delivery, making them highly effective for gene and drug delivery applications. Nanogels are emerging as powerful carriers for gene therapy, with ongoing advancements in their design and modification strategies to enhance transfection efficiency, reduce cytotoxicity, and achieve controlled, targeted delivery. These innovations hold great potential for improving therapeutic outcomes in the treatment of genetic disorders.

7.4 OTHER NANOPARTICLES

7.4.1 PLGA-Based Nanoparticles

PLGA nanoparticles have emerged as a powerful tool in the field of gene therapy, offering a unique blend of biocompatibility, biodegradability, and protection for genetic material during delivery [117]. As an FDA-approved polymer, PLGA breaks down into lactic acid and glycolic acid, which are naturally metabolized by the body, making it an exceptionally safe and versatile carrier for therapeutic applications. However, there are several challenges associated with using PLGA nanoparticles as gene carriers. While PLGA nanoparticles can protect encapsulated DNA from degradation in the body, the release of DNA tends to be slow, and the neutral charge of PLGA can hinder the incorporation and delivery of DNA. Additionally, during the preparation of these nanoparticles, DNA may be exposed to high shear forces and organic solvents, which can lead to its inactivation. To address these issues, PLGA nanoparticles can be modified with various agents to reduce cytotoxicity, improve delivery efficiency, and target specific tissues or cells more effectively. For example, modifications with cationic groups like chitosan, dendrimers, PEI, PLL, PAMAM, CTAB, DOTAP, etc. have been explored. For instance, chitosan-coated PLGA nanoparticles have been used for mRNA delivery in a mouse model of cystic fibrosis, resulting in increased lung accumulation and improved lung function after intravenous injection. Similarly, blending or grafting PEI with PLGA results in stable, cationic carriers that can simultaneously complex with large nucleic acids, such as pDNA, as well as peptides. These hybrid carriers have demonstrated improved transfection efficiency compared to using branched PEI alone.

The versatility of PLGA nanoparticles extends to their surface, which can be modified with various ligands to improve targeting and delivery efficiency. PEGylation can increase nanoparticle stability and help evade the immune system. Further surface modifications with antibodies, peptides, or aptamers allow the nanoparticles to hone in on specific cells or tissues, thereby enhancing the precision of gene delivery. Recently, PLGA nanoparticles surface-modified with Tween 80 have been utilized to load and deliver PAMAM-conjugated siRNA, achieving successful delivery across the blood-brain barrier [118]. One of the standout features of PLGA nanoparticles is their capacity for controlled and sustained release of genetic material. By tweaking the ratio of lactic acid to glycolic acid in the polymer, as well as adjusting the molecular weight of PLGA, the degradation rate of the nanoparticles can be fine-tuned. This precise control over the timing of gene release is crucial, as it maximizes therapeutic efficacy while minimizing potential side effects. Wang's group developed a cationic lipid-assisted nanoparticle (CLAN) system composed of PLGA, PEG-PLGA, and a cationic lipid called N-bis(2-hydroxyethyl)-N-methyl-N-(2-cholesteryloxycarbonyl aminoethyl) ammonium bromide (BHEM-Chol) [119]. This system was designed to deliver mRNA encoding antigens for cancer immunotherapy. Their findings demonstrated that CLAN nanoparticles loaded with mRNA significantly enhanced the maturation of dendritic cells (DCs) and promoted the proliferation of antigen-specific T cells, both in vitro and in vivo, showcasing the potential of PLGA-based systems in stimulating an immune response. Similarly, Yasar and colleagues created a hybrid nanoparticle system featuring a PLGA core coated with either cationic lipid N-[1-(2,3-dioleyloxy) propyl]-N,N,N-trimethylammonium chloride (DOTMA) or chitosan, followed by complexation with mCherry-encoding mRNA [120]. They observed that while both nanoparticles exhibited comparable cellular uptake efficiency, the PLGA-lipid hybrid nanoparticles had superior transfection efficiency compared to the PLGA-chitosan variants. Moreover, the PLGA core's ability to encapsulate hydrophobic adjuvants enabled the hybrid system to achieve multi-modal delivery, enhancing its versatility and efficacy. Further advancements were made by Yang et al., who developed another core-shell structured PLGA-lipid hybrid nanoparticle for the co-delivery of antigen mRNA and adjuvants [121]. This hybrid nanovaccine was shown to effectively promote DC maturation and elicit a strong T-cell response, thereby improving the overall efficacy of cancer treatments.

The potential applications of PLGA nanoparticles in gene therapy are vast and varied, spanning cancer treatment, genetic disorders, and regenerative medicine. In the realm of cancer therapy, PLGA nanoparticles can deliver genes that encode tumor-suppressing proteins or silence oncogenes through the use of siRNA. For example, PLGA nanoparticles loaded with siRNA targeting PD-L1 have shown promise in enhancing the immune response against tumors by blocking the PD-1/PD-L1 pathway, which many cancer cells exploit to evade immune detection [7]. Dendrimer-lipid hybrid systems have shown promise for mRNA delivery. The Siegwart group developed a system combining dendrimer (5A2-SC8) with liposomal components (DOPE, cholesterol, PEG-lipids) for protein replacement therapy. This system effectively delivered fumarylacetoacetate hydrolase (FAH) mRNA, leading to extended survival in a mouse model of hepatorenal tyrosinemia type I with minimal toxicity. A notable modification involved a PLGA core encapsulating a TLR7 adjuvant and a lipid shell carrying antigen-encoding mRNA, enabling multifunctional delivery [122]. These innovations underscore the potential of PLGA-based nanoparticles as versatile carriers for gene therapy, improving treatment outcomes in diverse applications.

PLGA nanoparticles offer a promising vehicle for delivering corrective genes or CRISPR/Cas9 components to treat genetic disorders like cystic fibrosis and muscular dystrophy [123], where precise delivery and controlled release are essential. In regenerative medicine, they deliver growth factors and genes that promote tissue regeneration, such as bone morphogenetic proteins (BMPs) for bone repair. However, challenges remain, including efficient endosomal escape and minimizing off-target effects. Solutions include incorporating endosome-disruptive agents, pH-sensitive coatings, and optimizing nanoparticle size and charge to improve cellular uptake. There is growing interest in combining PLGA with lipids or inorganic nanoparticles to create hybrid systems with enhanced properties. Additionally, personalized medicine is driving the development of PLGA-based nanoparticles tailored to individual patients, offering a more precise and effective approach to treatment. PLGA nanoparticles demonstrate significant potential in gene therapy, enabling the controlled and safe delivery of genetic material across various diseases.

7.4.2 Chitosan-Based Nanoparticles

Chitosan-based nanoparticles are gaining attention in gene therapy due to their natural origin, biocompatibility, and ability to deliver genetic material effectively. Derived from chitin in crustacean shells, chitosan's cationic nature enables it to interact with negatively charged nucleic acids like DNA, RNA, and siRNA, forming stable complexes that protect genetic material from degradation. Their mucoadhesive properties make them particularly suitable for non-invasive delivery methods, such as nasal or oral administration. Additionally, chitosan's ability to open tight junctions between epithelial cells enhances permeation, facilitating the efficient delivery of genetic material across cellular barriers.

Surface modifications, such as PEG coating, can improve the circulation time of chitosan nanoparticles in the bloodstream, while targeting ligands like antibodies or peptides can direct them to specific cells or tissues. Chitosan's ability to promote endosomal escape via the proton sponge effect is also a critical advantage, ensuring that the genetic material reaches its target within the cell. Although challenges remain, such as variability in chitosan's molecular weight and potential toxicity, ongoing research is refining its properties. Chitosan nanoparticles are being explored in cancer therapy, regenerative medicine, and genome editing, positioning them as a promising platform for future gene therapy applications.

7.5 MECHANISM OF PNPS TO OVERCOME THE PHYSIOLOGICAL BARRIERS

PNPs are designed to overcome physiological barriers such as the extracellular matrix and cell membranes, which hinder drug and gene delivery. Through their adjustable size, surface properties, and targeting capabilities, these nanoparticles enhance cellular uptake, avoid immune detection, and improve delivery efficiency. Their ability to respond to environmental cues further enables controlled and precise therapeutic release.

7.5.1 Nucleic Acid Protection

Nucleic acid delivery holds great promise for diagnostics and therapeutics, but unmodified NAs are prone to enzymatic degradation, reducing their effectiveness. Conventional nanotechnology approaches, like arranging oligonucleotides on gold nanoparticles (Au NPs) or packaging NAs with DNA origami, help preserve NA integrity. However, DNA origami uses large amounts of dsDNA, limiting hybridization, and Au NPs require a chemically uniform core, restricting diversity. PNPs offer a promising alternative by overcoming these limitations. For example, polymeric micellar nanoparticles are designed to tightly pack nucleic acids, making them resistant to nuclease digestion. This dense packing provides steric hindrance, reducing DNA accessibility to nucleases and thereby protecting the nucleic acids during delivery, enhancing their therapeutic potential [124]. PNPs serve as a versatile platform for gene therapy by encapsulating and safeguarding nucleic acids from degradation, efficiently delivering them into cells while minimizing toxicity [125]. Innovative delivery systems like polymeric-lipid hybrid nanoparticles (PLNs) combine the advantages of both PNPs and liposomes, enhancing therapeutic efficacy. These hybrid nanoparticles address challenges such as structural disintegration and material leakage, ensuring the stability of nucleic acids during delivery [126]. Additionally, degradable PNPs can self-assemble with pDNA to form stable complexes suitable for gene transfer applications, aiming to efficiently deliver nucleic acids into cells while reducing cytotoxicity [15]. Polymeric vehicles have been extensively studied for nucleic acid delivery, highlighting the crucial role of polymers in transporting genetic material [127]. In gene therapy, PNPs offer several advantages over traditional viral vectors, addressing safety concerns associated with viral methods. PEI and dendrimers provide safer alternatives, while polyester-based nanocarriers such as PLGA and PLA are promising due to their biocompatibility and biodegradability, which protect nucleic acids from degradation [112]. Targeted PNPs have also transformed cancer gene therapy [128] by improving the specificity and efficacy of gene delivery, allowing for better targeting of cancer cells and enhanced therapeutic outcomes [129]. Additionally, stimulus-sensitive PNPs have been developed for drug and gene delivery, offering precise control over the release of therapeutic agents. Incorporating stimuli-responsive elements into PNPs allows for controlled genetic material release, ensuring optimal therapeutic effects [130]. PNPs enhance gene therapy by preventing nucleic acid degradation, improving stability, resisting nuclease digestion, and enabling targeted delivery into cells.

7.5.2 Enhanced Blood Retention Time

To enhance blood retention time for successful gene therapy, PNPs employ several strategies to prolong their circulation in the bloodstream. One key approach is PEGylation, which reduces nonspecific interactions with blood proteins, evades immune system recognition, and extends circulation time, thereby enhancing therapeutic efficacy [131]. PEGylation prevents nanoparticle aggregation and supports targeted tissue accumulation, while shielding cationic particles with polyanions reduces nonspecific interactions and enhances circulation time. Hydrophilic polymer modification improves steric stability, and optimizing particle size helps avoid rapid renal filtration and immune clearance, prolonging bloodstream presence [132]. Incorporating specific ligands or targeting moieties on the surface of PNPs further extends their circulation time by enhancing interactions with biological targets. For instance, ligand-directed active tumor-targeting nanoparticles have shown significantly longer blood retention, increased tumor accumulation, and improved therapeutic outcomes compared to non-targeted nanoparticles [133]. The protein corona around PNPs affects their interaction with biological entities, influencing circulation time and biodistribution. Its composition can change the nanoparticles' synthetic identity, impacting retention and excretion rates [134]. By controlling protein corona formation, nanoparticles can be tailored for better blood retention and therapeutic outcomes in gene therapy. Overall, strategies like PEGylation, size optimization, targeting ligands, and protein corona modulation enhance nanoparticles' bioavailability and efficacy for gene delivery.

7.5.3 Targeting Strategies

Active and passive targeting are key strategies used by PNPs in gene therapy to improve specificity, efficacy, and therapeutic outcomes. *Active targeting* involves functionalizing nanoparticles with ligands or targeting moieties that bind to specific receptors or biomarkers on target cells, enhancing cellular uptake and intracellular delivery of genetic material [129]. For example, EGFR-targeted PNPs have demonstrated improved tumor-specific transfection and increased survival rates compared to non-targeted nanoparticles, highlighting the effectiveness of active targeting in gene therapy [129]. *Passive targeting* relies on the physicochemical properties of nanoparticles and the enhanced permeability and retention (EPR) effect at tumor sites, allowing selective accumulation in cancerous tissues [135]. PNPs use passive targeting to exploit tumors' leaky vasculature, improving drug accumulation and reducing off-target effects. Combining passive and active targeting, such as conjugating ligands to target cancer cell receptors, maximizes therapeutic efficacy by integrating both strategies [136].

- Designing PNPs with stimuli-responsive properties allows for precise gene delivery, responding to tumor-specific stimuli like pH, redox conditions, or enzymes to trigger genetic material release at the target site, enhancing specificity and reducing off-target effects. Macrophages, as antigen-presenting cells, are key targets for immunotherapy. M1 macrophages can be reprogrammed via targeted mRNA delivery to treat conditions like rheumatoid arthritis, while M2 macrophages (or tumor-associated macrophages, TAMs) involved in tumor progression can be reprogrammed for antitumor therapies [137]. For example, using PBAE-based nanocarriers with di-mannose ligands, the delivery of two mRNAs (IRF5 and IKKβ) reprogrammed 28% more TAMs in vitro compared to non-targeted nanocarriers. This approach was effective in three cancer models and in vitro with human macrophages, showing significant accumulation in organs like the spleen, liver, and lungs. The study also highlighted the need to assess potential side effects of repeated mRNA dosing [138].

Targeting T cells with PNPs can be achieved by incorporating ligands that interact with receptors like CD3 antibodies, facilitating targeted delivery and enhancing cellular uptake. Ligand-based designs can also exploit tumor-specific antigens like CD105 or αVβ3 integrins to improve localization and therapeutic impact within the tumor microenvironment. Optimizing polymeric carriers, such as tuning polyester-based carriers for organ-specific targeting, can further enhance the efficacy of T-cell therapies [126]. PNPs also effectively target DCs by functionalizing their surfaces with ligands like CD11c antibodies. DC-specific antigens, such as CD11c or mannose receptors, offer precise delivery options. PEI nanoparticles with surface-expressed mannose have shown potential in delivering antigens to DCs, a method already being explored in clinical trials for mRNA delivery. Optimizing carrier design to selectively target DCs can enhance immune modulation, with promising therapeutic applications. PNPs provide versatile platforms for targeting macrophages, T cells, and DCs by exploiting specific ligands, antigens, and tailored carrier designs, offering potential for improving immune responses and therapeutic outcomes across disease settings.

7.5.4 Immune System Evasion and Activation

PNPs enhance gene therapy efficacy through sophisticated immune evasion mechanisms. Surface modifications (PEG) or cell membrane-derived components effectively shield nanoparticles from immune recognition, prolonging systemic circulation and reducing immune clearance [139,140]. Additionally, functionalizing nanoparticles with specific ligands facilitates targeted interactions with cellular receptors, enhancing cellular uptake and intracellular delivery of genetic material while minimizing immune detection [129]. Stimuli-responsive nanoparticles further refine delivery precision by remaining inert in circulation and releasing their cargo in response to specific tumor microenvironmental triggers, thereby minimizing off-target effects and evading immune detection during circulation [141,142]. Furthermore, the integration of immune-modulating agents or RNA interference (RNAi) within nanoparticles can counteract immune evasion strategies of tumor cells. This approach can modulate immune checkpoint pathways and promote immune cell infiltration, enhancing the antitumor immune response and improving the therapeutic efficacy of gene delivery [143,144]. PNPs leverage immune evasion strategies, including surface functionalization, targeted delivery, stimuli-responsive release, and immune modulation, to optimize gene delivery and improve therapeutic outcomes.

7.6 ENDOLYSOSOMAL ESCAPE

Endolysosomal escape refers to the process by which substances, such as therapeutic drugs, nanoparticles, or viral particles, escape from the endosome or lysosome compartments within a cell into the cytoplasm. This escape is crucial for the effectiveness of many therapeutic strategies, as it allows the delivered molecules to reach their target sites within the cell and exert their intended effects. To avoid endolysosomal degradation, strategies can either enhance endolysosomal escape, bypass these organelles entirely, or evade lysosomal degradation. The endosome-lysosome pathway degrades nanoparticles, reducing the efficacy of encapsulated biologics. The goal is to escape these compartments quickly, with mechanisms involving movement across the endosomal/lysosomal membrane (Figure 7.4).

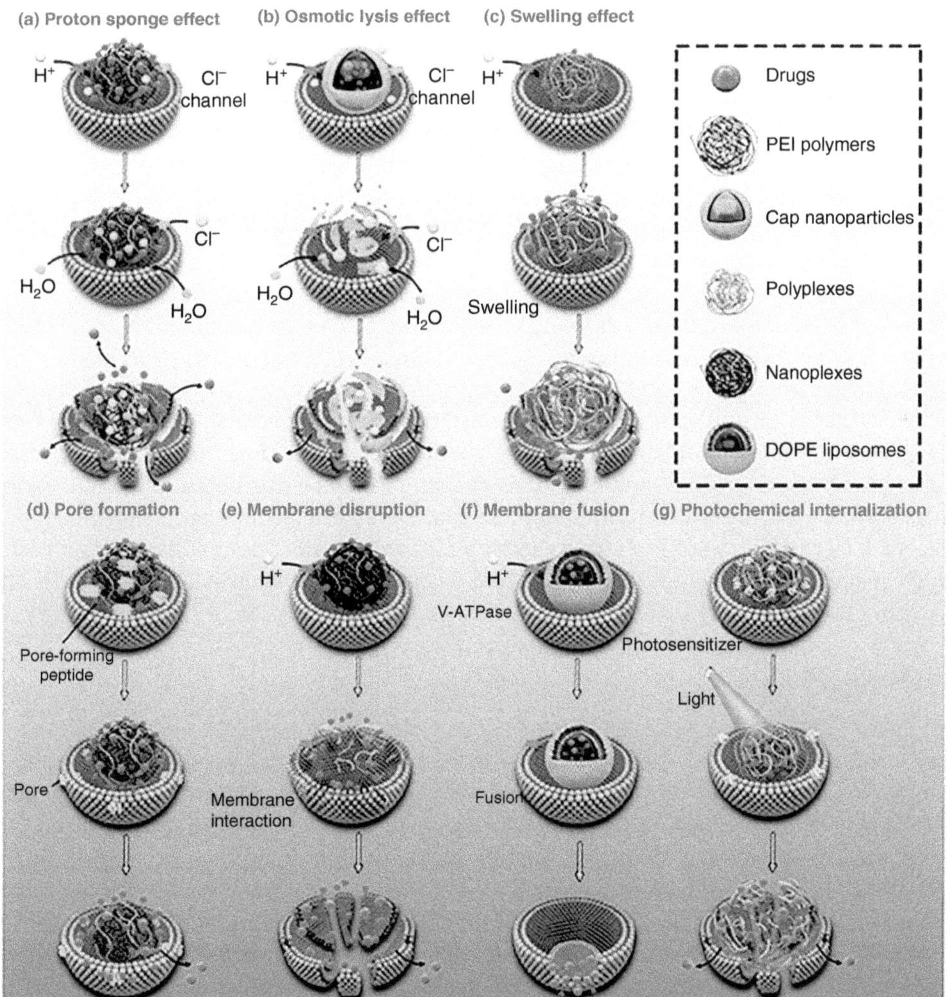

FIGURE 7.4 Schematic overview of mechanisms facilitating endosomal escape, including the proton sponge effect, osmotic lysis, swelling, pore formation, membrane disruption, membrane fusion, and photochemical internalization.

7.7 MECHANISMS FOR ENDOLYSOSOMAL ESCAPE

7.7.1 Proton Sponge Effect

This utilizes cationic materials with protonated amino groups to buffer within a physiological pH range. It leads to continuous proton pump activity, accumulation of chloride ions, water influx, swelling, and eventual rupture of lysosomes, releasing the nanocarriers [145]. The whole concept of this theory is based on the buffering effect and capacity of polycationic common materials including PEI [146], PLL [147,148], PAMAM dendrimers [149], urocanic acid-modified chitosan [150], and polymers composed of secondary or tertiary amines so that they can be protonated accordingly at low pH of endosomes/lysosomes.

Poly (histidine arginine) linked with chitosan shows strong lysosomal escape abilities. Triblock copolymers like PEG-PCL-PEI [151] and PAMAM/carbon dot nanohybrids [152] also enhance escape via this effect. Conjugation of ligand-mediated endocytosis via complexing pDNA with transferrin-conjugated PLL and gluconic acid helped in enhancing the DNA-mediated condensation and also a suitable ligand for facilitated endocytosis. Here the buffering capacity was provided by gluconic acid-modified polyhistidine that contains imidazole groups with pKa of 6.15 that enhanced the buffering capacity. Using histidyl groups for enhancing the endolysosomal escape ability of PLL was also explored to enhance the transfection efficiency. Lee et al. [152] developed rod-shaped nanoparticles by bundling Janus base nanotubes (JBNTs) with RNA payloads incorporated through charge interactions. These JBNTs/RNA nanoparticles demonstrated efficient cellular entry via macropinocytosis, similar to lipid nanoparticles. Additionally, due to their noncovalent structure and DNA-like chemistry, which enhance the proton sponge effect, JBNTs/RNA nanoparticles exhibited improved endosomal escape capabilities, akin to cationic polymers. Chen et al. [153] created metal-phenolic networks using tannic acid and FeIII or AlIII, providing versatile and non-toxic modifications to facilitate endosomal/lysosomal escape through the proton sponge effect. The efficiency of lysosomal escape was found to be proportional to the amount of material used [154]. Achieving effective transfection requires a substantial excess of polymers, often leading to dose-limiting toxicity in vivo.

The theory of the proton sponge effect in transfection is controversial. Evidence indicates that increasing amine groups to enhance buffering capacity can sometimes reduce transfection efficiency compared to the original polymer. This reduction may be attributed to limited endosomal escape, as adding a membrane disruption peptide can restore transfection efficiency. Further modifications, such as acetylation of PEI, have shown increased transfection efficiency despite reducing buffering capacity. This is believed to result from changes in vector unpacking, endocytic trafficking, or polymer lipophobicity.

7.7.2 Osmotic Lysis

Osmotic lysis occurs when pH-responsive nanoparticles disassemble in acidic lysosomal environments, leading to osmotic shock and membrane rupture. For example, the low acidic pH of endosomes was utilized for the disintegration of nanoparticle composed of diblock polymers like PMPC-*b*-PDPAEMA into its constituent monomers which subsequently led to the increase in osmotic pressure inside the endosome leading to their rupture and thus promoting the release of cargo. To facilitate from this mechanism of osmotic lysis ammonium-based nanoparticles were synthesized using quaternary triblock polymers for the delivery of siRNA [mPEG45-P(DPA50-co-DMAEMA56)-PT53] [155]. These nanoparticles switched from hydrophobic to hydrophilic under acidic pH due to protonation that led to their disintegration, thus releasing the siRNA and enhanced gene silencing activity. Calcium phosphate is a natural inorganic biomaterial that aids in osmotic lysis by the release of majorly Ca^+ and $H_3PO_4^-$ ions under acidic conditions that facilitates the release of cargo by altering the osmotic balance in lysosomes; however, CAP itself as a nanocarrier faces several challenges in the form of lack of tissue specificity, uncontrolled expansion in biological fluids, etc., and therefore natural polymers in the form of hyaluronic acid, chitosan, or else PEG have been incorporated along with CAP to enhance the transfection efficiency of the system as an ensemble [156,157]. Some of the manifestations of the above modification strategy involve alendronate-hyaluronic acid (AHA)-CAP-siRNA nanocarriers which involves AHA-coated CAP nanoparticles, where the coating is facilitated by chelation of calcium and phosphate ions. The mechanism of release of the internalized siRNA followed the same pattern where acidic pH was a trigger for the endosomal/lysosomal escape.

7.7.3 Swelling Effect

Nanoparticles designed to swell at low pH disrupt the lysosomal membrane through volumetric expansion. This effect has also been termed as "umbrella hypothesis" where the swelling nanoparticles are compared with a growing umbrella and the volumetric expansion of nanocarriers breaks open the lysosomal wall, promoting escape [158]. However, the exact reason of swelling is still not clear and the role of cross-linking density of polymers and considering polymers with a larger expansion coefficient should be considered. For example, nanoparticles synthesized using PEGDMA [159] as cross-linkers exhibit a two-fold increase under acidic conditions, mostly due to the electrostatic interactions followed by solvation of charged materials under the acidic pH conditions, releasing the encapsulated ovalbumin into the cytoplasm. Likewise, nanoparticles that can show about 100 times expansion were formulated and have been applied for delivering drugs to treat lung cancer. However, challenges exist as there lies an inverse relationship between cross-linking density and swelling, so a low cross-linking polymer has a better transfection efficiency which also means that higher cross-linking makes the nanoparticle stable so that it cannot react in a pH-dependent swelling manner, also the expansion coefficient is a crucial factor as it determines if the swelling of nanoparticles is enough to break open the lysosomes. All these factors must be considered while designing nanoparticles administering swelling effect.

7.7.4 Directly Evading Endolysosomal Pathways

Cell Membrane Penetration: Some nanocarriers evade endocytosis by directly merging with the cell membrane, entering the cytoplasm without interacting with endosomes or lysosomes, akin to viral transduction. For instance, siRNA nanocarriers can use porous silicon nanoparticles functionalized with fusogenic lipids to facilitate membrane fusion, or fusogenic exosomes modified with vesicular stomatitis virus fusion proteins to merge with the plasma membrane [160]. These fusogenic lipids enable fusion independently of receptor-mediated pathways, bypassing traditional endocytosis mechanisms.

Cell Membrane-Coated Nanoparticles: Coating nanoparticles with membranes derived from blood, bacterial, or tumor cells allows them to fuse with target cell membranes [161]. Examples include hydrophobic quantum dots coated with red blood cell membranes, silica nanoparticles coated with leukocyte membranes, or nanoparticles with cores made from PLGA or PCL [162,163].

Cell-Penetrating Peptides (CPPs): Utilized for their ability to penetrate membranes and facilitate direct cytoplasmic entry, various nanoparticles have been engineered for this purpose. For instance, nanoparticles incorporating polyarginine-rich motifs (R4 to R9) are designed for the direct cytosolic delivery of siRNA [164]. Although inorganic nanoparticles, such as Au NPs, are commonly employed, membrane modifications with tetrapeptides have also been used to enhance direct penetration beyond the cytosol and avoid endolysosomal degradation. However, the precise mechanism of these processes remains unclear, and it is uncertain whether the transfer exclusively occurs through membrane fusion. Examples include polyarginine-stabilized nano-capsules (NPSCs) for siRNA delivery and "MEND" carriers with tetrapeptides for pDNA delivery [165].

Endosome-Golgi/ER Pathway: Some nanoparticles exploit non-degradative pathways to avoid endosomal and lysosomal degradation. For example, KDEL is a peptide signal that facilitates translocation through the ER-Golgi membranes [166]. Au NPs containing siRNA have been engineered to express the retrograde transfer signal KDEL, directing them to the Golgi-ER complex. To enhance this process, nanoparticles derived from the ER membrane of cancer cells have been designed to mimic targeting strategies and evade the endosomal pathway. However, a significant challenge with this approach is scalability, as maintaining batch uniformity can be difficult, necessitating further research to address this issue. For instance, histone-targeted polyplexes utilize the endosome-Golgi/ER pathway for nuclear transport.

Various strategies for endolysosomal escape offer distinct advantages and limitations. While direct membrane penetration shows potential, it requires additional research to reduce cytotoxicity and improve specificity. Combining different approaches might yield the most effective results for nano-drug delivery and gene therapy applications. Interdisciplinary collaboration is crucial for designing advanced nanocarriers with high efficacy.

7.8 CLINICAL TRIALS INVOLVING PNPS

Approximately 2,000 clinical trials dedicated to gene therapy have been approved globally, with 38 therapies receiving global approval. Among these, 13 therapies were approved for in vivo gene expression to replace missing or faulty genes, including treatments like Gendicine, Oncorine, Rexin-G, Neovasculgen, Glybera, Imlygic, Luxturna, Collategene, Zolgensma, Comirnaty, Spikevax, Delytact, and Zycov-D. Additionally, 14 therapies were designed as in vivo gene interference systems primarily aimed at downregulating harmful genes, including Vitravene, Kynamro, Exondys 51, Spinraza, Apligen, Tegsedi, Onpattro, Vyvondys 53, Waylivra, Givlaari, Oxlumo, Viltepso, Leqvio, and Amondys 45. Furthermore, another 14 formulations are used for ex vivo cell therapies, such as Zalmoxis, Strimvelis, Kymriah, Yescarta, Invossa, Zynteglo, Tecartus, Libmeldy, Breyanzi, Abecma, ARI-001, Carteyva, Skysona, and Carvykti.

The data and trends indicate that most gene therapies are directed toward treating cancer, infectious diseases, or genetic disorders. Approximately 70% of these therapies use viral vectors, while the remaining 30% involve non-viral systems, typically manifested as naked/pDNA or lipid-based formulations. Clinical trials utilizing PNPs for gene therapy are at the forefront of cutting-edge research, offering promising pathways for advanced therapeutic interventions, particularly in cancer treatment and immunotherapy, notably for HIV. These trials focus on using nanoparticles to deliver genetic material, aiming to enhance the precision and effectiveness of gene-based therapies. Many of these trials are based on PEI systems, especially in cancer and HIV immunotherapy. A significant example is a Phase I trial conducted by Davis et al., which investigated the systemic administration of siRNA via targeted nanoparticle delivery in patients with solid tumors [167]. This study aimed to assess the safety and efficacy of siRNA delivery using nanoparticles, highlighting the growing interest in nanotechnology for gene therapy. However, the trial was terminated due to dose-limiting toxicities, including elevated creatinine and blood urea nitrogen levels, illustrating the challenges associated with this approach. There have been ten clinical studies that were terminated earlier than planned, with few or no participants, due to various reasons: recruitment issues (e.g., NCT01413087, NCT00614640), lack of efficiency (NCT03719300), or strategic business decisions (e.g., NCT00137865, NCT03065023, NCT03739138, NCT02828098, NCT04777708). Despite these setbacks, research into PEI-based clinical trials has continued, with 14 new trials initiated since 2018, though most results are still pending publication. Many of these trials explore pDNA systems using commercially available jetPEI, a cationic 22 kDa linear polymer.

Efforts in clinical trials are also exploring nanoparticle-based siRNA delivery for cancer therapy, demonstrating the broad potential of nanocarriers to improve therapeutic outcomes. However, the clinical success of these gene therapy strategies is often hindered by several challenges, including strong immune responses and hypersensitivity reactions, which are major factors in trial failures. The most commonly explored routes of administration in these trials are local, including intraperitoneal, intratumoral, intravesical, intramuscular, or topical delivery. Currently, only one formulation under clinical trial utilizes intravenous administration (NCT01435720). Among the various nanoparticle systems, several cationic polyethyleneimine (PEI)-based platforms, such as BC-819/PEI, BC-819, and DTA-H19, have been developed for clinical trials targeting different cancer types through local administration [168]. However, the substantial cytotoxicity observed with PEI polymers at the pre-clinical level has limited their clinical application, prompting the exploration of modified versions to mitigate these effects. One such modification involved the use of glycosylated JetPEI in CYL-02, designed to deliver plasmids encoding SSTR2 and DCK::UMK to suppress tumor cell proliferation and enhance tumor cell chemosensitivity to gemcitabine, respectively [169]. Notably, this approach resulted in only mild treatment-related toxicities [169].GEN-1 is a gene therapy for ovarian cancer that uses pDNA encoding IL-12 subunits, delivered via a non-viral lipopolymer vector [170]. This vector forms stable nanoparticles, enhancing nucleic acid delivery and stability. In animal models, GEN-1 extended survival and inhibited tumor growth. Clinical trials confirm its safety with mild side effects and show improved outcomes when combined with chemotherapy, especially in platinum-sensitive cases. Ongoing trials are testing its effectiveness with neoadjuvant chemotherapy and for second-look laparoscopy. DermaVir, a novel HIV treatment, utilizes pDNA encoding 15 HIV-1 proteins complexed with mannobiose-conjugated linear polyethylenimine (LPEI) of 22 kDa. This formulation, with a 3% grafting degree and an N/P ratio of three, forms stable nanoparticles under 200 nm, stabilized with 10% mannitol. Applied via the DermaPrep procedure to enhance transfection of Langerhans cells, DermaVir was well tolerated in Phase I (NCT00712530) and Phase I/II (NCT00270205) trials, showing increased HIV-specific memory T cells and sustained effects for up to a year. Further studies (NCT00711230, NCT00918840) demonstrated its safety and efficacy, with repeated doses leading to viral load reduction and improved immune responses in HIV-infected individuals. Genetic Immunity, the company developing DermaVir, announced plans for a Phase III clinical trial starting in 2021 in Russia, aiming to obtain marketing approval.

These examples highlight the potential and challenges of PNPs in gene therapy. Despite their promise for targeted gene delivery, issues such as cytotoxicity, immune responses, and the need for safety and efficacy enhancements remain critical hurdles. Similarly, lipid-based nanoparticles have shown versatility in clinical trials for chemo-immunotherapy, underscoring the broad potential of nanoparticle formulations in cancer treatment and the importance of evaluating various types for effective therapies. In ocular diseases, clinical trials are exploring supra-choroidal delivery of gene and cell therapies, demonstrating the diverse applications of nanotechnology beyond oncology.

However, the current number of clinical trials involving non-viral gene therapy nanocarriers remains limited, with few FDA-approved platforms. Ongoing trials, detailed in Table 7.1, reflect

TABLE 7.1
Overview of Clinical Trials Involving Nanovehicle Systems for Gene Delivery

Nanovehicle System	Cargo	Disease/Target Organ	Administration Route	Phase	Status	Identifier
CD NP with PEG	siRNA (RRM2)	Solid tumor	Systemic (IV)	I	Terminated	NCT00689065
PEI NP	pDNA (diphtheria toxin A)	Superficial bladder cancer	Local	II	Completed	NCT00595088
PEI NP	pDNA (diphtheria toxin A)	Superficial bladder cancer	Local	I	Completed	NCT01878188
PEI NP	pDNA (diphtheria toxin A)	Ovarian cancer	Systemic (IP)	I/II	Completed	NCT00826150

(*Continued*)

TABLE 7.1 (*Continued*)
Overview of Clinical Trials Involving Nanovehicle Systems for Gene Delivery

Nanovehicle System	Cargo	Disease/Target Organ	Administration Route	Phase	Status	Identifier
PEI NP	pDNA (diphtheria toxin A)	Pancreatic cancer	Local	II	Terminated	NCT01413087
PEI NP	pDNA (diphtheria toxin A)	Non-muscle invasive bladder cancer	Local	II	Active	NCT03719300
PEI NP	pDNA (diphtheria toxin A)	Superficial bladder cancer	Local	I/II	Completed	NCT00393809
PEI NP	pDNA (diphtheria toxin A)	Pancreatic neoplasms	Local	I/II	Completed	NCT00711997
JetPEI	pDNA (SSTR2 + DCK::UMK)	Pancreatic cancer	Local	I	Completed	NCT01274455
JetPEI	pDNA (SSTR2 + DCK::UMK)	Pancreatic cancer	Local	II	Recruiting	NCT02806687
JetPEI	RNA (DDX58 activator)	Solid tumor	Local	I	Active	NCT03739138
JetPEI	dsRNA (TLR-3, MDA5, RIG-I agonist)	Solid tumor	Local	I	Active	NCT02828098
PEG-PEI-cholesterol	pDNA (IL-12)	Ovarian cancer	Systemic (IP)	I	Terminated	NCT00137865
PEG-PEI-cholesterol	pDNA (IL-12)	Ovarian cancer	Systemic (IP)	I	Completed	NCT00473954
PEG-PEI-cholesterol	pDNA (IL-12)	Fallopian tube/ peritoneal/ ovarian cancer	Systemic (IP)	II	Completed	NCT01118052
PEG-PEI-cholesterol	pDNA (IL-12)	Fallopian tube/ peritoneal/ ovarian cancer	Systemic (IP)	I	Completed	NCT01489371
PEG-PEI-cholesterol	pDNA (IL-12)	Fallopian tube/ peritoneal/ ovarian cancer	Systemic (IP)	I	Active	NCT02480374
PLGA NP	siRNA (KRASG12D)	Pancreatic cancer	Local	I	Completed	NCT01188785
PLGA NPs	siRNA (KRASG12D)	Pancreatic cancer	Local	II	Recruiting	NCT01676259
PEI carrier	siRNA (eIF5A) pDNA (eIF5AK^{50R})	Myeloma/ lymphoma/ leukemia	Systemic (IV)	I/II	Unknown	NCT01435720

The table details various nanovehicle systems used in clinical trials, including their cargo, target diseases or organs, administration routes, clinical phases, trial statuses, and identifiers. It highlights the diversity of applications and ongoing research in using polymeric nanoparticles for targeted gene therapy.

progress but also emphasize the need for further research. Overall, the advancement of polymeric and lipid-based nanoparticles in gene therapy marks significant progress in personalized medicine. Continued research and clinical validation are crucial to fully realize the therapeutic potential of these nanoparticle-based delivery systems.

7.9 CONCLUSION

7.9.1 Challenges and Considerations

Despite advancements, several challenges need to be addressed to realize the full potential of PNPs in gene therapy. One major hurdle is the complexity of the biological environment, which can affect the stability and delivery efficiency of nanoparticles. Overcoming biological barriers such as the cellular membrane, endosomal escape, and avoiding immune detection are critical areas of ongoing research. For example, the protein corona on nanocarriers significantly impacts their physicochemical properties and delivery efficiency. The adsorption of proteins, like bovine serum albumin on PEI/mRNA complexes, can alter translation. The protein corona, being dynamic and environment-dependent, affects how polymeric nanocarriers interact with cells and their biodistribution in vivo. For instance, proteins on mRNA-loaded lipid nanoparticles influence their targeting to organs like the liver, spleen, or lungs. Understanding these effects can lead to improved delivery strategies. PMs, with minimal protein adsorption due to high PEG density, offer advantages in controlling biodistribution and targeting.

Improving delivery efficacy involves the development of more sophisticated targeting strategies. Ligand-receptor interactions, antibody conjugation, and aptamer-based targeting are some methods being explored to enhance specificity and reduce off-target effects. However, it is crucial to consider the risks of off-target effects that may arise due to variations in particle size, surface charge, or protein corona formation in the bloodstream. The current body of research on the use of targeting ligands in polymeric formulations for mRNA delivery is limited. Although there is significant interest in targeting therapeutic agents to the brain and studies have explored receptor-mediated drug uptake, there have been no reported systemic mRNA delivery studies using this method. Optimizing the requirements for ligands, such as their density or binding affinity, is essential for various applications. The development of in vitro models that can accurately predict the in vivo performance of ligand-equipped mRNA delivery systems is highly needed. Innovative organ-on-a-chip and body-on-a-chip systems hold promise for optimizing these delivery systems by evaluating their toxicity and efficacy. The increasing interest in mRNA-based therapies and the proven potential of targeting ligands and nanocarriers indicate that substantial advancements in delivery systems are likely in the near future. Additionally, the scale-up and reproducibility of nanoparticle synthesis remain significant challenges, requiring standardized manufacturing processes and rigorous quality control measures.

7.9.2 Regulatory and Safety Aspects

The clinical translation of PNPs in gene therapy necessitates careful consideration of regulatory and safety aspects. Regulatory bodies such as the FDA and EMA require comprehensive preclinical and clinical studies to assess the safety, efficacy, and quality of nanoparticle formulations. This includes evaluating the pharmacokinetics, biodistribution, immunogenicity, and potential long-term effects of the nanoparticles.

Addressing safety concerns involves ensuring the biodegradability and biocompatibility of the materials used, as well as minimizing any potential toxicity. Regulatory guidelines are also evolving to keep pace with the rapid advancements in nanomedicine, providing a framework for the development and approval of nanoparticle-based therapies. For example, polyplexes, despite their simpler structure compared to complex nano particulate systems, offer significant opportunities for modification to improve nucleic acid delivery. Key aspects that require fine-tuning include the molecular weight of the cationic polymer and the carrier-to-RNA ratio, which influence cytotoxicity and need to be tailored to the specific nucleic acid type. Many mRNA delivery systems lack proper carrier optimization. Reducing polymer toxicity through labile bonds and enhancing endosomal escape with ionizable groups or membrane-active peptides can improve transfection efficiency.

Adding surface ligands can enhance cell targeting and uptake, while hydrophilic modifications like PEG can stabilize colloidal formulations. Most systems utilize PEG or similar coatings for systemic administration stability.

7.9.3 Prospects

The future of nucleic acid-based therapies hinges on breakthroughs in delivery systems, particularly in the realm of PNPs. Innovations will focus on developing materials that excel at nucleic acid association, are less toxic and immunogenic, and demonstrate high efficiency in nucleic acid delivery both in vitro and in vivo. For instance, polymers like PLGA and PEG are currently valued for their biocompatibility and ability to stabilize and deliver genetic material effectively. However, to maximize the effectiveness of these systems and minimize side effects, it is crucial to elucidate the mechanisms by which these materials achieve successful delivery. This includes understanding the structure-function relationships of polymeric vectors and their interactions with cellular environments.

Future studies will likely explore how different polymers, such as PEI and PBAEs, can be optimized for specific applications by defining the requirements for optimal timing and longevity of genetic manipulation. As research progresses, insights into these mechanisms will guide the design of more efficient and safer delivery vehicles. With the rapid advancements in polymer chemistry and gene therapy technologies, nanoscale polymeric delivery systems are expected to play a pivotal role in the clinical translation of gene therapies, offering the potential for more effective and targeted treatments for a range of genetic disorders.

7.9.4 Summary

Polymeric nanoparticles hold immense potential in revolutionizing gene therapy by providing safer, more efficient, and targeted delivery systems. Innovations in nanoparticle design, driven by advances in nanotechnology and materials science, are paving the way for more effective therapies. However, overcoming biological barriers, ensuring reproducibility, and addressing regulatory and safety concerns are critical to translating these promising technologies into clinical applications. As research progresses, interdisciplinary collaboration and adherence to regulatory standards will be key to unlocking the full potential of polymeric nanoparticles in gene therapy, ultimately improving patient outcomes and advancing the field of genetic medicine.

REFERENCES

1. Gao, J.; Gunasekar, S.; Xia, Z.; Shalin, K.; Jiang, C.; Chen, H.; Lee, D.; Lee, S.; Pisal, N. D.; Luo, J. N.; et al. Gene Therapy for CNS Disorders: Modalities, Delivery and Translational Challenges. *Nature Reviews Neuroscience*, **2024**, 25 (8), 553–572. https://doi.org/10.1038/s41583-024-00829-7.
2. Wang, C.; Pan, C.; Yong, H.; Wang, F.; Bo, T.; Zhao, Y.; Ma, B.; He, W.; Li, M. Emerging Non-Viral Vectors for Gene Delivery. *Journal of Nanobiotechnology*, **2023**, 21 (1), 272. https://doi.org/10.1186/s12951-023-02044-5.
3. Prado, D. A.; Acosta-Acero, M.; Maldonado, R. S. Gene Therapy beyond Luxturna: A New Horizon of the Treatment for Inherited Retinal Disease. *Current Opinion in Ophthalmology*, **2020**, 31 (3), 147–154. https://doi.org/10.1097/ICU.0000000000000660.
4. Ogbonmide, T.; Rathore, R.; Rangrej, S. B.; Hutchinson, S.; Lewis, M.; Ojilere, S.; Carvalho, V.; Kelly, I. Gene Therapy for Spinal Muscular Atrophy (SMA): A Review of Current Challenges and Safety Considerations for Onasemnogene Abeparvovec (Zolgensma). *Cureus*, **2023**. https://doi.org/10.7759/cureus.36197.
5. Schuessler-Lenz, M.; Enzmann, H.; Vamvakas, S. Regulators' Advice Can Make a Difference: European Medicines Agency Approval of Zynteglo for Beta Thalassemia. *Clinical Pharmacology & Therapeutics*, **2020**, 107 (3), 492–494. https://doi.org/10.1002/cpt.1639.
6. Paunovska, K.; Loughrey, D.; Dahlman, J. E. Drug Delivery Systems for RNA Therapeutics. *Nature Reviews Genetics*, **2022**, 23 (5), 265–280. https://doi.org/10.1038/s41576-021-00439-4.

7. Ramezani, M.; Ebrahimian, M.; Hashemi, M. Current Strategies in the Modification of PLGA-Based Gene Delivery System. *Current Medicinal Chemistry*, **2017**, *24* (7), 728–739. https://doi.org/10.2174/0929867324666161205130416.
8. Breunig, M.; Lungwitz, U.; Liebl, R.; Goepferich, A. Breaking up the Correlation between Efficacy and Toxicity for Nonviral Gene Delivery. *Proceedings of the National Academy of Sciences*, **2007**, 104 (36), 14454–14459. https://doi.org/10.1073/pnas.0703882104.
9. Zhang, P.; Wagner, E. History of Polymeric Gene Delivery Systems. *Topics in Current Chemistry*, **2017**, *375* (2), 26. https://doi.org/10.1007/s41061-017-0112-0.
10. Itaka, K.; Harada, A.; Yamasaki, Y.; Nakamura, K.; Kawaguchi, H.; Kataoka, K. *In Situ* Single Cell Observation by Fluorescence Resonance Energy Transfer Reveals Fast Intra-cytoplasmic Delivery and Easy Release of Plasmid DNA Complexed with Linear Polyethylenimine. *Journal of Gene Medicine*, **2004**, 6 (1), 76–84. https://doi.org/10.1002/jgm.470.
11. Wightman, L.; Kircheis, R.; Rössler, V.; Carotta, S.; Ruzicka, R.; Kursa, M.; Wagner, E. Different Behavior of Branched and Linear Polyethylenimine for Gene Deliveryin Vitro Andin Vivo. *Journal of Gene Medicine*, **2001**, 3 (4), 362–372. https://doi.org/10.1002/jgm.187.
12. Kasturi, S.; Sachaphibulkij, K.; Roy, K. Covalent Conjugation of Polyethyleneimine on Biodegradable Microparticles for Delivery of Plasmid DNA Vaccines. *Biomaterials*, **2005**, 26 (32), 6375–6385. https://doi.org/10.1016/j.biomaterials.2005.03.043.
13. Chen, J.; Gao, X.; Hu, K.; Pang, Z.; Cai, J.; Li, J.; Wu, H.; Jiang, X. Galactose-Poly(Ethylene Glycol)-Polyethylenimine for Improved Lung Gene Transfer. *Biochemical and Biophysical Research Communications*, **2008**, 375 (3), 378–383. https://doi.org/10.1016/j.bbrc.2008.08.006.
14. Erbacher, P.; Zou, S.; Bettinger, T.; Steffan, A.; Remy, J. Chitosan-Based Vector/DNA Complexes for Gene Delivery: Biophysical Characteristics and Transfection Ability. *Pharmaceutical Research*, **1998**, 15 (9), 1332–1339. https://doi.org/10.1023/A:1011981000671.
15. Lynn, D. M.; Langer, R. Degradable Poly(β-Amino Esters): Synthesis, Characterization, and Self-Assembly with Plasmid DNA. *Journal of the American Chemical Society*, **2000**, 122 (44), 10761–10768. https://doi.org/10.1021/ja0015388.
16. Boyer, C.; Bulmus, V.; Davis, T. P.; Ladmiral, V.; Liu, J.; Perrier, S. Bioapplications of RAFT Polymerization. *Chemical Reviews*, **2009**, 109 (11), 5402–5436. https://doi.org/10.1021/cr9001403.
17. Zhou, J.; Liu, J.; Cheng, C. J.; Patel, T. R.; Weller, C. E.; Piepmeier, J. M.; Jiang, Z.; Saltzman, W. M. Biodegradable Poly(Amine-Co-Ester) Terpolymers for Targeted Gene Delivery. *Nature Materials*, **2012**, 11 (1), 82–90. https://doi.org/10.1038/nmat3187.
18. McCutchan, J. H.; Pagano, J. S. Enhancement of the Infectivity of Simian Virus 40 Deoxyribonucleic Acid with Diethylaminoethyl-Dextran. *Journal of the National Cancer Institute*, **1968**, *41* (2), 351–357.
19. Vaheri, A.; Pagano, J. S. Infectious Poliovirus RNA: A Sensitive Method of Assay. *Virology*, **1965**, 27 (3), 434–436. https://doi.org/10.1016/0042-6822(65)90126-1.
20. Wu, G. Y.; Wu, C. H. Receptor-Mediated Gene Delivery and Expression in Vivo. *Journal of Biological Chemistry*, **1988**, 263 (29), 14621–14624.
21. Wu, G. Y.; Wu, C. H. Receptor-Mediated In Vitro Gene Transformation by a Soluble DNA Carrier System. *Journal of Biological Chemistry*, **1987**, 262 (10), 4429–4432.
22. Wagner, E.; Zenke, M.; Cotten, M.; Beug, H.; Birnstiel, M. L. Transferrin-Polycation Conjugates as Carriers for DNA Uptake into Cells. *Proceedings of the National Academy of Sciences*, **1990**, 87 (9), 3410–3414. https://doi.org/10.1073/pnas.87.9.3410.
23. Cotten, M.; Längle-Rouault, F.; Kirlappos, H.; Wagner, E.; Mechtler, K.; Zenke, M.; Beug, H.; Birnstiel, M. L. Transferrin-Polycation-Mediated Introduction of DNA into Human Leukemic Cells: Stimulation by Agents That Affect the Survival of Transfected DNA or Modulate Transferrin Receptor Levels. *Proceedings of the National Academy of Sciences*, **1990**, 87 (11), 4033–4037. https://doi.org/10.1073/pnas.87.11.4033.
24. Ferkol, T.; Kaetzel, C. S.; Davis, P. B. Gene Transfer into Respiratory Epithelial Cells by Targeting the Polymeric Immunoglobulin Receptor. *Journal of Clinical Investigation*, **1993**, 92 (5), 2394–2400. https://doi.org/10.1172/JCI116845.
25. Luthman, H.; Magnusson, G. High Efficiency Polyoma DNA Transfection of Chloroquine Treated Cells. *Nucleic Acids Research*, **1983**, 11 (5), 1295–1308. https://doi.org/10.1093/nar/11.5.1295.
26. Erbacher, P.; Roche, A. C.; Monsigny, M.; Midoux, P. Putative Role of Chloroquine in Gene Transfer into a Human Hepatoma Cell Line by DNA/Lactosylated Polylysine Complexes. *Experimental Cell Research*, **1996**, 225 (1), 186–194. https://doi.org/10.1006/excr.1996.0169.

27. Cheng, J.; Zeidan, R.; Mishra, S.; Liu, A.; Pun, S. H.; Kulkarni, R. P.; Jensen, G. S.; Bellocq, N. C.; Davis, M. E. Structure–Function Correlation of Chloroquine and Analogues as Transgene Expression Enhancers in Nonviral Gene Delivery. *Journal of Medicinal Chemistry*, **2006**, *49* (22), 6522–6531. https://doi.org/10.1021/jm060736s.
28. Zauner, W.; Blaas, D.; Kuechler, E.; Wagner, E. Rhinovirus-Mediated Endosomal Release of Transfection Complexes. *Journal of Virology*, **1995**, 69 (2), 1085–1092. https://doi.org/10.1128/jvi.69.2.1085-1092.1995.
29. Cotten, M.; Wagner, E.; Zatloukal, K.; Birnstiel, M. L. Chicken Adenovirus (CELO Virus) Particles Augment Receptor-Mediated DNA Delivery to Mammalian Cells and Yield Exceptional Levels of Stable Transformants. *Journal of Virology*, **1993**, 67 (7), 3777–3785. https://doi.org/10.1128/jvi.67.7.3777-3785.1993.
30. Curiel, D. T.; Agarwal, S.; Wagner, E.; Cotten, M. Adenovirus Enhancement of Transferrin-Polylysine-Mediated Gene Delivery. *Proceedings of the National Academy of Sciences*, **1991**, 88 (19), 8850–8854. https://doi.org/10.1073/pnas.88.19.8850.
31. Wagner, E.; Zatloukal, K.; Cotten, M.; Kirlappos, H.; Mechtler, K.; Curiel, D. T.; Birnstiel, M. L. Coupling of Adenovirus to Transferrin-Polylysine/DNA Complexes Greatly Enhances Receptor-Mediated Gene Delivery and Expression of Transfected Genes. *Proceedings of the National Academy of Sciences*, **1992**, 89 (13), 6099–6103. https://doi.org/10.1073/pnas.89.13.6099.
32. Curiel, D. T.; Wagner, E.; Cotten, M.; Birnstiel, M. L.; Agarwal, S.; Li, C.-M.; Loechel, S.; Hu, P.-C. High-Efficiency Gene Transfer Mediated by Adenovirus Coupled to DNA–Polylysine Complexes. *Human Gene Therapy*, **1992**, 3 (2), 147–154. https://doi.org/10.1089/hum.1992.3.2-147.
33. Stingl, G.; Bröcker, E.-B.; Mertelsmann, R.; Wolff, K.; Schreiber, S.; Kämpgen, E.; Schneeberger, A.; Dummer, W.; Brennscheid, U.; Veelken, H.; et al. Phase I Study to the Immunotherapy of Metastatic Malignant Melanoma by a Cancer Vaccine Consisting of Autologous Cancer Cells Transfected with the Human IL-2 Gene. University of Vienna, Austria. *Human Gene Therapy*, **1996**, *7* (4), 551–563. https://doi.org/10.1089/hum.1996.7.4-551.
34. Schreiber, S.; Kampgen, E.; Wagner, E.; Pirkhammer, D.; Trcka, J.; Korschan, H.; Lindemann, A.; Dorffner, R.; Kittler, H.; Kasteliz, F.; et al. Immunotherapy of Metastatic Malignant Melanoma by a Vaccine Consisting of Autologous Interleukin 2-Transfected Cancer Cells: Outcome of a Phase I Study. *Human Gene Therapy*, **1999**, *10* (6), 983–993. https://doi.org/10.1089/10430349950018382.
35. Saito, G.; Amidon, G. L.; Lee, K.-D. Enhanced Cytosolic Delivery of Plasmid DNA by a Sulfhydryl-Activatable Listeriolysin O/Protamine Conjugate Utilizing Cellular Reducing Potential. *Gene Therapy*, **2003**, 10 (1), 72–83. https://doi.org/10.1038/sj.gt.3301859.
36. Gottschalk, S.; Tweten, R. K.; Smith, L. C.; Woo, S. L. Efficient Gene Delivery and Expression in Mammalian Cells Using DNA Coupled with Perfringolysin O. *Gene Therapy*, **1995**, *2* (7), 498–503.
37. Wagner, E.; Plank, C.; Zatloukal, K.; Cotten, M.; Birnstiel, M. L. Influenza Virus Hemagglutinin HA-2 N-Terminal Fusogenic Peptides Augment Gene Transfer by Transferrin-Polylysine-DNA Complexes: Toward a Synthetic Virus-like Gene-Transfer Vehicle. *Proceedings of the National Academy of Sciences*, **1992**, 89 (17), 7934–7938. https://doi.org/10.1073/pnas.89.17.7934.
38. Plank, C.; Zatloukal, K.; Cotten, M.; Mechtler, K.; Wagner, E. Gene Transfer into Hepatocytes Using Asialoglycoprotein Receptor Mediated Endocytosis of DNA Complexed with an Artificial Tetra-Antennary Galactose Ligand. *Bioconjugate Chemistry*, **1992**, 3 (6), 533–539. https://doi.org/10.1021/bc00018a012.
39. Kichler, A.; Leborgne, C.; März, J.; Danos, O.; Bechinger, B. Histidine-Rich Amphipathic Peptide Antibiotics Promote Efficient Delivery of DNA into Mammalian Cells. *Proceedings of the National Academy of Sciences*, **2003**, 100 (4), 1564–1568. https://doi.org/10.1073/pnas.0337677100.
40. Midoux, P.; Kichler, A.; Boutin, V.; Maurizot, J.-C.; Monsigny, M. Membrane Permeabilization and Efficient Gene Transfer by a Peptide Containing Several Histidines. *Bioconjugate Chemistry*, **1998**, 9 (2), 260–267. https://doi.org/10.1021/bc9701611.
41. Gottschalk, S.; Sparrow, J. T.; Hauer, J.; Mims, M. P.; Leland, F. E.; Woo, S. L.; Smith, L. C. A Novel DNA-Peptide Complex for Efficient Gene Transfer and Expression in Mammalian Cells. *Gene Therapy*, **1996**, 3 (5), 448–457.
42. Wyman, T. B.; Nicol, F.; Zelphati, O.; Scaria, P. V.; Plank, C.; Szoka, F. C. Design, Synthesis, and Characterization of a Cationic Peptide That Binds to Nucleic Acids and Permeabilizes Bilayers. *Biochemistry*, **1997**, 36 (10), 3008–3017. https://doi.org/10.1021/bi9618474.
43. Haensler, J.; Szoka, F. C. Polyamidoamine Cascade Polymers Mediate Efficient Transfection of Cells in Culture. *Bioconjugate Chemistry*, **1993**, 4 (5), 372–379. https://doi.org/10.1021/bc00023a012.

44. Kloeckner, J.; Prasmickaite, L.; HØgset, A.; Berg, K.; Wagner, E. Photochemically Enhanced Gene Delivery of EGF Receptor-Targeted DNA Polyplexes. *Journal of Drug Targeting*, **2004**, 12 (4), 205–213. https://doi.org/10.1080/10611860410001723090.
45. de Bruin, K. G.; Fella, C.; Ogris, M.; Wagner, E.; Ruthardt, N.; Bräuchle, C. Dynamics of Photoinduced Endosomal Release of Polyplexes. *Journal of Controlled Release*, **2008**, 130 (2), 175–182. https://doi.org/10.1016/j.jconrel.2008.06.001.
46. Berg, K.; Weyergang, A.; Prasmickaite, L.; Bonsted, A.; Høgset, A.; Strand, M.-T. R.; Wagner, E.; Selbo, P. K. *Photochemical Internalization (*PCI*): A Technology for Drug Delivery*, 2010, pp 133–145. https://doi.org/10.1007/978-1-60761-697-9_10.
47. Remy, J.-S.; Sirlin, C.; Vierling, P.; Behr, J.-P. Gene Transfer with a Series of Lipophilic DNA-Binding Molecules. *Bioconjugate Chemistry*, **1994**, 5 (6), 647–654. https://doi.org/10.1021/bc00030a021.
48. Behr, J. P.; Demeneix, B.; Loeffler, J. P.; Perez-Mutul, J. Efficient Gene Transfer into Mammalian Primary Endocrine Cells with Lipopolyamine-Coated DNA. *Proceedings of the National Academy of Sciences*, **1989**, 86 (18), 6982–6986. https://doi.org/10.1073/pnas.86.18.6982.
49. Zou, S.-M.; Erbacher, P.; Remy, J.-S.; Behr, J.-P. Systemic Linear Polyethylenimine (L-PEI)-Mediated Gene Delivery in the Mouse. *Journal of Gene Medicine*, **2000**, 2 (2), 128–134. https://doi.org/10.1002/(SICI)1521-2254(200003/04)2:2<128::AID-JGM95>3.0.CO;2-W.
50. Coll, J.-L.; Chollet, P.; Brambilla, E.; Desplanques, D.; Behr, J.-P.; Favrot, M. In Vivo Delivery to Tumors of DNA Complexed with Linear Polyethylenimine. *Human Gene Therapy*, **1999**, 10 (10), 1659–1666. https://doi.org/10.1089/10430349950017662.
51. Behr, J.-P. The Proton Sponge: A Trick to Enter Cells the Viruses Did Not Exploit. *Chimia*, **1997**, *51* (1–2), 34. https://doi.org/10.2533/chimia.1997.34.
52. Boussif, O.; Lezoualc'h, F.; Zanta, M. A.; Mergny, M. D.; Scherman, D.; Demeneix, B.; Behr, J. P. A Versatile Vector for Gene and Oligonucleotide Transfer into Cells in Culture and in Vivo: Polyethylenimine. *Proceedings of the National Academy of Sciences*, **1995**, 92 (16), 7297–7301. https://doi.org/10.1073/pnas.92.16.7297.
53. Boeckle, S.; von Gersdorff, K.; van der Piepen, S.; Culmsee, C.; Wagner, E.; Ogris, M. Purification of Polyethylenimine Polyplexes Highlights the Role of Free Polycations in Gene Transfer. *Journal of Gene Medicine*, **2004**, 6 (10), 1102–1111. https://doi.org/10.1002/jgm.598.
54. Grandinetti, G.; Ingle, N. P.; Reineke, T. M. Interaction of Poly(Ethylenimine)–DNA Polyplexes with Mitochondria: Implications for a Mechanism of Cytotoxicity. *Molecular Pharmaceutics*, **2011**, 8 (5), 1709–1719. https://doi.org/10.1021/mp200078n.
55. Moghimi, S. M.; Symonds, P.; Murray, J. C.; Hunter, A. C.; Debska, G.; Szewczyk, A. A Two-Stage Poly(Ethylenimine)-Mediated Cytotoxicity: Implications for Gene Transfer/Therapy. *Molecular Therapy*, **2005**, 11 (6), 990–995. https://doi.org/10.1016/j.ymthe.2005.02.010.
56. Plank, C.; Mechtler, K.; Szoka, F. C.; Wagner, E. Activation of the Complement System by Synthetic DNA Complexes: A Potential Barrier for Intravenous Gene Delivery. *Human Gene Therapy*, **1996**, *7* (12), 1437–1446. https://doi.org/10.1089/hum.1996.7.12-1437.
57. Bulmus, V. A New PH-Responsive and Glutathione-Reactive, Endosomal Membrane-Disruptive Polymeric Carrier for Intracellular Delivery of Biomolecular Drugs. *Journal of Controlled Release*, **2003**, 93 (2), 105–120. https://doi.org/10.1016/j.jconrel.2003.06.001.
58. Murthy, N.; Robichaud, J. R.; Tirrell, D. A.; Stayton, P. S.; Hoffman, A. S. The Design and Synthesis of Polymers for Eukaryotic Membrane Disruption. *Journal of Controlled Release*, **1999**, 61 (1–2), 137–143. https://doi.org/10.1016/S0168-3659(99)00114-5.
59. Rozema, D. B.; Lewis, D. L.; Wakefield, D. H.; Wong, S. C.; Klein, J. J.; Roesch, P. L.; Bertin, S. L.; Reppen, T. W.; Chu, Q.; Blokhin, A. V.; et al. Dynamic PolyConjugates for Targeted *in Vivo* Delivery of SiRNA to Hepatocytes. *Proceedings of the National Academy of Sciences*, **2007**, 104 (32), 12982–12987. https://doi.org/10.1073/pnas.0703778104.
60. Wakefield, D. H.; Klein, J. J.; Wolff, J. A.; Rozema, D. B. Membrane Activity and Transfection Ability of Amphipathic Polycations as a Function of Alkyl Group Size. *Bioconjugate Chemistry*, **2005**, 16 (5), 1204–1208. https://doi.org/10.1021/bc050067h.
61. Böttger, M.; Vogel, F.; Platzer, M.; Kiessling, U.; Grade, K.; Strauss, M. Condensation of Vector DNA by the Chromosomal Protein HMG1 Results in Efficient Transfection. *Biochimica et Biophysica Acta (BBA) - Gene Structure and Expression*, **1988**, 950 (2), 221–228. https://doi.org/10.1016/0167-4781(88)90014-0.
62. Zaitsev, S.; Haberland, A.; Otto, A.; Vorob'ev, V.; Haller, H.; Böttger, M. H1 and HMG17 Extracted from Calf Thymus Nuclei Are Efficient DNA Carriers in Gene Transfer. *Gene Therapy*, **1997**, 4 (6), 586–592. https://doi.org/10.1038/sj.gt.3300433.

63. Chen, J.; Stickles, R. J.; Daichendt, K. A. Galactosylated Histone-Mediated Gene Transfer and Expression. *Human Gene Therapy*, **1994**, 5 (4), 429–435. https://doi.org/10.1089/hum.1994.5.4-429.
64. Dong, L.; Li, Y.; Cong, H.; Yu, B.; Shen, Y. A Review of Chitosan in Gene Therapy: Developments and Challenges. *Carbohydrate Polymers*, **2024**, *324*, 121562. https://doi.org/10.1016/j.carbpol.2023.121562.
65. Hwang, S. J.; Bellocq, N. C.; Davis, M. E. Effects of Structure of β-Cyclodextrin-Containing Polymers on Gene Delivery. *Bioconjugate Chemistry*, **2001**, 12 (2), 280–290. https://doi.org/10.1021/bc0001084.
66. Pun, S. H.; Davis, M. E. Development of a Nonviral Gene Delivery Vehicle for Systemic Application. *Bioconjugate Chemistry*, **2002**, 13 (3), 630–639. https://doi.org/10.1021/bc0155768.
67. Altman, G. H.; Diaz, F.; Jakuba, C.; Calabro, T.; Horan, R. L.; Chen, J.; Lu, H.; Richmond, J.; Kaplan, D. L. Silk-Based Biomaterials. *Biomaterials*, **2003**, 24 (3), 401–416. https://doi.org/10.1016/S0142-9612(02)00353-8.
68. Li, L.; Puhl, S.; Meinel, L.; Germershaus, O. Silk Fibroin Layer-by-Layer Microcapsules for Localized Gene Delivery. *Biomaterials*, **2014**, 35 (27), 7929–7939. https://doi.org/10.1016/j.biomaterials.2014.05.062.
69. Elzoghby, A.; Freag, M.; Mamdouh, H.; Elkhodairy, K. Zein-Based Nanocarriers as Potential Natural Alternatives for Drug and Gene Delivery: Focus on Cancer Therapy. *Current Pharmaceutical Design*, **2018**, *23* (35). https://doi.org/10.2174/1381612823666170622111250.
70. Karthikeyan, K.; Krishnaswamy, V. R.; Lakra, R.; Kiran, M. S.; Korrapati, P. S. Fabrication of Electrospun Zein Nanofibers for the Sustained Delivery of SiRNA. *Journal of Materials Science: Materials in Medicine*, **2015**, *26* (2), 101. https://doi.org/10.1007/s10856-015-5439-x.
71. Hu, Y.; Li, Y.; Xu, F.-J. Versatile Functionalization of Polysaccharides via Polymer Grafts: From Design to Biomedical Applications. *Accounts of Chemical Research*, **2017**, 50 (2), 281–292. https://doi.org/10.1021/acs.accounts.6b00477.
72. Singh, B.; Maharjan, S.; Park, T.; Jiang, T.; Kang, S.; Choi, Y.; Cho, C. Tuning the Buffering Capacity of Polyethylenimine with Glycerol Molecules for Efficient Gene Delivery: Staying In or Out of the Endosomes. *Macromolecular Bioscience*, **2015**, 15 (5), 622–635. https://doi.org/10.1002/mabi.201400463.
73. Wu, P.; Chen, H.; Jin, R.; Weng, T.; Ho, J. K.; You, C.; Zhang, L.; Wang, X.; Han, C. Non-Viral Gene Delivery Systems for Tissue Repair and Regeneration. *Journal of Translational Medicine*, **2018**, 16 (1), 29. https://doi.org/10.1186/s12967-018-1402-1.
74. Akinc, A.; Anderson, D. G.; Lynn, D. M.; Langer, R. Synthesis of Poly(β-Amino Ester)s Optimized for Highly Effective Gene Delivery. *Bioconjugate Chemistry*, **2003**, 14 (5), 979–988. https://doi.org/10.1021/bc034067y.
75. Lim, Y.; Kim, S.; Suh, H.; Park, J. Biodegradable, Endosome Disruptive, and Cationic Network-Type Polymer as a Highly Efficient and Nontoxic Gene Delivery Carrier. *Bioconjugate Chemistry*, **2002**, 13 (5), 952–957. https://doi.org/10.1021/bc025541n.
76. Anderson, D. G.; Lynn, D. M.; Langer, R. Semi-Automated Synthesis and Screening of a Large Library of Degradable Cationic Polymers for Gene Delivery. *Angewandte Chemie International Edition*, **2003**, *42* (27), 3153–3158. https://doi.org/10.1002/anie.200351244.
77. Akinc, A.; Lynn, D. M.; Anderson, D. G.; Langer, R. Parallel Synthesis and Biophysical Characterization of a Degradable Polymer Library for Gene Delivery. *Journal of the American Chemical Society*, **2003**, 125 (18), 5316–5323. https://doi.org/10.1021/ja034429c.
78. Lynn, D. M.; Anderson, D. G.; Putnam, D.; Langer, R. Accelerated Discovery of Synthetic Transfection Vectors: Parallel Synthesis and Screening of a Degradable Polymer Library. *Journal of the American Chemical Society*, **2001**, 123 (33), 8155–8156. https://doi.org/10.1021/ja016288p.
79. Wang, X.; Liow, S. S.; Wu, Q.; Li, C.; Owh, C.; Li, Z.; Loh, X. J.; Wu, Y. Codelivery for Paclitaxel and Bcl-2 Conversion Gene by PHB-PDMAEMA Amphiphilic Cationic Copolymer for Effective Drug Resistant Cancer Therapy. *Macromolecular Bioscience*, **2017**, *17* (11). https://doi.org/10.1002/mabi.201700186.
80. Lin, D.; Jiang, Q.; Cheng, Q.; Huang, Y.; Huang, P.; Han, S.; Guo, S.; Liang, Z.; Dong, A. Polycation-Detachable Nanoparticles Self-Assembled from MPEG-PCL-g-SS-PDMAEMA for in Vitro and in Vivo SiRNA Delivery. *Acta Biomaterialia*, **2013**, 9 (8), 7746–7757. https://doi.org/10.1016/j.actbio.2013.04.031.
81. Shi, H.; Sun, S.; Xu, H.; Zhao, Z.; Han, Z.; Jia, J.; Wu, D.; Lu, J.; Liu, H.; Yu, R. Combined Delivery of Temozolomide and SiPLK1 Using Targeted Nanoparticles to Enhance Temozolomide Sensitivity in Glioma. *International Journal of Nanomedicine*, 2020, 15, 3347–3362. https://doi.org/10.2147/IJN.S243878.
82. Fröhlich, E. The Role of Surface Charge in Cellular Uptake and Cytotoxicity of Medical Nanoparticles. *International Journal of Nanomedicine*, **2012**, 5577. https://doi.org/10.2147/IJN.S36111.

83. Zhao, Z.-X.; Gao, S.-Y.; Wang, J.-C.; Chen, C.-J.; Zhao, E.-Y.; Hou, W.-J.; Feng, Q.; Gao, L.-Y.; Liu, X.-Y.; Zhang, L.-R.; et al. Self-Assembly Nanomicelles Based on Cationic MPEG-PLA-b-Polyarginine(R15) Triblock Copolymer for SiRNA Delivery. *Biomaterials*, **2012**, *33* (28), 6793–6807. https://doi.org/10.1016/j.biomaterials.2012.05.067.
84. Kara, A.; Ozturk, N.; Esendagli, G.; Ozkose, U. U.; Gulyuz, S.; Yilmaz, O.; Telci, D.; Bozkir, A.; Vural, I. Development of Novel Self-Assembled Polymeric Micelles from Partially Hydrolysed Poly(2-Ethyl-2-Oxazoline)- *Co* -PEI-b-PCL Block Copolymer as Non-Viral Vectors for Plasmid DNA *in Vitro* Transfection. *Artificial Cells, Nanomedicine, and Biotechnology*, **2018**, *46* (sup3), 264–273. https://doi.org/10.1080/21691401.2018.1491478.
85. Wu, T.; Wang, L.; Ding, S.; You, Y. Fluorinated PEG-Polypeptide Polyplex Micelles Have Good Serum-Resistance and Low Cytotoxicity for Gene Delivery. *Macromolecular Bioscience*, **2017**, *17* (8). https://doi.org/10.1002/mabi.201700114.
86. Gaspar, V. M.; Gonçalves, C.; de Melo-Diogo, D.; Costa, E. C.; Queiroz, J. A.; Pichon, C.; Sousa, F.; Correia, I. J. Poly(2-Ethyl-2-Oxazoline)–PLA-g–PEI Amphiphilic Triblock Micelles for Co-Delivery of Minicircle DNA and Chemotherapeutics. *Journal of Controlled Release*, **2014**, 189, 90–104. https://doi.org/10.1016/j.jconrel.2014.06.040.
87. Uchida, S.; Kinoh, H.; Ishii, T.; Matsui, A.; Tockary, T. A.; Takeda, K. M.; Uchida, H.; Osada, K.; Itaka, K.; Kataoka, K. Systemic Delivery of Messenger RNA for the Treatment of Pancreatic Cancer Using Polyplex Nanomicelles with a Cholesterol Moiety. *Biomaterials*, **2016**, 82, 221–228. https://doi.org/10.1016/j.biomaterials.2015.12.031.
88. Lomas, H.; Canton, I.; MacNeil, S.; Du, J.; Armes, S. P.; Ryan, A. J.; Lewis, A. L.; Battaglia, G. Biomimetic PH Sensitive Polymersomes for Efficient DNA Encapsulation and Delivery. *Advanced Materials*, **2007**, *19* (23), 4238–4243. https://doi.org/10.1002/adma.200700941.
89. Huang, Z.; Teng, W.; Liu, L.; Wang, L.; Wang, Q.; Dong, Y. Efficient Cytosolic Delivery Mediated by Polymersomes Facilely Prepared from a Degradable, Amphiphilic, and Amphoteric Copolymer. *Nanotechnology*, **2013**, *24* (26), 265104. https://doi.org/10.1088/0957-4484/24/26/265104.
90. Gao, M.; Zhu, X.; Wu, L.; Qiu, L. Cationic Polyphosphazene Vesicles for Cancer Immunotherapy by Efficient in Vivo Cytokine IL-12 Plasmid Delivery. *Biomacromolecules*, **2016**, 17 (6), 2199–2209. https://doi.org/10.1021/acs.biomac.6b00433.
91. Matini, T.; Francini, N.; Battocchio, A.; Spain, S. G.; Mantovani, G.; Vicent, M. J.; Sanchis, J.; Gallon, E.; Mastrotto, F.; Salmaso, S.; et al. Synthesis and Characterization of Variable Conformation PH Responsive Block Co-Polymers for Nucleic Acid Delivery and Targeted Cell Entry. *Polymer Chemistry.*, **2014**, 5 (5), 1626–1636. https://doi.org/10.1039/C3PY00744H.
92. Kim, H.; Kim, E.; An, Y.; Choi, J.; Jang, E.; Choi, E. B.; Kukreja, A.; Kim, M.; Kang, B.; Kim, D.; et al. A Biodegradable Polymersome Containing Bcl-xL SiRNA and Doxorubicin as a Dual Delivery Vehicle for a Synergistic Anticancer Effect. *Macromolecular Bioscience*, **2013**, 13 (6), 745–754. https://doi.org/10.1002/mabi.201200448.
93. Wang, F.; Gao, J.; Xiao, J.; Du, J. Dually Gated Polymersomes for Gene Delivery. *Nano Letters*, **2018**, 18 (9), 5562–5568. https://doi.org/10.1021/acs.nanolett.8b01985.
94. Kim, Y.; Tewari, M.; Pajerowski, J. D.; Cai, S.; Sen, S.; Williams, J.; Sirsi, S.; Lutz, G.; Discher, D. E. Polymersome Delivery of SiRNA and Antisense Oligonucleotides. *Journal of Controlled Release*, **2009**, 134 (2), 132–140. https://doi.org/10.1016/j.jconrel.2008.10.020.
95. Ge, X.; Zhang, Q.; Cai, Y.; Duan, S.; Chen, S.; Lv, N.; Jin, T.; Chen, Y.; Yuan, W. PEG–PCL–DEX Polymersome–Protamine Vector as An Efficient Gene Delivery System Via PEG-Guided Self-Assembly. *Nanomedicine*, **2014**, *9* (8), 1193–1207. https://doi.org/10.2217/nnm.13.83.
96. Espuche, B.; Moya, S. E.; Calderón, M. Nanogels: Smart Tools to Enlarge the Therapeutic Window of Gene Therapy. *International Journal of Pharmaceutics*, **2024**, 653, 123864. https://doi.org/10.1016/j.ijpharm.2024.123864.
97. Du, Z.; Chen, M.; He, Q.; Zhou, Y.; Jin, T. Polymerized Spermine as a Novel Polycationic Nucleic Acid Carrier System. *International Journal of Pharmaceutics*, **2012**, 434 (1–2), 437–443. https://doi.org/10.1016/j.ijpharm.2012.05.065.
98. Azzam, T.; Eliyahu, H.; Makovitzki, A.; Domb, A. J. Dextran-spermine Conjugate: An Efficient Vector for Gene Delivery. *Macromolecular Symposia*, **2003**, 195 (1), 247–262. https://doi.org/10.1002/masy.200390130.
99. Agarwal, S.; Zhang, Y.; Maji, S.; Greiner, A. PDMAEMA Based Gene Delivery Materials. *Materials Today*, **2012**, 15 (9), 388–393. https://doi.org/10.1016/S1369-7021(12)70165-7.

100. Guo, P.; Gu, W.; Chen, Q.; Lu, H.; Han, X.; Li, W.; Gao, H. Dual Functionalized Amino Poly(Glycerol Methacrylate) with Guanidine and Schiff-Base Linked Imidazole for Enhanced Gene Transfection and Minimized Cytotoxicity. *Journal of Materials Chemistry B*, **2015**, *3* (34), 6911–6918. https://doi.org/10.1039/C5TB01291K.
101. Li, R.-Q.; Wu, W.; Song, H.-Q.; Ren, Y.; Yang, M.; Li, J.; Xu, F.-J. Well-Defined Reducible Cationic Nanogels Based on Functionalized Low-Molecular-Weight PGMA for Effective PDNA and SiRNA Delivery. *Acta Biomaterialia*, **2016**, 41, 282–292. https://doi.org/10.1016/j.actbio.2016.06.006.
102. Xiao, F.; Chen, Z.; Wei, Z.; Tian, L. Hydrophobic Interaction: A Promising Driving Force for the Biomedical Applications of Nucleic Acids. *Advanced Science*, **2020**, *7* (16). https://doi.org/10.1002/advs.202001048.
103. Mok, H.; Park, T. G. PEG-Assisted DNA Solubilization in Organic Solvents for Preparing Cytosol Specifically Degradable PEG/DNA Nanogels. *Bioconjugate Chemistry*, **2006**, *17* (6), 1369–1372. https://doi.org/10.1021/bc060119i.
104. Lei, H.; Fan, D. A Combination Therapy Using Electrical Stimulation and Adaptive, Conductive Hydrogels Loaded with Self-Assembled Nanogels Incorporating Short Interfering RNA Promotes the Repair of Diabetic Chronic Wounds. *Advanced Science*, **2022**, *9* (30). https://doi.org/10.1002/advs.202201425.
105. Jena, S.; Dutta, J.; Tulsiyan, K. D.; Sahu, A. K.; Choudhury, S. S.; Biswal, H. S. Noncovalent Interactions in Proteins and Nucleic Acids: Beyond Hydrogen Bonding and π-Stacking. *Chemical Society Reviews*, **2022**, 51 (11), 4261–4286. https://doi.org/10.1039/D2CS00133K.
106. Ding, F.; Huang, X.; Gao, X.; Xie, M.; Pan, G.; Li, Q.; Song, J.; Zhu, X.; Zhang, C. A Non-Cationic Nucleic Acid Nanogel for the Delivery of the CRISPR/Cas9 Gene Editing Tool. *Nanoscale*, **2019**, 11 (37), 17211–17215. https://doi.org/10.1039/C9NR05233J.
107. Gao, X.; Yao, L.; Song, Q.; Zhu, L.; Xia, Z.; Xia, H.; Jiang, X.; Chen, J.; Chen, H. The Association of Autophagy with Polyethylenimine-Induced Cytotoxity in Nephritic and Hepatic Cell Lines. *Biomaterials*, **2011**, 32 (33), 8613–8625. https://doi.org/10.1016/j.biomaterials.2011.07.047.
108. Yaroslavov, A. A.; Melik-Nubarov, N. S.; Menger, F. M. Polymer-Induced Flip-Flop in Biomembranes. *Acc Chem Res*, **2006**, 39 (10), 702–710. https://doi.org/10.1021/ar050078q.
109. Lin, C.-W.; Jan, M.-S.; Kuo, J.-H. S.; Hsu, L.-J.; Lin, Y.-S. Protective Role of Autophagy in Branched Polyethylenimine (25K)- and Poly(L-Lysine) (30–70K)-Induced Cell Death. *European Journal of Pharmaceutical Sciences*, **2012**, 47 (5), 865–874. https://doi.org/10.1016/j.ejps.2012.09.007.
110. Hall, A.; Parhamifar, L.; Lange, M. K.; Meyle, K. D.; Sanderhoff, M.; Andersen, H.; Roursgaard, M.; Larsen, A. K.; Jensen, P. B.; Christensen, C.; et al. Polyethylenimine Architecture-Dependent Metabolic Imprints and Perturbation of Cellular Redox Homeostasis. *Biochimica et Biophysica Acta (BBA) - Bioenergetics*, **2015**, *1847* (3), 328–342. https://doi.org/10.1016/j.bbabio.2014.12.002.
111. Eslami, P.; Rossi, F.; Fedeli, S. Hybrid Nanogels: Stealth and Biocompatible Structures for Drug Delivery Applications. *Pharmaceutics*, **2019**, *11* (2), 71. https://doi.org/10.3390/pharmaceutics11020071.
112. Kunzmann, A.; Andersson, B.; Thurnherr, T.; Krug, H.; Scheynius, A.; Fadeel, B. Toxicology of Engineered Nanomaterials: Focus on Biocompatibility, Biodistribution and Biodegradation. *Biochimica et Biophysica Acta (BBA) - General Subjects*, **2011**, *1810* (3), 361–373. https://doi.org/10.1016/j.bbagen.2010.04.007.
113. Knipe, J. M.; Strong, L. E.; Peppas, N. A. Enzyme- and PH-Responsive Microencapsulated Nanogels for Oral Delivery of SiRNA to Induce TNF-α Knockdown in the Intestine. *Biomacromolecules*, **2016**, 17 (3), 788–797. https://doi.org/10.1021/acs.biomac.5b01518.
114. Wang, Y.; Zheng, C.; Wu, Y.; Zhang, B.; Hu, C.; Guo, C.; Kong, Q.; Wang, Y. An Injectable and Self-Strengthening Nanogel Encapsuled Hydrogel Gene Delivery System Promotes Degenerative Nucleus Pulposus Repair. *Composites Part B: Engineering*, **2023**, *250*, 110469. https://doi.org/10.1016/j.compositesb.2022.110469.
115. Luten, J.; van Nostrum, C. F.; De Smedt, S. C.; Hennink, W. E. Biodegradable Polymers as Non-Viral Carriers for Plasmid DNA Delivery. *Journal of Controlled Release*, **2008**, 126 (2), 97–110. https://doi.org/10.1016/j.jconrel.2007.10.028.
116. Subhash, D.; Mody, H.; Banerjee, R.; Bahadur, D.; Srivastava, R. Poly(N-Isopropylacrylamide) Based Polymer Nanogels for Drug Delivery Applications. In *2011 11th IEEE International Conference on Nanotechnology*; IEEE, 2011, pp 1741–1744. https://doi.org/10.1109/NANO.2011.6144388.
117. Danhier, F.; Ansorena, E.; Silva, J. M.; Coco, R.; Le Breton, A.; Préat, V. PLGA-Based Nanoparticles: An Overview of Biomedical Applications. *Journal of Controlled Release*, **2012**, 161 (2), 505–522. https://doi.org/10.1016/j.jconrel.2012.01.043.

118. Li, W.; Qiu, J.; Li, X.-L.; Aday, S.; Zhang, J.; Conley, G.; Xu, J.; Joseph, J.; Lan, H.; Langer, R.; et al. BBB Pathophysiology–Independent Delivery of SiRNA in Traumatic Brain Injury. *Science Advances*, **2021**, *7* (1). https://doi.org/10.1126/sciadv.abd6889.
119. Fan, Y.-N.; Li, M.; Luo, Y.-L.; Chen, Q.; Wang, L.; Zhang, H.-B.; Shen, S.; Gu, Z.; Wang, J. Cationic Lipid-Assisted Nanoparticles for Delivery of MRNA Cancer Vaccine. *Biomaterials Science*, **2018**, *6* (11), 3009–3018. https://doi.org/10.1039/C8BM00908B.
120. Yasar, H.; Biehl, A.; De Rossi, C.; Koch, M.; Murgia, X.; Loretz, B.; Lehr, C.-M. Kinetics of MRNA Delivery and Protein Translation in Dendritic Cells Using Lipid-Coated PLGA Nanoparticles. *J Nanobiotechnology*, **2018**, 16 (1), 72. https://doi.org/10.1186/s12951-018-0401-y.
121. Yang, J.; Arya, S.; Lung, P.; Lin, Q.; Huang, J.; Li, Q. Hybrid Nanovaccine for the Co-Delivery of the MRNA Antigen and Adjuvant. *Nanoscale*, **2019**, 11 (45), 21782–21789. https://doi.org/10.1039/C9NR05475H.
122. Yan, Y.; Xiong, H.; Zhang, X.; Cheng, Q.; Siegwart, D. J. Systemic MRNA Delivery to the Lungs by Functional Polyester-Based Carriers. *Biomacromolecules*, **2017**, 18 (12), 4307–4315. https://doi.org/10.1021/acs.biomac.7b01356.
123. Sirsi, S. R.; Schray, R. C.; Wheatley, M. A.; Lutz, G. J. Formulation of Polylactide-Co-Glycolic Acid Nanospheres for Encapsulation and Sustained Release of Poly(Ethylene Imine)-Poly(Ethylene Glycol) Copolymers Complexed to Oligonucleotides. *J Nanobiotechnology*, **2009**, 7 (1), 1. https://doi.org/10.1186/1477-3155-7-1.
124. Rush, A. M.; Thompson, M. P.; Tatro, E. T.; Gianneschi, N. C. Nuclease-Resistant DNA *via* High-Density Packing in Polymeric Micellar Nanoparticle Coronas. *ACS Nano*, **2013**, 7 (2), 1379–1387. https://doi.org/10.1021/nn305030g.
125. Spirescu, V. A.; Chircov, C.; Grumezescu, A. M.; Andronescu, E. Polymeric Nanoparticles for Antimicrobial Therapies: An Up-to-Date Overview. *Polymers*, **2021**, *13* (5), 724. https://doi.org/10.3390/polym13050724.
126. Sivadasan, D.; Sultan, M. H.; Madkhali, O.; Almoshari, Y.; Thangavel, N. Polymeric Lipid Hybrid Nanoparticles (PLNs) as Emerging Drug Delivery Platform—A Comprehensive Review of Their Properties, Preparation Methods, and Therapeutic Applications. *Pharmaceutics*, **2021**, *13* (8), 1291. https://doi.org/10.3390/pharmaceutics13081291.
127. Piotrowski-Daspit, A. S.; Kauffman, A. C.; Bracaglia, L. G.; Saltzman, W. M. Polymeric Vehicles for Nucleic Acid Delivery. *Advanced Drug Delivery Reviews*, **2020**, 156, 119–132. https://doi.org/10.1016/j.addr.2020.06.014.
128. Piperno, A.; Sciortino, M. T.; Giusto, E.; Montesi, M.; Panseri, S.; Scala, A. Recent Advances and Challenges in Gene Delivery Mediated by Polyester-Based Nanoparticles. *International Journal of Nanomedicine*, 2021, V*olume* 16, 5981–6002. https://doi.org/10.2147/IJN.S321329.
129. Kim, J.; Wilson, D. R.; Zamboni, C. G.; Green, J. J. Targeted Polymeric Nanoparticles for Cancer Gene Therapy. *Journal of Drug Targeting*, **2015**, 23 (7–8), 627–641. https://doi.org/10.3109/1061186X.2015.1048519.
130. Li, Y.; Gao, G. H.; Lee, D. S. Stimulus-Sensitive Polymeric Nanoparticles and Their Applications as Drug and Gene Carriers. *Advanced Healthcare Materials*, **2013**, 2 (3), 388–417. https://doi.org/10.1002/adhm.201200313.
131. Elsabahy, M.; Wooley, K. L. Design of Polymeric Nanoparticles for Biomedical Delivery Applications. *Chemical Society Reviews*, **2012**, 41 (7), 2545. https://doi.org/10.1039/c2cs15327k.
132. Yang, J.; Luly, K. M.; Green, J. J. Nonviral Nanoparticle Gene Delivery into the CNS for Neurological Disorders and Brain Cancer Applications. *WIREs Nanomedicine and Nanobiotechnology*, **2023**, *15* (2). https://doi.org/10.1002/wnan.1853.
133. Zhong, Y.; Meng, F.; Deng, C.; Zhong, Z. Ligand-Directed Active Tumor-Targeting Polymeric Nanoparticles for Cancer Chemotherapy. *Biomacromolecules*, **2014**, *15* (6), 1955–1969. https://doi.org/10.1021/bm5003009.
134. Kenry; Yeo, T.; Manghnani, P. N.; Middha, E.; Pan, Y.; Chen, H.; Lim, C. T.; Liu, B. Mechanistic Understanding of the Biological Responses to Polymeric Nanoparticles. *ACS Nano*, **2020**, 14 (4), 4509–4522. https://doi.org/10.1021/acsnano.9b10195.
135. Goodall, S.; Jones, M. L.; Mahler, S. Monoclonal Antibody-targeted Polymeric Nanoparticles for Cancer Therapy – Future Prospects. *Journal of Chemical Technology & Biotechnology*, **2015**, 90 (7), 1169–1176. https://doi.org/10.1002/jctb.4555.
136. Xiang, Y.; Huang, W.; Huang, C.; Long, J.; Zhou, Y.; Liu, Y.; Tang, S.; He, D.; Tan, X.; Wei, H.; et al. Facile Fabrication of Nanoparticles with Dual-Targeting Ligands for Precise Hepatocellular Carcinoma Therapy *In Vitro* and *In Vivo*. *Molecular Pharmaceutics*, **2020**, 17 (9), 3223–3235. https://doi.org/10.1021/acs.molpharmaceut.0c00327.

137. Hu, G.; Guo, M.; Xu, J.; Wu, F.; Fan, J.; Huang, Q.; Yang, G.; Lv, Z.; Wang, X.; Jin, Y. Nanoparticles Targeting Macrophages as Potential Clinical Therapeutic Agents Against Cancer and Inflammation. *Frontiers in Immunology*, **2019**, *10*. https://doi.org/10.3389/fimmu.2019.01998.
138. Zhang, F.; Parayath, N. N.; Ene, C. I.; Stephan, S. B.; Koehne, A. L.; Coon, M. E.; Holland, E. C.; Stephan, M. T. Genetic Programming of Macrophages to Perform Anti-Tumor Functions Using Targeted MRNA Nanocarriers. *Nature Communications*, **2019**, 10 (1), 3974. https://doi.org/10.1038/s41467-019-11911-5.
139. Chen, Z.; Zhao, P.; Luo, Z.; Zheng, M.; Tian, H.; Gong, P.; Gao, G.; Pan, H.; Liu, L.; Ma, A.; et al. Cancer Cell Membrane–Biomimetic Nanoparticles for Homologous-Targeting Dual-Modal Imaging and Photothermal Therapy. *ACS Nano*, **2016**, 10 (11), 10049–10057. https://doi.org/10.1021/acsnano.6b04695.
140. Zhang, M.; Cheng, S.; Jin, Y.; Zhang, N.; Wang, Y. Membrane Engineering of Cell Membrane Biomimetic Nanoparticles for Nanoscale Therapeutics. *Clinical and Translational Medicine*, **2021**, *11* (2). https://doi.org/10.1002/ctm2.292.
141. Seelam, M. L.; Yarraguntla, S. R.; Paravastu, V. K. K.; Vurukuti, S. S.; Mylavarapu, S. S. V. Polymeric Nanoparticles with Stimuli-Responsive Properties for Drug Delivery. *GSC Biological and Pharmaceutical Sciences*, **2022**, 20 (1), 044–055. https://doi.org/10.30574/gscbps.2022.20.1.0259.
142. Deng, K.; Yang, D.; Zhou, Y. Nanotechnology-Based SiRNA Delivery Systems to Overcome Tumor Immune Evasion in Cancer Immunotherapy. *Pharmaceutics*, **2022**, *14* (7), 1344. https://doi.org/10.3390/pharmaceutics14071344.
143. Ganesh, S.; Shui, X.; Craig, K. P.; Park, J.; Wang, W.; Brown, B. D.; Abrams, M. T. RNAi-Mediated β-Catenin Inhibition Promotes T Cell Infiltration and Antitumor Activity in Combination with Immune Checkpoint Blockade. *Molecular Therapy*, **2018**, 26 (11), 2567–2579. https://doi.org/10.1016/j.ymthe.2018.09.005.
144. Matsuda, A.; Ishiguro, K.; Yan, I. K.; Patel, T. Extracellular Vesicle-Based Therapeutic Targeting of B-Catenin to Modulate Anticancer Immune Responses in Hepatocellular Cancer. *Hepatology Communications*, **2019**, 3 (4), 525–541. https://doi.org/10.1002/hep4.1311.
145. Wang, H.; Qin, L.; Zhang, X.; Guan, J.; Mao, S. Mechanisms and Challenges of Nanocarriers as Non-Viral Vectors of Therapeutic Genes for Enhanced Pulmonary Delivery. *Journal of Controlled Release*, **2022**, 352, 970–993. https://doi.org/10.1016/j.jconrel.2022.10.061.
146. Neuberg, P.; Kichler, A. Recent developments in nucleic acid delivery with polyethylenimines. In *Advances in Genetics*, 2014, pp. 263–288. https://doi.org/10.1016/B978-0-12-800148-6.00009-2.
147. Dhandapani, R. K.; Gurusamy, D.; Palli, S. R. Development of Catechin, Poly- l -Lysine, and Double-Stranded RNA Nanoparticles. *ACS Applied Bio Materials*, **2021**, 4 (5), 4310–4318. https://doi.org/10.1021/acsabm.1c00109.
148. Chen, J.; Ding, J.; Wang, Y.; Cheng, J.; Ji, S.; Zhuang, X.; Chen, X. Sequentially Responsive Shell-Stacked Nanoparticles for Deep Penetration into Solid Tumors. *Advanced Materials*, **2017**, *29* (32). https://doi.org/10.1002/adma.201701170.
149. Bober, Z.; Bartusik-Aebisher, D.; Aebisher, D. Application of Dendrimers in Anticancer Diagnostics and Therapy. *Molecules*, **2022**, *27* (10), 3237. https://doi.org/10.3390/molecules27103237.
150. Xiao, B.; Ma, P.; Viennois, E.; Merlin, D. Urocanic Acid-Modified Chitosan Nanoparticles Can Confer Anti-Inflammatory Effect by Delivering CD98 SiRNA to Macrophages. *Colloids and Surfaces B: Biointerfaces*, **2016**, 143, 186–193. https://doi.org/10.1016/j.colsurfb.2016.03.035.
151. Endres, T.; Zheng, M.; Kılıç, A.; Turowska, A.; Beck-Broichsitter, M.; Renz, H.; Merkel, O. M.; Kissel, T. Amphiphilic Biodegradable PEG-PCL-PEI Triblock Copolymers for FRET-Capable *in Vitro* and *in Vivo* Delivery of SiRNA and Quantum Dots. *Molecular Pharmaceutics*, **2014**, 11 (4), 1273–1281. https://doi.org/10.1021/mp400744a.
152. Lee, J.; Sands, I.; Zhang, W.; Zhou, L.; Chen, Y. DNA-Inspired Nanomaterials for Enhanced Endosomal Escape. *Proceedings of the National Academy of Sciences*, **2021**, *118* (19). https://doi.org/10.1073/pnas.2104511118.
153. Chen, J.; Li, J.; Zhou, J.; Lin, Z.; Cavalieri, F.; Czuba-Wojnilowicz, E.; Hu, Y.; Glab, A.; Ju, Y.; Richardson, J. J.; et al. Metal–Phenolic Coatings as a Platform to Trigger Endosomal Escape of Nanoparticles. *ACS Nano*, **2019**, 13 (10), 11653–11664. https://doi.org/10.1021/acsnano.9b05521.
154. Mahajan, S.; Tang, T. Polyethylenimine–DNA Nanoparticles under Endosomal Acidification and Implication to Gene Delivery. *Langmuir*, **2022**, 38 (27), 8382–8397. https://doi.org/10.1021/acs.langmuir.2c00952.
155. Massignani, M.; Canton, I.; Sun, T.; Hearnden, V.; MacNeil, S.; Blanazs, A.; Armes, S. P.; Lewis, A.; Battaglia, G. Enhanced Fluorescence Imaging of Live Cells by Effective Cytosolic Delivery of Probes. *PLoS One*, **2010**, *5* (5), e10459. https://doi.org/10.1371/journal.pone.0010459.

156. Pittella, F.; Zhang, M.; Lee, Y.; Kim, H. J.; Tockary, T.; Osada, K.; Ishii, T.; Miyata, K.; Nishiyama, N.; Kataoka, K. Enhanced Endosomal Escape of SiRNA-Incorporating Hybrid Nanoparticles from Calcium Phosphate and PEG-Block Charge-Conversional Polymer for Efficient Gene Knockdown with Negligible Cytotoxicity. *Biomaterials*, **2011**, *32* (11), 3106–3114. https://doi.org/10.1016/j.biomaterials.2010.12.057.
157. Lee, M. S.; Lee, J. E.; Byun, E.; Kim, N. W.; Lee, K.; Lee, H.; Sim, S. J.; Lee, D. S.; Jeong, J. H. Target-Specific Delivery of SiRNA by Stabilized Calcium Phosphate Nanoparticles Using Dopa–Hyaluronic Acid Conjugate. *Journal of Controlled Release*, **2014**, 192, 122–130. https://doi.org/10.1016/j.jconrel.2014.06.049.
158. Nguyen, J.; Szoka, F. C. Nucleic Acid Delivery: The Missing Pieces of the Puzzle? *Accounts of Chemical Research*, **2012**, 45 (7), 1153–1162. https://doi.org/10.1021/ar3000162.
159. Hu, Y.; Litwin, T.; Nagaraja, A. R.; Kwong, B.; Katz, J.; Watson, N.; Irvine, D. J. Cytosolic Delivery of Membrane-Impermeable Molecules in Dendritic Cells Using PH-Responsive Core–Shell Nanoparticles. *Nano Letters*, **2007**, 7 (10), 3056–3064. https://doi.org/10.1021/nl071542i.
160. Yang, Y.; Hong, Y.; Nam, G.; Chung, J. H.; Koh, E.; Kim, I. Virus-Mimetic Fusogenic Exosomes for Direct Delivery of Integral Membrane Proteins to Target Cell Membranes. *Advanced Materials*, **2017**, *29* (13). https://doi.org/10.1002/adma.201605604.
161. Chen, H.-Y.; Deng, J.; Wang, Y.; Wu, C.-Q.; Li, X.; Dai, H.-W. Hybrid Cell Membrane-Coated Nanoparticles: A Multifunctional Biomimetic Platform for Cancer Diagnosis and Therapy. *Acta Biomaterialia*, **2020**, 112, 1–13. https://doi.org/10.1016/j.actbio.2020.05.028.
162. Rao, L.; Bu, L.; Xu, J.; Cai, B.; Yu, G.; Yu, X.; He, Z.; Huang, Q.; Li, A.; Guo, S.; et al. Red Blood Cell Membrane as a Biomimetic Nanocoating for Prolonged Circulation Time and Reduced Accelerated Blood Clearance. *Small*, **2015**, *11* (46), 6225–6236. https://doi.org/10.1002/smll.201502388.
163. Xuan, M.; Shao, J.; Zhao, J.; Li, Q.; Dai, L.; Li, J. Magnetic Mesoporous Silica Nanoparticles Cloaked by Red Blood Cell Membranes: Applications in Cancer Therapy. *Angewandte Chemie International Edition*, **2018**, *57* (21), 6049–6053. https://doi.org/10.1002/anie.201712996.
164. Allolio, C.; Magarkar, A.; Jurkiewicz, P.; Baxová, K.; Javanainen, M.; Mason, P. E.; Šachl, R.; Cebecauer, M.; Hof, M.; Horinek, D.; et al. Arginine-Rich Cell-Penetrating Peptides Induce Membrane Multilamellarity and Subsequently Enter via Formation of a Fusion Pore. *Proceedings of the National Academy of Sciences*, **2018**, 115 (47), 11923–11928. https://doi.org/10.1073/pnas.1811520115.
165. Deng, H.; Zhao, X.; He, D.; Guo, W.; Yang, K.; Dong, A.; Liang, X.-J. One-Step Gene Delivery into the Cytoplasm in a Fusion-Dependent Manner Based on a New Membrane Fusogenic Lipid. *Chemical Communications*, **2016**, 52 (46), 7406–7408. https://doi.org/10.1039/C6CC01996J.
166. Wang, G.; Norton, A. S.; Pokharel, D.; Song, Y.; Hill, R. A. KDEL Peptide Gold Nanoconstructs: Promising Nanoplatforms for Drug Delivery. *Nanomedicine*, **2013**, 9 (3), 366–374. https://doi.org/10.1016/j.nano.2012.09.002.
167. Davis, M. E.; Zuckerman, J. E.; Choi, C. H. J.; Seligson, D.; Tolcher, A.; Alabi, C. A.; Yen, Y.; Heidel, J. D.; Ribas, A. Evidence of RNAi in Humans from Systemically Administered SiRNA via Targeted Nanoparticles. *Nature*, **2010**, *464* (7291), 1067–1070. https://doi.org/10.1038/nature08956.
168. Gulino, A. Nanoparticle-Based Delivery of Small Interfering RNA: Challenges for Cancer Therapy. *International Journal of Nanomedicine*, **2012**, 3637. https://doi.org/10.2147/IJN.S23696.
169. Buscail, L.; Bournet, B.; Vernejoul, F.; Cambois, G.; Lulka, H.; Hanoun, N.; Dufresne, M.; Meulle, A.; Vignolle-Vidoni, A.; Ligat, L.; et al. First-in-Man Phase 1 Clinical Trial of Gene Therapy for Advanced Pancreatic Cancer: Safety, Biodistribution, and Preliminary Clinical Findings. *Molecular Therapy*, **2015**, 23 (4), 779–789. https://doi.org/10.1038/mt.2015.1.
170. Thaker, P. H.; Borys, N.; Fewell, J.; Anwer, K. GEN-1 Immunotherapy for the Treatment of Ovarian Cancer. *Future Oncology*, **2019**, 15 (4), 421–438. https://doi.org/10.2217/fon-2018-0423.

8 Cancer Nanotherapeutics
Trends and Challenges

Neelam Vishwakarma[1,2,3] *and Suman Singh*[1,2]
[1]Applied Materials & Instrumentation, CSIR-Central Scientific Instruments Organisation, Chandigarh, India
[2]Academy of Scientific and Innovative Research, Ghaziabad, India
[3]RMIT University, Melbourne, Australia

8.1 INTRODUCTION

Nanotechnology has emerged as one of the most fascinating and ubiquitous fields of the century so far, and every researcher and scientist is eager to explore novel potentials of various nanomaterials, owing to their unique molecular and atomic properties. Though the advent of nanomaterials and their applications seems like a new technology, evidence of its existence can be tracked back up to 4th-century Lycurgus cups and 17th-century Damascene swords [1]. Nanotechnology can be defined as the preparation and modification of materials on nanoscale molecular structures with sizes varying in the range of 1–100 nm in order to alter their intrinsic properties compared to their bulk counterparts and tailor the new structure for their desired applications. Any structure with at least one dimension in 1–100 nm range can be described as a nanomaterial and will follow the laws of quantum physics [2,3].

Modern medicine has undergone a significant evolutionary journey since the days of traditional medicine, thriving in areas such as surgery, drug delivery, diagnostics, laser treatments, and more [4]. Even now, new and improved technologies are explored diligently to enhance the efficacy of these treatments and mitigate their associated toxic side effects. Discovering targeted medicine solutions with precision medicine, with effective drug delivery vectors, had been the preferred topic of interests for inventors and researchers.

Nanotherapeutics, a fairly recent technology, revolves around the adaptation and modification of nanomaterials to enhance the pharmacological effects of medicine and treatments for any disorder [5]. Nanotherapeutics has two significant components as nanomedicine and nanodiagnostics. Nanomedicine primarily involves the integration of nanomaterials with already established medical methods for improved treatment efficacy of diseases [6,7]. These nanomaterials may be designed to enhance drug delivery, target specific tissues or cells, etc., to enhance the effectiveness and safety of medical treatments. On the other hand, nanodiagnostics revolves around nanosensors and diagnostics tools using nanomaterial, with special emphasis on point-of-care diagnostic devices [8]. This may include nanosensors for detecting disease biomarkers, nanoscale imaging techniques for high-resolution imaging of tissues or cells, or the development of point-of-care diagnostic devices that utilize nanomaterials for rapid and sensitive detection of diseases. Nanodiagnostics aims to improve disease detection, monitoring, and prognosis through the development of highly sensitive and specific diagnostic tools [9,10].

Cancer is irrefutably one of the deadliest diseases in the world today with over 19.3 million cases in 2020 alone with 10 million fatalities [11,12]. Cancer could affect people of all age group, ethnicities, and lifestyles. Despite extensive research, determining the root cause of cancer cell growth remains a formidable challenge [13]. While certain risk factors, such as genetic predisposition, exposure to carcinogens, unhealthy lifestyle choices, and environmental factors, have been

 DOI: 10.1201/9781003473015-8

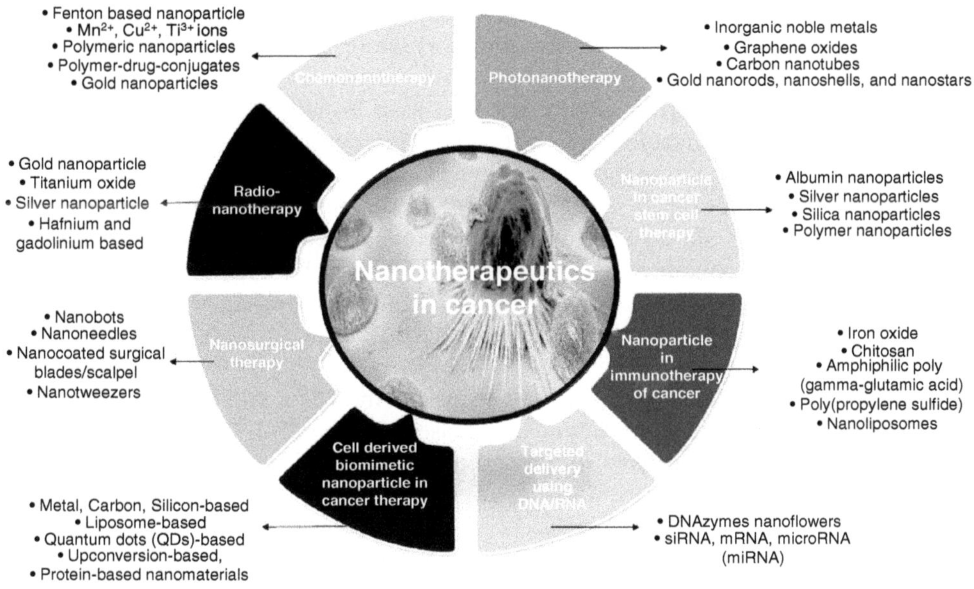

FIGURE 8.1 Nanoparticles in different types of cancer therapies [16]. (Reprinted with permission.)

identified, the exact mechanisms underlying cancer development in each individual case are often complex and multifaceted [14,15].

Given the alarming statistics and limited ability to diagnose and treat various cancer disorders, numerous researchers and scientists have been tirelessly working to devise new and efficient ways for early detection, risk stratification, efficient and precise treatment, and monitoring of the medicine. In these efforts nanotechnology has proved to be a great tool with many diverse applications like nanodrug carriers, nanorobots, nanosensors, nanoparticle (NP) vaccines, genetic therapy, medical imaging, etc. Figure 8.1 shows various kinds of NPs preferred for different therapies related to cancer diagnosis and treatment strategies.

8.2 EVOLUTION OF CANCER NANOTHERAPEUTICS

Even though the first ever known case of cancer in humans can be pointed back to Egypt 3000 BC, it still took almost 25 centuries before humans finally started to gain some understanding of the disease [17]. The Greeks and Romans were the first to come forward with terminology like 'oncos' meaning swelling, or 'carcinos', translated to crab. It was later in the 16th century when the term 'cachexia' came forward in Greek Lexicon and was linked to 'loss of energy', a prominent symptom in the majority of cancer cases [18]. The birth of modern oncology in the 18th and 19th centuries, with advanced scientific procedures, surgeries, and modern microscopy inventions, finally led to a break in understanding, diagnosing, and treating cancer in patients [19].

The very first evidence of using nanomaterials in medicine can be observed in early 1990s when colloidal NP-based drug delivery systems found some success due to their unique morphology [20]. The term 'Nanomedicine' was first presented by Robert A. Freitas in 1999, and has gained widespread use in technical literature [21].

Nanotherapeutics is a recent scientific endeavor that has very quickly attracted the attention of world healthcare systems. Nanotechnology itself hasn't been around for a very long while and the coalition of nanotechnology with biotechnology and modern medicine has been a venture of early 21st century. With the advent of the electron microscope in the 1930s by Max Knoll and Ernst Ruska and the introduction of nanotechnology by Richard Feynman in 1959, a whole new world of observing and manipulating nanostructures emerged, paving the way for numerous new possibilities. Figure 8.2 shows a timeline view for the evolution of nanomaterials in respect of cancer medicine and therapies.

In the last few decades, cancer nanotherapeutics have evolved significantly owing to rapid advancements in the fields of nanotechnology, targeted therapeutic strategies, and diagnostic platform development methods. During the 1970s, the introduction of advanced nanomaterials started in cancer treatment with liposomes and phospholipid-based vesicles designed for drug encapsulation. In the 1980s, liposomal drug delivery was revolutionized by Prof. Gregory Gregoriadis, who founded the cancer nanotherapeutics field [22]. During the 1990s, first Food and Drug Administration (FDA) approval was given to Doxil, a PEGylated liposomal doxorubicin formulation which worked on the pharmacokinetics, lowering toxicity while improving tumor targeting through the enhanced permeability and retention (EPR) effect [23]. In 2005, a major milestone in targeted cancer nanotherapeutics was observed when Abraxane, an albumin-bound paclitaxel NP, was approved to decrease cytotoxicity and increase solubility [24]. During this time, gold and other metallic NPs were also explored for photothermal therapies for tumor cells and superparamagnetic iron oxide nanoparticles (SPIONs) enabled magnetic resonance imaging (MRI)-guided diagnostics and magnetic hyperthermia for localized cancer therapies [25,26]. As time progressed, with advancement in cancer theragnostic areas, other NPs (silica-based, graphene-based, etc.) also gained popularity due to their drug-carrying and therapeutic capabilities [27]. RNA-based nanotherapeutics paved the way for lipid NPs, which later played a critical part in COVID-19 mRNA vaccines and has great potential for cancer gene silencing therapies [28,29].

In the last few years, artificial intelligence (AI)-aided medicine designing has laid firm foundations for personalized and precision medicine development. Gold and silver NPs are still preferred materials for precise photoacoustic imaging and targeted photothermal therapy, while carbon-based nanomaterials (e.g., graphene, carbon nanotubes) have been focused on drug delivery and biosensing areas [30,31]. The advent of nanobots and nanochips for applications in vivo and in vitro has enabled several advanced methods for nanotherapeutics on cancer.

In the regulatory body and government initiatives, the 20th and early 21st centuries saw a rise in various missions, which were explicitly initiated to cancer, its prevention and innovation of

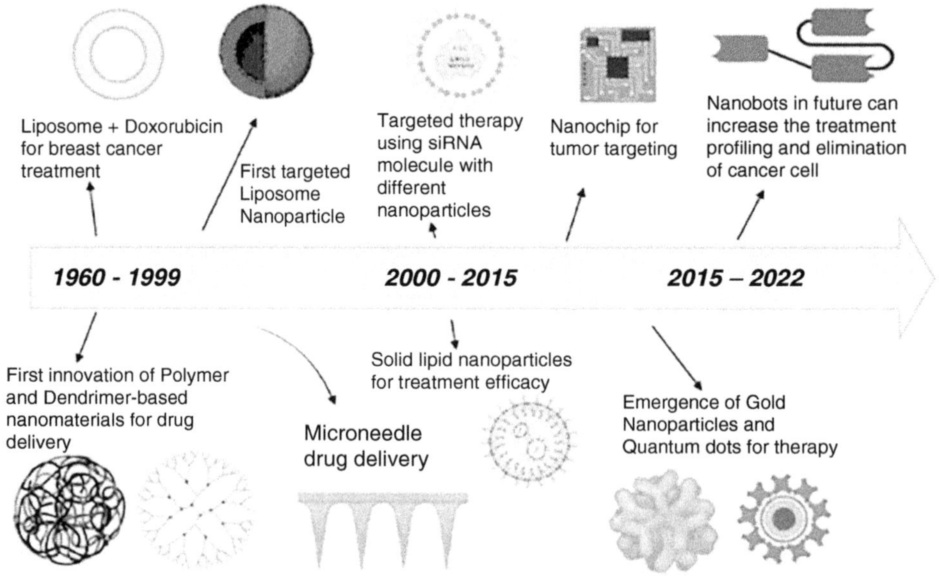

FIGURE 8.2 Timeline of cancer nanomedicine [21]. (Reprinted with permission.)

new technologies for treatment [32–34]. However, despite extensive research efforts, the current landscape of cancer mortality and morbidity remains daunting for everyone involved. The global economic burden of cancer from 2020 to 2050 was estimated to be around USD 25.2 trillion which poses a great risk to the sustainability and health of people with an unfairly distributed burden across various income groups, countries, and low-income regions [35].

8.3 NANOTECHNOLOGY IN MEDICINE

Nanotechnology has found its purpose in a variety of fields, including medicine, particularly in the development of drug delivery systems for complex diseases. Nanomedicine is the branch of nanotechnology that deals particularly with creating powerful and effective methods for treatment, prevention, and efficient drug delivery vectors for diseases, injuries, and elevation of overall wellness [36]. The correct and adequate delivery of drug compounds is one of the crucial factors for any disease management, and nanomedicines focus on providing competent delivery methods for drugs, antibodies, proteins, etc., through painless, precise, and proficient methods to various parts of the body [37–39]. Navigating drug molecules through barriers like the blood-brain and blood-placenta is a common challenge traditional medicine faces, which nanomedicine aims to address. NPs, such as liposomes, polymeric micelles, and albumin NPs, are efficient carriers for anticancer drugs. Their small size and tailored surface properties enable EPR effects, leading to improved accumulation within tumors while minimizing systemic toxicity [40].

8.3.1 Targeting Strategies for Drug Delivery

Targeting strategies in NP delivery involve directing NPs specifically to diseased cells or tissues while minimizing their interaction with healthy cells. These strategies aim to enhance the efficacy and reduce the side effects of therapeutic agents encapsulated within NPs. By combining and altering these targeting strategies, various efficient NP delivery systems can be designed and tested which can efficiently deliver therapeutic agents to diseased tissues or cells, improving treatment outcomes and minimizing side effects [41]. Figure 8.3 discusses two of the most prominent targeting mechanisms for drug delivery using NPs.

8.3.1.1 Passive Targeting

Passive targeting exploits the distinct physiological traits of tumors, namely the leaky vasculature and compromised lymphatic drainage of tumor cells, to bolster the accumulation of NPs within tumor tissues via the EPR effect [42]. Through this mechanism, NPs, carefully tailored in terms of size and surface properties, can traverse leaky blood vessels and amass within the tumor interstitium.

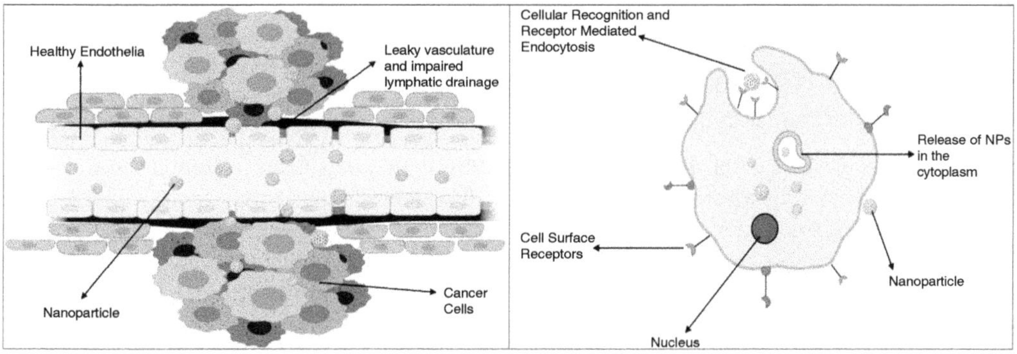

FIGURE 8.3 Pictorial representation: passive targeting mechanism (left) and active targeting mechanism (right) [46]. (Reprinted with permission.)

This phenomenon occurs due to the diminished lymphatic drainage in tumor regions, facilitating the retention of NPs and culminating in elevated drug concentrations at the tumor site. As a result, passive targeting serves as a valuable strategy for improving the localization and efficacy of therapeutic agents within tumors while potentially mitigating systemic side effects [43].

8.3.1.2 Active Targeting

This type of targeting mechanism represents a sophisticated approach in NP delivery systems, characterized by the attachment of ligands onto NPs that exhibit specificity toward receptors or biomarkers overexpressed on the surface of diseased cells [44]. These targeting ligands encompass a variety of molecules, such as antibodies, peptides, aptamers, or small molecules, each possessing high affinity and selectivity for their respective targets. Upon administration, these targeted NPs selectively bind to the receptors present on the surface of diseased cells, a process facilitated by receptor-mediated endocytosis [45]. Subsequently, the internalization of these targeted NPs into the diseased cells enhances the delivery of encapsulated therapeutic agents to the intended site, thereby amplifying the efficacy of treatment while potentially reducing off-target effects. Active targeting thus holds immense promise for precision medicine by ensuring the precise localization of therapeutic payloads to diseased tissues or cells, ultimately optimizing therapeutic outcomes.

8.3.1.3 Cellular and Subcellular Targeting

Cellular targeting endeavors to deliver NPs to particular cell types within tissues or organs, offering a tailored approach to therapy. NPs can be engineered to zero in on immune cells, stem cells, or specific cell populations implicated in disease progression. By selecting targeting ligands that recognize cell surface markers or receptors selectively expressed on the desired cell types, precise delivery of therapeutic agents becomes achievable [47]. On the other hand, subcellular targeting involves guiding NPs to distinct organelles or intracellular compartments within cells. Through functionalization with organelle-targeting peptides or proteins, NPs can navigate their way to locations such as the nucleus, mitochondria, or endoplasmic reticulum. This subcellular precision enables the effective delivery of therapeutic agents to intracellular targets, thereby enhancing therapeutic efficacy while potentially minimizing off-target effects [48].

8.3.1.4 Stimuli-Responsive Targeting

Stimuli-responsive targeting harnesses alterations in the microenvironment of diseased tissues, like variations in pH, temperature, or enzyme activity, as cues for NP activation and targeting [49]. Engineered NPs can be programmed to undergo structural or chemical modifications upon encountering these specific stimuli, resulting in amplified accumulation and release of therapeutic agents precisely at the target site. By offering spatiotemporal control over drug delivery, stimuli-responsive targeting strategies pave the way for precision therapy while potentially mitigating systemic toxicity. This dynamic approach holds promise for enhancing therapeutic outcomes and minimizing adverse effects in the treatment of various diseases [50].

8.3.2 Nanoformulations

Today, approximately 40% of the drug compounds face limitations in solubility, stability, and absorption efficiency when interacting with smaller biomolecules. These limitations paved the way for the exploration of nanoformulations. Nanoformulations represent a significant advancement in the field of cancer therapy, offering improved chemical stability, reproducibility, and biocompatibility compared to conventional methods due to their protective coatings, which enhance drug stability [51]. Nanoformulations can be prepared with various nanomaterials, such as liposomes, polymeric NPs, micelles, dendrimers, and carbon nanotubes [52]. These structures may be used to encapsulate drugs, proteins, nucleic acids, or imaging agents, allowing for targeted delivery to specific tissues or cells [53]. A clear overview of the various nanoformulations used in drug delivery applications is presented in Figure 8.4.

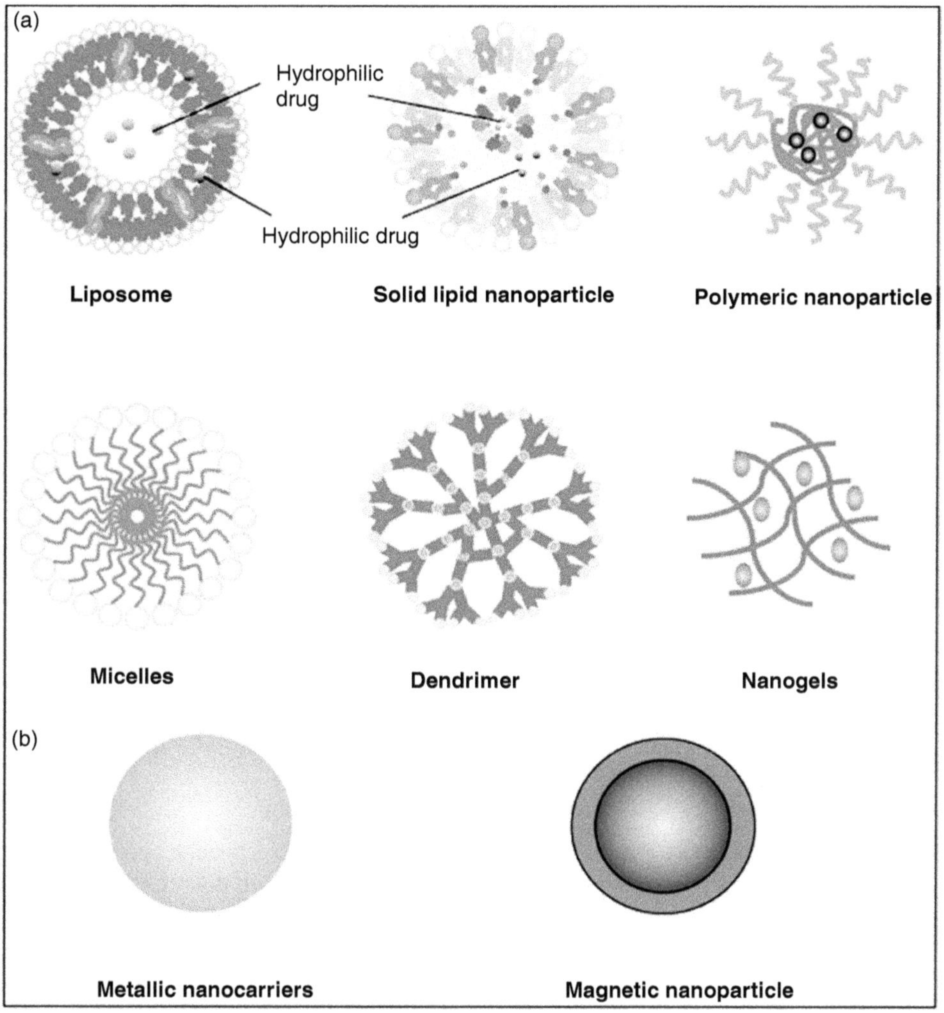

FIGURE 8.4 Various nanocarriers used for drug delivery: (a) organic nanocarriers and (b) inorganic nanoparticle carriers [83]. (Reprinted with permission.)

8.3.2.1 Liposomes

Liposomes, one of the oldest NPs to find their application in cancer therapy, are defined as spherical vesicular structures with one or more lipid bilayers and an aqueous core [54]. Liposomes provide enhanced biocompatibility, adaptability, and stability in biological environments and are, therefore, one of the most popular choices for drug-carrying vectors. The liposomes are used for encapsulation of therapeutic agents like drug or protein molecules and can be functionalized to target specific sites, providing precision medicine and reducing off-target effects [55]. These encapsulated structures can vary in size from 50 to 300nm and provide a shield to the drug molecules from unfavorable conditions before reaching their target [56].

As per reports, more than 1,800 cancer-related clinical studies using liposomes had been conducted. Liposomes like Doxil® (for doxorubicin delivery), Vyxeos® (used in cytarabine and daunorubicin delivery), and Onivyde® (in irinotecan drug delivery) have already gained FDA approvals [57].

8.3.2.2 Dendrimers

Dendrimers are highly branched, tree-like molecules with a well-defined structure composed of repeating units radiating from a central core [58]. These structures are made from polymeric nanostructures and characterized by their precisely controlled size, shape, and surface functionality. Dendrimers hold multiple active sites on their outer layer, allowing functional groups or drug molecules to be attached. They contain three distinct zones in their structure: the multivalent core, interior, and periphery, which enable a variety of advantages for transporting multiple classes of therapeutic and imaging agents [59,60]. Drug molecules and imaging agents can be covalently attached to surface sites or encapsulated within the core, facilitating solubilization of hydrophobic anticancer drugs. Various dendrimer structures have been studied to deliver therapeutic substances successfully, for example, polyamidoamine (PAMAM) and poly(propylene imine) (PPI), exhibiting promising potential for anticancer applications [61]. These structures enhance flexibility and binding efficiency due to their defined particle sizes, numerous functional groups for drug conjugation, and interior voids for drug encapsulation.

The drug carried through dendrimers has been deeply investigated via various ingestion routes like oral, skin, and nasal pathways. These structures also provide freedom of structure modifications, which could aid in eliminating any negative side effects, such as toxicity.

Few studies have demonstrated the delivery of polyethylene glycol (PEG)-based dendrimers and PAMAM-based dendrimers successfully across the blood-brain barrier and to cancerous cells, both in vitro and in vivo [62–64]. Folic acid-conjugated dendrimers effectively target tumor cells by exploiting overexpressed folate receptors [65]. Researchers also observe that dendrimers loaded with imaging agents enable improved monitoring of tumor angiogenesis and help to overcome challenges associated with traditional cancer treatments, including poor bioavailability and drug resistance [66–68].

8.3.2.3 Metallic NPs

Metal NPs or inorganic NPs can either encapsulate or disperse the therapeutic agents. NPs prepared from various inorganic materials, such as gold, silver, carbon quantum dots (CQDs), and magnetic particles, are extensively utilized in cancer treatment. These NPs offer precise targeting, good pharmacokinetics, and the ability to encapsulate poorly soluble drugs [69]. Gold and silver NPs deliver small and large drug molecules to tumor sites, mainly through EPR effects and tumor microenvironmental properties like changing pH and redox potential. Despite their potential, issues like aggregation and cytotoxicity to healthy cells limit their use unless combined with polymers like PEG. Magnetic NPs, typically made from metals or oxides, are employed for hyperthermic cancer therapy, allowing localized heating of tumors using external sources like microwaves [70]. Due to their superparamagnetic properties, they also find applications in theranostics, photodynamic therapy, and MRI. CQDs are fluorescent carbon NPs with excellent targeting capabilities and low toxicity. They are promising for bio-imaging, drug delivery, and diagnostics owing to their biocompatibility and ease of functionalization [71]. Overall, these inorganic NPs hold significant potential for advancing cancer treatment through targeted drug delivery and diagnostic applications.

8.3.2.4 Nanocapsules

Nanoemulsions are fine oil dispersion/water systems stabilized by a thin layer of artificial surfactants, with droplet size ranging from 20 to 600 nm. They can be oil-in-water, water-in-oil, or in a bicontinuous state and are generally transparent in nature due to their small size [72]. Nanoemulsions mask unpleasant tastes from oily liquids while introducing stability from hydrolysis and oxidation and are biocompatible, making them material of interest for drug delivery. They utilize passive targeting via the EPR effect and active targeting through surface functionalization [73]. Various targeting methods, including peptides and antibodies, enhance the specificity of tumor sites. They have advantages such as versatility in drug loading, overcoming multidrug resistance, reduced toxicity, and potential use without additional need for carriers [21]. Research has shown promising results, such as folate-targeted theranostic nanoemulsions reducing ovarian cancer tumor growth [74]. Overall, nanoemulsions present intriguing options for cancer therapy due to their unique properties and targeting capabilities.

8.3.2.5 Solid Lipid NPs

Solid lipid nanoparticles (SLNs) are colloidal drug delivery systems with liquid lipids replaced by solid lipids, emulsifiers, and water [75]. Triglycerides, waxes, steroids, fatty acids, and partial glycerides are some common examples of lipids used. They can be administered via topical, rectal, oral, or parental pathways [76,77]. SLNs exhibit a high level of drug delivery owing to their large surface area and uniform drug distribution, facilitated by lipid carrier crystallization behavior [78]. They employ passive, active, and co-delivery mechanisms for targeted drug delivery, utilizing EPR effects and receptor recognition on tumor cells. Vorinostat-loaded SLNs have demonstrated enhanced pharmacokinetics and efficacy against multidrug-resistant cancer cells like MCF-7, MDA-MB-231, and A549 [79]. SLNs offer advantages such as high biocompatibility, scalability, good bioavailability, and controlled drug release, although limitations like drug expulsion and low drug incorporation capacity exist. Novel synthesis methods, such as ultrasonic melting-emulsification, improve SLN properties.

8.3.2.6 Nanosponges

Nanosponges are garnering attention as a versatile drug formulation and delivery system capable of loading both hydrophilic and lipophilic compounds [80]. They possess a spongy colloid-like structure with various voids for incorporating pharmaceutically active substances. Typically prepared using beta-cyclodextrins and cross-linking agents like hexamethylene diisocyanate, nanosponges are insoluble in water and most carbon-based solvents. They exhibit inherent sterilization properties, a pH range of 2–11, and stability up to 300°C [81]. These characteristics make nanosponges promising candidates for drug delivery applications [82].

8.3.3 Drug Loading and Release Mechanisms

Drug loading and release mechanisms are crucial aspects of NP-based drug delivery systems in cancer nanotherapeutics. These mechanisms determine how efficiently therapeutic agents are encapsulated within NPs and subsequently released at the target site [84,85].

8.3.3.1 Drug Loading

Drug loading refers to the process of incorporating therapeutic agents, such as chemotherapy drugs or biological molecules, into NPs. This step is essential for ensuring the efficacy of the nanotherapeutic system [86]. Each loading method offers unique advantages and challenges, depending on the drug's and NPs' properties, desired release kinetics, and intended application. There are several methods for loading drugs into NPs, including:

i. *Encapsulation*: In this method, drugs are physically entrapped within the matrix of NPs during their synthesis or assembly. This can involve simple mixing of drugs with NP precursors followed by self-assembly or encapsulation during NP formation [87].
ii. *Chemical Conjugation*: Drugs can be chemically conjugated or attached to the surface or interior of NPs through covalent bonding or other chemical reactions [86]. This approach ensures stable drug loading and controlled release.
iii. *Adsorption*: Drugs can be adsorbed onto the surface of NPs through weak interactions such as electrostatic forces, hydrophobic interactions, or van der Waals forces. Although relatively simple, this method may result in less controlled drug release [86].
iv. *Incorporation during NP Formation*: Drugs can be incorporated into NPs during their synthesis process, such as during the formation of polymer NPs or lipid-based vesicles. This ensures a homogeneous distribution of drugs within the NP matrix [88].

8.3.3.2 Drug Release Mechanisms

Once loaded into NPs, drugs must be released in a controlled manner at the target site to achieve therapeutic efficacy while minimizing off-target effects. These can be classified into four categories: (i) diffusion-controlled release, (ii) degradation-controlled release, (iii) stimuli-responsive release, and (iv) triggered release [89]. In a diffusion-controlled release, drugs diffuse through the NP matrix or across its surface, driven by concentration gradients. Factors such as NP size, porosity, and drug hydrophobicity influence the rate of diffusion and release kinetics. Some NP materials, such as biodegradable polymers or lipids, undergo degradation or erosion in biological environments, releasing encapsulated drugs. Degradation-controlled release offers temporal control over drug release, as the degradation rate can be tailored by modifying NP composition. Stimuli-responsive NPs can release drugs in response to specific environmental cues, such as pH, temperature, enzymes, or light. These NPs are designed to undergo structural or chemical changes in response to external stimuli, triggering drug release at the desired site. In triggered release mechanisms, drugs are released in response to external stimuli, such as magnetic fields, ultrasound, or electrical signals. These stimuli can be applied externally to the body, allowing spatial and temporal control over drug release.

8.4 TARGETED THERAPIES AND PRECISION MEDICINE

Targeted therapies and precision medicine represent a paradigm shift in cancer treatment, focusing on tailoring treatments to individual patients based on their unique genetic, molecular, and clinical characteristics [90]. Rather than employing a one-size-fits-all approach, personalized medicine in cancer treatment involves identifying specific molecular alterations driving tumor growth and selecting therapies that target these aberrations. By targeting key pathways or molecules involved in cancer development and progression, targeted therapies aim to disrupt tumor growth while minimizing damage to healthy tissues. Precision medicine approaches have led to the development of novel therapies that demonstrate improved efficacy and reduced toxicity compared to traditional chemotherapy, offering new hope for patients with various types of cancer [91].

8.4.1 Personalized Medicine Approaches in Cancer Treatment

Personalized medicine approaches in cancer treatment encompass a range of strategies aimed at tailoring therapies to the individual characteristics of each patient and their tumor. This includes utilizing molecular profiling techniques, such as genomic sequencing and proteomic analysis, to identify specific genetic mutations, biomarkers, or other molecular signatures associated with the patient's cancer [92]. Armed with this information, clinicians can select targeted therapies or immunotherapies most likely effective for that particular patient. Personalized medicine also encompasses the use of predictive biomarkers to monitor treatment response and adjust therapy as needed, optimizing outcomes while minimizing side effects.

8.4.2 Targeted Nanotherapies for Specific Cancer Types

Targeted nanotherapies represent a promising approach to precision cancer medicine, leveraging the unique properties of NPs to deliver therapeutic agents specifically to cancer cells while sparing healthy tissues. These nanotherapies can be designed to target specific molecular markers or pathways that are overexpressed or dysregulated in particular cancer types. For example, NPs can be functionalized with targeting ligands, such as antibodies or peptides, that recognize and bind to receptors on the surface of cancer cells [93,94]. This targeted approach enhances drug delivery to the tumor site, increasing therapeutic efficacy while reducing systemic toxicity. Targeted nanotherapies have shown promise in the treatment of various cancer types, including breast cancer, lung cancer, and melanoma, among others [95].

8.4.3 Challenges in Achieving Precision Medicine with Nanotherapeutics

Despite the potential benefits of targeted nanotherapies in precision cancer medicine, several challenges must be addressed to realize their full potential. These challenges include overcoming biological barriers to NP delivery, such as the tumor microenvironment, which can impede NP penetration and hinder therapeutic efficacy [96]. Additionally, issues related to NP stability, toxicity, and manufacturing scalability must be addressed to facilitate clinical translation. Furthermore, the heterogeneity of tumors presents a significant challenge, as different patients may respond differently to the same therapy based on their tumor subtype or molecular profile. Overcoming these challenges requires interdisciplinary collaboration among researchers, clinicians, engineers, and regulatory agencies to develop innovative solutions and advance the field of precision cancer medicine [97].

8.4.4 Biological Barriers in Nanomedicine

Biological barriers hinder the effective delivery of nanotherapeutics to diseased sites, impacting treatment efficacy in conditions like cancer and inflammation [98]. Overcoming biological barriers in NP-based drug delivery to tumors is imperative for enhancing therapeutic efficacy and improving outcomes in cancer treatment. The intricate tumor microenvironment presents formidable challenges, characterized by a dense extracellular matrix, aberrant blood vessel architecture, and elevated interstitial fluid pressure, collectively impeding the efficient accumulation and penetration of NPs into tumor tissues. Additionally, systemic clearance mechanisms, such as the reticuloendothelial system (RES), pose further hurdles by rapidly eliminating NPs from circulation before they can reach the tumor site, thus reducing their bioavailability [17]. To address these challenges, the development of diverse strategies has been explored for enhancing tumor penetration and accumulation of NPs. These strategies encompass optimizing the physicochemical properties of NPs, including size, shape, surface charge, and surface modifications, to improve their circulation half-life and tumor-targeting capabilities.

The incorporation of targeting ligands, such as antibodies, peptides, or aptamers, enhances the specific binding of NPs to tumor cells, facilitating their internalization and enhancing therapeutic efficacy [99]. Stimuli-responsive NPs, which undergo structural or chemical changes in response to tumor-specific cues like pH or enzyme activity, offer an additional avenue to enhance tumor penetration and accumulation. The engineered NPs can leverage physical forces, such as ultrasound or magnetic fields, to improve their distribution within tumor tissues. Beyond tumor-specific barriers, addressing immune and physiological barriers is crucial for optimizing NP-based drug delivery to tumors [100]. Strategies aimed at modulating the immune response, such as immunomodulatory NPs or combination therapies with immunotherapeutic agents, can overcome immune evasion mechanisms employed by tumors and enhance the anti-tumor immune response.

8.4.5 Artificial Intelligence in Nanomedicine

AI emerges as a transformative tool to address the challenges in nanomedicine by globally optimizing drug and dose selection, dynamically adjusting treatment regimens, and predicting treatment outcomes based on individual patient characteristics [101]. A crucial aspect of optimizing combination therapy lies in identifying synergistic drug combinations and determining the appropriate dosages to maximize efficacy while minimizing toxicity. AI offers a systematic and data-driven approach to exploring this complex landscape, leveraging computational algorithms to analyze large datasets and identify optimal treatment strategies. Recent studies have demonstrated the ability of AI platforms to identify effective drug combinations that outperform conventional treatments, leading to improved patient outcomes and reduced treatment-related toxicity [102]. Also, the dynamic nature of drug interaction and patient responses throughout treatment presents additional challenges that

AI can help address. By continuously monitoring patient data and adapting treatment regimens in real time, AI-guided therapies could optimize dosing strategies to maintain efficacy and minimize adverse effects [103]. This dynamic approach to combination therapy ensures that treatment remains responsive to changes in patient physiology and disease progression, maximizing the likelihood of successful outcomes. AI can also play a crucial role in optimizing drug targeting and localization parameters, leveraging computational models to design NPs that maximize therapeutic efficacy while minimizing off-target effects [102].

8.5 NANOTECHNOLOGY IN DIAGNOSTICS

Nanotechnology emerges as a transformative force in diagnostics, offering the ability to detect cancer in its earliest stages, pinpoint disease subtypes, and precisely deliver therapy where it's most effective [104]. Operating on a scale of a few nanometers, nanodevices harness unique properties distinct from bulk materials, such as self-assembly and quantum effects. These traits enable the development of novel imaging agents and biosensors that capitalize on NPs like magnetic particles and quantum dots, providing enhanced stability, targeting, and contrast compared to conventional methods. NPs deliver contrast agents or probes inside cells without disruption, enabling highly sensitive and multiplexed sensors capable of detecting various signatures [104]. Integrating targeting, imaging, sensing, and therapeutic delivery functionalities into multifunctional NPs lays the foundation for intelligent platforms capable of identifying, detecting, and treating tumors.

8.5.1 In Vivo Diagnostics: NP-Based Imaging

NP-based imaging is a cutting-edge approach within in vivo diagnostics that employs NPs as contrast agents or imaging probes to visualize and analyze biological structures and processes at the molecular and cellular levels. NPs used in imaging applications are engineered to possess unique properties that enhance their interaction with biological tissues and enable precise imaging. These NPs can be functionalized with targeting ligands to bind to specific biomarkers associated with disease selectively, improving the specificity of imaging [105]. NPs can also be designed to emit signals, such as fluorescence or magnetic resonance, allowing them to be detected and visualized using specialized imaging equipment. The use of NP-based imaging offers several advantages over traditional imaging methods like increased sensitivity and resolution, allowing for the detection of smaller lesions or abnormalities at earlier stages of disease progression [106].

8.5.1.1 Nanodiagnostics Using Contrast Imaging

Traditional techniques like MRI use contrast agents, which, even though effective, often rely on broad physiological characteristics to distinguish between tissues, limiting their sensitivity and specificity. NP-based contrast agents, however, hold the potential to detect subtle biochemical differences between tissues before gross anatomical features are apparent. The NPs, such as liposomes, dendrimers, and nanotubes, can be loaded with imaging agents like paramagnetic metals or radionuclides [107]. By targeting tumor cells either passively or actively with specific antibodies or aptamers, these NPs can enhance the sensitivity and specificity of imaging, enabling noninvasive detection and characterization of diseases at earlier stages.

Innovative NP formulations, such as gado-nanotubes encapsulating gadolinium atoms, have demonstrated significantly improved sensitivity compared to conventional contrast agents [108]. These novel formulations enhance image resolution and reduce the toxicity associated with metal-based contrast agents. Moreover, nanobubbles composed of polymer-based materials have shown promise in contrast-enhanced ultrasound lymphography, facilitating more efficient transport to regional lymphatics and enabling imaging of lymphatic structures with high contrast enhancement [109]. These advancements underscore the potential of nanotechnology to revolutionize medical imaging, enabling more accurate and sensitive diagnosis of diseases like cancer and improving patient outcomes.

8.5.1.2 Optical Imaging Nanomaterials

Quantum dots and semiconductor nanocrystals offer an innovative approach to biological labeling and optical imaging, serving as alternatives to traditional fluorophore dyes [110,111]. These nanomaterials, composed of a semiconductor core surrounded by an inorganic and organic shell, exhibit broad absorption spectra and emit a wide range of colors, enabling the creation of thousands of unique signatures. Developed microbeads embedding quantum dots can theoretically achieve a multiplex capacity of up to one million [112]. Intravenously injected quantum dots have demonstrated successful in vivo imaging of targeted tumor tissues, leveraging both EPR at tumor sites and specific antibody binding to cancer-specific biomarkers. Efforts in material development have expanded to include various semiconductor families, enabling emission across a broad spectrum of wavelengths. Near-infrared-emitting quantum dots have particularly shown promise in overcoming tissue autofluorescence, allowing for deep-tissue imaging. In extensive animal studies, these quantum dots have facilitated intraoperative mapping of sentinel lymph nodes located up to 1 cm below the surface within minutes of injection [113]. Quantum dots have proven effective for intracellular binding and imaging of inner cell components and activity, with methods developed to promote their uptake into cells through endocytosis or specific peptide recognition. For instance, quantum dots labeled with cancer markers have successfully stained cellular structures such as actin and microtubule fibers and nuclear antigens, demonstrating their potential for cellular imaging and diagnostics.

8.5.1.3 Imaging Functional Activity

NPs offer a versatile platform for imaging functional activity within tissues and cells, allowing for studying dynamic cellular events and biochemical activities indicative of early precancerous or cancerous states. For instance, MRI of angiogenic vasculature, a marker for cancer recognition, has been achieved using liposome NPs targeting $\alpha_v\beta_3$ integrin, highly expressed in neovascular endothelial cells. This approach has enabled high-resolution imaging of melanoma in its earliest growth phase by visualizing $\alpha_v\beta_3$ integrin expression on the neovasculature of minute solid tumors [114,115].

NPs conjugated to annexin-V have been utilized to monitor apoptosis, providing insight into the success of therapeutic treatments by binding to phosphatidyl serine exposed during cell membrane breakdown [116]. NPs have been explored to image intracellular enzymatic activity, offering a glimpse into cellular processes at the molecular level. Nanoprobes utilizing sequestered gadolinium atoms have been developed to detect enzymatic activity, where cleavage of an active site exposes gadolinium to water, enhancing image contrast [117].

Imaging nanoprobes consisting of a gold NP attached to a quantum dot via a peptide sequence have been devised to track a broad range of enzymatic activity in vivo. This innovative approach allows for simultaneous tracking of multiple proteases' activity by tuning the emission spectrum of the quantum dot and varying the peptide sequence. These advancements highlight the potential of NP-based imaging in exposing intricate cellular mechanisms and disease progression.

8.5.2 In Vitro Diagnostics: Biosensors

To meet the demands of early cancer detection, biosensors with high specificity and sensitivity detect nucleic acids and proteins at extremely low concentrations. The platforms should enable label-free detection, eliminating the need for target tagging, and support homogeneous assays for continuous signal monitoring [118]. Multiplex capability, allowing recognition of numerous molecular signatures simultaneously, is also essential. Nanotechnology plays a crucial role in advancing biosensor capabilities, with nanocomponents enhancing sensor design and implementation. Integrated sample preparation further enhances these sensors, facilitating their use in clinical settings closer to patients for more timely diagnostic information and improved medical decision-making [119]. Figure 8.5 provides a brief overview of various nanostructures used for in vitro and in vivo early diagnostic applications in cancer, along with the detection mechanisms employed.

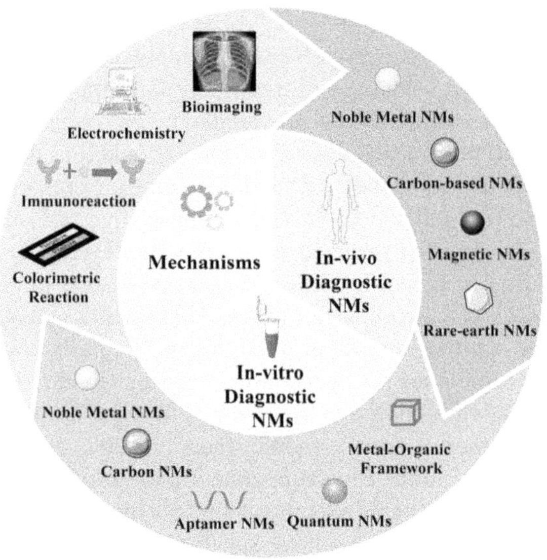

FIGURE 8.5 Nanomaterials in early diagnosis of cancer for in vitro and in vivo analysis and their detecting mechanisms [120]. (Reprinted with permission.)

8.5.2.1 Nanoarray Sensors

Nanoarrays have emerged as powerful tools for cancer biomarker detection and post-therapy monitoring, enabled by advancements in manufacturing techniques borrowed from the semiconductor industry. These nanoarrays comprise nucleic acid and protein probes, offering massive multiplexing capabilities to simultaneously detect numerous binding events. Innovations include lithography-based arrays and more straightforward fabrication methods utilizing microelectromechanical system micromirrors or carbon nanotube sites for higher sensitivity and electronic readout [121]. Exotic concepts like nanogap capacitors and dip-pen lithography are also being explored, pushing the boundaries of array density and probe site recognition.

8.5.2.2 Electromechanical Sensors

Electromechanical sensors, such as micro- and nanocantilevers, offer label-free detection and direct recognition approaches, simplifying assays. These sensors, exemplified by their application in monitoring prostate-specific antigen and DNA binding, show promise for highly sensitive detection, potentially eliminating the need for DNA amplification [122]. Similarly, nanowires and carbon nanotubes integrated into transistor devices offer label-free detection with high sensitivity, paving the way for large arrays capable of detecting binding events with precision.

8.5.2.3 NP Sensors

These sensors leverage distinct signatures of nano-objects, like quantum dots and metallic NPs, for multiplexed assays and direct recognition of binding events. Gold NPs, for instance, enable sensitive detection of DNA through conductivity changes across electrode gaps [123]. Innovations like gold nanoshells for immunoassays and DNA barcodes attached to magnetic particles further enhance sensitivity and selectivity, promising detection at atto- to femtomolar levels for both nucleic acids and proteins. These advancements hold significant potential for improving data acquisition in large-scale population studies and enhancing cancer biomarker detection in clinical settings.

8.5.3 Toxicity and Fate of NPs in the Human Body

Nanotechnology and NPs have significantly advanced various fields, including healthcare, pharmaceuticals, therapeutics, and environmental science, to name a few. However, being a relatively newer field, it isn't easy to judge the long-term effects of nanomaterials, especially in in vitro applications. The major concerns are potential toxicity, ADMET properties, and ultimate fate within the human body. These effects could result from the physicochemical properties of NPs like dimensions, charge, morphology, composition, etc. These properties question the cellular uptake and the final destination of these particles in the body. NPs have been observed to induce oxidative stress and reactive oxygen species (ROS) generation, which result in high risks of cell damage, apoptosis, inflammation, etc. Metal-based NPs like silver and titanium dioxide have been reported to generate ROS-damaging proteins, lipids, and nucleic acid materials [124].

Carbon-based NPs like carbon nanotubes, graphene oxide activates immune cells by interacting with macrophages and other immune cells, leading to chronic inflammation. Polymeric (PLGA, PEG) and lipid-based NPs (liposomes) have also been reported to provoke immune reactions, influencing nanomedicine safety and efficacy [125]. Metal and metal oxide NPs have been shown to induce genotoxic effects by directly interacting with DNA or through secondary oxidative stress pathways [126].

With such concerns, the final fate of NPs in the human body remains questionable. Due to the limited availability of long-term data, the route of exposure, interactions with biological barriers, and excretion capability of nanomaterials are still major concerns [127]. The absorption and accumulation of NPs begin through inhalation, ingestion, skin contact, or intravenous administration [128]. Once inside the body, if they successfully cross biological barriers, the repercussions could be systemic, especially in the case of the placental or blood-brain barriers [129]. Metabolism and clearance depend on NP composition—some undergo enzymatic degradation, while others resist metabolism and accumulate in tissues [130]. Organic NPs, such as lipid-based and polymeric formulations, are more biodegradable than inorganic NPs like gold or silica [131]. Excretion pathways include renal clearance for smaller, hydrophilic NPs and hepatobiliary excretion for larger or hydrophobic NPs. Research on magnetic nanostructures for cancer theranostic applications (Current Pathobiology Reports) suggests that surface modifications can enhance NP clearance, thereby reducing toxicity risks [132]. Understanding these mechanisms is crucial for designing safer and more effective nanomedicine applications.

8.5.4 Challenges in Nanodiagnostics

The pursuit of early cancer detection through nanotechnology presents a dual challenge. While it promises to revolutionize diagnostics and improve treatment outcomes, it also necessitates careful consideration of safety and regulatory concerns. Nanotechnology enables the detection of early-stage cancers, but determining the appropriate course of treatment remains a complex issue, particularly for indolent tumors that may not progress or cause harm. Nanotechnology-based in vivo sensing holds the potential for analyzing lesions based on biomarker signatures, offering insights into personalized treatment decisions.

However, safety concerns surrounding nanomaterials, such as quantum dots, raise questions about toxicity and regulatory oversight. Efforts are underway to address these issues, with studies assessing in vitro and in vivo safety and exploring modifications to render NPs nontoxic. Regulatory protocols must adapt to the unique challenges posed by multifunctional NPs, streamlining approval processes without compromising safety. Collaboration between regulatory agencies and research institutions is crucial to develop standardized toxicity testing protocols and ensure the timely translation of nanodiagnostics into clinical practice [133].

Despite these challenges, the impact of early cancer detection on survival rates underscores the importance of advancing nanotechnology in diagnostics. Nanodiagnostics offer enhanced sensitivity, spatial resolution, and real-time therapeutic efficacy monitoring, paving the way for personalized medicine tailored to individual patient's genetic and molecular profiles. Interdisciplinary collaboration and training are essential to bridge the gap between biological research and engineering, driving innovation in nanotechnology solutions for cancer diagnosis and treatment. Initiatives like the National Cancer Institute's Alliance for Nanotechnology in Cancer and the National Science Foundation's Integrative Graduate Education and Research Traineeship Program aim to foster collaboration and develop common platforms for data integration, accelerating progress in the field of nanodiagnostics [134].

8.6 FUTURE PROSPECTS AND CONCLUSION

The discussion highlights the transformative potential of nanotherapeutics in cancer diagnostics and treatment by integrating multiple functionalities into a single platform, enabling personalized and targeted therapy. Nanotherapeutics facilitate real-time monitoring of treatment efficacy and guided drug delivery, promising enhanced clinical outcomes. Key aspects include co-encapsulation of chemotherapeutics and imaging agents for simultaneous diagnostic imaging and therapeutic applications. With unique properties such as surface modifications for enhanced targeting and customizable size distribution, nanotherapeutics can exploit tumor microenvironments for efficient drug delivery while minimizing systemic toxicity.

Despite their immense potential, nanotherapeutics face challenges related to the tumor microenvironment, biological barriers, and regulatory approval processes. Addressing these challenges requires interdisciplinary collaboration among researchers from engineering, sciences, the pharmaceutical industry, and medicine. Moreover, comprehensive training programs in translational nanomedicine are essential to prepare the next generation of scientists and clinicians for advancing this field. The development of nanotherapeutics necessitates overcoming hurdles in clinical trial design, regulatory approval, and cost-effectiveness. Innovative approaches such as virtual R&D, information technology-guided clinical trials, and public-private partnerships can expedite the translation of nanotherapeutics from bench to bedside. Moreover, regulatory agencies like the FDA play a crucial role in providing guidance and support for nanomedicine research and development. Looking ahead, nanotherapeutics hold immense promise for improving cancer diagnosis, monitoring, and treatment. As the global market for nanomedicine continues to grow, investments in research, education, and collaborative partnerships will be pivotal in realizing the full potential of nanotherapeutics in clinical practice. Ultimately, nanotherapeutics represents a significant advancement in precision medicine and personalized cancer care, with far-reaching implications for improving patient outcomes in the years to come.

REFERENCES

1. Deshmukh, K., Nanotechnology in ancient era. In Menka Khoobchandani and Arpita Saxena (Eds.), *Biotechnology Products in Everyday Life*, 2019: p. 3–14.
2. Nasrollahzadeh, M., et al., An introduction to nanotechnology. In Arthur T. Hubbard (Ed.), *Interface Science and Technology*. 2019: p. 1–27, Elsevier.
3. Wolf, E.L., *Nanophysics and Nanotechnology: An Introduction to Modern Concepts in Nanoscience*. 2015, John Wiley & Sons.
4. Rai, P. and S.A. Morris, *Nanotheranostics for Cancer Applications*. 2019. Springer link
5. Zaidi, S., L. Misba, and A.U. Khan, Nano-therapeutics: A revolution in infection control in post antibiotic era. *Nanomedicine: Nanotechnology, Biology and Medicine*, 2017. 13(7): p. 2281–2301.
6. Logothetidis, S., Nanomedicine: The medicine of tomorrow. In Stergios Logothetidis (Ed.), *Nanomedicine and Nanobiotechnology*. 2011: p. 1–26, Springer.
7. Bhowmik, D., et al., Nanomedicine-an overview. *International Journal of PharmTech Research*, 2010. 2(4): p. 2143–2151.
8. Alharbi, K.K. and Y.A. Al-Sheikh, Role and implications of nanodiagnostics in the changing trends of clinical diagnosis. *Saudi Journal of Biological Sciences*, 2014. 21(2): p. 109–117.

9. Wang, Y., et al., Application of nanodiagnostics in point-of-care tests for infectious diseases. *International Journal of Nanomedicine*, 2017: p. 4789–4803.
10. Jain, K.K., Role of nanodiagnostics in personalized cancer therapy. *Clinics in Laboratory Medicine*, 2012. 32(1): p. 15–31.
11. Ferlay, J., et al., Cancer statistics for the year 2020: An overview. *International Journal of Cancer*, 2021. 149(4): p. 778–789.
12. Sung, H., et al., Global cancer statistics 2020: GLOBOCAN estimates of incidence and mortality worldwide for 36 cancers in 185 countries. *CA: A Cancer Journal for Clinicians*, 2021. 71(3): p. 209–249.
13. Blackadar, C.B., Historical review of the causes of cancer. *World Journal of Clinical Oncology*, 2016. 7(1): p. 54.
14. Meijers, W.C. and R.A. de Boer, Common risk factors for heart failure and cancer. *Cardiovascular Research*, 2019. 115(5): p. 844–853.
15. Stein, C. and G. Colditz, Modifiable risk factors for cancer. *British Journal of Cancer*, 2004. 90(2): p. 299–303.
16. Ojha, A., et al., Nanoparticles and nanomaterials-based recent approaches in upgraded targeting and management of cancer: A review. *Cancers*, 2022. 15(1): p. 162.
17. Ediriwickrema, A. and W.M. Saltzman, Nanotherapy for cancer: Targeting and multifunctionality in the future of cancer therapies. *ACS Biomaterials Science & Engineering*, 2015. 1(2): p. 64–78.
18. Hartshorn, C.M. and S.A. Morris, Theranostics: A historical perspective of cancer nanotechnology paving the way for simultaneous use applications. *Nanotheranostics for Cancer Applications*, 2019: p. 91–105.
19. Falzone, L., S. Salomone, and M. Libra, Evolution of cancer pharmacological treatments at the turn of the third millennium. *Frontiers in Pharmacology*, 2018. 9: p. 421926.
20. Rasool, B.K.A., et al., Advances in vaccine delivery strategies to promote effective immunization. *Journal of Applied Pharmaceutical Science*, 2022. 12(5): p. 001–026.
21. Nirmala, M.J., et al., Cancer nanomedicine: A review of nano-therapeutics and challenges ahead. *RSC Advances*, 2023. 13(13): p. 8606–8629.
22. Demetzos, C., *Nanotechnology in Therapeutics: Basics and Trends*. 2024, John Wiley & Sons.
23. Barenholz, Y.C., Doxil®—The first FDA-approved nano-drug: Lessons learned. *Journal of Controlled Release*, 2012. 160(2): p. 117–134.
24. Desai, N., Nanoparticle albumin-bound paclitaxel (Abraxane®). In *Albumin in Medicine: Pathological and Clinical Applications*. 2016: p. 101–119, Springer.
25. Wu, M., et al., Nanocluster of superparamagnetic iron oxide nanoparticles coated with poly (dopamine) for magnetic field-targeting, highly sensitive MRI and photothermal cancer therapy. *Nanotechnology*, 2015. 26(11): p. 115102.
26. Subhan, M.A. and M. Muzibur Rahman, Recent development in metallic nanoparticles for breast cancer therapy and diagnosis. *The Chemical Record*, 2022. 22(7): p. e202100331.
27. Chaturvedi, V.K., et al., Cancer nanotechnology: A new revolution for cancer diagnosis and therapy. *Current Drug Metabolism*, 2019. 20(6): p. 416–429.
28. Serpico, L., et al., Lipid nanoparticles-based RNA therapies for breast cancer treatment. *Drug Delivery and Translational Research*, 2024. 14(10): p. 2823–2844.
29. Gedefaw, L., et al., Targeting inflammasome activation in COVID-19: Delivery of RNA interference-based therapeutic molecules. *Biomedicines*, 2021. 9(12): p. 1823.
30. Liu, Y., et al., Photothermal therapy and photoacoustic imaging via nanotheranostics in fighting cancer. *Chemical Society Reviews*, 2019. 48(7): p. 2053–2108.
31. Kumar, D., I. Mutreja, and A. Kaushik, Recent advances in noble metal nanoparticles for cancer nanotheranostics. *Journal of Nanotheranostics*, 2023. 4(2): p. 150–170.
32. Erren, T.C., et al., *What Do We Know 40 Years after Nixon Declared the 'War on Cancer'? On the Origin, Prevention and Treatment of Cancer*. 2012: p. 597–600, Springer.
33. International Agency for Research on Cancer, *IARC's Mission: Cancer Research for Cancer Prevention*. Available from: https://www.iarc.fr/cards_page/aboutiarc, 2020.
34. EU, C.M.B. *Cancer Mission*. Available from: https://www.healthncp.net/cancer-mission#:~:text=What%20are%20the%20goals%20and,to%20live%20longer%20and%20better.
35. Chen, S., et al., Estimates and projections of the global economic cost of 29 cancers in 204 countries and territories from 2020 to 2050. *JAMA Oncology*, 2023. 9(4): p. 465–472.
36. Bawa, R., The future of nanomedicine. In *Hopes and Visions for the 21st Century*, 2007: p. 266–283. World Future Society.
37. De Jong, W.H. and P.J. Borm, Drug delivery and nanoparticles: Applications and hazards. *International Journal of Nanomedicine*, 2008. 3(2): p. 133–149.

38. Moghimi, S.M., A.C. Hunter, and J.C. Murray, Nanomedicine: Current status and future prospects. *The FASEB Journal*, 2005. 19(3): p. 311–330.
39. Pardeshi, S.R., et al., Importance of nanomedicine in human health. In Tariq Altalhi, Inamuddin (Ed.), *Green Sustainable Process for Chemical and Environmental Engineering and Science*. 2023: p. 3–33, Elsevier.
40. Loureiro, A., et al., Albumin-based nanodevices as drug carriers. *Current Pharmaceutical Design*, 2016. 22(10): p. 1371–1390.
41. Grant, J., et al., Engineering multifunctional nanomedicine platforms for drug delivery and imaging. *Nanotheranostics for Cancer Applications*, 2019: p. 319–344.
42. Durymanov, M., et al., Exploiting passive nanomedicine accumulation at sites of enhanced vascular permeability for non-cancerous applications. *Journal of Controlled Release*, 2017. 261: p. 10–22.
43. Elkhodiry, M.A., et al., Synergistic nanomedicine: Passive, active, and ultrasound-triggered drug delivery in cancer treatment. *Journal of Nanoscience and Nanotechnology*, 2016. 16(1): p. 1–18.
44. Torchilin, V.P., Passive and active drug targeting: Drug delivery to tumors as an example. *Drug Delivery*, 2010: p. 3–53.
45. Cho, K., et al., Therapeutic nanoparticles for drug delivery in cancer. *Clinical Cancer Research*, 2008. 14(5): p. 1310–1316.
46. Gavas, S., S. Quazi, and T.M. Karpiński, Nanoparticles for cancer therapy: Current progress and challenges. *Nanoscale Research Letters*, 2021. 16(1): p. 173.
47. Ma, X., et al., Future of nanotherapeutics: Targeting the cellular sub-organelles. *Biomaterials*, 2016. 97: p. 10–21.
48. Nag, O.K. and J.B. Delehanty, Active cellular and subcellular targeting of nanoparticles for drug delivery. *Pharmaceutics*, 2019. 11(10): p. 543.
49. Qiao, Y., et al., Stimuli-responsive nanotherapeutics for precision drug delivery and cancer therapy. *Wiley Interdisciplinary Reviews: Nanomedicine and Nanobiotechnology*, 2019. 11(1): p. e1527.
50. Song, Y., et al., Recent advances in targeted stimuli-responsive nano-based drug delivery systems combating atherosclerosis. *Chinese Chemical Letters*, 2022. 33(4): p. 1705–1717.
51. Jeevanandam, J., Y. San Chan, and M.K. Danquah, Nano-formulations of drugs: Recent developments, impact and challenges. *Biochimie*, 2016. 128: p. 99–112.
52. Kumar, A., et al., Nanotherapeutics: A novel and powerful approach in modern healthcare system. In *Nanotechnology in Modern Animal Biotechnology*. 2019: p. 149–161, Elsevier.
53. Koo, O.M., I. Rubinstein, and H. Onyuksel, Role of nanotechnology in targeted drug delivery and imaging: A concise review. *Nanomedicine: Nanotechnology, Biology and Medicine*, 2005. 1(3): p. 193–212.
54. Lasic, D., Liposomes. *American Scientist*, 1992. 80(1): p. 20–31.
55. Gu, W., et al., Actively targeted nanomedicines for precision cancer therapy: Concept, construction, challenges and clinical translation. *Journal of Controlled Release*, 2021. 329: p. 676–695.
56. Rommasi, F. and N. Esfandiari, Liposomal nanomedicine: Applications for drug delivery in cancer therapy. *Nanoscale Research Letters*, 2021. 16(1): p. 95.
57. Tezcan, T. and C.-H. Hsu, Nanotechnology in healthcare: Nanoparticles for diagnostic and therapy. In Debmalya Barh (ED.), *Biotechnology in Healthcare*. 2022: p. 55–69, Elsevier.
58. Tomalia, D.A., J.B. Christensen, and U. Boas, *Dendrimers, Dendrons, and Dendritic Polymers: Discovery, Applications, and the Future*. 2012, Cambridge University Press.
59. Singh, J., et al., Dendrimers in anticancer drug delivery: Mechanism of interaction of drug and dendrimers. *Artificial Cells, Nanomedicine, and Biotechnology*, 2016. 44(7): p. 1626–1634.
60. Kesharwani, P., *Dendrimer-Based Nanotherapeutics*. 2021, Academic Press.
61. Chis, A.A., et al., Applications and limitations of dendrimers in biomedicine. *Molecules*, 2020. 25(17): p. 3982.
62. Zaręba, M., et al., Mixed-generation PAMAM G3-G0 megamer as a drug delivery system for nimesulide: Antitumor activity of the conjugate against human squamous carcinoma and glioblastoma cells. *International Journal of Molecular Sciences*, 2019. 20(20): p. 4998.
63. Bae, Y., et al., Polyplexes of functional PAMAM dendrimer/apoptin gene induce apoptosis of human primary glioma cells in vitro. *Polymers*, 2019. 11(2): p. 296.
64. Choi, J., et al., Telodendrimers for physical encapsulation and covalent linking of individual or combined therapeutics. *Molecular Pharmaceutics*, 2017. 14(8): p. 2607–2615.
65. Fatima, M., et al., Folic acid conjugated poly (amidoamine) dendrimer as a smart nanocarriers for tracing, imaging, and treating cancers over-expressing folate receptors. *European Polymer Journal*, 2022. 170: p. 111156.

66. Garrigue, P., et al., Self-assembling supramolecular dendrimer nanosystem for PET imaging of tumors. *Proceedings of the National Academy of Sciences*, 2018. 115(45): p. 11454–11459.
67. Qiao, Z. and X. Shi, Dendrimer-based molecular imaging contrast agents. *Progress in Polymer Science*, 2015. 44: p. 1–27.
68. Ding, L., et al., Dendrimer-based magnetic resonance imaging agents for brain cancer. *Science China Materials*, 2018. 61(11): p. 1420–1443.
69. Ghosh, P., et al., Gold nanoparticles in delivery applications. *Advanced Drug Delivery Reviews*, 2008. 60(11): p. 1307–1315.
70. Farzin, A., et al., Magnetic nanoparticles in cancer therapy and diagnosis. *Advanced Healthcare Materials*, 2020. 9(9): p. 1901058.
71. Santhosh, P.B. and N.P. Ulrih, Multifunctional superparamagnetic iron oxide nanoparticles: Promising tools in cancer theranostics. *Cancer Letters*, 2013. 336(1): p. 8–17.
72. Mahato, R., Nanoemulsion as targeted drug delivery system for cancer therapeutics. *Journal of Pharmaceutical Sciences and Pharmacology*, 2017. 3(2): p. 83–97.
73. Kim, B., C.D. Pena, and D.T. Auguste, Targeted lipid nanoemulsions encapsulating epigenetic drugs exhibit selective cytotoxicity on $CDH1^{-}$/$FOXM1^{+}$ triple negative breast cancer cells. *Molecular Pharmaceutics*, 2019. 16(5): p. 1813–1826.
74. Patel, N.R., et al., *In Vitro* and *In Vivo* evaluation of a novel folate-targeted theranostic nanoemulsion of docetaxel for imaging and improved anticancer activity against ovarian cancers. *Cancer Biology & Therapy*, 2018. 19(7): p. 554–564.
75. Müller, R.H., K. Mäder, and S. Gohla, Solid lipid nanoparticles (SLN) for controlled drug delivery–A review of the state of the art. *European Journal of Pharmaceutics and Biopharmaceutics*, 2000. 50(1): p. 161–177.
76. Dingler, A., et al., Solid lipid nanoparticles (SLNTM/LipopearlsTM) a pharmaceutical and cosmetic carrier for the application of vitamin E in dermal products. *Journal of Microencapsulation*, 1999. 16(6): p. 751–767.
77. Sznitowska, M., et al., Bioavailability of diazepam from aqueous-organic solution, submicron emulsion and solid lipid nanoparticles after rectal administration in rabbits. *European Journal of Pharmaceutics and Biopharmaceutics*, 2001. 52(2): p. 159–163.
78. Bezbaruah, R., et al., Nanoparticle-based delivery systems for vaccines. *Vaccines*, 2022. 10(11): p. 1946.
79. Akanda, M., et al., Bioconjugated solid lipid nanoparticles (SLNs) for targeted prostate cancer therapy. *International Journal of Pharmaceutics*, 2021. 599: p. 120416.
80. Trotta, F. and R. Cavalli, Characterization and applications of new hyper-cross-linked cyclodextrins. *Composite Interfaces*, 2009. 16(1): p. 39–48.
81. Selvamuthukumar, S., et al., Nanosponges: A novel class of drug delivery system-review. *Journal of Pharmacy & Pharmaceutical Sciences*, 2012. 15(1): p. 103–111.
82. Ahmed, R.Z., G. Patil, and Z. Zaheer, Nanosponges–a completely new nano-horizon: Pharmaceutical applications and recent advances. *Drug Development and Industrial Pharmacy*, 2013. 39(9): p. 1263–1272.
83. Feng, X., P. Jia, and D. Zhang, Nanocarrier drug delivery system: Promising platform for targeted depression therapy. *Frontiers in Pharmacology*, 2024. 15: p. 1435133.
84. Parhi, R. and P. Suresh, Production of solid lipid nanoparticles-drug loading and release mechanism. *Journal of Chemical and Pharmaceutical Research*, 2010. 2(1): p. 211–27.
85. Tran, S., et al., Cancer nanomedicine: A review of recent success in drug delivery. *Clinical and Translational Medicine*, 2017. 6: p. 1–21.
86. Liu, Y., et al., Development of high-drug-loading nanoparticles. *ChemPlusChem*, 2020. 85(9): p. 2143–2157.
87. Reis, C.P., et al., Nanoencapsulation I. Methods for preparation of drug-loaded polymeric nanoparticles. *Nanomedicine: Nanotechnology, Biology and Medicine*, 2006. 2(1): p. 8–21.
88. Singh, R. and J.W. Lillard Jr, Nanoparticle-based targeted drug delivery. *Experimental and Molecular Pathology*, 2009. 86(3): p. 215–223.
89. Wong, P.T. and S.K. Choi, Mechanisms of drug release in nanotherapeutic delivery systems. *Chemical Reviews*, 2015. 115(9): p. 3388–3432.
90. La Thangue, N.B. and D.J. Kerr, Predictive biomarkers: A paradigm shift towards personalized cancer medicine. *Nature Reviews Clinical Oncology*, 2011. 8(10): p. 587–596.
91. Wang, Y., et al., Nanomaterials for cancer precision medicine. *Advanced Materials*, 2018. 30(17): p. 1705660.

92. Hoeben, A., E.A. Joosten, and M.H. van den Beuken-van Everdingen, Personalized medicine: Recent progress in cancer therapy. *Cancers*, 2021. 13(2): p. 242.
93. Marques, A., et al., Functionalizing nanoparticles with cancer-targeting antibodies: A comparison of strategies. *Journal of Controlled Release*, 2020. 320: p. 180–200.
94. Yu, B., et al., Receptor-targeted nanocarriers for therapeutic delivery to cancer. *Molecular Membrane Biology*, 2010. 27(7): p. 286–298.
95. Friedman, D. A., Claypool, S. E., and Liu, R., The smart targeting of nanoparticles. *Current Pharmaceutical Design*, 2013. 19(35): p. 6315–6329.
96. Zhang, C., et al., Progress, challenges, and future of nanomedicine. *Nano Today*, 2020. 35: p. 101008.
97. Kaur, J., et al., Trends in precision medicine. In Mukesh Verma and Debmalya Barh (Eds.), *Progress and Challenges in Precision Medicine*. 2017: p. 269–299, Elsevier.
98. Blanco, E., H. Shen, and M. Ferrari, Principles of nanoparticle design for overcoming biological barriers to drug delivery. *Nature Biotechnology*, 2015. 33(9): p. 941–951.
99. Elsabahy, M. and K.L. Wooley, Design of polymeric nanoparticles for biomedical delivery applications. *Chemical Society Reviews*, 2012. 41(7): p. 2545–2561.
100. Yao, Y., et al., Nanoparticle-based drug delivery in cancer therapy and its role in overcoming drug resistance. *Frontiers in Molecular Biosciences*, 2020. 7: p. 193.
101. Ho, D., P. Wang, and T. Kee, Artificial intelligence in nanomedicine. *Nanoscale Horizons*, 2019. 4(2): p. 365–377.
102. Adir, O., et al., Integrating artificial intelligence and nanotechnology for precision cancer medicine. *Advanced Materials*, 2020. 32(13): p. 1901989.
103. Siddique, A., Leveraging AI in medical engineering for targeted cancer therapy delivery. *Journal Environmental Sciences and Technology*, 2024. 3(1): p. 261–281.
104. Han, L. and X. Zhou, Synthesis and characterization of liposomes nano-composite-particles with hydrophobic magnetite as a MRI probe. *Applied Surface Science*, 2016. 376: p. 252–260.
105. He, X., K. Wang, and Z. Cheng, In vivo near-infrared fluorescence imaging of cancer with nanoparticle-based probes. *Wiley Interdisciplinary Reviews: Nanomedicine and Nanobiotechnology*, 2010. 2(4): p. 349–366.
106. Wu, Y., K. Briley, and X. Tao, Nanoparticle-based imaging of inflammatory bowel disease. *Wiley Interdisciplinary Reviews: Nanomedicine and Nanobiotechnology*, 2016. 8(2): p. 300–315.
107. Chakraborty, D., et al., Nano-diagnostics as an emerging platform for oral cancer detection: Current and emerging trends. *Wiley Interdisciplinary Reviews: Nanomedicine and Nanobiotechnology*, 2023. 15(1): p. e1830.
108. Sitharaman, B., et al., Superparamagnetic gadonanotubes are high-performance MRI contrast agents. *Chemical Communications*, 2005. (31): p. 3915–3917.
109. Wisner, E.R., et al., Sentinel node detection using contrast-enhanced power Doppler ultrasound lymphography. *Investigative Radiology*, 2003. 38(6): p. 358–365.
110. Alivisatos, A.P., Semiconductor clusters, nanocrystals, and quantum dots. *Science*, 1996. 271(5251): p. 933–937.
111. Lim, Y.T., et al., Selection of quantum dot wavelengths for biomedical assays and imaging. *Molecular Imaging*, 2003. 2(1): p. 15353500200302163.
112. Chan, W.C., et al., Luminescent quantum dots for multiplexed biological detection and imaging. *Current Opinion in Biotechnology*, 2002. 13(1): p. 40–46.
113. Kim, S., et al., Near-infrared fluorescent type II quantum dots for sentinel lymph node mapping. *Nature Biotechnology*, 2004. 22(1): p. 93–97.
114. Winter, P.M., et al., Molecular imaging of angiogenesis in nascent Vx-2 rabbit tumors using a novel $\alpha_v\beta_3$-targeted nanoparticle and 1.5 tesla magnetic resonance imaging. *Cancer Research*, 2003. 63(18): p. 5838–5843.
115. Anderson, S.A., et al., Magnetic resonance contrast enhancement of neovasculature with $\alpha_v\beta_3$-targeted nanoparticles. *Magnetic Resonance in Medicine: An Official Journal of the International Society for Magnetic Resonance in Medicine*, 2000. 44(3): p. 433–439.
116. Gao, X., W.C. Chan, and S. Nie, Quantum-dot nanocrystals for ultrasensitive biological labeling and multicolor optical encoding. *Journal of Biomedical Optics*, 2002. 7(4): p. 532–537.
117. Chang, E., et al., Protease-activated quantum dot probes. *Biochemical and Biophysical Research Communications*, 2005. 334(4): p. 1317–1321.
118. Fritz, J., et al., Translating biomolecular recognition into nanomechanics. *Science*, 2000. 288(5464): p. 316–318.

119. Liu, R.H., et al., Self-contained, fully integrated biochip for sample preparation, polymerase chain reaction amplification, and DNA microarray detection. *Analytical Chemistry*, 2004. 76(7): p. 1824–1831.
120. Guo, Y., et al., Application of nanomaterials in early diagnosis of cancer. *Nanotechnology Reviews*, 2023. 12(1): p. 20230116.
121. Li, J., et al., Carbon nanotube nanoelectrode array for ultrasensitive DNA detection. *Nano Letters*, 2003. 3(5): p. 597–602.
122. Arntz, Y., et al., Label-free protein assay based on a nanomechanical cantilever array. *Nanotechnology*, 2002. 14(1): p. 86.
123. Jin, S., et al., Scalable interconnection and integration of nanowire devices without registration. *Nano Letters*, 2004. 4(5): p. 915–919.
124. Das, B., et al., Current knowledge on toxicity of nanomaterials: Toxicity assessment and impact. In Hemant Kumar Daima, S. L. Kothari, Bhargava Suresh Kumar Eds.), *Nanotoxicology*, 2021: p. 339–375. CRC Press, Taylor & Francis.
125. Liu, J., et al., The interaction between nanoparticles and immune system: Application in the treatment of inflammatory diseases. *Journal of Nanobiotechnology*, 2022. 20(1): p. 127.
126. Kundu, D., et al., Environmental impact and econanotoxicity of engineered nanomaterials. *Nanotoxicology and Nanoecotoxicology*, 2021, 1: p. 287–312.
127. Gogoi, M., Magnetic nanostructures for cancer theranostic applications. *Current Pathobiology Reports*, 2021. 9: p. 71–78.
128. De Matteis, V., Exposure to inorganic nanoparticles: Routes of entry, immune response, biodistribution and in vitro/in vivo toxicity evaluation. *Toxics*, 2017. 5(4): p. 29.
129. Mahato, M., S. Patra, and M. Gogoi, Herbal nanocarriers for cancer therapy. *Nanopharmaceuticals: Principles and Applications*, 2021. 2: p. 41–75.
130. Wang, B., et al., Metabolism of nanomaterials in vivo: Blood circulation and organ clearance. *Accounts of Chemical Research*, 2013. 46(3): p. 761–769.
131. Ulises, A. and A. Sharma, Drug-delivery using inorganic and organic nanoparticles. In Ashutosh Sharma and Goldie Oza (Eds.), *Nanochemistry: Synthesis, Characterization and Applications*, 2023: p. 194. CRC Press.
132. Sharma, A., A.K. Goyal, and G. Rath, Recent advances in metal nanoparticles in cancer therapy. *Journal of Drug Targeting*, 2018. 26(8): p. 617–632.
133. Ferrari, M. and G. Downing, Medical nanotechnology: Shortening clinical trials and regulatory pathways? *BioDrugs*, 2005. 19: p. 203–210.
134. Buetow, K.H., Cyberinfrastructure: Empowering a "third way" in biomedical research. *Science*, 2005. 308(5723): p. 821–824.

9 Engineered Nanomaterials for the Treatment of Neglected Tropical Diseases

Abutwaibe KA[1], Sherilraj PM[1], Kanika Arora[1], and Shyam Lal Mudavath[1,2]

[1]Infectious Disease Biology Laboratory, Institute of Nanoscience and Technology, Mohali, India
[2]Department of Animal Biology, School of Life Sciences, University of Hyderabad, Hyderabad, India

TOC

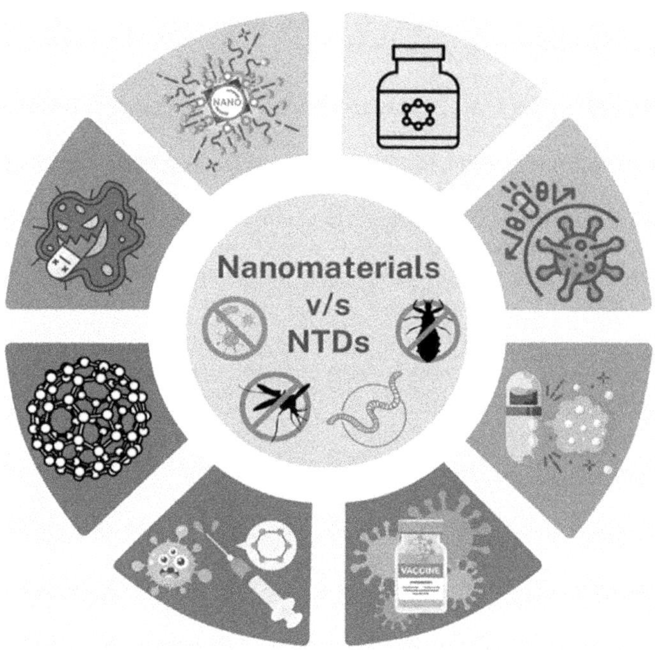

Nanomaterials in Action: Combating Neglected Tropical Diseases

9.1 INTRODUCTION

Neglected tropical diseases (NTDs) represent a group of diverse infections that primarily afflict populations in low-resource regions, often overlooked by mainstream healthcare systems. Despite concerted efforts to combat these diseases, challenges such as limited access to effective treatments, drug resistance, and the absence of vaccines continue to impede progress. These diseases often receive little attention from the global health community and lack adequate resources for research, prevention, and treatment. The World Health Organization (WHO) has identified 20 NTDs,

 DOI: 10.1201/9781003473015-9

encompassing infections caused by various pathogens such as viruses, bacteria, fungi, and protozoa. These diseases collectively threaten the health of over 1.4 billion individuals living in extreme poverty, predominantly in developing nations. Despite the significant morbidity associated with these diseases and the substantial expenses incurred for treatment and hospitalization, it is apparent that the private sector shows limited interest in funding programs aimed at combating many of these NTDs ("Global Report on Neglected Tropical Diseases 2023" n.d.).

Engineered nanomaterials (ENMs) have emerged as promising tools in the fight against NTDs, offering innovative approaches for diagnosis, treatment, and prevention. These nanomaterials, engineered at the nanoscale, possess unique physical and chemical properties that make them highly effective in addressing the challenges associated with NTDs (Santos-Valle et al. 2019). In diagnostics, nanomaterial-based platforms enable the development of sensitive and specific detection methods for NTD-causing pathogens. Nanoparticle-based biosensors, for example, can detect biomarkers of diseases such as malaria or dengue fever with high sensitivity, facilitating early diagnosis and prompt treatment initiation (Deroco, Junior, and Kubota 2021). In therapeutics, ENMs play a crucial role in enhancing drug delivery and efficacy. By encapsulating therapeutic agents within nanoparticles, researchers can improve drug stability, solubility, and bioavailability, while also enabling targeted delivery to the site of infection. This targeted approach reduces systemic toxicity and enhances treatment outcomes, particularly in cases of drug-resistant NTDs (Pandian et al. 2021)·(Şenel and Yüksel 2020). Also, nanomaterials can serve as platforms for the development of novel vaccines against NTDs. Nanoparticle-based vaccine delivery systems enhance the immunogenicity of antigens, leading to stronger and longer-lasting immune responses. This can be especially beneficial for diseases like Chagas disease or schistosomiasis, where traditional vaccine approaches have faced challenges. ENMs offer opportunities for vector control and environmental remediation, addressing key aspects of NTD transmission and persistence. Nanoparticle-based insecticides or larvicides can effectively target disease vectors while minimizing environmental impact, contributing to vector-borne disease control efforts (Barry et al. 2016). The versatility and efficacy of ENMs hold great promise for addressing the complex challenges posed by NTDs. Continued research and innovation in this field have the potential to revolutionize NTD diagnosis, treatment, and prevention strategies, ultimately improving health outcomes and reducing the burden of these diseases on vulnerable populations worldwide.

This chapter explores the potential of ENMs in tackling NTDs, providing insights into their design principles, mechanisms of action, and applications in disease management. By leveraging the interdisciplinary intersection of nanotechnology, medicine, and biology, researchers are pioneering innovative strategies to overcome the challenges posed by NTDs and improve healthcare outcomes for vulnerable populations.

Through a comprehensive review of recent advancements and case studies, this chapter aims to elucidate the role of ENMs in revolutionizing the landscape of NTD therapeutics. By shedding light on their potential benefits, limitations, and future directions, it seeks to inspire further exploration and collaboration in harnessing nanotechnology for the eradication of NTDs, ultimately advancing global health equity and justice.

9.2 CHALLENGES OF CURRENT THERAPY

The current treatment options available for NTDs come with several disadvantages, which pose significant challenges in effectively managing these diseases, particularly in resource-limited settings. Some of the key drawbacks are given in the following sections.

9.2.1 Limited Efficacy

Many existing treatments for NTDs have limited efficacy, especially against drug-resistant strains of pathogens. For example, in the case of malaria, the widespread emergence of drug-resistant

Plasmodium strains has rendered some antimalarial drugs ineffective, leading to treatment failures and increased morbidity and mortality rates.

9.2.2 High Cost

Some NTD treatments are prohibitively expensive, making them inaccessible to the populations most affected by these diseases. For instance, drugs used to treat diseases like Chagas or leishmaniasis can be costly, placing a financial burden on both patients and healthcare systems in low-resource settings.

9.2.3 Long Treatment Duration

Several NTD treatments require prolonged courses of therapy, which can be challenging for patients to adhere to, particularly in regions with limited access to healthcare services. For example, the treatment regimen for tuberculosis, an NTD caused by *Mycobacterium tuberculosis*, typically lasts 6 months or longer, posing challenges for patient compliance and increasing the risk of treatment failure or relapse.

9.2.4 Adverse Effects

Many NTD medications can cause significant adverse effects, ranging from mild to severe. For instance, some anti-parasitic drugs used to treat diseases like schistosomiasis or lymphatic filariasis can cause nausea, vomiting, and neurological symptoms, leading to treatment discontinuation or reluctance among patients to seek treatment.

9.2.5 Lack of Accessibility

In remote or underserved areas, access to essential NTD treatments may be limited or non-existent due to factors such as inadequate healthcare infrastructure, drug stockouts, or geographical barriers. This lack of accessibility further exacerbates the burden of NTDs and contributes to ongoing transmission and morbidity in affected communities.

9.2.6 Development of Resistance

Overreliance on certain medications for NTD treatment can lead to the development of drug resistance among pathogens, diminishing the effectiveness of available treatments over time. This is a significant concern, particularly in diseases like visceral leishmaniasis, where resistance to antileishmanial drugs has been reported in some regions, posing challenges for disease control efforts.

The drawbacks of the current NTD treatment choices, taken as a whole, highlight the critical need for ongoing research and innovation to produce more accessible, inexpensive, and effective medicines that can handle the intricate problems these diseases present.

9.3 ENMS TO COMBAT NTDS

ENMs include a wide variety of nanoscale materials crafted to have specific properties and functions, making them particularly useful in the treatment and diagnosis of NTDs. These nanomaterials can be created from different substances such as metals, metal oxides, polymers, carbon-based materials, and hybrid composites, allowing for customized approaches to address the unique challenges posed by NTDs (Albalawi et al. 2021). By adjusting the size, shape, surface chemistry, and structure of ENMs, researchers can precisely tailor their physicochemical properties for specific applications. In the context of NTDs, these customizations allow ENMs to be utilized effectively for drug delivery, diagnostics, imaging, and therapeutic purposes. For instance, nanocarriers such as liposomes, polymeric micelles, dendrimers, and inorganic materials like gold nanoparticles (GNPs) and quantum dots (QDs) have shown great potential in creating targeted drug delivery systems. These nanoparticles are designed to deliver treatments directly to infection sites, improving therapeutic outcomes for NTDs while minimizing unwanted side effects (B. Das et al. 2018; A. Kumar et al. 2014). By functionalizing their surfaces with targeting ligands, such as antibodies or peptides, ENMs can selectively deliver drugs to specific cells or tissues, minimizing off-target effects and enhancing therapeutic efficacy (Abbasi et al. 2023). Moreover, the unique optical, magnetic, and electronic properties exhibited by certain ENMs make them valuable tools for imaging and diagnostic purposes. QDs, for example, possess tunable fluorescence properties that enable high-resolution imaging of biological structures and processes (Gubala et al. 2018). Magnetic nanoparticles (MNPs), on the other hand, can be used as contrast agents for magnetic resonance imaging (MRI) or for magnetic hyperthermia in cancer therapy, where localized heating is induced in tumor tissues by an alternating magnetic field (Farzin et al. 2020).

In the context of NTDs, ENMs offer innovative solutions to address the challenges associated with diagnosis, treatment, and prevention (Engels and Zhou 2020). For instance, in the case of parasitic infections such as malaria, leishmaniasis, or schistosomiasis, ENMs such as liposomes, polymeric micelles, and dendrimers can be utilized to develop more effective anti-parasitic drugs with enhanced bioavailability and targeted delivery to infected tissues (Bao, Mitragotri, and Tong 2013). Furthermore, nanotechnology-based diagnostic platforms hold promise for rapid and sensitive detection of NTD pathogens (Thwala et al. 2023), enabling early intervention and control measures in resource-limited settings where conventional diagnostic methods may be impractical or inaccessible. Beyond healthcare, ENMs find applications in environmental remediation, energy storage, catalysis, and electronics, among others (Hajizade et al. 2023). For instance, nanomaterial-based catalysts exhibit higher catalytic activity and selectivity compared to bulk counterparts, making them attractive for industrial processes such as fuel production, pollutant degradation, and hydrogen generation (Chaturvedi, Dave, and Shah 2012). However, despite their immense potential, the widespread adoption of ENMs raises concerns regarding their safety, biocompatibility, and environmental impact (Pandian et al. 2021). Therefore, comprehensive studies are essential to understand the potential risks associated with ENMs and to develop appropriate regulatory frameworks to ensure their safe and responsible use (Kabanov and Gendelman 2007). In summary, ENMs represent a versatile and promising class of materials with transformative potential across various sectors, including healthcare, environmental sustainability, and energy. Through interdisciplinary research and collaboration, ENMs continue to advance and offer novel solutions to address pressing global challenges, including NTDs, paving the way for a brighter and more sustainable future.

9.3.1 Nanoparticle-Based Anti-Parasitic Drugs

Nanoparticle-based anti-parasitic drugs represent a novel approach to combating parasitic infections, offering advantages such as improved drug delivery, enhanced efficacy, reduced side effects, and potential strategies to overcome drug resistance (Bajwa et al. 2022). Parasitic diseases, including malaria, leishmaniasis, trypanosomiasis, schistosomiasis, and others, pose significant global health burdens, particularly in resource-limited regions where access to effective treatments may be limited. The development of nanoparticle-based therapeutics presents a promising avenue to address these challenges (Y. Sun et al. 2019). One of the primary advantages of nanoparticle-based anti-parasitic drugs is their ability to enhance drug delivery to target sites within the body (Patra et al. 2018). Nanoparticles can be engineered to encapsulate or conjugate with anti-parasitic drugs, protecting them from degradation and facilitating their transport to specific tissues or cells where the parasites reside. This targeted delivery approach minimizes drug exposure to healthy tissues, reducing systemic toxicity and improving therapeutic outcomes (Verdan et al. 2023). Nanoparticle platforms offer opportunities for the co-delivery of multiple anti-parasitic drugs or combination therapies, allowing for synergistic effects and overcoming drug resistance (Y. Sun et al. 2019). Surface modification of nanoparticles with targeting ligands, such as antibodies, peptides, or carbohydrates, enables specific recognition and binding to parasite-infected cells or tissues (Yetisgin et al. 2020). This targeted delivery approach enhances the accumulation of anti-parasitic drugs at the site of infection, maximizing therapeutic efficacy while minimizing off-target effects on healthy tissues (Abdelkawi et al. 2023).

One prominent example involves the utilization of polymeric nanoparticles for the delivery of anti-parasitic agents. Polymeric nanoparticles, such as poly(lactic-co-glycolic acid) (PLGA) nanoparticles, have gained attention due to their biocompatibility, tunable properties, and ability to encapsulate a wide range of drugs (Lu et al. 2023). In the context of anti-parasitic therapy, PLGA nanoparticles have been investigated for the delivery of drugs targeting parasites such as *Plasmodium* spp. (causative agents of malaria) and *Trypanosoma cruzi* (causative agent of Chagas disease) (Makadia and Siegel 2011). Similarly, PLGA nanoparticles have been explored for the delivery of benznidazole, a frontline drug for the treatment of Chagas disease (Gomes et al. 2023). By encapsulating benznidazole within PLGA nanoparticles, researchers aim to overcome the limitations associated with its poor aqueous solubility and high toxicity (Choudhury 2021). This nanoparticle-based approach enhances drug stability, facilitates sustained release, and promotes selective accumulation at the site of infection, thereby improving the therapeutic outcome and reducing the risk of adverse effects.

PLGA nanoparticles have emerged as a promising approach for improving the treatment of malaria (Dauda et al. 2017). These nanoparticles serve as efficient carriers for antimalarial drugs, such as artemisinin, due to their biocompatibility and biodegradability. By encapsulating artemisinin within PLGA nanoparticles, its solubility and stability are significantly enhanced, leading to improved bioavailability and therapeutic efficacy (Heidari, Golenser, and Greiner 2022). PLGA nanoparticles enable targeted drug delivery to infection sites, ensuring higher drug concentrations at the parasitic targets while reducing systemic exposure. They are readily taken up by macrophages, which are key in malaria pathogenesis. These nanoparticles can passively target infected red blood cells and accumulate in organs such as the liver and spleen, where the malaria parasite is primarily found. By delivering antimalarial drugs directly to the infected cells, PLGA nanoparticles increase drug concentration at the site of infection, which may help in overcoming drug resistance (Gogoi 2017). The controlled release kinetics of artemisinin from PLGA nanoparticles further ensures sustained therapeutic levels, reducing the need for frequent dosing and enhancing patient compliance (Hines and Kaplan 2013). Overall, PLGA nanoparticles hold great promise for optimizing the treatment of malaria by overcoming the limitations associated with conventional drug formulations.

In the realm of Chagas disease treatment, PLGA nanoparticles offer a versatile platform for delivering benznidazole, a key anti-parasitic drug. Encapsulation of benznidazole within PLGA nanoparticles enhances drug stability and improves its aqueous solubility, addressing critical challenges associated with its formulation (Quezada et al. 2019). This nanoparticle-based approach enables targeted delivery of benznidazole to the site of infection, maximizing drug accumulation in tissues harboring *T. cruzi* parasites while minimizing exposure to healthy tissues (Tiwari et al. 2023). Additionally, the sustained release profile of benznidazole from PLGA nanoparticles prolongs its therapeutic effect, potentially reducing the frequency of administration and improving patient compliance (Guo et al. 2023). By leveraging the unique properties of PLGA nanoparticles, such as biocompatibility and tunable release kinetics, this innovative drug delivery system holds promise for enhancing the efficacy and safety of Chagas disease treatment strategies (Alsaab et al. 2022).

Another noteworthy example involves the use of lipid-based nanoparticles, such as solid lipid nanoparticles (SLNs) and nanostructured lipid carriers (NLCs), for anti-parasitic drug delivery. These lipid-based nanoparticles offer advantages such as biocompatibility, controlled release, and enhanced drug-loading capacity, making them promising candidates for targeted therapy against parasitic infections. SLNs are composed of a solid lipid core that encapsulates the drug, offering protection from degradation and enhancing bioavailability. Upon administration, they can passively target infection sites due to their small size and interaction with the host's immune cells. SLNs are taken up by macrophages, where many parasites reside, allowing for targeted delivery of anti-parasitic drugs and reduced systemic toxicity (Singh et al. 2020). SLNs loaded with amphotericin B, a potent anti-fungal agent effective against *Leishmania* parasites, have demonstrated significant promise for the treatment of visceral leishmaniasis. Encapsulation of amphotericin B within SLNs improves its aqueous solubility, bioavailability, and retention at the site of infection, thereby enhancing its therapeutic efficacy while reducing the risk of systemic toxicity (Mishra et al. 2018). Moreover, the sustained release of amphotericin B from SLNs ensures prolonged drug exposure to the parasites, leading to improved treatment outcomes. NLCs represent another lipid-based nanoparticle formulation that offers advantages such as enhanced drug-loading capacity and improved drug release kinetics (Viegas et al. 2023). Both SLNs and NLCs are biocompatible and can be engineered for targeted delivery through surface modifications, enhancing drug accumulation at parasitic infection sites while minimizing side effects. By harnessing the unique properties of lipid nanoparticles, including their ability to encapsulate hydrophobic drugs and target specific tissues, these lipid-based nanocarriers present a promising strategy for combating parasitic diseases. This approach is particularly valuable in the development of effective and safe treatments for visceral leishmaniasis, where targeted drug delivery and sustained release profiles can significantly improve therapeutic outcomes (Elmowafy and Al-Sanea 2021).

9.3.2 Nanoformulations for Antiviral Therapies

Nanoformulations represent a cutting-edge approach in the development of antiviral therapies, offering targeted drug delivery, enhanced drug stability, and improved pharmacokinetics (A. K. Mahor et al. 2023). Within the context of NTDs, where viral infections pose significant health challenges, nanoformulations hold promise for overcoming treatment barriers and improving patient outcomes. Nanotechnology enables the design and engineering of nanoparticles tailored for antiviral drug delivery (Lembo et al. 2018). These nanoparticles can be composed of various materials, including lipids, polymers, or inorganic substances, each offering unique advantages in terms of drug encapsulation, biocompatibility, and controlled release. By encapsulating antiviral drugs within nano-sized carriers, such as liposomes, polymeric nanoparticles, or lipid-based nanocarriers, researchers aim to enhance drug solubility, prolong drug circulation time, and achieve targeted delivery to viral reservoirs (Lembo et al. 2018). Furthermore, nanoparticle-based vaccine delivery systems represent a promising strategy for preventing viral infections in neglected tropical regions. Nanoparticle carriers can encapsulate viral antigens or nucleic acid-based vaccines, improving their stability, immunogenicity, and targeted delivery to immune cells (Arora et al. 2022). These nanoformulations enable controlled release of antigens, modulation of immune responses, and potential induction of long-lasting protective immunity against viral pathogens.

9.3.2.1 Lipid-Based Nanoparticles for Antiretroviral Therapy (HIV/AIDS)

Lipid nanoparticles, such as liposomes or lipid-based nanocarriers, have been explored for the delivery of antiretroviral drugs in the treatment of HIV/AIDS (Faria et al. 2021). These nanoparticles can cross biological barriers, such as the blood-brain barrier, ensuring drug delivery to HIV reservoirs in the central nervous system, which are typically challenging to treat with conventional formulations. By targeting these reservoirs, lipid nanoparticles help inhibit viral replication and reduce the chances of viral latency or rebound. Surface modifications of lipid nanoparticles can be engineered to enhance targeting to specific receptors on HIV-infected cells, allowing for more efficient drug delivery with reduced systemic toxicity (Mondal and Ghosh 2023; Cunha et al. 2021; Mahajan et al. 2021). For example, liposomal formulations of protease inhibitors or nucleoside analogs have demonstrated improved drug stability and bioavailability, leading to enhanced efficacy and reduced toxicity compared to conventional drug formulations. These lipid-based nanoformulations enable targeted delivery to HIV-infected cells, prolong drug circulation time, and minimize systemic side effects, thereby improving treatment outcomes for patients with HIV/AIDS in neglected tropical regions (Mallipeddi and Rohan 2010).

9.3.2.2 Virus-Like Particle Vaccines for Dengue Fever

Virus-like particles (VLPs) represent an innovative vaccine platform for preventing viral infections such as dengue fever, which is endemic in many tropical regions (Nooraei et al. 2021). VLP-based vaccines mimic the structure of the virus but lack the viral genome, making them safe and immunogenic. VLPs can be engineered to display viral antigens, eliciting potent immune responses against dengue virus (Castilho et al. 2022). The mechanism behind VLP vaccines involves their ability to elicit a strong immune response by mimicking the natural virus's external structure. When administered, VLPs stimulate the body's immune system to recognize the viral proteins as foreign, leading to the production of neutralizing antibodies. These antibodies can then target and neutralize the real dengue virus upon subsequent exposure, preventing infection (Daniel et al. 2024; Warner and Frietze 2021). VLPs are non-replicating and cannot cause disease, they provide a safer alternative to live-attenuated vaccines. Additionally, VLP vaccines can present antigens from multiple dengue virus serotypes, offering broad protection against the various strains responsible for dengue fever. This strategy holds significant potential for effective and safe vaccination against dengue, especially in endemic regions. Nanoformulations of VLP vaccines offer advantages such as enhanced stability, controlled antigen release, and targeted delivery to immune cells, leading to improved vaccine efficacy and potentially offering long-lasting protection against dengue fever in neglected tropical areas.

9.3.2.3 GNPs for Antiviral Therapy

GNPs have gained attention as potential antiviral agents due to their unique physicochemical properties and biocompatibility. These nanoparticles can be functionalized with antiviral compounds or modified to directly interact with viral particles, inhibiting viral attachment, entry, or replication processes (Sarkar et al. 2022). GNPs have shown broad-spectrum antiviral activity against various viral pathogens, including HIV, hepatitis B virus (HBV), influenza virus, and herpes simplex virus (HSV), among others (Chen and Liang 2020). In the context of NTDs, GNPs hold promise for combating viral infections prevalent in resource-limited settings. These nanoparticles can be engineered to target specific viral proteins or structures, disrupting viral replication and reducing viral load (Babaei et al. 2021). Additionally, GNPs can be conjugated with targeting ligands to enhance their specificity for infected cells or tissues, minimizing off-target effects and improving therapeutic outcomes.

9.3.2.4 Silver Nanoparticles for Antiviral Therapy

Silver nanoparticles have emerged as potent antiviral agents due to their broad-spectrum activity against a wide range of viral pathogens (Galdiero et al. 2011). These nanoparticles possess unique physicochemical properties, such as high surface area-to-volume ratio and inherent antimicrobial activity, making them effective against viruses by disrupting viral membranes, inhibiting viral replication, or interfering with viral attachment and entry processes. In NTDs, silver nanoparticles offer a promising approach for combating viral infections prevalent in resource-limited regions. These nanoparticles can be applied topically or systemically to treat viral skin infections, respiratory viral infections, or sexually transmitted viral diseases (Sharmin et al. 2021). Additionally, silver nanoparticles can be incorporated into medical devices, personal protective equipment, or antiviral coatings to prevent viral transmission and reduce the spread of infectious diseases in vulnerable populations.

9.3.3 Nanomaterials for Vector Control Strategies

Nanomaterials offer innovative solutions for vector control strategies aimed at reducing the transmission of NTDs by targeting disease-carrying vectors such as mosquitoes, ticks, and sandflies (Nie et al. 2023). Leveraging the unique properties of nanomaterials, researchers are exploring novel approaches to disrupt disease transmission cycles and protect vulnerable populations. Nanotechnology plays a crucial role in the development of insecticidal formulations with improved efficacy and reduced environmental impact. Nanoemulsion-based insecticides represent one example, wherein insecticidal compounds are encapsulated within nanoscale droplets of oil and water stabilized by surfactants (Manjesh et al. 2022). These nanoemulsions enhance the stability and bioavailability of insecticides, facilitating their penetration through the insect cuticle and prolonged residual activity (Mustafa and Hussein 2020). For instance, nanoemulsion formulations containing pyrethroids or organophosphates have shown promise in controlling mosquito populations and reducing the spread of diseases such as malaria and dengue fever (Rahman et al. 2019). Additionally, nanotechnology-enabled traps offer innovative solutions for vector surveillance and control. Nanomaterials such as graphene oxide (GO) or carbon nanotubes (CNTs) can be incorporated into traps to enhance their sensitivity and selectivity for capturing disease vectors (A. Mahor et al. 2021). These nanomaterial-based traps can detect and monitor vector populations in real time, providing valuable data for targeted vector control interventions. Moreover, traps incorporating photothermal or photoluminescent nanomaterials can attract and kill insect vectors using light-based strategies, offering environmentally friendly alternatives to chemical insecticides (Figure 9.1).

9.3.3.1 Nanoemulsion-Based Insecticides

Nanoemulsions are colloidal dispersions composed of nanoscale oil droplets dispersed in water, stabilized by surfactants or emulsifiers. This unique formulation offers several advantages for insecticidal applications. Firstly, nanoemulsions provide enhanced stability and solubilization of insecticidal compounds, such as pyrethroids or organophosphates, which are commonly used to target mosquitoes and other disease-carrying vectors (Pavoni et al. 2019). By encapsulating these active ingredients within nanoscale oil droplets, nanoemulsions prevent their premature degradation, ensuring sustained efficacy over time. This stability is crucial for maintaining the potency of

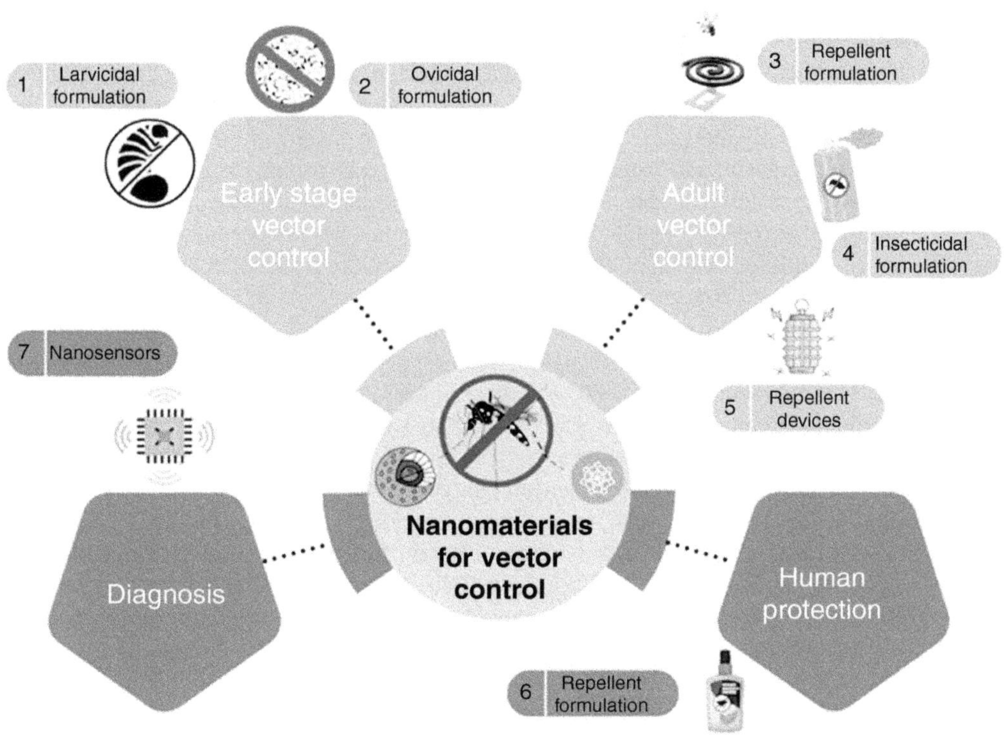

FIGURE 9.1 Different ways of vector control by nanomaterials.

insecticides during storage and application, especially in tropical environments where temperature fluctuations can degrade conventional formulations. Secondly, nanoemulsion-based insecticides improve the bioavailability and penetration of active ingredients through the insect cuticle, enhancing their insecticidal effects (Mustafa and Hussein 2020). The nanoscale droplets in nanoemulsions provide a larger surface area for contact with insects, facilitating the absorption of insecticidal compounds into the insect's body. This enhanced penetration enables more efficient targeting of physiological processes crucial for insect survival, such as nerve function or muscle contraction, leading to rapid paralysis and death of the vector. Moreover, nanoemulsions offer prolonged residual activity on treated surfaces, providing sustained protection against disease vectors (Preeti et al. 2023). The small droplet size and uniform distribution of nanoemulsions allow for better adhesion to surfaces, such as foliage or mosquito breeding sites, resulting in longer-lasting insecticidal effects. This prolonged residual activity reduces the need for frequent reapplication of insecticides, thereby optimizing resource utilization and minimizing environmental impact (Feng et al. 2018). Furthermore, nanoemulsion-based insecticides exhibit reduced environmental impact compared to conventional formulations. The use of nanotechnology enables the formulation of insecticides with lower concentrations of active ingredients while maintaining or even enhancing their efficacy (Jaiswal, Dudhe, and Sharma 2015). This reduction in active ingredient concentration reduces the overall environmental load of insecticides, mitigating potential ecological risks and minimizing adverse effects on non-target organisms.

In summary, nanoemulsion-based insecticides offer a promising approach for vector control, with improved stability, bioavailability, penetration, and residual activity compared to conventional formulations (Hikal et al. 2023). By harnessing the unique properties of nanoscale emulsions, these insecticidal formulations contribute to the effective control of mosquito populations and the prevention of mosquito-borne diseases in endemic regions (Mapossa et al. 2021). Continued research and development in this field are essential to optimize the efficacy, safety, and sustainability of nanoemulsion-based insecticides for vector control applications.

9.3.3.2 Nanotechnology-Enabled Traps

Nanotechnology-enabled traps represent a novel and innovative approach in vector control strategies, aimed at improving the efficiency and effectiveness of capturing disease vectors such as mosquitoes, ticks, and sandflies. By integrating nanomaterials into trap designs, researchers aim to enhance the sensitivity, selectivity, and functionality of these traps, thereby contributing to the reduction of NTDs transmitted by vectors (Campos et al. 2020). One example of nanotechnology-enabled traps involves the incorporation of GO or CNTs into trap surfaces. These nanomaterials possess unique properties such as high surface area, excellent conductivity, and strong adsorption capabilities. When integrated into trap surfaces, GO (Hoseini-Ghahfarokhi et al. 2020) or CNTs enhance the sensitivity and selectivity of traps for capturing disease vectors. These nanomaterial-modified traps can effectively attract, capture, and retain target vectors, providing valuable data for surveillance and control efforts (Bhattacharya et al. 2016). Furthermore, nanomaterial-based traps with photothermal or photoluminescent properties offer innovative solutions for vector control. These traps utilize nanomaterials that can absorb or emit light in specific wavelength ranges, allowing for targeted attraction and elimination of insect vectors (Doughty et al. 2019). For example, nanomaterials with photothermal properties can generate heat upon exposure to light, attracting insects through thermal cues and leading to their immobilization or death. Similarly, nanomaterials with photoluminescent properties can emit light, acting as visual attractants for insect vectors. By harnessing light-based strategies, these nanotechnology-enabled traps offer sustainable alternatives to chemical insecticides, minimizing environmental impact while effectively controlling vector populations (Duan et al. 2023).

All things considered, traps enabled by nanotechnology offer useful instruments for identifying, keeping an eye on, and managing disease vectors in endemic areas. Through the utilization of nanomaterials' distinct characteristics, including their large surface area, electrical conductivity, and behavior in response to light, these traps improve the efficacy and efficiency of vector control treatments. In addition, the information gathered from these traps advances our knowledge of vector populations and the dynamics of transmission, allowing for more focused vector control measures and ultimately a decrease in the number of neglected tropical illnesses spread by vectors. More research and development in this area is required to optimize the design, functionality, and sustainability of nanotechnology-enabled traps for vector control applications.

In conclusion, the utilization of ENMs holds significant promise in the fight against NTDs. These materials offer a multifaceted approach, addressing various aspects including drug delivery, diagnostics, and therapeutic interventions. By leveraging the unique properties of nanomaterials, such as their small size, high surface area-to-volume ratio, and tunable surface chemistry, researchers can overcome the limitations of traditional treatments for NTDs, such as poor drug solubility, bioavailability, and delivery barriers (Pandian et al. 2021). Additionally, ENMs enable targeted delivery to specific sites within the body, reducing systemic toxicity and enhancing treatment efficacy. Despite the considerable progress made in this field, challenges remain, including ensuring the safety and biocompatibility of nanomaterials, scaling up production for widespread use, and addressing regulatory hurdles (Patra et al. 2018). Collaborative efforts among researchers, policymakers, and healthcare providers are essential to further harness the potential of ENMs for combating NTDs and improving global health outcomes.

9.3.4 Diagnostic Nanomaterials for NTDs Detection

Diagnostic nanomaterials refer to nanoscale materials that are specifically designed and utilized for diagnostic purposes in healthcare. These materials play a crucial role in various diagnostic techniques, including medical imaging, biosensors, and point-of-care testing (Malik, Muhammad, and Waheed 2023). Diagnostic nanomaterials have shown promise in detecting NTDs by offering enhanced sensitivity, specificity, and portability in diagnostic assays (Gedda et al. 2021). Here are some examples of diagnostic nanomaterials used for NTD detection:

9.3.4.1 Gold Nanoparticles

GNPs are frequently utilized in lateral flow assays (LFAs) to detect NTDs like malaria, dengue, and Chagas disease (Medina-Rivera et al. 2022). These GNPs, when functionalized, can attach to disease-specific biomarkers, resulting in visible color changes that signify the presence of the disease. LFAs employing GNPs offer rapid results, are cost-effective, and are well suited for point-of-care testing in settings with limited resources (Rong-Hwa et al. 2010).

a. *Functionalization:* GNPs can be functionalized with specific ligands such as antibodies, aptamers, or peptides that target biomarkers associated with NTDs. For example, antibodies can be conjugated to GNPs to target antigens from pathogens like *Plasmodium* (malaria), Dengue virus, or *T. cruzi* (Chagas disease) (Schmidt et al. 2014). This functionalization allows for selective binding and detection of disease-specific molecules (Li et al. 2019).
b. *Lateral Flow Assays:* GNPs are commonly used as labels or reporters in LFAs, which are simple and rapid diagnostic tests suitable for point-of-care settings. In LFA for NTD detection, a sample containing the NTD biomarker (e.g., pathogen antigen or antibody) is applied to the test strip. The strip typically consists of several zones, including a sample pad, conjugate pad (containing GNPs conjugated with detection molecules), nitrocellulose membrane (with capture molecules), and an absorbent pad.
c. *Detection Principle:* When the sample flows along the strip, the GNPs carrying the detection molecules migrate and bind to the target biomarker if present in the sample. This binding event forms a complex that continues to migrate along the strip until it reaches the capture zone. In the capture zone, the complex is captured by immobilized capture

molecules, resulting in a visible signal (e.g., colored line) that indicates a positive result for the NTD.

d. *Signal Amplification:* GNPs provide signal amplification in LFAs due to their large surface area-to-volume ratio and unique optical properties (e.g., plasmon resonance) (Ye et al. 2020). This amplifies the detection signal, allowing for sensitive and reliable detection of even low concentrations of NTD biomarkers. The color change or line intensity in the test zone is proportional to the concentration of the target biomarker in the sample.
e. *Advantages:* The use of GNPs in LFAs for NTD detection offers several advantages, including rapid results (typically within minutes), minimal sample preparation, ease of use without specialized equipment, and cost-effectiveness. These features make GNP-based LFAs suitable for resource-limited settings where access to sophisticated laboratory infrastructure is limited.

9.3.4.2 Quantum Dots

QDs are semiconductor nanocrystals with unique optical properties that enable sensitive detection of NTD biomarkers (Shao, Gao, and Yan 2011). They can be conjugated with antibodies or aptamers to target specific antigens or nucleic acids associated with NTD pathogens. QD-based assays offer high sensitivity and multiplexing capabilities, allowing simultaneous detection of multiple NTDs in a single sample.

a. *Functionalization:* QDs can be functionalized with specific recognition molecules such as antibodies, aptamers, or peptides that target NTD-related antigens or nucleic acids. This functionalization allows QDs to selectively bind to the target biomarkers, enhancing the specificity of the diagnostic assay (Mohkam et al. 2023).
b. *Multiplexing Capability:* One of the key advantages of QDs is their ability to emit light at different wavelengths depending on their size and composition (Barroso 2011). This property enables multiplexed detection, where multiple NTD biomarkers can be simultaneously detected in a single sample using QD-based assays. Multiplexing enhances the efficiency and throughput of NTD diagnostics.
c. *Detection Techniques:* QDs can be incorporated into various detection platforms, including fluorescence-based assays and immunoassays (Zhang et al. 2009). In fluorescence-based assays, QDs emit specific wavelengths of light upon excitation, allowing for sensitive and quantitative detection of NTD biomarkers. Immunoassays using QDs as labels can detect the presence of NTD antigens or antibodies with high sensitivity and specificity.
d. *Applications in NTD Detection:* QDs have been used in the detection of NTDs such as malaria, dengue, leishmaniasis, and schistosomiasis. For example, QD-based assays can detect malaria antigens or antibodies in blood samples with high sensitivity, aiding in early diagnosis and monitoring of the disease (Plucinski, Aidoo, and Rogier 2021). Similarly, QDs have been employed in multiplexed assays for simultaneous detection of multiple NTDs, providing a comprehensive diagnostic approach.
e. *Advantages:* The use of QDs in NTD detection offers several advantages, including high sensitivity, multiplexing capability, rapid detection, and compatibility with various detection platforms. QD-based assays are suitable for point-of-care testing and surveillance programs for NTDs in resource-limited settings.

9.3.4.3 Carbon Nanotubes

CNTs are utilized in electrochemical biosensors for detecting NTD-related biomolecules such as proteins, DNA, and enzymes (Jacobs, Peairs, and Venton 2010). Functionalized CNTs enhance the electron transfer rate, leading to improved sensor performance in terms of sensitivity and selectivity (Nishimura et al. 2019). CNT-based biosensors are suitable for detecting NTDs like leishmaniasis, schistosomiasis, and lymphatic filariasis (Ghorai 2023).

a. *Sensing Mechanism:* CNTs can act as highly sensitive transducers in biosensing platforms due to their excellent electrical and mechanical properties (Sireesha et al. 2018). When functionalized with specific recognition elements such as antibodies, aptamers, or peptides, CNTs can selectively bind to NTD biomarkers, enabling the detection of disease-specific molecules.
b. *Electrochemical Biosensors:* CNTs are commonly used in electrochemical biosensors designed for NTD detection. In these biosensors, CNTs serve as the sensing element that interacts with the target biomarkers. Upon binding to the biomarkers, changes in the electrical properties of CNTs occur, which can be measured and quantified, providing a rapid and sensitive detection method for NTDs.
c. *Enhanced Sensitivity:* Functionalized CNTs exhibit enhanced electron transfer rates, leading to improved sensitivity in detecting NTD-related biomolecules such as proteins, DNA, and enzymes. This enhanced sensitivity allows for the detection of low concentrations of NTD biomarkers, which is crucial for early diagnosis and monitoring of diseases.
d. *Selectivity:* The functionalization of CNTs with specific recognition molecules ensures high selectivity in NTD detection. By targeting NTD-related antigens or nucleic acids, CNT-based biosensors can distinguish between different pathogens or disease stages, providing accurate diagnostic information.
e. *Applications in NTDs:* For example, CNT-based biosensors can detect specific proteins or genetic markers associated with these diseases in patient samples, facilitating early diagnosis and treatment.

9.3.4.4 Magnetic Nanoparticles

MNPs are employed in MRI and magnetic separation techniques for NTD diagnosis (C. Sun, Lee, and Zhang 2008). Functionalized MNPs can target and isolate NTD pathogens or biomarkers from biological samples, enabling their detection and characterization (Farinha et al. 2021). MNPs are particularly useful in diagnosing NTDs with low pathogen concentrations or complex sample matrices.

a. *Magnetic Resonance Imaging:* MNPs are used as contrast agents in MRI scans for visualizing anatomical structures and detecting abnormalities associated with NTDs. Functionalized MNPs can target specific tissues, organs, or biomarkers related to NTDs, enhancing the sensitivity and specificity of MRI diagnosis. For example, in cases of cerebral malaria or neurocysticercosis, MNPs can be targeted to areas of inflammation or parasite localization, providing detailed imaging insights for accurate disease diagnosis and monitoring (Rasalkar et al. 2011).
b. *Magnetic Separation Techniques:* MNPs are employed in magnetic separation techniques for isolating NTD pathogens or biomarkers from complex biological samples such as blood, serum, or tissue extracts (Tang et al. 2020). Functionalized MNPs are designed to specifically bind to NTD-related molecules, allowing for their selective extraction from the sample matrix. This magnetic separation process enables the concentration and purification of NTD biomarkers, facilitating their detection and characterization in subsequent analytical assays.
c. *Targeting and Isolation:* Functionalized MNPs can target and isolate various components relevant to NTD diagnosis, including pathogens (e.g., *Plasmodium* spp. in malaria, *T. cruzi* in Chagas disease), disease-specific antigens, antibodies, nucleic acids (DNA/RNA), or metabolic biomarkers. MNPs conjugated with specific ligands such as antibodies, aptamers, or peptides ensure the selective binding and capture of the target molecules, enhancing the accuracy and reliability of NTD diagnostics.
d. *Enhanced Sensitivity:* MNPs offer enhanced sensitivity in NTD diagnosis, particularly for cases with low pathogen concentrations or complex sample matrices. The magnetic

properties of MNPs allow for efficient concentration and enrichment of target biomarkers, improving the detection limits of analytical techniques such as polymerase chain reaction (PCR), enzyme-linked immunosorbent assay (ELISA) (Sue et al. 2014), or nucleic acid amplification tests (NAATs).

e. *Applications in NTDs:* MNPs have been applied in the diagnosis of various NTDs. For example, in malaria diagnosis, MNPs can be functionalized to target *Plasmodium* antigens or nucleic acids, enabling their isolation and detection in blood samples (Slater et al. 2022). Similarly, in Chagas disease, MNPs can target *T. cruzi* parasites or specific antibodies, aiding in disease diagnosis and monitoring.
f. *Advantages:* MNPs offer several advantages in NTD diagnosis, including rapid and selective targeting, enhanced sensitivity, compatibility with various analytical techniques, and the ability to process complex biological samples. Their use facilitates early and accurate diagnosis of NTDs, leading to improved patient outcomes and targeted interventions.

9.3.4.5 Nanowires and Nanoporous Materials

Nanowires and nanoporous materials are employed in biosensors and nanodevices for capturing and detecting NTD-related analytes with high sensitivity (Naresh and Lee 2021). Their large surface areas and unique properties enhance the binding kinetics and signal amplification, improving the accuracy of NTD diagnostics.

a. *Large Surface Area:* Nanowires and nanoporous materials possess a large surface-to-volume ratio, providing a significant surface area for interactions with target analytes. This large surface area allows for increased binding sites, enhancing the chances of capturing NTD-related biomolecules present in biological samples.
b. *Enhanced Binding Kinetics:* The unique structure of nanowires and nanoporous materials promotes rapid and efficient binding kinetics with NTD biomarkers. Functionalized surfaces of these materials can be tailored with specific recognition elements such as antibodies, aptamers, or peptides, enabling selective and high-affinity binding to target analytes.
c. *Signal Amplification:* Nanowires and nanoporous materials offer signal amplification capabilities in biosensing platforms. Upon binding of NTD-related analytes, the signal generated (e.g., electrical, optical, or electrochemical) can be amplified due to the enhanced interaction and accumulation of target molecules on the sensor surface. This signal amplification leads to improved sensitivity and detection limits in NTD diagnostics.
d. *Versatility in Detection Methods:* Nanowires and nanoporous materials can be integrated into various detection methods, including electrochemical, optical, and mass-sensitive techniques. For instance, in electrochemical biosensors, nanowires can serve as conductive elements that facilitate electron transfer during the detection process, while nanoporous materials can act as matrices for immobilizing recognition molecules and enhancing analyte capture.
e. *Applications in NTDs:* Nanowires and nanoporous materials have been utilized in the detection of diverse NTDs, including malaria, dengue, Chagas disease, leishmaniasis, schistosomiasis, and lymphatic filariasis. Functionalized nanowires and nanoporous surfaces can selectively capture disease-specific antigens, antibodies, nucleic acids, or metabolites, enabling accurate diagnosis and monitoring of NTDs.

The utilization of diagnostic nanomaterials has revolutionized the detection and management of NTDs as shown in Figure 9.2. GNPs in LFAs, QDs with their optical properties, CNTs in electrochemical biosensors, MNPs in MRI, and nanowires/nanoporous materials in biosensors collectively offer enhanced sensitivity, specificity, and portability in NTD diagnostics. These nanomaterials enable rapid, cost-effective, and point-of-care testing, particularly crucial in resource-limited settings where NTDs are prevalent. The integration of these advanced technologies into NTD

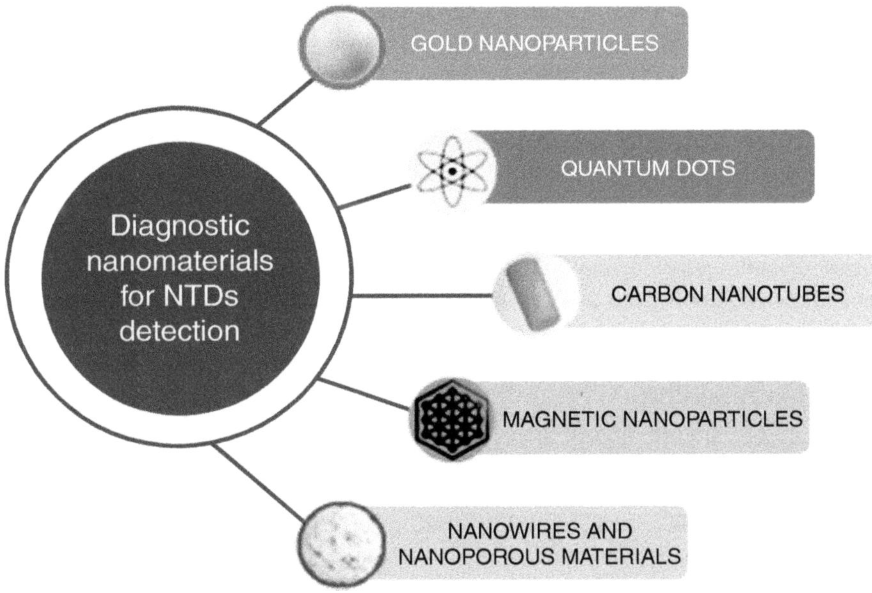

FIGURE 9.2 Different diagnostic nanomaterials for detection of NTDs.

detection platforms has significantly improved early diagnosis, surveillance, and monitoring of NTDs, ultimately leading to better patient outcomes and more effective disease control efforts. Furthermore, their compatibility with portable and cost-effective devices makes them suitable for use in decentralized healthcare settings, addressing the challenges posed by endemic regions. Overall, diagnostic nanomaterials represent a promising frontier in the fight against NTDs, offering hope for improved healthcare delivery and disease management worldwide.

9.3.5 Nanostructured Vaccines for NTDs

In recent years, there has been a growing recognition of the urgent need to address NTDs comprehensively and effectively. One promising avenue of research and innovation in this regard is the development of nanostructured vaccines tailored specifically for combating NTDs (Weng, Chen, and Wang 2018). Nanostructured vaccines refer to vaccines that incorporate nanotechnology-based components or features to enhance their efficacy, stability, and targeting capabilities (Bezbaruah et al. 2022). Nanostructured vaccines hold great promise for addressing NTDs due to improved immune responses, increased vaccine stability, and enabled targeted delivery to specific cells or tissues (Tiwari et al. 2023). The intricate design of nanostructured vaccines allows for the incorporation of multiple antigenic components, mimicking the complex nature of pathogens causing NTDs. This multifaceted approach enhances the immune system's ability to recognize and combat these pathogens, leading to stronger and more durable immune responses compared to traditional vaccine formulations (Ghattas et al. 2021). Moreover, nanostructured vaccines can be engineered to withstand challenging environmental conditions, such as lack of refrigeration or exposure to heat, ensuring their efficacy in resource-limited settings where NTDs are most prevalent. Furthermore, nanostructured vaccines offer the flexibility to incorporate adjuvant properties directly into their structure, reducing the need for additional adjuvants and simplifying vaccine formulations. This streamlined approach not only enhances vaccine efficacy but also streamlines production and administration processes, making these vaccines more accessible to vulnerable populations. Additionally, the modular design of nanostructured vaccines facilitates rapid adaptation to evolving NTD strains or emerging pathogens, ensuring continued effectiveness in the face of dynamic disease challenges. Combined with targeted delivery mechanisms that concentrate vaccine activity at the site of infection or immune response, nanostructured vaccines hold immense promise for revolutionizing NTD prevention and control efforts on a global scale (Dourado et al. 2024; Morilla, Ghosal, and Romero 2024; Tambe et al. 2024).

Nanostructured vaccines offer several innovative ways to address NTDs effectively. Here are some key strategies in which these vaccines can be utilized:

i. *Enhanced Immune Response*: Nanostructured vaccines can be designed to mimic the structure of pathogens causing NTDs or carry specific antigenic components, leading to enhanced recognition by the immune system (Ghattas et al. 2021). This can result in stronger and longer-lasting immune responses compared to conventional vaccines, crucial for diseases like malaria and dengue fever where robust immunity is essential for protection (Amanna and Slifka 2020).
ii. *Stability in Challenging Conditions*: Many NTDs are prevalent in regions with limited access to refrigeration and healthcare infrastructure. Nanostructured vaccines can be engineered to be stable at ambient temperatures or withstand temperature fluctuations, ensuring their efficacy during storage and transport in resource-limited settings.
iii. *Targeted Delivery*: Nanoparticles can be functionalized to target specific cells, tissues, or organs relevant to NTDs, such as immune cells or sites of infection. This targeted delivery enhances vaccine uptake and immune activation at the desired locations, potentially improving efficacy while minimizing off-target effects.
iv. *Adjuvant Properties*: Some nanomaterials possess inherent adjuvant properties, reducing the need for additional adjuvants in vaccine formulations. This simplifies vaccine design and administration while still eliciting robust immune responses against NTD pathogens.
v. *Combination Vaccines*: Nanostructured platforms allow for the incorporation of multiple antigens or therapeutic agents into a single vaccine formulation. This enables the development of combination vaccines targeting multiple NTDs simultaneously or addressing co-infections common in affected populations.
vi. *Modular Design for Flexibility*: Nanostructured vaccines can be designed with modular components, allowing for rapid customization and adaptation to evolving NTD strains or emerging pathogens. This flexibility is crucial for staying ahead of disease challenges in endemic regions.
vii. *Oral Vaccine Delivery*: Nanoparticles can be engineered for oral delivery, a particularly promising approach for NTDs like cholera and intestinal parasites. This route of administration can improve vaccine accessibility and compliance, especially in settings with limited access to healthcare facilities.
viii. *Immune Modulation*: Nanoparticles can modulate immune responses, potentially addressing immunosuppressive factors associated with chronic NTD infections. This immune modulation can enhance vaccine efficacy and contribute to long-term protection against these diseases.

By leveraging these strategies, nanostructured vaccines have the potential to significantly improve the prevention, control, and eventual elimination of NTDs, ultimately benefiting the health and well-being of vulnerable populations worldwide. Table 9.1 showcases list of nanostructured vaccines against some NTDs.

9.4 APPLICATIONS AND ADVANTAGES OF NANOMATERIALS FOR NTDS

Nanomaterials have shown great promise in the detection and treatment of NTDs due to their unique properties and versatility (Volpedo et al. 2019). Nanomaterials have revolutionized the approach to NTDs by offering a range of sophisticated applications and substantial advantages.

TABLE 9.1
List of Nanostructured Vaccine Formulation for NTDs

Type of Nanomaterial	Vaccine Antigen	Disease	Ref
Gold nanoparticles	CHrPfs-25 peptide	Malaria	R. Kumar et al. (n.d.)
PLGA nanoparticles	*Plasmodium vivax* circumsporozoite protein VMP001	Malaria	Moon, Suh, Polhemus, et al. (2012)
Liposomes	*Plasmodium vivax* circumsporozoite protein VMP001	Malaria	Moon, Suh, Li, et al. (2012)
Liposomes (AS01)	RTS,S (Mosqurix®)	Malaria	Wang, Chen, and Wang (2019)
PLGA nanoparticles	*Trypanosoma cruzi* Tc24 antigen	Chagas disease	Barry et al. (2016)
PLGA nanoparticles	Autoclaved *Leishmania* antigen	Visceral leishmaniasis	Tosyali et al. (2021)
Virus-like particle	Fusion protein (KMP-11, LJM-11, Leish F3)	Visceral leishmaniasis	Cecílio et al. (2017)
Solid lipid nanoparticles	cpc DNA and protein	Visceral leishmaniasis	Doroud et al. (2010)
Liposomes	*Leishmania donovani* CPA, CPB, CPC protein cocktail	Visceral leishmaniasis	A. Das and Ali (2014)
Liposomes	*Leishmania donovani* cpc DNA	Visceral leishmaniasis	A. Das et al. (2018)
Liposomes	*Leishmania donovani* elongation factor EF1-α protein	Visceral leishmaniasis	Sabur et al. (2018)

These applications span diagnostics, therapeutics, imaging, and monitoring, each contributing significantly to the fight against these often devastating diseases.

1. *Diagnostic Applications*: Nanomaterial-based diagnostic applications represent a groundbreaking advancement in the realm of NTDs compared to current treatment strategies. These innovative approaches harness the unique properties of nanomaterials to deliver rapid, sensitive, and multiplexed testing capabilities, revolutionizing the landscape of disease diagnosis and management. Unlike traditional methods that may be time-consuming, labor-intensive, and reliant on specialized equipment and expertise, nanomaterial-based assays offer a streamlined and accessible alternative. They empower healthcare providers in resource-limited settings to conduct point-of-care testing with ease, facilitating early detection of infections, comprehensive biomarker profiling, and tailored treatment approaches. This transformative impact extends to improving patient outcomes, optimizing healthcare resource allocation, and strengthening public health interventions against NTDs on a global scale.

   Nanomaterials have greatly enhanced the speed and accuracy of NTD diagnosis (Thwala et al. 2023). One notable example is the use of GNPs in LFAs. These assays leverage the unique properties of GNPs to enable rapid and on-site detection of NTDs like malaria, dengue, and Chagas disease. The incorporation of functionalized GNPs allows for specific binding to disease biomarkers, leading to visible color changes that indicate the presence of the disease. This rapid and sensitive detection capability is invaluable in resource-limited settings where timely diagnosis is crucial for effective treatment. Furthermore, nanomaterials such as QDs and nanowires offer high sensitivity in detecting disease biomarkers, even at extremely low concentrations. This not only facilitates early disease detection but also enables multiplexed assays, allowing for the simultaneous analysis of multiple disease markers in a single sample. The ability to conduct comprehensive diagnostics efficiently is a significant advancement in managing NTDs effectively.

2. *Therapeutic Applications*: Nanomaterials play a pivotal role in improving the efficacy and safety of NTD treatments. Nanoparticles like CNTs and MNPs can be engineered to deliver drugs directly to infected cells or tissues, enhancing targeted therapy while minimizing adverse effects on healthy cells. Nanomaterial-based therapeutic applications mark a revolutionary departure from current treatment paradigms for NTDs, heralding a new era of precision medicine and targeted therapy. These cutting-edge approaches leverage the unique properties of nanomaterials to enhance drug delivery, improve treatment efficacy, and minimize adverse effects. Traditional treatment strategies often face challenges such as limited drug bioavailability (Bhalani et al. 2022), non-specific targeting, and potential toxicity, which can hamper therapeutic outcomes and patient well-being. In contrast, nanomaterial-based drug delivery systems, such as nanoparticle carriers and functionalized nanotubes, offer tailored solutions that address these challenges comprehensively. By encapsulating drugs within nanoparticles or attaching them to nanocarriers, nanomaterials enable targeted delivery to specific cells or tissues, ensuring optimal drug concentrations at the site of action while minimizing off-target effects (Ezike et al. 2023). Moreover, the controlled release capabilities of nanomaterials allow for sustained drug release over time, leading to prolonged therapeutic effects and reduced dosing frequency (Javaid et al. 2024). This precision and control in drug delivery not only improve treatment outcomes but also enhance patient compliance and quality of life. Furthermore, nanomaterials facilitate the development of combination therapies and synergistic drug formulations, unlocking new possibilities for combating drug-resistant strains and enhancing therapeutic efficacy against NTDs. By harnessing the potential of nanotechnology in therapeutics, healthcare providers can offer personalized and optimized treatment regimens tailored to individual patient needs, ultimately driving advancements in NTD management, reducing disease burden, and improving global health outcomes.
3. *Imaging and Monitoring*: Nanomaterial-based imaging and monitoring applications herald a paradigm shift in the realm of NTDs, revolutionizing disease diagnosis, treatment monitoring, and patient care. MNPs serve as effective contrast agents in MRI, enabling healthcare professionals to visualize NTD-related complications with high resolution (Caspani et al. 2020). This capability is crucial for accurate diagnosis, monitoring disease progression, and assessing the effectiveness of treatment interventions. Traditional imaging techniques often face limitations such as low resolution, limited sensitivity, and the inability to provide real-time feedback, which can impact the accuracy of disease assessment and treatment outcomes. In contrast, nanomaterial-based imaging agents, such as MNPs and QDs, offer unparalleled capabilities in terms of precision, sensitivity, and real-time monitoring. MNPs, for instance, serve as highly effective contrast agents in MRI, enabling healthcare professionals to visualize NTD-related complications with unprecedented clarity and detail. This enhanced imaging resolution facilitates accurate diagnosis, treatment planning, and disease monitoring, leading to improved patient outcomes. Similarly, QDs and other fluorescent nanomaterials enable precise visualization of cellular and molecular processes, allowing for real-time monitoring of disease biomarkers, treatment responses, and therapeutic efficacy. The ability to track disease progression, assess treatment effectiveness, and detect early signs of recurrence empowers healthcare providers to make informed clinical decisions, tailor treatment regimens, and optimize patient care. Moreover, nanomaterial-based imaging and monitoring technologies offer the potential for theranostic applications, where diagnostic imaging and therapeutic interventions are seamlessly integrated, further enhancing the precision and effectiveness of NTD management. By harnessing the power of nanotechnology in imaging and monitoring, healthcare providers can achieve unprecedented levels of accuracy, efficiency, and personalized care in combating NTDs, ultimately advancing global health outcomes and reducing disease burden.

9.5 CHALLENGES AND CONSIDERATIONS

Using ENMs to combat NTDs presents both exciting opportunities and daunting challenges. While nanotechnology offers innovative solutions for diagnosing, treating, and preventing NTDs, we need to approach this with caution. One of the main challenges we face is ensuring that these ENMs are safe for human use. Despite their potential benefits, there are concerns about their potential toxicity and long-term effects on our health and the environment. It's vital that we rigorously test and understand these materials to minimize any risks and ensure they're safe for use in addressing NTDs.

Another important aspect to consider is whether these nanotechnology-based solutions can be scaled up and made affordable for those who need them most. While they show promise in improving the effectiveness of NTD treatments, making them accessible to resource-limited settings remains a significant hurdle. We need to focus on developing cost-effective manufacturing methods and strategies for large-scale production to ensure that everyone who needs these treatments can access them. Also, navigating the regulatory and ethical landscape is crucial in translating these nanotechnology-based interventions from the lab to clinical practice. The rules and guidelines for evaluating the safety and efficacy of these materials are still evolving, requiring collaboration between researchers, policymakers, and regulatory agencies to ensure they meet the necessary standards. Meanwhile, we must address the socioeconomic and logistical challenges of implementing these interventions in NTD-endemic regions. Limited access to healthcare infrastructure, trained personnel, and resources could hinder the adoption of these innovative technologies in low-resource settings. We need to develop strategies for capacity building, technology transfer, and community engagement to ensure the successful integration of nanotechnology into NTD control programs.

9.6 GLOBAL INITIATIVE AND FUTURE PERSPECTIVE TO COMBAT NTDS

In order to address the burden of NTDs worldwide, governments, non-governmental organizations, academic institutions, and international agencies have joined forces to create the global initiative for the management and prevention of NTDs. This program includes several tactics to lessen the incidence and effects of NTDs, with an emphasis on underprivileged and marginalized groups in low-resource environments. The initiative's core is its dedication to integrated approaches, which blend initiatives to boost community engagement and strengthen health systems with preventive measures like mass drug administration (MDA), vector control, improved sanitation, and health education. Through the simultaneous targeting of several NTDs and the utilization of pre-existing infrastructure and resources, this method optimizes both the efficacy and affordability of disease control initiatives.

Key stakeholders collaborate through various platforms and partnerships, including the WHO NTD Roadmap, the London Declaration on NTDs, and the Expanded Special Project for Elimination of NTDs (ESPEN). These initiatives provide frameworks for strategic planning, resource mobilization, and monitoring progress toward NTD control and elimination goals. The WHO has a 2030 global target to reduce the number of people requiring treatment for NTDs by 90%, reduce disability-adjusted life years (DALYs) related to NTDs by 75%, and eliminate at least one NTD in at least 100 countries. The WHO also has other targets, such as eradicating two diseases, dracunculiasis and yaws, and focusing on multisectoral coordination, universal health coverage, and country ownership ("Neglected Tropical Diseases -- GLOBAL" n.d.). The Global Network for Neglected Tropical Diseases is a movement dedicated to advocating for increased awareness, funding, and governmental support to combat and eradicate the prevalent NTDs. Formulated by the WHO in the early 2000s, a comprehensive strategy was developed focusing on five key public health interventions: enhanced and innovative disease management, widespread preventive treatments, integrated vector control measures, and initiatives targeting veterinary public health(Engels and Zhou 2020). Back in 2006, the United States Agency for International Development (USAID) set up the NTD Control Program. Its aim was to support national efforts targeting the control or elimination of diseases like lymphatic filariasis, onchocerciasis, schistosomiasis, soil-transmitted helminthiasis, and blinding trachoma (King 2011). The Bill & Melinda Gates Foundation has prioritized the fight against NTDs, ensuring their investments align with donor governments and developing countries' efforts, which provide the majority of funding for NTD control. They target areas with limited resources where their support can catalyze change, committing over US$1.02 billion in grants to develop innovative tools and delivery methods. Advocating for increased international funding, they focus on diseases with significant social and economic burdens in developing nations, aiming for elimination or eradication through strategic interventions. Their efforts are directed at the ten NTDs outlined in the London Declaration, tailoring approaches to address each disease's unique challenges ("Neglected Tropical Diseases | Bill & Melinda Gates Foundation" n.d.). The Indian initiative to eliminate NTDs has shown significant progress, particularly through the Accelerated Plan for Elimination of Lymphatic Filariasis (APELF) launched in 2018. This initiative, supported by the WHO and regional alliances with Bangladesh and Nepal, aims to enhance early diagnosis and treatment, as well as improve disease surveillance and vector control efforts, notably targeting sandfly populations for Kala-Azar control (Engels and Zhou 2020). India has already achieved success in eliminating several NTDs, such as guinea worm, trachoma, and yaws. Key strategies include MDA rounds providing anti-filarial medicines to at-risk communities and Indoor Residual Spraying to prevent sandfly breeding. Additionally, the government prioritizes morbidity management and disability prevention for those affected by lymphedema and hydrocele, along with introducing wage compensation schemes for Kala-Azar patients and individuals with Post-Kala-Azar Dermal Leishmaniasis. These comprehensive efforts underscore India's commitment to NTD elimination and improving public health outcomes for its population (WHO 2020).

Looking ahead, the future perspective for combating NTDs is promising but requires concerted efforts and innovative approaches. As like advancements in nanotechnology, genomics, artificial intelligence hold immense potential for accelerating progress in NTD research, diagnosis, and treatment. These technologies enable the development of more precise diagnostics, targeted therapies, and novel interventions, thereby enhancing our ability to tackle NTDs more effectively. Strengthening health systems and increasing access to key medicines and healthcare services are critical to ensuring fair distribution of NTD interventions, particularly in marginalized and distant populations. To boost the reach and effectiveness of NTD programs, more investment is needed in healthcare facilities, personnel development, and supply chain management. Advocacy and political commitment are also crucial for mobilizing resources and raising awareness about the burden of NTDs. By elevating NTDs on the global health agenda and promoting cross-sectoral collaboration, policymakers can drive sustainable investments and foster innovation in NTD control efforts. Community engagement and empowerment are critical components of NTD prevention and management. Empowering communities through health education, community-based interventions, and participatory approaches promotes ownership and sustainability of NTD programs, resulting in better health outcomes and a higher quality of life for afflicted populations. Despite the considerable obstacles in the fight against neglected tropical illnesses, there is hope for the future thanks to the implementation of integrated strategies, advances in technology, improved health systems, greater governmental support, and community involvement. We can achieve the ultimate aim of eradicating NTDs and enhancing health equity for all by utilizing these tactics and encouraging cooperation at all levels.

9.7 CONCLUSION

The exploration of ENMs for combating NTDs represents a pivotal advancement in global health research and intervention strategies. By addressing the limitations of current treatment approaches and leveraging the unique properties of nanomaterials, such as targeted drug delivery, enhanced efficacy, and improved diagnostics, we have the potential to revolutionize NTD management and control. From nanoparticle-based anti-parasitic drugs to nanostructured vaccines and diagnostic nanomaterials, the applications and advantages of nanotechnology offer promising avenues for more effective and sustainable NTD interventions. However, significant challenges and considerations, including safety, scalability, regulatory hurdles, and socioeconomic factors, must be carefully addressed to ensure the successful translation of nanotechnology-based solutions into clinical practice. Moving forward, collaborative efforts, global initiatives, and sustained investments are essential to harnessing the full potential of ENMs in the fight against NTDs, ultimately advancing health equity and improving the lives of millions worldwide.

ACKNOWLEDGMENTS

This work is supported by the Government of India for funding under DST-SERB (EEQ/2020/000563) and ICMR (DDR/IIRP23/3052).

REFERENCES

Abbasi, Reza, Ghazal Shineh, Mohammadmahdi Mobaraki, Sarah Doughty, and Lobat Tayebi. 2023. "Structural Parameters of Nanoparticles Affecting Their Toxicity for Biomedical Applications: A Review." *Journal of Nanoparticle Research* 25 (3). https://doi.org/10.1007/S11051-023-05690-W.

Abdelkawi, Abdullah, Aliyah Slim, Zaineb Zinoune, and Yashwant Pathak. 2023. "Surface Modification of Metallic Nanoparticles for Targeting Drugs." *Coatings* 13 (9): 1660. https://doi.org/10.3390/COATINGS13091660.

Albalawi, Fahad, Mohd Zobir Hussein, Sharida Fakurazi, and Mas Jaffri Masarudin. 2021. "Engineered Nanomaterials: The Challenges and Opportunities for Nanomedicines." *International Journal of Nanomedicine* 16: 161. https://doi.org/10.2147/IJN.S288236.

Alsaab, Hashem O., Fatima D. Alharbi, Alanoud S. Alhibs, Nouf B. Alanazi, Bayan Y. Alshehri, Marwa A. Saleh, Fahad S. Alshehri, et al. 2022. "PLGA-Based Nanomedicine: History of Advancement and Development in Clinical Applications of Multiple Diseases." *Pharmaceutics* 14 (12). https://doi.org/10.3390/PHARMACEUTICS14122728.

Amanna, Ian J., and Mark K. Slifka. 2020. "Successful Vaccines." *Current Topics in Microbiology and Immunology* 428: 1. https://doi.org/10.1007/82_2018_102.

Arora, Kanika, Aakriti Singh, Aaqib Javaid, and Shyam Lal Mudavath. 2022. "Promising Functional Supramolecules in Antiviral Drugs." *Pharmaceutical Applications of Supramolecules*, January, 135–55. https://doi.org/10.1007/978-3-031-21900-9_6.

Babaei, Abouzar, Seyed Mahmoud Mousavi, Marzie Ghasemi, Neda Pirbonyeh, Masoud Soleimani, and Afagh Moattari. 2021. "Gold Nanoparticles Show Potential in Vitro Antiviral and Anticancer Activity." *Life Sciences* 284: 119652. https://doi.org/https://doi.org/10.1016/j.lfs.2021.119652.

Bajwa, Hammad Ur Rehman, Muhammad Kasib Khan, Zaheer Abbas, Roshan Riaz, Tauseef Ur Rehman, Rao Zahid Abbas, Muhammad Tahir Aleem, et al. 2022. "Nanoparticles: Synthesis and Their Role as Potential Drug Candidates for the Treatment of Parasitic Diseases." *Life* 12 (5): 750. https://doi.org/10.3390/LIFE12050750.

Bao, Gang, Samir Mitragotri, and Sheng Tong. 2013. "Multifunctional Nanoparticles for Drug Delivery and Molecular Imaging." *Annual Review of Biomedical Engineering* 15 (July): 253–82. https://doi.org/10.1146/ANNUREV-BIOENG-071812-152409.

Barroso, Margarida M. 2011. "Quantum Dots in Cell Biology." *Journal of Histochemistry and Cytochemistry* 59 (3): 237–51. https://doi.org/10.1369/0022155411398487.

Barry, Meagan A, Qian Wang, Kathryn M Jones, Michael J Heffernan, Munir H Buhaya, Coreen M Beaumier, Brian P Keegan, et al. 2016. "A Therapeutic Nanoparticle Vaccine against Trypanosoma Cruzi in a BALB/c Mouse Model of Chagas Disease." *Human Vaccines & Immunotherapeutics* 12 (4): 976–87. https://doi.org/10.1080/21645515.2015.1119346.

Bezbaruah, Rajashri, Vivek P. Chavda, Lawandashisha Nongrang, Shahnaz Alom, Kangkan Deka, Tutumoni Kalita, Farak Ali, Bedanta Bhattacharjee, and Lalitkumar Vora. 2022. "Nanoparticle-Based Delivery Systems for Vaccines." *Vaccines* 10 (11). https://doi.org/10.3390/vaccines10111946.

Bhalani, Dixit V., Bhingaradiya Nutan, Avinash Kumar, and Arvind K. Singh Chandel. 2022. "Bioavailability Enhancement Techniques for Poorly Aqueous Soluble Drugs and Therapeutics." *Biomedicines* 10 (9). https://doi.org/10.3390/biomedicines10092055.

Bhattacharya, Kunal, Sourav P. Mukherjee, Audrey Gallud, Seth C. Burkert, Silvia Bistarelli, Stefano Bellucci, Massimo Bottini, Alexander Star, and Bengt Fadeel. 2016. "Biological Interactions of Carbon-Based Nanomaterials: From Coronation to Degradation." *Nanomedicine: Nanotechnology, Biology and Medicine* 12 (2): 333–51. https://doi.org/10.1016/J.NANO.2015.11.011.

Campos, Estefânia Vangelie Ramos, Jhones Luiz de Oliveira, Daniele Carvalho Abrantes, Carolina Barbára Rogério, Carolina Bueno, Vanessa Regina Miranda, Renata Aparecida Monteiro, and Leonardo Fernandes Fraceto. 2020. "Recent Developments in Nanotechnology for Detection and Control of Aedes Aegypti-Borne Diseases." *Frontiers in Bioengineering and Biotechnology* 8 (February): 515164. https://doi.org/10.3389/FBIOE.2020.00102/BIBTEX.

Caspani, Sofia, Ricardo Magalhães, João Pedro Araújo, and Célia Tavares Sousa. 2020. "Magnetic Nanomaterials as Contrast Agents for MRI." *Materials* 13 (11). https://doi.org/10.3390/ma13112586.

Castilho, Leda R., Nathalia R. Mattos, Wallace S. Abreu, and Melissa L. E. Gutarra. 2022. "Virus-Like Particles (VLPs) as Important Tools for Flavivirus Vaccine Development." *Biologics* 2 (4): 226–42. https://doi.org/10.3390/BIOLOGICS2040018.

Cecílio, Pedro, Begoña Pérez-Cabezas, Laura Fernández, Javier Moreno, Eugenia Carrillo, José M. Requena, Epifanio Fichera, et al. 2017. "Pre-Clinical Antigenicity Studies of an Innovative Multivalent Vaccine for Human Visceral Leishmaniasis." *PLOS Neglected Tropical Diseases* 11 (11): e0005951. https://doi.org/10.1371/JOURNAL.PNTD.0005951.

Chaturvedi, Shalini, Pragnesh N. Dave, and N. K. Shah. 2012. "Applications of Nano-Catalyst in New Era." *Journal of Saudi Chemical Society* 16 (3): 307–25. https://doi.org/10.1016/J.JSCS.2011.01.015.

Chen, Lu, and Jiangong Liang. 2020. "An Overview of Functional Nanoparticles as Novel Emerging Antiviral Therapeutic Agents." *Materials Science and Engineering C* 112 (March). https://doi.org/10.1016/j.msec.2020.110924.

Choudhury, Satabdi Datta. 2021. "Nano-Medicines a Hope for Chagas Disease!" *Frontiers in Molecular Biosciences* 8 (June): 655435. https://doi.org/10.3389/FMOLB.2021.655435/BIBTEX.

Cunha, Rita F, Sandra Simões, Manuela Carvalheiro, José M Azevedo Pereira, Quirina Costa, and Andreia Ascenso. 2021. "Novel Antiretroviral Therapeutic Strategies for HIV." *Molecules* 26 (17). https://doi.org/10.3390/molecules26175305.

Daniel, Thoresen, Matsuda Kenta, Urakami Akane, Ngwe Tun Mya Myat, Nomura Takushi, Moi Meng Ling, Watanabe Yuri, et al. 2024. "A Tetravalent Dengue Virus-like Particle Vaccine Induces High Levels of Neutralizing Antibodies and Reduces Dengue Replication in Non-Human Primates." *Journal of Virology* 98 (5): e00239–24. https://doi.org/10.1128/jvi.00239-24.

Das, Amrita, and Nahid Ali. 2014. "Combining Cationic Liposomal Delivery with MPL-TDM for Cysteine Protease Cocktail Vaccination against Leishmania Donovani : Evidence for Antigen Synergy and Protection." *PLoS Neglected Tropical Diseases* 8 (8). https://doi.org/10.1371/JOURNAL.PNTD.0003091.

Das, Amrita, Mohammad Asad, Abdus Sabur, Nicky Didwania, and Nahid Ali. 2018. "Monophosphoryl Lipid A Based Cationic Liposome Facilitates Vaccine Induced Expansion of Polyfunctional T Cell Immune Responses against Visceral Leishmaniasis." *ACS Applied Bio Materials* 1 (4): 999–1018. https://doi.org/10.1021/ACSABM.8B00184.

Das, Bhaskar, Manashjit Gogoi, Satakshi Hazra, and Sanjukta Patra. 2018. "Nanocarrier-Assisted Drug Delivery for Neglected Tropical Diseases." In *Nanoconjugate Nanocarriers for Drug Delivery*, edited by Keservani Raj K and Sharma Anil K, 1st ed., 34. Apple Academy Press, Taylor & Francis Group.

Dauda, Kabiru, Zulaikha Busari, Olajumoke Morenikeji, Funmilayo Afolayan, Oyetunde Oyeyemi, Jairam Meena, Debasis Sahu, and Amulya Panda. 2017. "Poly(D,L-Lactic-Co-Glycolic Acid)-Based Artesunate Nanoparticles: Formulation, Antimalarial and Toxicity Assessments." *Journal of Zhejiang University. Science. B* 18 (11): 977–85. https://doi.org/10.1631/JZUS.B1600389.

Deroco, Patricia Batista, Dagwin Wachholz Junior, and Lauro Tatsuo Kubota. 2021. "Recent Advances in Point-of-Care Biosensors for the Diagnosis of Neglected Tropical Diseases." *Sensors and Actuators B: Chemical* 349: 130821. https://doi.org/https://doi.org/10.1016/j.snb.2021.130821.

Doroud, Delaram, Alireza Vatanara Vatanara, Farnaz Zahedifard, Elham Gholami, Rouhollah Vahabpour, Abdolhossein Rouholamini Najafabadi, and Sima Rafati. 2010. "Cationic Solid Lipid Nanoparticles Loaded by Cysteine Proteinase Genes as a Novel Anti-Leishmaniasis DNA Vaccine Delivery System: Characterization and in Vitro Evaluations." *Journal of Pharmacy & Pharmaceutical Sciences : A Publication of the Canadian Society for Pharmaceutical Sciences, Societe Canadienne Des Sciences Pharmaceutiques* 13 (3): 320–35. https://doi.org/10.18433/J3R30T.

Doughty, Austin C.V., Ashley R. Hoover, Elivia Layton, Cynthia K. Murray, Eric W. Howard, and Wei R. Chen. 2019. "Nanomaterial Applications in Photothermal Therapy for Cancer." *Materials* 12 (5). https://doi.org/10.3390/MA12050779.

Dourado, Douglas, Thayse Silva Medeiros, Éverton do Nascimento Alencar, Edijane Matos Sales, and Fábio Rocha Formiga. 2024. "Curcumin-Loaded Nanostructured Systems for Treatment of Leishmaniasis: A Review." *Beilstein Journal of Nanotechnology* 15: 37–50. https://doi.org/10.3762/bjnano.15.4.

Duan, Shufan, Yanling Hu, Ying Zhao, Kaiyuan Tang, Zhijing Zhang, Zilu Liu, Ying Wang, et al. 2023. "Nanomaterials for Photothermal Cancer Therapy." *RSC Advances* 13 (21): 14443. https://doi.org/10.1039/D3RA02620E.

Elmowafy, Mohammed, and Mohammad M. Al-Sanea. 2021. "Nanostructured Lipid Carriers (NLCs) as Drug Delivery Platform: Advances in Formulation and Delivery Strategies." *Saudi Pharmaceutical Journal : SPJ* 29 (9): 999. https://doi.org/10.1016/J.JSPS.2021.07.015.

Engels, Dirk, and Xiao Nong Zhou. 2020. "Neglected Tropical Diseases: An Effective Global Response to Local Poverty-Related Disease Priorities." *Infectious Diseases of Poverty* 9 (1). https://doi.org/10.1186/S40249-020-0630-9.

Ezike, Tobechukwu Christian, Ugochukwu Solomon Okpala, Ufedo Lovet Onoja, Chinenye Princess Nwike, Emmanuel Chimeh Ezeako, Osinachi Juliet Okpara, Charles Chinkwere Okoroafor, et al. 2023. "Advances in Drug Delivery Systems, Challenges and Future Directions." *Heliyon* 9 (6): e17488. https://doi.org/10.1016/j.heliyon.2023.e17488.

Faria, Maria J., Carla M. Lopes, José Das Neves, and Marlene Lúcio. 2021. "Lipid Nanocarriers for Anti-HIV Therapeutics: A Focus on Physicochemical Properties and Biotechnological Advances." *Pharmaceutics* 13 (8): 1294. https://doi.org/10.3390/PHARMACEUTICS13081294.

Farinha, Pedro, João M.P. Coelho, Catarina Pinto Reis, and Maria Manuela Gaspar. 2021. "A Comprehensive Updated Review on Magnetic Nanoparticles in Diagnostics." *Nanomaterials* 11 (12): 11. https://doi.org/10.3390/NANO11123432/S1.

Farzin, Ali, Seyed Alireza Etesami, Jacob Quint, Adnan Memic, and Ali Tamayol. 2020. "Magnetic Nanoparticles in Cancer Therapy and Diagnosis." *Advanced Healthcare Materials* 9 (9): e1901058. https://doi.org/10.1002/ADHM.201901058.

Feng, Jianguo, Qi Zhang, Qi Liu, Zhengxi Zhu, David Julian McClements, and Seid Mahdi Jafari. 2018. "Application of Nanoemulsions in Formulation of Pesticides." *Nanoemulsions: Formulation, Applications, and Characterization*, March, 379–413. https://doi.org/10.1016/B978-0-12-811838-2.00012-6.

Galdiero, Stefania, Annarita Falanga, Mariateresa Vitiello, Marco Cantisani, Veronica Marra, and Massimiliano Galdiero. 2011. "Silver Nanoparticles as Potential Antiviral Agents." *Molecules* 16 (10): 8894. https://doi.org/10.3390/MOLECULES16108894.

Gedda, Mallikarjuna Rao, Prasoon Madhukar, Ashish Shukla, Shyam Lal Mudavath, Onkar Nath Srivastava, Om Prakash Singh, and Shyam Sundar. 2021. "Nanodiagnostics in Leishmaniasis: A New Frontiers for Early Elimination." *Wiley Interdisciplinary Reviews. Nanomedicine and Nanobiotechnology* 13 (2): e1675. https://doi.org/10.1002/WNAN.1675.

Ghattas, Majed, Garima Dwivedi, Marc Lavertu, and Mohamad Gabriel Alameh. 2021. "Vaccine Technologies and Platforms for Infectious Diseases: Current Progress, Challenges, and Opportunities." *Vaccines* 9 (12): 1–31. https://doi.org/10.3390/vaccines9121490.

Ghorai, Suvankar. 2023. "Editorial: Reviews in Neglected Tropical Infectious Diseases." *Frontiers in Microbiology* 14: 2019–21. https://doi.org/10.3389/fmicb.2023.1196838.

"Global Report on Neglected Tropical Diseases 2023." n.d. Accessed April 4, 2024. https://www.who.int/teams/control-of-neglected-tropical-diseases/global-report-on-neglected-tropical-diseases-2023.

Gogoi, Manashjit. 2017. "Recent Advances in Nanomedicine for Antimalarial Drug Delivery." *Biomedical Research Journal* 4 (2): 151. https://doi.org/10.4103/2349-3666.240598.

Gomes, Daniele Cavalcante, Thayse Silva Medeiros, Eron Lincoln Alves Pereira, João Felipe Oliveira da Silva, Johny W. de Freitas Oliveira, Matheus de Freitas Fernandes-Pedrosa, Marcelo de Sousa da Silva, and Arnóbio Antônio da Silva-Júnior. 2023. "From Benznidazole to New Drugs: Nanotechnology Contribution in Chagas Disease." *International Journal of Molecular Sciences* 24 (18). https://doi.org/10.3390/IJMS241813778.

Gubala, Vladimir, Linda J. Johnston, Ziwei Liu, Harald Krug, Colin J. Moore, Christopher K. Ober, Michael Schwenk, and Michel Vert. 2018. "Engineered Nanomaterials and Human Health: Part 1. Preparation, Functionalization and Characterization (IUPAC Technical Report)." *Pure and Applied Chemistry* 90 (8): 1283–1324. https://doi.org/10.1515/PAC-2017-0101.

Guo, Xiaoping, Xu Zuo, Zhengjie Zhou, Yinuo Gu, Haoyu Zheng, Xinlei Wang, Guoqiang Wang, Caina Xu, and Fang Wang. 2023. "PLGA-Based Micro/Nanoparticles: An Overview of Their Applications in Respiratory Diseases." *International Journal of Molecular Sciences* 24 (5): 24. https://doi.org/10.3390/IJMS24054333.

Hajizade, Abbas, Gholamreza Ahmadian, Kelong Fan, Mingzhao Zhu, and Ayyoob Arpanaei. 2023. "Editorial: Nanotechnology-Based Detection, Prevention and Treatment of Infectious Diseases." *Frontiers in Microbiology* 14 (June): 1224727. https://doi.org/10.3389/FMICB.2023.1224727/BIBTEX.

Heidari, Mina, Jacob Golenser, and Andreas Greiner. 2022. "Meeting the Needs of a Potent Carrier for Malaria Treatment: Encapsulation of Artemisone in Poly(Lactide-Co-Glycolide) Micro- and Nanoparticles." *Particle and Particle Systems Characterization* 39 (5). https://doi.org/10.1002/ppsc.202100152.

Hikal, Wafaa M., Mohamed M. Baz, Mohammed Ali Alshehri, Omar Bahattab, Rowida S. Baeshen, Abdelfattah M. Selim, Latifah Alhwity, Rabaa Bousbih, Maha Suleiman Alshourbaji, and Hussein A.H.Said Al Ahl. 2023. "Sustainable Pest Management Using Novel Nanoemulsions of Honeysuckle and Patchouli Essential Oils against the West Nile Virus Vector, Culex Pipiens, under Laboratory and Field Conditions." *Plants* 12 (21): 3682. https://doi.org/10.3390/PLANTS12213682/S1.

Hines, Daniel J., and David L. Kaplan. 2013. "Poly (Lactic-Co-Glycolic Acid) Controlled Release Systems: Experimental and Modeling Insights." *Critical Reviews in Therapeutic Drug Carrier Systems* 30 (3): 257. https://doi.org/10.1615/CRITREVTHERDRUGCARRIERSYST.2013006475.

Hoseini-Ghahfarokhi, Mojtaba, Soroush Mirkiani, Naeimeh Mozaffari, Mohamad Amin Abdolahi Sadatlu, Amir Ghasemi, Somayeh Abbaspour, Mohsen Akbarian, Fatemeh Farjadian, and Mahdi Karimi. 2020. "Applications of Graphene and Graphene Oxide in Smart Drug/Gene Delivery: Is the World Still Flat?" *International Journal of Nanomedicine* 15: 9469. https://doi.org/10.2147/IJN.S265876.

Jacobs, Christopher B., M. Jennifer Peairs, and B. Jill Venton. 2010. "Review: Carbon Nanotube Based Electrochemical Sensors for Biomolecules." *Analytica Chimica Acta* 662 (2): 105–27. https://doi.org/10.1016/J.ACA.2010.01.009.

Jaiswal, Manjit, Rupesh Dudhe, and P. K. Sharma. 2015. "Nanoemulsion: An Advanced Mode of Drug Delivery System." *3 Biotech* 5 (2): 123. https://doi.org/10.1007/S13205-014-0214-0.

Javaid, Aaqib, Krishana Kumar Sharma, Abutwaibe Ka, Anurag Verma, and Shyam Lal Mudavath. 2024. "Therapeutic Potential of Molsidomine-Loaded Liquid Crystal Nanoparticles for the Treatment and Management of Niacin-Induced Varicose Veins: In Vitro and In Vivo Studies." *ACS Applied Bio Materials*, September. https://doi.org/10.1021/acsabm.4c00980.

Kabanov, A. V., and H. E. Gendelman. 2007. "Nanomedicine in the Diagnosis and Therapy of Neurodegenerative Disorders." *Progress in Polymer Science* 32 (8–9): 1054. https://doi.org/10.1016/J.PROGPOLYMSCI.2007.05.014.

King, Charles H. 2011. "The Causes and Impacts of Neglected Tropical and Zoonotic Diseases : Opportunities for Integrated Intervention Strategies." *Nature*. National Academies Press (US); 2011. A15. Available from: https://www.ncbi.nlm.nih.gov/books/NBK62515/

Kumar, Arun, Prashant Kumar, Ananthitha Anandan, Teresa F. Fernandes, Godwin A. Ayoko, and George Biskos. 2014. "Engineered Nanomaterials: Knowledge Gaps in Fate, Exposure, Toxicity, and Future Directions." *Journal of Nanomaterials* 2014. https://doi.org/10.1155/2014/130198.

Kumar, Rajesh, Paresh C Ray, Dibyadyuti Datta, Geetha P Bansal, Evelina Angov, and Nirbhay Kumar. n.d. "Nanovaccines for Malaria Using Plasmodium Falciparum Antigen Pfs25 Attached Gold Nanoparticles." https://doi.org/10.1016/j.vaccine.2015.08.025.

Lembo, David, Manuela Donalisio, Andrea Civra, Monica Argenziano, and Roberta Cavalli. 2018. "Nanomedicine Formulations for the Delivery of Antiviral Drugs: A Promising Solution for the Treatment of Viral Infections." *Expert Opinion on Drug Delivery* 15 (1): 93–114. https://doi.org/10.1080/17425247.2017.1360863.

Li, Lele, Hang Xing, Jingjing Zhang, and Yi Lu. 2019. "Functional DNA Molecules Enable Selective and Stimuli-Responsive Nanoparticles for Biomedical Applications." *Accounts of Chemical Research* 52 (9): 2415. https://doi.org/10.1021/ACS.ACCOUNTS.9B00167.

Lu, Yue, Dongfang Cheng, Baohua Niu, Xiuzhi Wang, Xiaxia Wu, and Aiping Wang. 2023. "Properties of Poly (Lactic-Co-Glycolic Acid) and Progress of Poly (Lactic-Co-Glycolic Acid)-Based Biodegradable Materials in Biomedical Research." *Pharmaceuticals* 16 (3). https://doi.org/10.3390/PH16030454.

Mahajan, Supreeti, Shweta Choudhary, Pravindra Kumar, and Shailly Tomar. 2021. "Antiviral Strategies Targeting Host Factors and Mechanisms Obliging +ssRNA Viral Pathogens." *Bioorganic & Medicinal Chemistry* 46: 116356. https://doi.org/https://doi.org/10.1016/j.bmc.2021.116356.

Mahor, Alok Kumar, Prem Prakash Singh, Rishikesh Gupta, Peeyush Bhardwaj, Priyanka Rathore, Ankita Kishore, Rohit Goyal, et al. 2023. "Nanostructured Lipid Carriers for Improved Delivery of Therapeutics via the Oral Route." *Journal of Nanotechnology* 2023. https://doi.org/10.1155/2023/4687959.

Mahor, Alok, Prem Prakash Singh, Peeyush Bharadwaj, Neeraj Sharma, Surabhi Yadav, Jessica M. Rosenholm, and Kuldeep K. Bansal. 2021. "Carbon-Based Nanomaterials for Delivery of Biologicals and Therapeutics: A Cutting-Edge Technology." *C* 7 (1): 19. https://doi.org/10.3390/C7010019.

Makadia, Hirenkumar K., and Steven J. Siegel. 2011. "Poly Lactic-Co-Glycolic Acid (PLGA) as Biodegradable Controlled Drug Delivery Carrier." *Polymers* 3 (3): 1377. https://doi.org/10.3390/POLYM3031377.

Malik, Shiza, Khalid Muhammad, and Yasir Waheed. 2023. "Emerging Applications of Nanotechnology in Healthcare and Medicine." *Molecules* 28 (18): 6624. https://doi.org/10.3390/MOLECULES28186624.

Mallipeddi, Rama, and Lisa Cencia Rohan. 2010. "Progress in Antiretroviral Drug Delivery Using Nanotechnology." *International Journal of Nanomedicine* 5 (1): 533.

Manjesh, Keerthiraj, Aditi Kundu, Anirban Dutta, Supradip Saha, and Bhagyasree Sira Neelakanthaiah. 2022. "Bio-Insecticidal Nanoemulsions of Essential Oil and Lipid-Soluble Fractions of Pogostemon Cablin." *Frontiers in Plant Science* 13 (April): 874221. https://doi.org/10.3389/FPLS.2022.874221/BIBTEX.

Mapossa, António B., Walter W. Focke, Robert K. Tewo, René Androsch, and Taneshka Kruger. 2021. "Mosquito-repellent Controlled-release Formulations for Fighting Infectious Diseases." *Malaria Journal* 20 (1): 1–33. https://doi.org/10.1186/S12936-021-03681-7.

Medina-Rivera, Melisa, Washington B. Cárdenas, David Erickson, and Saurabh Mehta. 2022. "Gold Nanoshells-Based Lateral Flow Assay for the Detection of Chagas Disease at the Point-of-Care." *American Journal of Tropical Medicine and Hygiene* 107 (2): 323–27. https://doi.org/10.4269/AJTMH.21-1119.

Mishra, Vijay, Kuldeep K. Bansal, Asit Verma, Nishika Yadav, Sourav Thakur, Kalvatala Sudhakar, and Jessica M. Rosenholm. 2018. "Solid Lipid Nanoparticles: Emerging Colloidal Nano Drug Delivery Systems." *Pharmaceutics* 10 (4). https://doi.org/10.3390/PHARMACEUTICS10040191.

Mohkam, Milad, Mohammad Sadraeian, Antonio Lauto, Ahmad Gholami, Seyed Hesamodin Nabavizadeh, Hossein Esmaeilzadeh, and Soheila Alyasin. 2023. "Exploring the Potential and Safety of Quantum Dots in Allergy Diagnostics." *Microsystems and Nanoengineering* 9 (1). https://doi.org/10.1038/s41378-023-00608-x.

Mondal, Sourav, and Sourish Ghosh. 2023. "Liposome-Mediated Anti-Viral Drug Delivery across Blood-Brain Barrier: Can Lipid Droplet Target Be Game Changers?" *Cellular and Molecular Neurobiology* 44 (1): 9. https://doi.org/10.1007/s10571-023-01443-4.

Moon, James J., Heikyung Suh, Adrienne V. Li, Christian F. Ockenhouse, Anjali Yadava, and Darrell J. Irvine. 2012. "Enhancing Humoral Responses to a Malaria Antigen with Nanoparticle Vaccines That Expand Tfh Cells and Promote Germinal Center Induction." *Proceedings of the National Academy of Sciences of the United States of America* 109 (4): 1080–85. https://doi.org/10.1073/PNAS.1112648109.

Moon, James J, Heikyung Suh, Mark E Polhemus, Christian F Ockenhouse, Anjali Yadava, and Darrell J Irvine. 2012. "Antigen-Displaying Lipid-Enveloped PLGA Nanoparticles as Delivery Agents for a Plasmodium Vivax Malaria Vaccine." *PLoS One* 7 (2): e31472. https://doi.org/10.1371/journal.pone.0031472.

Morilla, Maria Jose, Kajal Ghosal, and Eder Lilia Romero. 2024. "Nanomedicines against Chagas Disease: A Critical Review." *Beilstein Journal of Nanotechnology* 15 (Cd): 333–49. https://doi.org/10.3762/bjnano.15.30.

Mustafa, Isshadiba Faikah, and Mohd Zobir Hussein. 2020. "Synthesis and Technology of Nanoemulsion-Based Pesticide Formulation." *Nanomaterials* 10 (8): 1–26. https://doi.org/10.3390/NANO10081608.

Naresh, Varnakavi, and Nohyun Lee. 2021. "A Review on Biosensors and Recent Development of Nanostructured Materials-Enabled Biosensors." *Sensors* 21 (4): 1–35. https://doi.org/10.3390/s21041109.

"Neglected Tropical Diseases -- GLOBAL." n.d. Accessed April 4, 2024. https://www.who.int/health-topics/neglected-tropical-diseases#tab=tab_1.

"Neglected Tropical Diseases | Bill & Melinda Gates Foundation." n.d. Accessed April 4, 2024. https://www.gatesfoundation.org/our-work/programs/global-health/neglected-tropical-diseases.

Nie, Danyue, Jiaqiao Li, Qinghua Xie, Lele Ai, Changqiang Zhu, Yifan Wu, Qiyuan Gui, Lingling Zhang, and Weilong Tan. 2023. "Nanoparticles: A Potential and Effective Method to Control Insect-Borne Diseases." *Bioinorganic Chemistry and Applications* 2023. https://doi.org/10.1155/2023/5898160.

Nishimura, Keita, Takuya Ushiyama, Nguyen Xuan Viet, Masafumi Inaba, Shigeru Kishimoto, and Yutaka Ohno. 2019. "Enhancement of the Electron Transfer Rate in Carbon Nanotube Flexible Electrochemical Sensors by Surface Functionalization." *Electrochimica Acta* 295 (February): 157–63. https://doi.org/10.1016/J.ELECTACTA.2018.10.147.

Nooraei, Saghi, Howra Bahrulolum, Zakieh Sadat Hoseini, Camellia Katalani, Abbas Hajizade, Andrew J Easton, and Gholamreza Ahmadian. 2021. "Virus-like Particles: Preparation, Immunogenicity and Their Roles as Nanovaccines and Drug Nanocarriers." *Journal of Nanobiotechnology* 19 (1): 59. https://doi.org/10.1186/s12951-021-00806-7.

Pandian, Sureshbabu Ram Kumar, Theivendren Panneerselvam, Parasuraman Pavadai, Saravanan Govindaraj, Vigneshwaran Ravishankar, Ponnusamy Palanisamy, Muthukumar Sampath, Murugesan Sankaranarayanan, and Selvaraj Kunjiappan. 2021. "Nano Based Approach for the Treatment of Neglected Tropical Diseases." *Frontiers in Nanotechnology* 3 (June): 1–21. https://doi.org/10.3389/fnano.2021.665274.

Patra, Jayanta Kumar, Gitishree Das, Leonardo Fernandes Fraceto, Estefania Vangelie Ramos Campos, Maria Del Pilar Rodriguez-Torres, Laura Susana Acosta-Torres, Luis Armando Diaz-Torres, et al. 2018. "Nano Based Drug Delivery Systems: Recent Developments and Future Prospects." *Journal of Nanobiotechnology* 16 (1): 1–33. https://doi.org/10.1186/S12951-018-0392-8.

Pavoni, Lucia, Roman Pavela, Marco Cespi, Giulia Bonacucina, Filippo Maggi, Valeria Zeni, Angelo Canale, Andrea Lucchi, Fabrizio Bruschi, and Giovanni Benelli. 2019. "Green Micro- and Nanoemulsions for Managing Parasites, Vectors and Pests." *Nanomaterials* 9 (9): 1285. https://doi.org/10.3390/NANO9091285.

Plucinski, Mateusz, Michael Aidoo, and Eric Rogier. 2021. "Laboratory Detection of Malaria Antigens: A Strong Tool for Malaria Research, Diagnosis, and Epidemiology." *Clinical Microbiology Reviews* 34 (3): 1–20. https://doi.org/10.1128/CMR.00250-20.

Preeti, Sharda Sambhakar, Rohit Malik, Saurabh Bhatia, Ahmed Al Harrasi, Chanchal Rani, Renu Saharan, Suresh Kumar, Geeta, and Renu Sehrawat. 2023. "Nanoemulsion: An Emerging Novel Technology for Improving the Bioavailability of Drugs." *Scientifica* 2023. https://doi.org/10.1155/2023/6640103.

Quezada, Christian Quijia, Clênia S. Azevedo, Sébastien Charneau, Jaime M. Santana, Marlus Chorilli, Marcella B. Carneiro, and Izabela Marques Dourado Bastos. 2019. "Advances in Nanocarriers as Drug Delivery Systems in Chagas Disease." *International Journal of Nanomedicine* 14: 6407. https://doi.org/10.2147/IJN.S206109.

Rahman, Khaista, Shahid Ullah Khan, Shah Fahad, Ming Xian Chang, Aqleem Abbas, Wasim Ullah Khan, Lutfur Rahman, Zaheer Ul Haq, Ghulam Nabi, and Dilfaraz Khan. 2019. "Nano-Biotechnology: A New Approach to Treat and Prevent Malaria." *International Journal of Nanomedicine* 14: 1401. https://doi.org/10.2147/IJN.S190692.

Rasalkar, Darshana D., B. K. Paunipagar, D. Sanghvi, B. D. Sonawane, and P. Loniker. 2011. "Magnetic Resonance Imaging in Cerebral Malaria: A Report of Four Cases." *British Journal of Radiology* 84 (1000): 380–85. https://doi.org/10.1259/BJR/85759874.

Rong-Hwa, Shyu, Tang Shiao-Shek, Chiao Der-Jiang, and Hung Yao-Wen. 2010. "Gold Nanoparticle-Based Lateral Flow Assay for Detection of Staphylococcal Enterotoxin B." *Food Chemistry* 118 (2): 462–66. https://doi.org/https://doi.org/10.1016/j.foodchem.2009.04.106.

Sabur, Abdus, Sudipta Bhowmick, Rudra Chhajer, Sarfaraz Ahmad Ejazi, Nicky Didwania, Mohammad Asad, Anirban Bhattacharyya, Utsa Sinha, and Nahid Ali. 2018. "Liposomal Elongation Factor-1α Triggers Effector CD4 and CD8 T Cells for Induction of Long-Lasting Protective Immunity against Visceral Leishmaniasis." *Frontiers in Immunology* 9 (JAN). https://doi.org/10.3389/FIMMU.2018.00018.

Santos-Valle, Ana Beatriz C, Gabriela R R Souza, Camila Q Paes, Takuya Miyazaki, Adny Henrique Silva, Maria J Altube, Maria J Morilla, et al. 2019. "Nanomedicine Strategies for Addressing Major Needs in Neglected Tropical Diseases." *Annual Reviews in Control* 48: 423–41. https://doi.org/https://doi.org/10.1016/j.arcontrol.2019.08.001.

Sarkar, Joy, Sunandana Das, Sahasrabdi Aich, Prithu Bhattacharyya, and Krishnendu Acharya. 2022. "Antiviral Potential of Nanoparticles for the Treatment of Coronavirus Infections." *Journal of Trace Elements in Medicine and Biology* 72 (July): 126977. https://doi.org/10.1016/J.JTEMB.2022.126977.

Schmidt, Michael, Wolf Jochen Geilenkeuser, Walid Sireis, Erhard Seifried, and Kai Hourfar. 2014. "Emerging Pathogens – How Safe Is Blood?" *Transfusion Medicine and Hemotherapy* 41 (1): 10. https://doi.org/10.1159/000358017.

Şenel, Sevda, and Selin Yüksel. 2020. "Chitosan-Based Particulate Systems for Drug and Vaccine Delivery in the Treatment and Prevention of Neglected Tropical Diseases." *Drug Delivery and Translational Research* 10 (6): 1644–74. https://doi.org/10.1007/s13346-020-00806-4.

Shao, Lijia, Yanfang Gao, and Feng Yan. 2011. "Semiconductor Quantum Dots for Biomedical Applications." *Sensors* 11 (12): 11736–51. https://doi.org/10.3390/s111211736.

Sharmin, Shabnam, Md Mizanur Rahaman, Chandan Sarkar, Olubunmi Atolani, Mohammad Torequl Islam, and Oluyomi Stephen Adeyemi. 2021. "Nanoparticles as Antimicrobial and Antiviral Agents: A Literature-Based Perspective Study." *Heliyon* 7 (3): e06456. https://doi.org/10.1016/J.HELIYON.2021.E06456.

Singh, Aakriti, Ganesh Yadagiri, Shabi Parvez, Om Prakash Singh, Anurag Verma, Shyam Sundar, and Shyam Lal Mudavath. 2020. "Formulation, Characterization and in Vitro Anti-Leishmanial Evaluation of Amphotericin B Loaded Solid Lipid Nanoparticles Coated with Vitamin B(12)-Stearic Acid Conjugate." *Materials Science & Engineering. C, Materials for Biological Applications* 117 (December): 111279. https://doi.org/10.1016/j.msec.2020.111279.

Sireesha, Merum, Veluru Jagadeesh Babu, A. Sandeep Kranthi Kiran, and Seeram Ramakrishna. 2018. "A Review on Carbon Nanotubes in Biosensor Devices and Their Applications in Medicine." *Nanocomposites* 4 (2): 36–57. https://doi.org/10.1080/20550324.2018.1478765.

Slater, Lucinda, Shoaib Ashraf, Osama Zahid, Qasim Ali, Muhammad Oneeb, Muhammad Haroon Akbar, Muhammad Ilyas Riaz, Kiran Afshan, Neil Sargison, and Umer Chaudhry. 2022. "Current Methods for the Detection of Plasmodium Parasite Species Infecting Humans." *Current Research in Parasitology and Vector-Borne Diseases* 2 (March): 100086. https://doi.org/10.1016/j.crpvbd.2022.100086.

Sue, Mei Jean, Swee Keong Yeap, Abdul Rahman Omar, and Sheau Wei Tan. 2014. "Application of PCR-ELISA in Molecular Diagnosis." *BioMed Research International* 2014. https://doi.org/10.1155/2014/653014.

Sun, Conroy, Jerry S.H. Lee, and Miqin Zhang. 2008. "Magnetic Nanoparticles in MR Imaging and Drug Delivery." *Advanced Drug Delivery Reviews* 60 (11): 1252. https://doi.org/10.1016/J.ADDR.2008.03.018.

Sun, Yuzhu, Dongmei Chen, Yuanhu Pan, Wei Qu, Haihong Hao, Xu Wang, Zhenli Liu, and Shuyu Xie. 2019. "Nanoparticles for Antiparasitic Drug Delivery." *Drug Delivery* 26 (1): 1206. https://doi.org/10.1080/10717544.2019.1692968.

Tambe, Srushti, Sagnik Nag, Shivani R. Pandya, Rohit Kumar, Kalpana Balakrishnan, Ranvijay Kumar, Sandeep Kumar, Purnima Amin, and Piyush Kumar Gupta. 2024. "Revolutionizing Leishmaniasis Treatment with Cutting Edge Drug Delivery Systems and Nanovaccines: An Updated Review." *ACS Infectious Diseases* 10 (6): 1871–89. https://doi.org/10.1021/acsinfecdis.4c00010.

Tang, Congli, Ziyu He, Hongmei Liu, Yuyue Xu, Hao Huang, Gaojian Yang, Ziqi Xiao, et al. 2020. "Application of Magnetic Nanoparticles in Nucleic Acid Detection." *Journal of Nanobiotechnology* 18 (1): 62. https://doi.org/10.1186/S12951-020-00613-6.

Thwala, Lungile Nomcebo, Sphumelele Colin Ndlovu, Kelvin Tafadzwa Mpofu, Masixole Yvonne Lugongolo, and Patience Mthunzi-Kufa. 2023. "Nanotechnology-Based Diagnostics for Diseases Prevalent in Developing Countries: Current Advances in Point-of-Care Tests." *Nanomaterials* 13 (7): 1–19. https://doi.org/10.3390/nano13071247.

Tiwari, Rahul, Rohit P. Gupta, Vishal K. Singh, Awnish Kumar, None Rajneesh, Prasoon Madhukar, Shyam Sundar, Vibhav Gautam, and Rajiv Kumar. 2023. "Nanotechnology-Based Strategies in Parasitic Disease Management: From Prevention to Diagnosis and Treatment." *ACS Omega* 8 (45): 42014–27. https://doi.org/10.1021/acsomega.3c04587.

Tosyali, Ozlem Ayse, Adil Allahverdiyev, Melahat Bagirova, Emrah Sefik Abamor, Mehmet Aydogdu, Sahar Dinparvar, Tayfun Acar, Zeynep Mustafaeva, and Serap Derman. 2021. "Nano-Co-Delivery of Lipophosphoglycan with Soluble and Autoclaved Leishmania Antigens into PLGA Nanoparticles: Evaluation of in Vitro and in Vivo Immunostimulatory Effects against Visceral Leishmaniasis." *Materials Science & Engineering. C, Materials for Biological Applications* 120 (January). https://doi.org/10.1016/J.MSEC.2020.111684.

Verdan, Mariana, Igor Taveira, Flávia Lima, Fernanda Abreu, and Dirlei Nico. 2023. "Drugs and Nanoformulations for the Management of Leishmania Infection: A Patent and Literature Review (2015–2022)." *Expert Opinion on Therapeutic Patents* 33 (3): 137–50. https://doi.org/10.1080/13543776.2023.2201431.

Viegas, Cláudia, Ana B. Patrício, João M. Prata, Akhtar Nadhman, Pavan Kumar Chintamaneni, and Pedro Fonte. 2023. "Solid Lipid Nanoparticles vs. Nanostructured Lipid Carriers: A Comparative Review." *Pharmaceutics* 15 (6). https://doi.org/10.3390/PHARMACEUTICS15061593.

Volpedo, Greta, Lourena Costa, Nathan Ryan, Gregory Halsey, Abhay Satoskar, and Steve Oghumu. 2019. "Nanoparticulate Drug Delivery Systems for the Treatment of Neglected Tropical Protozoan Diseases." *Journal of Venomous Animals and Toxins Including Tropical Diseases* 25: 1–14. https://doi.org/10.1590/1678-9199-jvatitd-1441-18.

Wang, Ning, Minnan Chen, and Ting Wang. 2019. "Liposomes Used as a Vaccine Adjuvant-Delivery System: From Basics to Clinical Immunization." *Journal of Controlled Release : Official Journal of the Controlled Release Society* 303 (June): 130–50. https://doi.org/10.1016/J.JCONREL.2019.04.025.

Warner, Nikole L, and Kathryn M Frietze. 2021. "Development of Bacteriophage Virus-Like Particle Vaccines Displaying Conserved Epitopes of Dengue Virus Non-Structural Protein 1." *Vaccines* 9 (7). https://doi.org/10.3390/vaccines9070726.

Weng, Hong Bo, Hai Xia Chen, and Ming Wei Wang. 2018. "Innovation in Neglected Tropical Disease Drug Discovery and Development." *Infectious Diseases of Poverty* 7 (1): 1–9. https://doi.org/10.1186/s40249-018-0444-1.

WHO. 2020. *Ending the Neglect to Attain the Sustainable Development Goals: A Road Map for Neglected Tropical Diseases 2021–2030*. WHO, Geneva, Switzerland.

Ye, Haihang, Yaning Liu, Li Zhan, Yilin Liu, and Zhenpeng Qin. 2020. "Signal Amplification and Quantification on Lateral Flow Assays by Laser Excitation of Plasmonic Nanomaterials." *Theranostics* 10 (10): 4359–73. https://doi.org/10.7150/thno.44298.

Yetisgin, Abuzer Alp, Sibel Cetinel, Merve Zuvin, Ali Kosar, and Ozlem Kutlu. 2020. "Therapeutic Nanoparticles and Their Targeted Delivery Applications." *Molecules* 25 (9). https://doi.org/10.3390/MOLECULES25092193.

Zhang, Bingbo, Xiaofei Liang, Lijuan Hao, Jing Cheng, Xiaoqun Gong, Xuhui Liu, Guiping Ma, and Jin Chang. 2009. "Quantum Dots/Particle-Based Immunofluorescence Assay: Synthesis, Characterization and Application." *Journal of Photochemistry and Photobiology B: Biology* 94 (1): 45–50. https://doi.org/10.1016/j.jphotobiol.2008.09.008.

10 Nanotechnology-Based Approach for Diabetes Management

Naba Jyoti Deka[1], Prasanta Chabukdhara[2], Ankita Gogoi[3], and Dhruba Jyoti Kalita[1]
[1]Department of Veterinary Biochemistry, College of Veterinary Science, AAU, Guwahati, India
[2]Department of Veterinary Physiology and Biochemistry, Lakhimpur College of Veterinary Science, AAU, North Lakhimpur, India
[3]Department of Animal Genetics & Breeding, College of Veterinary Science, AAU, Khanapara, Guwahati, India

10.1 INTRODUCTION

The International Diabetes Federation (IDF) has reported that the South-East Asia (SEA) region that consists of India, Sri Lanka, Bangladesh, Bhutan, Mauritius, and the Maldives had a diabetic adult population exceeding 72 million in 2013, with projections indicating an increase beyond 123 million by 2035. The current trend suggests that over 60% of the global diabetic population will be concentrated in Asia (Ramachandran et al. 2014).

In recent decades, India has undergone a rapidly growing diabetes epidemic. Currently, the country has the second-highest diabetic population globally after China. India has 72.9 million individuals with diabetes in 2017, a figure expected to reach 134.3 million by 2045. The prevalence of diabetes in urban India, particularly in major metropolitan areas, has surged from 2% in the 1970s to over 20% today, with rural areas also witnessing a significant rise (ICMR 2018).

Diabetes is a chronic metabolic disorder that occurs when the β-cells of the pancreas fails to produce sufficient insulin or when the body is unable to utilize it efficiently (insulin resistance). It is characterized by persistent hyperglycemia accompanied by disturbances in the metabolism of carbohydrate, fat, and protein due to impairments in insulin secretion, function, or both and over time it causes serious damage to various bodily systems, particularly affecting the nerves and blood vessels (World Health Organization 2024).

According to the American Diabetes Association (ADA) and the World Health Organization, diabetes is categorized into four main types such as type 1 diabetes (T1D), type 2 diabetes (T2D), gestational diabetes, and other types of diabetes (monogenic diabetes, pancreatic diabetes, drug-induced diabetes, etc.) (ICMR 2018). T1D occurs due to autoimmune destruction of the β-cells within the pancreatic islets of Langerhans, resulting in complete deficiency of insulin. Although the prevalence of T1D is increasing, the total number of affected individuals in India remains relatively low. In contrast, T2D accounts for 90%–95% of all diabetes cases and is marked by insulin resistance and impaired insulin secretion, either of which may predominate (ICMR 2018). T2D predominantly impacts middle-aged and elderly individuals, whereas T1D is more frequently observed in children and adolescents (Gromada et al. 2018, Bastaki 2005). In both the situations, the disruption of homeostatic control mechanisms chronically may result in hyperglycemia or hypoglycemia (Ross et al. 2004).

DOI: 10.1201/9781003473015-10

In most cases, the management of diabetes mellitus and the prevention of its complications involve dietary regulation, physical activity, administration of antidiabetic medications, or a combination of these approaches. According to ADA, a dietary plan may consist of 25–30 g of fiber daily, with protein contributing 15%–20% of the total daily energy intake. Carbohydrates should primarily come from sources such as fruits, vegetables, whole grains, legumes, and low-fat dairy products. Healthy fats can be incorporated through at least two servings of fish per week. Engaging in 90–150 minutes of physical activity per week is also advised to help enhance blood glucose regulation. The primary treatment for T1D typically involves the administration of exogenous insulin. A newer drug, Pramlintide, has been approved by the U.S. Food and Drug Administration (FDA) for T1D (Mehanna 2013). However, insulin-based therapy has certain limitations such as the need of multiple injections and the risk of hypoglycemia if dosages are not accurately adjusted. Moreover, the currently available oral drugs for the management of T2D include sulfonylureas, meglitinides, metformin (a biguanide), thiazolidinediones (TZDs), alpha-glucosidase inhibitors, dipeptidyl peptidase-IV (DPP-4) inhibitors, bile acid sequestrants, dopamine agonists, sodium-glucose transport protein 2 (SGLT2) inhibitors, and oral glucagon-like peptide 1 (GLP-1) receptor agonists. Conversely, GLP-1 receptor agonists, dual GLP-1 receptor and glucose-dependent insulinotropic polypeptide (GIP) receptor agonists, and pramlintide are administered via injection (Feingold 2024). The standard care for both types of diabetes involves frequent finger prick to draw blood for estimation of blood glucose level, daily insulin administration through subcutaneous route or insulin pumps. Nevertheless, various factors such as discomfort and the repetitive tiresome daily procedure leads to infrequent blood glucose monitoring and noncompliance with prescribed treatment regimen (American Diabetes Association 2019). This drives to fluctuating insulin dosages that could result in hyperglycemia or hypoglycemia, and in severe cases, may cause seizures, unconsciousness, or even fatality (Schulman et al. 2014). Therefore, there is a great need of improved strategies in diabetes management. Recent developments in nanomedicine have substantially enhanced treatment strategies for various disease conditions including autoimmune diseases, inflammatory and fibrotic disorders and are now being actively investigated for their potential in diabetes management (Zaid and Ariel 2024, Lemmerman et al. 2020). The current definitions of nanomedicine are defined by the National Institutes of Health of the United States and the European Science Foundation which describe it as the science that employs nanomaterials to the development of diagnostic tools, therapies, and preventive strategies for specific medical applications (Cancino-Bernardi et al. 2017). The primary objective of using nanomedicine is to deliver drug-encapsulated nanomaterials or nanocarriers to target tissue more precisely with controlled release through different mechanisms under diverse environmental conditions (Jahangirian et al. 2017). A nanomaterial refers to any substance engineered to have dimensions ranging from 1 to 100 nm in at least one direction (Deka 2017). The distinctive physicochemical characteristics of nanoparticles (NPs) offer notable advantages vis-à-vis enhanced biocompatibility, precise targeting, efficient cellular absorption, and improved bioavailability (Sarkhel et al. 2024). In the context of diabetes, NPs provide effective insulin release that responds to the changes of blood glucose levels, thereby minimizing risk of hypoglycemia. Furthermore, NPs reportedly protect insulin from degradation in the gastrointestinal tract, thereby enabling oral delivery and avoiding the need of daily injections (Patra et al. 2018). The nano-based drug delivery system can also be employed for gene and cell therapy in the management of diabetes. The oligonucleotides can be encapsulated inside the NPs for expression of insulin genes or repression of defective genes for transduction in pancreatic or stem cells (Khoshnevisan and Sajjadi-Jazi 2023). This chapter addresses the recent advances in the field of NP-based drug delivery system for efficient management of diabetes.

10.2 NANOPARTICLES

NPs are biocompatible and biodegradable particles in the range of 100 to 300 nm in diameter in which a therapeutic or biological agents such as peptides and oligonucleotides are encapsulated or chemically coupled. Depending on the type of NPs, both oral and injectable routes can be utilized for administration. NPs can enhance the stability and solubility of encapsulated cargos, facilitate membrane transport, prolong the circulation times to boost safety and efficacy, and release their drug at the target cell in response to external stimuli (Mitchell et al. 2021, Andreadi et al. 2024).

10.3 CLASSIFICATION OF NPS

NPs can be classified as lipid-based, polymeric, and inorganic NPs (Figure 10.1). Each category includes various subclasses bearing numerous individual advantages and disadvantages in regard to its cargo, delivery, and therapeutic response (Mitchell et al. 2021). Lipid-based NPs are spherical structures consisting of one or more lipid bilayers that enclose at least one internal aqueous compartment. It provides several benefits as a drug delivery system such as simple formulation parameters, self-assembly, biocompatibility, high bioavailability, and large payload capacity. Liposomes, lipid nanoparticles (LNPs) are two subsets of lipid-based NPs. Polymeric NPs are solid polymer-based structure that distributes drugs uniformly. On the other hand, inorganic NPs consist of nanostructured material that are engineered by using inorganic materials such as gold, silver, and zinc for various drug delivery applications. Iron oxide NPs constitute the majority of inorganic nanomedicines approved by the FDA (Mitchell et al. 2021, Bobo et al. 2016).

The major class of NPs utilized in diabetes therapy include polymeric NPs, liposomes, LNPs, and inorganic NPs (Bobo et al. 2016).

10.3.1 Polymeric NPs

The widely used polymeric NPs are nanocapsules, which are hollow structures enclosed by a polymer shell and nanospheres, which are solid matrix systems. They are derived either from natural sources like polysaccharides, proteins or synthetic such as polylactic acid (PLA), poly lactic-co-glycolic acid (PLGA), and polyethyleneimine (PEI) and are engineered using different methodologies such as emulsification (solvent displacement or diffusion), nanoprecipitation, ionic gelation, and microfluidics (Brown et al. 2019, Zhang et al. 2019, Le et al. 2018, He et al. 2020, Zhang et al. 2020). Therapeutics are incorporated within the NPs core, chemically linked to the polymer matrices or bound to the NPs surface. This makes NPs an ideal delivery vehicle for both hydrophobic and hydrophilic compounds as well as biological macromolecule like proteins. Polymeric nanocapsules can encapsulate proteins which need to be cross-linked to avoid solubilization in the aqueous environment at the site of administration. Albumin nanocapsules carry hydrophobic liquids such as vegetable oils, making them ideal for encapsulating lipophilic drugs. When the outer polymer shell is made of PLA or PLGA, the inner core of the nanocapsules is aqueous. Thus, they are suitable for incorporating hydrophilic drug like insulin (Andreadi et al. 2024). Besides the two primary groups under polymeric NPs, NPs are further categorized into structural forms like polymersomes, micelles, and dendrimers. Polymersomes, also known as polymeric vesicles, are synthetic NPs with membranes formed by the self-assembly process of amphiphilic block copolymers capable of carrying hydrophilic moiety in the aqueous core and hydrophobic part in the membrane (Fonseca et al. 2024).

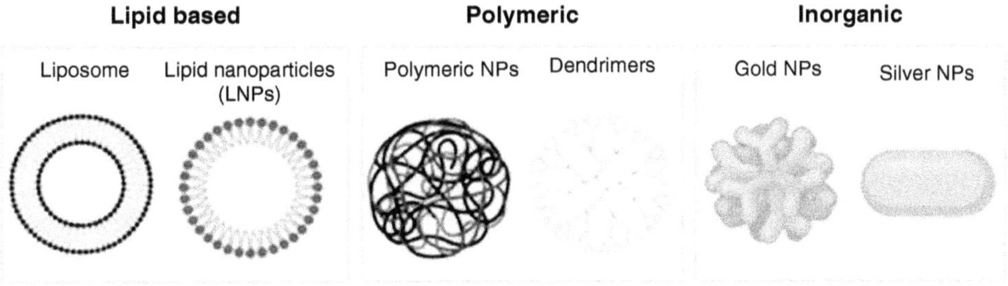

FIGURE 10.1 Classification of nanoparticles. (The image was created using BioRender.com.)

10.3.2 Liposomes

They are typically unilamellar and multilamellar vesicular structures composed of phospholipid bilayers that encapsulate an aqueous environment (Andreadi et al. 2024). They exhibit diversified capabilities such as ability to deliver hydrophilic, hydrophobic, and lipophilic drugs within the same formulations. The stability of the NPs is largely influenced by its size, surface charge, lipid bilayer composition, and surface modification. Surface modification with ligands or polymer may be required as the reticuloendothelial system can take up the NPs rapidly (Sarfraz et al. 2018, Sedighi et al. 2019).

10.3.3 Lipid Nanoparticles

These class of nanocarriers are liposome-like structures mostly used for the delivery of protein and nucleic acids. They differ from the conventional liposomes as they possess single micellar structure within the NP core. They consist of four major lipid components: ionizable lipids that bind and encapsulate negatively charged genetic material, phospholipids for NP structural support, cholesterol for stability and integrity, and PEGylated lipids to improve stability and blood circulation time (Andreadi et al. 2024, Jung et al. 2022). The amount of loaded PEGylated lipids is also crucial as it affects the size and zeta potential of the NPs (Ryals et al. 2020).

10.3.4 Inorganic NPs

10.3.4.1 Gold NPs (AuNPs)

Due to the physiochemical properties like small size with larger surface area, shape, surface charge, biologically non-reactive, and simple synthetic protocol, AuNPs have received great interest for use as therapeutic agent in the treatment of diabetes and its complications (Alomari et al. 2021, Almohmadi et al. 2025). They contain unbound electrons at their outermost shell which undergo continuous oscillation based on their size and shape, imparting them with photothermal capabilities (Wang et al. 2020). It was documented that AuNPs with a size of 50 nm synthesized using *Bacillus licheniformis* exhibited anti-hyperglycemic properties by promoting regeneration of β-cells of pancreas, lowering the blood glucose level on streptozotocin-induced diabetic mice. The NPs also showed good antioxidant effects that inhibit the formation of reactive oxygen species (ROS) and scavenge free radicals (Barathmanikanth et al. 2010).

10.3.4.2 Zinc Oxide NPs (ZnO NPs)

Another potent nano-drug delivery system is ZnO NPs. Due to its small size and high surface area, these are often used in biomedical applications as well as daily appliances like toothpaste, sunscreens, packaging material, and food additives (Almohmadi et al. 2025). ZnO NPs demonstrated antihyperglycemic effects in diabetic rats following daily oral administration for a varying length of time. It was also successful in treating diabetes-induced injury in pancreas as well as restoring the blood glucose and serum insulin homeostasis following the therapy (Mocchegiani et al. 2008).

10.3.4.3 Silver NPs (AgNPs)

Among the various metal NPs that are developed by green synthetic protocol, AgNPs are considered as the most efficient due to its safety, non-toxicity, antimicrobial, antidiabetic, and antioxidant activity. Plant-mediated synthesis of NPs is an easy green chemistry approach that connects technology with plants eliminating the need of microbial culture (Almohmadi et al. 2025, Deka et al. 2021). It is evident that AgNPs can aid in better regulation of blood glucose levels and protect the pancreatic β-cells from oxidative stress, which is crucial in the management of diabetes (Rahuman et al. 2022, Wahab et al. 2022). AgNPs synthesized using *Azadirachta indica* seed extract showed remarkable dose-dependent antidiabetic activity, resulting in substantial reduction in blood glucose levels along with the regeneration of pancreatic and hepatic cells (Rehman et al. 2023).

10.4 DELIVERY AND DISTRIBUTION

During delivery and distribution, NPs face some biological barriers which depend on the route of administration, disease condition, and progression. During circulation, various factors such as excretion, blood flow, and phagocytic cells can lower the stability of NPs and thus its delivery in the targeted site. For example, NPs smaller than 10 nm are rapidly excreted by the renal system while those larger than 200 nm may trigger activation of the complement system in the body. Incorporating polyethylene glycol (PEG) as stealth coating in the NPs can alter its size and stability, and protects from enzymes and antibodies that may cause disruption and rapid excretion. However, immune cells like macrophage can recognize PEG that may result in the synthesis of anti-PEG antibodies and subsequently induction of rapid renal excretion (McSweeney et al. 2018, Yang et al. 2016).

10.5 INSULIN RELEASE

NPs are fabricated in such a way that it responds to the variation of blood glucose levels as that of body's natural response. The glucose-responsive nano-drug delivery system has shown to achieve efficient blood glucose regulation compared to traditional subcutaneous route of injecting insulin frequently in a day. Presently, the primary glucose-sensitive drugs used in nano delivery system are phenylboronic acid (PBA) and its derivatives, concanavalin A (Con A) and glucose oxidase (GOD). In most of the nanocarrier delivery system, glucose-dependent insulin release primarily depends on reversible binding capacity of PBA with glucose molecules. NPs conjugated with PBA and polysaccharide possess molecular interactions between glucose and PBA for a stable polymeric structure. Whenever there is elevated glucose level in the bodily fluids, the exogenous glucose undergoes competitive binding to PBA, enters the polymeric matrix, disrupts the structural integrity, and induces the release of insulin (Andreadi et al. 2024). Higher the glucose concentration, quicker the insulin release rate, and larger the release amount. The controlled release of drugs (insulin) is due to the competitive response of PBA. PBA-linked polymers such as 3-aminoPBA, alginate, chitosan 3-fluoro-4-carboxyl PBA have been reported to exhibit promising result as glucose-responsive systems for oral insulin delivery (Wang et al. 2024). The most important limitation with PBA is that it has low specificity for glucose and can bind to other biomolecules such as fructose, nucleic acids, and catechol (Matsumoto et al. 2004, Ma et al. 2021). Additionally, Con A, a glucose-binding lectin protein, shows strong affinity toward non-reducing sugar like a-D-mannose, a-D-glucose, and polysaccharide with unmodified hydroxyl groups at C-3, C-4, and C-6 position. It can attach to polysaccharide-loaded NPs, forming multiple interactions that stabilize their core structure. As that of PBA, elevated glucose level in the bodily fluids induce competitive binding of exogenous glucose to Con A leading to disruption and release of insulin (Andreadi et al. 2024, Wu and Zhou 2013). Another insulin delivery method for controlled and sustained release involves using the enzyme GOD in NPs containing pH-sensitive polymers which converts glucose into gluconic acid, creating an acidic environment in a hyperglycemic condition. The glucose decreases the pH, causing protonation of the polymers that results in repulsive environment causing disruption in the structural integrity and release of insulin (Andreadi et al. 2024). Most studied pH-sensitive polymers are chitosan, dextran, poly 2-(dimethylamino) ethyl methacrylate, and poly(ethylenimine). However, more exploration on clinical trials is needed for reliable use of these systems.

10.6 NPS FOR ORAL DELIVERY OF INSULIN

Successful oral delivery of insulin enhances the quality of life of the diabetic patient who takes multiple injections in a day to maintain the blood glucose level. Additionally, it is the most convenient, simple, and physiological way as it simulates the endogenous insulin secretion. Physiologically, insulin undergoes first-pass regulation through hepatic portal system in the liver so that an appropriate level of insulin is present in the systemic circulation and thus maintaining euglycemia in the body (Figure 10.2).

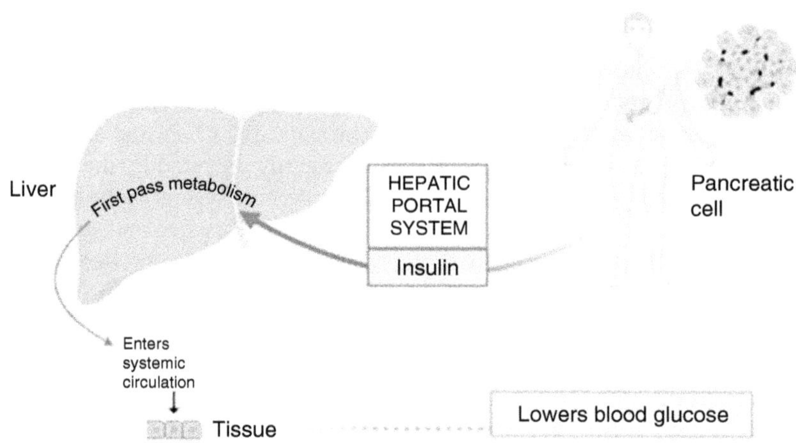

FIGURE 10.2 Insulin entry into hepatic portal system. (The image was created using BioRender.com.)

However, this route of administration encounters a few difficulties such as degradation by proteolytic gastrointestinal enzymes, lower absorption, wide pH range, lower bioavailability, and short half-life (Damgé et al. 2007). Nanocarrier-based drug delivery system offers an optimal solution to overcome these difficulties. The delivery system can modify the permeability of the intestinal mucosa to peptides, allowing paracellular uptake of insulin by opening the tight junctions between epithelial cells, improve its intestinal absorption, increase bioavailability, protect from degradation, and subsequently its controlled release. In one study, lectin-modified lipid nanocarrier delivery system showed relative bioavailability of insulin after oral administration of between 4.99% and 7.11% in comparison to subcutaneous insulin injection (Bakhru et al. 2013). In another study, insulin-loaded NPs fabricated to target neonatal Fc receptor, a potential mediator in transport of IgG across the epithelium, have shown effective transportation across the epithelial barriers in both in vitro and in vivo models in mice. The targeted NPs containing insulin, after oral administration at a dose of 1.1 U/kg orally, induce longer hypoglycemic effect in wild-type mice (Pridgen et al. 2013). Chitosan-based NP is another promising oral delivery system of insulin in diabetic mice, showing higher bioavailability, better efficacy, and comparable tissue distribution to subcutaneous administration (Hunt et al. 2024). The polysaccharide-based natural polymers used in the formulation of NPs are chitosan, hyaluronic acid, sodium alginate, starch while the synthetic category includes PLA, PLGA, and PEG. Polysaccharide-based NPs have shown better absorption, adhesion, and higher bioavailability after oral administration. However, despite encouraging in vitro results in most of the studies, suboptimal in vivo results have highlighted the need for more exploration in the formulation of oral insulin nano delivery system to meet the therapeutic need of diabetic patients (Barfar et al. 2024).

10.7 NANOMEDICINE IN DIABETIC GENE THERAPY

Gene therapy is an innovative approach that aims not only to add a missing gene but also to treat, cure, or prevent the effects of a defective gene by incorporating DNA, RNA, or small interfering RNA (siRNA) to enhance or mitigate the function of defective genes. There are about 75 genetic loci identified involved in the pathogenesis of T1D. This has paved the way for further exploitation in therapeutic applications. NPs using PEI have been found to enhance the production of insulin by pancreatic β-cells by encapsulating the gene responsible for the GLP-1 receptor (Oh et al. 2003). However, LNPs have been shown to normalize blood glucose homeostasis by increasing plasma glucagon levels through the use of siRNA in a mouse model study of diabetes (Neumann et al. 2017). In obese diabetic patients, inflammation of adipose tissue is common and lipid NPs have been found to silence the genes responsible for inflammation (Andreadi et al. 2024). The genetic loci that downregulate the expression of the nucleotide binding oligomerization domain-like receptor protein 3 (NLRP3) inflammasome have been shown to reduce inflammation by interfering with NLRP3 inflammasome activation. In this context, chitosan-based NPs have been used for the targeted delivery of a plasmid encoding interleukin-4 (IL-4) and interleukin-10 (IL-10) to reduce the pancreatic inflammation. Although numerous preclinical studies have shown promising results, this strategy is still far from being part of standard therapeutic protocol (Vallianou et al. 2025).

10.8 NANOMEDICINE IN CELLULAR THERAPY

Cellular therapy in diabetes involves transplantation of functioning pancreatic cells into the pancreas of the diabetic individual. Conventionally, this approach has been highly associated with many adverse effects such as immunosuppression, sophisticated procedure to isolate pancreatic cells from suitable donor. In the year 2023, the FDA approved Lantidra, the first allogeneic (donor) pancreatic islet cellular therapy for treatment of T1D patients. However, there has been report of varied adverse effects in each patient after administration. It includes nausea, fatigue, anemia, diarrhea and abdominal pain. Moreover, there is need of administration of immunosuppressive drugs to maintain the islet cell viability (Andreadi et al. 2024, Vallianou et al. 2025). Under these circumstances, nanomedicine offers an alternative for simplifying the isolation of stem cells. The use of pluripotent or multipotent stem cells to derive surrogate β-cells for transplantation is relatively less complex (Andreadi et al. 2024). Technology advancement such as clustered regularly interspaced short palindromic repeats/CRISPR-associated protein 9 (CRISPR/Cas9) or the transfection of stem cells with plasmids has facilitated enhanced gene editing. The modified genes are then encapsulated within lecithin-based or cationic lipid-assisted PEG/PLGA NPs. This strategy helps to mitigate foreign body response against these cells and thus protects the transplanted cells from immune response facilitating insulin homeostasis.

10.9 NANOMEDICINE FOR WOUND HEALING

Diabetic wound is one of the most troublesome complications in diabetic patients. It may lead to development of chronic intractable ulcer due to infections. Inadequate blood supply and higher oxygen consumption induce hypoxia in the diabetic wound. The oxygen supply is hindered due to vascular dysfunction and neuropathy. Moreover, diabetic wound does not heal through normal process but progresses to chronic inflammation with accumulation of macrophages. Hypoxia-inducible factor 1 alpha (HIF-1α) plays a pivotal role in angiogenesis and tissue repair due to its beneficial effects on cellular responses to hypoxic condition. Localized infiltration of HIF-1α at the wound has been shown as a promising therapeutic strategy to promote wound healing. However, its function is impaired in T1D patients (Vallianou et al. 2025). Angiogenic mediator and growth factors such as vascular endothelial growth factor (VEGF) and epidermal growth factor (EGF) influence wound closure and tissue repair activity. In the case of diabetic wound, the EGF and its receptor are lacking. Inorganic NPs like AgNPs, AuNPs are currently used in wound healing. AgNP is highly effective due to its anti-inflammatory properties and can act against both natural and nosocomial strains of multidrug-resistant (MDR) microorganisms, aiding the healing process (Bai et al. 2020). NPs based on PLGA containing EGF and carboxymethyl chitosan have also been demonstrated to improve efficacy in tissue repair. Moreover, curcumin-loaded chitosan-based NPs have shown better efficacy in granulation tissue formation and VEGF production in diabetic wound (Meng et al. 2013). However, there is urgent need of exploration to use nanomaterials locally at the diabetic wound.

10.10 CONCLUSIONS

The use of nanomedicine in the management of diabetes is of paramount importance. Currently, nanomaterials are being explored for diagnostic, therapeutic, and preventive application. The primary objective is to deliver an encapsulated antidiabetic drug through a nano delivery system more precisely at the targeted site with controlled release under various bodily situations. NPs have also shown great prospects in glucose sensing and monitoring. However, there is urgent and indispensable requirement to focus on safety protocols in the fabrication of NP-based formulations. By resolving the existing issues and exploiting future technologies, glucose-sensitive insulin release nano-formulation offers substantial strategy to significantly advance the current paradigm of diabetes treatment. Therefore, nanotechnology-based therapeutic approach in diabetes management and treatment demands comprehensive interdisciplinary collaborative approach for a successful clinical application.

REFERENCES

Almohmadi, N. H. S., Tiwari, A., Chaudhary, T., Sindhu, R. K., Babu, M. A., Yassen, A. S., Alexiou, A., Papadakis, M. and Batiha, G. E. S. 2025. Nanocarrier-based drug delivery systems: A way to effective diabetes management. *BioNanoScience* 15 (2):1–15.

Alomari, G., Hamdan, S. and Al-Trad, B. 2021. Gold nanoparticles as a promising treatment for diabetes and its complications: Current and future potentials. *Brazilian Journal of Pharmaceutical Sciences* 57: e19040.

American Diabetes Association. 2019. Classification and diagnosis of diabetes: Standards of medical care in diabetes 2019. *Diabetes Care* 42 (Suppl. S1): S13–S28.

Andreadi, A., Lodeserto, P., Todaro, F., Meloni, M., Romano, M., Minasi, A., Bellia, A., Lauro, D. 2024. Nanomedicine in the treatment of diabetes. *International Journal of Molecular Science* 25: 7028. https://doi.org/10.3390/ijms25137028

Bai, Q., Han, K., Dong, K., Zheng, C., Zhang, Y., Long, Q. and Lu, T. 2020. Potential applications of nanomaterials and technology for diabetic wound healing. *International Journal of Nanomedicine* 9717–9743.

Bakhru, S. H., Furtado, S., Morello, A. P. and Mathiowitz, E. 2013. Oral delivery of proteins by biodegradable nanoparticles, *Advanced Drug Delivery Reviews* 65(6): 811–821 https://doi.org/10.1016/j.addr.2013.04.006

Barathmanikanth, S., Kalishwaralal, K., Sriram, M., Pandian, S. R., Youn, H. S., Eom, S. and Gurunathan, S. 2010. Anti-oxidant effect of gold nanoparticles restrains hyperglycemic conditions in diabetic mice. *Journal of Nanotechnology* 8(1):16.

Barfar, A., Alizadeh, H., Masoomzadeh, S. and Javadzadeh, Y. 2024. Oral insulin delivery: A review on recent advancements and novel strategies. *Current Drug Delivery*. 21(6): 887–900.

Bastaki, S. 2005. Diabetes mellitus and its treatment. *Journal of Diabetes & Metabolism* 13: 111–134. https://doi.org/10.1159/000497580

Bobo, D., Robinson, K. J., Islam, J., Thurecht, K. J. and Corrie, S. R. 2016. Nanoparticle- based medicines: A review of FDA- approved materials and clinical trials to date. *Pharmaceutical Research* 33: 2373–2387.

Brown, S. B., Wang, L., Jungels, R. R. and Sharma, B. 2019. Effects of cartilage- targeting moieties on nanoparticle biodistribution in healthy and osteoarthritic joints. *Acta Biomaterialia* 101: 469–483.

Cancino-Bernardi, J., Marangoni, V. S. and Zucolotto, V. 2017. Nanomedicine. In *Nanoscience and Its Applications*, eds. A. L. Da Róz., M. Ferreira., F. de Lima Leite and O. N. Oliveira, 71–92. William Andrew Publishing.

Damgé, C., Maincent, P. and Ubrich, N. 2007. Oral delivery of insulin associated to polymeric nanoparticles in diabetic rats. *Journal of Controlled Release* 117(2): 163–170.

Deka, N. J. 2017. Green synthesis and characterization of silver nanoparticles and assessment of its antioxidant & antimicrobial activity. MVSc thesis submitted to Assam Agricultural University, Jorhat.

Deka, N. J., Nath, R., Tamuly, T, Pegu, S. R. and Deka, S. M. 2021. Green synthesis and characterization of silver nanoparticles using leaves extract of Neem (*Azadirachta indica* L.) and assessment of its in vitro antioxidant and antibacterial activity. *Annals of Phytomedicine* 10(1): 171–177.

Feingold, K. R. 2024. Oral and injectable (non-insulin) pharmacological agents for the treatment of type 2 diabetes. Endotext. https://www.ncbi.nlm.nih.gov/books/NBK279141/

Fonseca, M., Jarak, I., Victor, F., Domingues, C., Veiga, F. and Figueiras, A. 2024. Polymersomes as the next attractive generation of drug delivery systems: Definition, synthesis and applications. *Materials* 17(2): 319. https://doi.org/10.3390/ma17020319

Gromada, J., Chabosseau, P. and Rutter, G. A. 2018. The α-cell in diabetes mellitus. *Nature Reviews Endocrinology*, 14(12): 694–704. https://doi.org/10.1038/s41574-018-0097-y

He, C., Yue, H., Xu, L., Liu, Y., Song, Y., Tang, C. and Yin, C. 2020. siRNA release kinetics from polymeric nanoparticles correlate with RNAi efficiency and inflammation therapy via oral delivery. *Acta Biomaterialia*. 103: 213–222.

Hunt, N. J., Lockwood, G. P., Heffernan, S. J., Daymond, J., Ngu, M., Narayanan, R. K. and Cogger, V. C. 2024. Oral nanotherapeutic formulation of insulin with reduced episodes of hypoglycaemia. *Nature Nanotechnology* 19(4): 534–544.

ICMR. 2018. Technical ICMR guidelines for management of type 2 diabetes. https://www.icmr.gov.in/icmrobject/custom_data/pdf/resourceguidelines/ICMR_GuidelinesType2diabetes2018_0.pdf

Jahangirian, H., Lemraski, E. G., Webster, T. J., Rafiee-Moghaddam, R. and Abdollahi, Y. A. 2017. Review of drug delivery systems based on nanotechnology and green chemistry: Green nanomedicine. *International Journal of Nanomedicine*. 12:2957.

Jung, H. N., Lee, S. Y., Lee, S., Youn, H. and Im, H. J. 2022. Lipid nanoparticles for delivery of RNA therapeutics: Current status and the role of in vivo imaging. *Theranostics* 12(17), 7509–7531. https://doi.org/10.7150/thno.77259

Khoshnevisan, K. and Sajjadi-Jazi, S. M. 2023. Diabetic stem cell therapy and nanomedicine: Advancements in treating diabetes. *Journal of Diabetes & Metabolic Disorders* 22: 1805–1807.

Le, Z., Chen, Y., Han, H., Tian, H., Zhao, P., Yang, C., He, Z., Liu, L., Leong, K.W., Mao, H. Q., Liu, Z. and Chen, Y. 2018. Hydrogen- bonded tannic acid- based anticancer nanoparticle for enhancement of oral chemotherapy. *ACS Applied Materials & Interfaces.* 10: 42186–42197.

Lemmerman, L.R., Das, D., Higuita-Castro, N., Mirmira, R.G. and Gallego-Perez, D. 2020. Nanomedicine-based strategies for diabetes: Diagnostics, monitoring, and treatment. *Trends in Endocrinology and Metabolism* 31: 448–458.

Ma, Q., Zhao, X., Shi, A., & Wu, J. 2021. Bioresponsive functional phenylboronic acid-based delivery system as an emerging platform for diabetic therapy. *International Journal of Nanomedicine* 16: 297–314 https://doi.org/10.2147/IJN.S284357.

Matsumoto, A., Yoshida, R. and Kataoka, K. 2004. Glucose-responsive polymer gel bearing phenylborate derivative as a glucose-sensing moiety operating at the physiological pH. *Biomacromolecules* 5: 1038–1045.

McSweeney, M. D., Wessler, T., Price, L. S. L. Ciociola, E. C., Herity, L. B., Piscitelli, J. A., Zamboni, W. C., Forest, M. G., Cao, Y. and Lai, S. K. 2018. A minimal physiologically based pharmacokinetic model that predicts anti- PEG IgG- mediated clearance of PEGylated drugs in human and mouse. *Journal of Controlled Release* 284: 171–178.

Mehanna, A. (2013). Antidiabetic agents: Past, present and future. *Future Medicinal Chemistry* 5(4): 411–430 https://doi.org/10.4155/fmc.13.13

Meng, B., Li, J. and Cao, H. 2013. Antioxidant and antiinflammatory activities of curcumin on diabetes mellitus and its complications. *Current Pharmaceutical Design* 19: 2101–2113.

Mitchell, M. J., Billingsley, M. M., Haley, R. M. Wechsler, M. E., Peppas, N. A. and Langer, R. 2021. Engineering precision nanoparticles for drug delivery. *Nature Reviews Drug Discovery* 20: 101–124. https://doi.org/10.1038/s41573-020-0090-8

Mocchegiani, E., Giacconi, R. and Malavolta, M. 2008. Zinc signalling and subcellular distribution: Emerging targets in type 2 diabetes. *Trends in Molecular Medicine* 14(10): 419–28. https://doi.org/10.1016/j.molmed.2008.08.002

Neumann, U. H., Ho, J. S., Chen, S., Tam, Y. Y. C., Cullis, P. R. and Kieffer, T. J. 2017. Lipid nanoparticle delivery of glucagon receptor siRNA improves glucose homeostasis in mouse models of diabetes. *Molecular Metabolism* 6(10): 1161–1172.

Oh, S., Lee, M., Ko, K. S., Choi, S. and Kim, S. W. 2003 GLP-1 gene delivery for the treatment of type 2 diabetes. *Molecular Therapy* 7: 478–483.

Patra, J. K., Das, G., Fraceto, L. F., Campos, E. V. R., Rodriguez-Torres, M. D. P., Acosta-Torres, L. S., Diaz-Torres, L. A., Grillo, R., Swamy, M. K., Sharma, S. and Habtemariam, S. 2018. Nano based drug delivery systems: Recent developments and future prospects. *Journal of Nanobiotechnology* 16: 71. https://doi.org/10.1186/s12951-018-0392-8

Pridgen, E. M., Alexis, F., Kuo, T. T., Levy-Nissenbaum, E., Karnik, R., Blumberg, R. S., Farokhzad, O. C. 2013. Transepithelial transport of Fc-targeted nanoparticles by the neonatal Fc receptor for oral delivery. *Science Translational Medicine* 5(213): 213ra167. https://doi.org/10.1126/scitranslmed.3007049

Rahuman, H. B. H., Dhandapani, R., Narayanan, S., Palanivel, V., Paramasivam, R., Subbarayalu, R., Thangavelu, S. and Muthupandian, S. 2022. Medicinal plants mediated the green synthesis of silver nanoparticles and their biomedical applications. *Institution of Engineering and Technology Nanobiotechnology* 16:115–144.

Ramachandran, A., Snehalatha, C. and Ma, R. C. W. 2014. Diabetes in south-east Asia: An update. *Diabetes Research and Clinical Practice* 103(2): 231–237. https://doi.org/10.1016/j.diabres.2013.11.011

Rehman, G., Umar, M., Shah, N., Hamayun, M., Ali, A., Khan, W., Khan, A., Ahmad, S., Alrefaei, A. F., Almutairi, M. H. and Moon, Y. S. 2023. Green synthesis and characterization of silver nanoparticles using *Azadirachta indica* seeds extract: In vitro and in vivo evaluation of anti-diabetic activity. *Pharmaceuticals* 16: 1677.

Ross, S. A., Gulve, E. A. and Wang, M. 2004. Chemistry and biochemistry of type 2 diabetes. *Chemical Reviews* 104: 1255–1282.

Ryals, R. C., Patel, S., Acosta, C., McKinney, M., Pennesi, M. E. and Sahay, G. 2020. The effects of PEGylation on LNP based mRNA delivery to the eye. *PLoS One* 15: e0241006. https://doi.org/10.1371/journal.pone.0241006

Sarfraz, M., Afzal, A., Yang, T., Gai, Y., Raza, S. M., Khan, M. W., Cheng, Y., Ma, X. and Xiang, G. 2018. Development of dual drug loaded nanosized liposomal formulation by a reengineered ethanolic injection method and its pre-clinical pharmacokinetic studies. *Pharmaceutics* 10(3): 151. https://doi.org/10.3390/pharmaceutics10030151

Sarkhel, S., Shuvo, S.M., Ansari, M.A., Mondal, S., Kapat, P., Ghosh, A., Sarkar, T., Biswas, R., Atanase, L. I. and Carauleanu, A. 2024. Nanotechnology-based approaches for the management of diabetes mellitus: An innovative solution to long-lasting challenges in antidiabetic drug delivery. *Pharmaceutics* 16: 1572. https://doi.org/10.3390/pharmaceutics16121572

Schulman, R. C., Moshier, E. L., Rho, L., Casey, M. F., Godbold, J. H. and Mechanick, J. I. 2014. Association of glycemic control parameters with clinical outcomes in chronic critical illness. *Endocrine Practice* 20: 884–893.

Sedighi, M., Sieber, S., Rahimi, F., Shahbazi, M. A., Rezayan, A. H., Huwyler, J. and Witzigmann, D. 2019. Rapid optimization of liposome characteristics using a combined microfluidics and design-of-experiment approach. *Drug Delivery and Translational Research* 9(1): 404–413. https://doi.org/10.1007/s13346-018-0587-4

Vallianou, N. G., Dalamaga, M., Pavlou, A., Rebelos, E., Karamanolis, N. N., Papachristoforou, E., Mavrothalassitis, E., Eleftheriadou, I., Tentolouris, N. and Kounatidis, D. 2025. The transformative role of nanotechnology in the management of diabetes mellitus: Insights from current research. *Biomolecules* 15(5): 653. https://doi.org/10.3390/biom15050653

Wahab, M., Bhatti, A. and John, P. 2022. Evaluation of antidiabetic activity of biogenic silver nanoparticles using *Thymus serpyllum* on streptozotocin-induced diabetic BALB/c mice. *Polymers* 14: 3138.

Wang, J., Potocny, A. M., Rosenthal, J. and Day, E. S. 2020. Gold nanoshell- linear tetrapyrrole conjugates for near infrared- activated dual photodynamic and photothermal therapies. *ACS Omega* 5: 926–940.

Wang, X., Sun, H. and Mu, T. 2024. Materials and structure of polysaccharide-based delivery carriers for oral insulin: A review. *Carbohydrate Polymers* 323: 121364.

World Health Organization 2024. Diabetes (key facts). https://www.who.int/news-room/fact-sheets/detail/diabetes.

Wu, W. and Zhou, S. 2013. Responsive materials for self- regulated insulin delivery. *Macromolecular Bioscience* 13: 1464–1477.

Yang, Q., Jacobs, T. M., McCallen, J. D., Moore, D. T., Huckaby, J. T., Edelstein, J. N. and Lai, S. K. 2016. Analysis of pre-existing IgG and IgM antibodies against polyethylene glycol (PEG) in the general population. *Analytical Chemistry* 88(23): 11804–11812. https://doi.org/10.1021/acs.analchem.6b03437.

Zaid, A. and Ariel, A. 2024. Harnessing anti-inflammatory pathways and macrophage nano delivery to treat inflammatory and fibrotic disorders. *Advanced Drug Delivery Reviews* 207: 115204.

Zhang, C. X., Cheng, Y., Liu, D. Z., Liu, M., Cui, H., Zhang, B. L., Mei, Q. B. and Zhou, S. Y. 2019. Mitochondria-targeted cyclosporin A delivery system to treat myocardial ischemia reperfusion injury of rats. *Journal of Nanobiotechnology* 17: 18. https://doi.org/10.1186/s12951-019-0451-9.

Zhang, L., Beatty, A., Lu, L., Abdalrahman, A., Makris, T. M., Wang, G. and Wang, Q. 2020 Microfluidic-assisted polymer-protein assembly to fabricate homogeneous functional nanoparticles. *Materials Science and Engineering: C - Materials for Biological Applications* 111: 110768. https://doi.org/10.1016/j.msec.2020.110768

11 Nanomedicine
A Boon for Precision Medicine

Basu Bhattacharjee, Kavipriya Murugaiyan, Sunjeet Saha, Sunil Venkanna Pogu, and Aravind Kumar Rengan
Department of Biomedical Engineering, Indian Institute of Technology Hyderabad, Kandi, Telangana, India

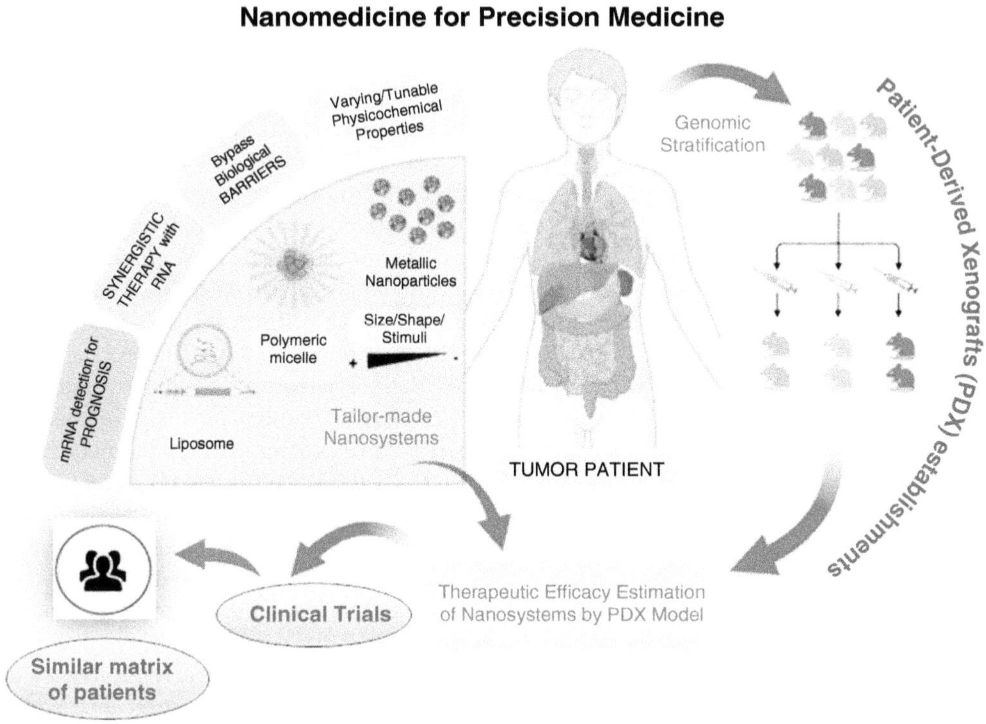

SCHEME 11.1 A concept representation of cancer precision therapy mediated by tailor-made nanomaterials. (The schematic has been designed using Biorender.)

Nanomedicine has become a vital tool in advancing personalized medicine by facilitating molecularly targeted delivery, unlike traditional systemic delivery methods that often lead to undesirable side effects, drug resistance development, and most importantly treatment failures. A diverse array of nanocarriers, including polymeric nanoparticles, liposomes, and inorganic or metallic nanoparticles (MNPs), have been engineered to precisely control the targeted molecular transport. These nanocarriers can alter various aspects of a drug's performance, including pharmacokinetics (PK/PD), stability, absorption, and exposure to both tumors and healthy tissues. They also support the administration of synergistic drug combinations, thereby enhancing the overall efficacy of therapeutic interventions. These nanoparticles can be tailor-made based on individual patient requirements through modifications in size, morphology, or functionalization with therapeutic molecules and targeting moieties, thus creating customized drug delivery systems (DDSs). In the

DOI: 10.1201/9781003473015-11

realm of cancer precision therapy, nanomedicine plays a crucial role in enhancing the delivery of noncoding RNAs that specifically target and regulate oncogenes responsible for certain types of cancers (Scheme 11.1).

According to the National Institutes of Health (NIH), precision medicine involves a customized medical approach that takes into account patient-related specific information, such as any gene mutations, biomarker presence/absence, or metabolite concentrations. Therapeutic interventions can then be devised to address individual genetic factors that augment the healing effects. The establishment of patient-derived xenograft (PDX) models is particularly prominent in cancer therapy due to their ability to mimic the tumor microenvironment (TME) or niche and more importantly genetic map/footprint of the patient. Comparable models are under development for other diseases. Owing to intelligent nanoparticle designs that have heightened efficacy and site-directed specificity/activity combined with PDX models, precision medicine can thereby drastically improve the overall patient treatment strategies.

11.1 INTRODUCTION

Nanomedicine is an interdisciplinary field comprising of nanoscience, nanoengineering, and nanotechnology which can act as effective modalities to diagnose, treat, repair, and regenerate biological systems (Pelaz et al., 2017; Liz-Marzán et al., 2022). Nanomedicines have the potential to enter into clinics once the regulatory, safety, and ethical requirements are satisfied (Pelaz et al., 2017). They have empowered the field of biosensors, microfluidics, and drug delivery. The development of nanomedicines can be divided into three stages. The first stage sets back around 1964–1995, during which the structure of liposomes was discovered and the approval of US Food and Drug Administration (FDA) was given to the first ever nanomedicine – doxorubicin-loaded liposomes (doxil, adriamycin, and lipodox now generally known by their brand names). The second stage was based on commercialization and validation of nanomedicines which span almost around 1995–2007. The third stage deals with the development of modern nanomedicines, significantly smart nanomedicines which started since 2008. Nanomedicines have greater efficacy than conventional drugs due to its smaller size in nanometer range, large specificity, and ability to be surface functionalized which helps to reach the targeted tissues (C. Zhang et al., 2020). Owing to their smaller size they have unique physiochemical properties such as mechanical, magnetic, electrical, and biological properties based on their composition. They can be designed to have prolonged circulation times due to their increased bioavailability. Controlled or sustained release of drugs from such nanoparticles helps us to reduce the dosage and also its adverse effects (Patra et al., 2018; R. Singh & Lillard, 2009). Combination of nanoparticles with natural bioactive compounds has recently been studied due to its lower toxicity (P. Patel et al., 2024; Han et al., 2022). The biomolecular interactions of the nanoparticles are based on surface engineering using peptide, antibodies, aptamers, cationic molecules, drugs, and folic acid (Díez-Pascual, 2022). Modification using nanotopography on the surface of titanium implants affected the behavior of endothelial cells and showed rapid re-endothelialization (Cherian et al., 2022). Modifying the surface of nanoparticles or simply using nanotopography could enhance the performance of the designed nanosystems with desired treatment outcome (Finbloom et al., 2023; W. Zhang et al., 2021). In the field of cancer, multidrug resistance is an ongoing challenge and targeted nanoparticles contribute in overcoming the condition due to its characteristic features of increased cellular uptake, passive targeting, and evading the efflux pumps (Bar-Zeev et al., 2017). Thus, nanomedicine because of its unique properties is becoming a potential alternative to traditional medicine (Germain et al., 2020). As of 2021, hundreds of nanomedicines have already been marketed, and currently, 563 nanomedicines are in the clinical trials or in the other stages (Thapa & Kim, 2023).

The term *Precision medicine* is an analog or often used interchangeably to personalized medicine. According to the US National Genomic Research Institute, precision medicine is an innovative approach that utilizes the genetic and lifestyle information of the patient to accurately design the diagnosis, prevention, and treatment modalities for a patient (Delpierre & Lefèvre, 2023). In 2011, Hood and Friend introduced the concept of P4 medicine – which includes predictive, personalized, preventive, and participatory medicine. P4 medicine is based on the huge amount of omics data. Considerable scientific and societal barriers are expected. It poses a challenge for the scientists to build new ways to bring ideal partnerships which foster the shared coherent objectives (Hood & Friend, 2011). The emergence of precision medicine basically occurred when the practice of medicine underwent a paradigm shift from reactive medicine to proactive medicine, slowly treating a disease concentrated more on the personalized data acquired from individual patients. Precision medicine has clearly originated due to the understandings from the Human Genome Project. Precision medicine utilizes computational models to thoroughly understand the mechanism of the disease via both clinic and basic research. The roadblocks to precision medicine still remain such as alterations in the genetic targets, resistance to therapies, lack of awareness among clinicians, the cost and accessibility to genomic sequencing (Duffy, 2016; Kiran et al., 2024). Precision medicine research on marginalized communities that are isolated from the normal social, economic, or cultural life poses an urgent requirement for health data justice to prevent intensification of health inequities (Shaw et al., 2024; Sevelius et al., 2020). By empowering both the clinicians as well as patients with user-friendly tools, precision medicine can bring the participatory component of P4 medicine into clinics (Duffy, 2016).

Conducting clinical research in stratified patient populations can get us an overview of uniform treatment response which will increase the efficient role of nanomedicines in the field of precision medicine. The current role of nanotechnology is limited to diagnostic applications such as identification of early biomarkers, and nanomedicines are yet to see the horizon in clinics due to the heterogeneity of biological barriers overshadowing the efficacy among successfully treated smaller subpopulation. Smart nanomedicines given to stratified patients along with genetic profiling can contribute to the success of precision medicine (Mitchell et al., 2021).

11.2 MODIFICATIONS AND IMPLICATIONS OF NANOMEDICINE FOR PRECISION APPROACHES

The field of precision medicine has undergone a paradigm change as a result of the modifications and implications of nanomedicine. Unsurpassed opportunities exist in nanotechnology to precisely control pharmacokinetics, biodistribution, and therapeutic efficacy in DDSs. Nanoparticles can be engineered to selectively interact with biological targets by means of surface changes and functionalization. This allows for the precise delivery of medicines to disease locations while reducing the likelihood of off-target effects. Furthermore, personalized medical approaches – where medications are tailored based on unique patient features, such as genetic makeup and disease profile – have been made possible by advances in nanomedicine. Precision medicine is a new era of personalized healthcare that can improve treatment outcomes, improve patient safety, and lessen the burden of side effects by utilizing nanotechnology (Sandbhor et al., 2024; Ashkarran et al., 2024).

11.2.1 Metal Nanoparticles for Drug Delivery

MNPs have demonstrated a wide range of characteristics in the field of nanotechnology, opening up numerous new avenues, particularly in targeted medication delivery systems. MNPs are widely used as drug delivery vehicles for a variety of therapeutic agents, including peptides, chemotherapeutic medicines, antibodies, and nucleic acids (Ahmad et al., 2010). The majority of MNPs, including copper, zinc, titanium, gold, palladium, silver, and gold nanoparticles, have improved, with adjustable optical qualities. Furthermore, conjugating targeted agents and active biomolecules via H-bonding, covalent bonding, and electrostatic interactions is a simple way to functionalize their surface. MNPs are derived from their ability to repress or completely eradicate rapid renal drug excretion, lengthen the duration that pharmaceuticals circulate in the blood, and increase the water solubility of hydrophobic pharmacological compounds. Metal nanoparticles provided a model to achieve three goals: directing the therapeutic agent to the site of action, reducing the drug's negative effects on healthy tissues or organs, and managing the drug's release to prevent the traditional overdosing/underdosing cycle (Chandrakala et al., 2022).

11.2.2 Polymer-Based Drug Delivery Vehicles

During the past 20 years, polymer-based DDSs have attracted a lot of attention due to their capacity to precisely target tumor tissues and greatly extend the therapy opportunity. Delivery systems or formulations based on polymers that can transfer medicines into the body with the primary goal of improving bioavailability, safety, and efficacy are known as polymer-based DDSs. The best way to get around the drawbacks of chemotherapy as a cancer treatment is to employ polymer-based DDSs. They accomplish this by controlling the drug's rate of release and guiding it to particular biological locations. The utilization of biodegradable and bioabsorbable polymers, which offer a safe framework for delivering medicines without harming the body, is a crucial component of polymer-based DDSs (Ghosh, 2004; Ding et al., 2024).

For many years, natural polymers such as chitosan, arginine, cellulose, hyaluronic acid (HA), and polysaccharides have been used to improve the effectiveness of drug administration. Novel biomaterials for applications involving controlled drug delivery have been created by modifying these naturally occurring polymers (Guo et al., 2016). Furthermore, because of their bioresponsiveness and bioactivity as well as how easily their structures may be changed, synthetic polymers are gaining popularity. In DDSs, aliphatic polyesters are most frequently used as components. Examples include poly(ethylene glycol) (PEG), poly(glycolic acid) (PGA), poly(lactic acid) (PLA), or poly(lactic-co-glycolic acid) (PLGA), poly (caprolactone), polyurethane, and polydioxanone (Saha et al., 2024).

11.2.3 Protein-Based Drug Delivery Vehicles

Protein nanomaterials are distinct, hollow protein nanoparticles that include ferritin, heat shock proteins, chaperonins, virus-like particles, and many other substances. As drug delivery vehicles, protein-based nanomaterials exhibit many desirable characteristics such as being appropriately sized for endocytosis, nontoxic, biocompatible, and biodegradable (MaHam et al., 2009).

11.2.4 Hydrogel-Based Drug Delivery Vehicles

Hydrogels have become highly effective biomaterials for drug delivery because of their special qualities, which include high water content, biocompatibility, and mechanical properties that may be adjusted. This section offers a thorough review of hydrogel-based drug delivery methods, emphasizing current developments, obstacles, and potential paths forward in this quickly developing subject.

Hydrogels are three-dimensional networks of hydrophilic polymers capable of absorbing and retaining large amounts of water. They can be classified based on their origin (natural or synthetic) and mode of cross-linking (physical or chemical). Natural hydrogels, such as alginate, chitosan, and HA, offer inherent biocompatibility and bioactivity, while synthetic hydrogels provide precise control over mechanical properties and degradation kinetics. The properties of hydrogels, including porosity, swelling behavior, and degradation rate, can be tailored to suit specific drug delivery applications (Vashist et al., 2014).

DDSs based on hydrogels provide flexible platforms for loading and regulating the release of different treatments, including proteins, nucleic acids, and small compounds. Chemical conjugation, affinity interactions, or physical encapsulation can all be used to incorporate drugs into the hydrogel matrix. Diffusion, degradation, and environmental stimuli control the release kinetics of

TABLE 11.1
Therapeutic Applications of Nanomaterials Developed from Various Inorganic and Organic Precursors

Nanomaterial Precursors	Application	Ref.
Copper	Cardiac mitochondrial function	Qu et al. (2024)
Silver	Colon cancer treatment	Taati et al. (2024)
Gold	Breast cancer treatment	He et al. (2024)
Palladium	Colon cancer treatment	Golestannezhad et al. (2024)
PLA	Tissue engineering	Alam et al. (2023)
PEG	Antimicrobial treatment	Appidi et al. (2021)
PCL	Breast cancer treatment	Espinoza et al. (2020)
Chondroitin sulfate	Colon cancer treatment	Luo et al. (2020)
PLA	Tissue engineering	Alam et al. (2023)
PEG	Antimicrobial treatment	Appidi et al. (2021)
PCL	Breast cancer treatment	Espinoza et al. (2020)
Chondroitin sulfate	Colon cancer treatment	Luo et al. (2020)
Ferritin	Ischemic stroke	Qi et al. (2024)
HSP	Alveolar adenocarcinoma	Ibrahim et al. (2024)
Albumin	Breast cancer and lung cancer treatment	Ghazy & Hanafy (2024)
Collagen	Periodontal regeneration	Takallu et al. (2024)
Collagen	Wound healing	S. Li et al. (2024)
Alginate	Antibacterial agent	Dai et al. (2024)
Chitosan	Bone infection	Wassif et al. (2024)
Hyaluronic acid	Wound healing	F. Zhang et al. (2024)
Collagen	Wound healing	S. Li et al. (2024)
Alginate	Antibacterial agent	Dai et al. (2024)
Chitosan	Bone infection	Wassif et al. (2024)
Hyaluronic acid	Wound healing	F. Zhang et al. (2024)

encapsulated pharmaceuticals, enabling sustained or stimulus-responsive drug release customized to the intended treatment plan.

In the fields of tissue engineering, wound healing, cancer treatment, and regenerative medicine, hydrogel-based drug delivery methods are widely used. Hydrogels play a crucial role in regenerative medicine by acting as scaffolds for tissue regeneration and cell encapsulation. They also facilitate the targeted administration of bioactive substances that aid in the healing process. Hydrogels minimize systemic toxicity during the targeted delivery of chemotherapeutic drugs to tumor locations in cancer therapy. Furthermore, by retaining moisture, having antibacterial qualities, and allowing for the regulated release of therapeutic drugs, hydrogel-based dressings provide cutting-edge wound care options (Table 11.1).

11.3 ADVANCEMENTS IN PRECISION MEDICINE

Precision medicine involves the molecular profiling of individual diseases along with the pre-established clinical-pathological indexes (Naithani et al., 2021; Buljan & Wick, 2022). It ascertains the individual patient's diagnostic and prognostic risk profile in real time. Thus, disease-specific treatment plans can be devised which are tailored for individual patients. It helps in improving the rapidly changing clinical stratification and places each patient at the center of a customized treatment plan for therapy against diseases like cancer. Customized treatment plans are essential due to the diversity among patients and diseases, aiming to reduce unnecessary drug exposure and mitigate the risks of side effects without therapeutic dividends. Contemporary medical professionals are slowly moving away from classical treatment approaches and gravitating toward personalized care that addresses the unique needs of each individual. Achieving comprehensive personalized medicine requires thorough knowledge of patients' genetic, phenotypic, and metabolomic profiles, along with the classification of psychological and epigenetic characteristics. PDX models also help in circumventing the pitfalls of conventional cancer therapy. This approach also considers environmental and lifestyle factors to enhance drug efficacy and safety, benefiting both healthcare systems and individual patients (Elzagallaai et al., 2023; Shrestha et al., 2022). Precision medicine leverages technological innovations and data analytics to tailor medical treatment for individual patients (Gaur et al., 2022). Some of them are mentioned in this section (Figure 11.1).

11.3.1 Tailoring Personalized Therapies for Various Diseases

Tailoring personalized therapies for various diseases is the cornerstone of precision medicine, aiming to optimize treatment outcomes while minimizing adverse effects. Personalized therapy, rooted in the concept of tailoring medical care to individual patients, is advancing across various disease domains. Precision medicine can be crucial for diabetes mitigation due to the disease's heterogeneity, with responses to antidiabetic drugs varying based on genetic and epigenetic factors, necessitating tailored drug treatments (Rizvi et al., 2022). Furthermore, personalized medicine, encompassing individualized approaches based on genomic profiles, holds the potential to predict safe and effective medical therapies for specific patients, leading to improved well-being, longevity, and reduced costs (A. K. Singh et al., 2023). The integration of deep learning algorithms, such as Convolutional Neural Networks and Recurrent Neural Networks, in personalized therapy is enhancing disease classifications and treatment recommendations based on detailed patient data,

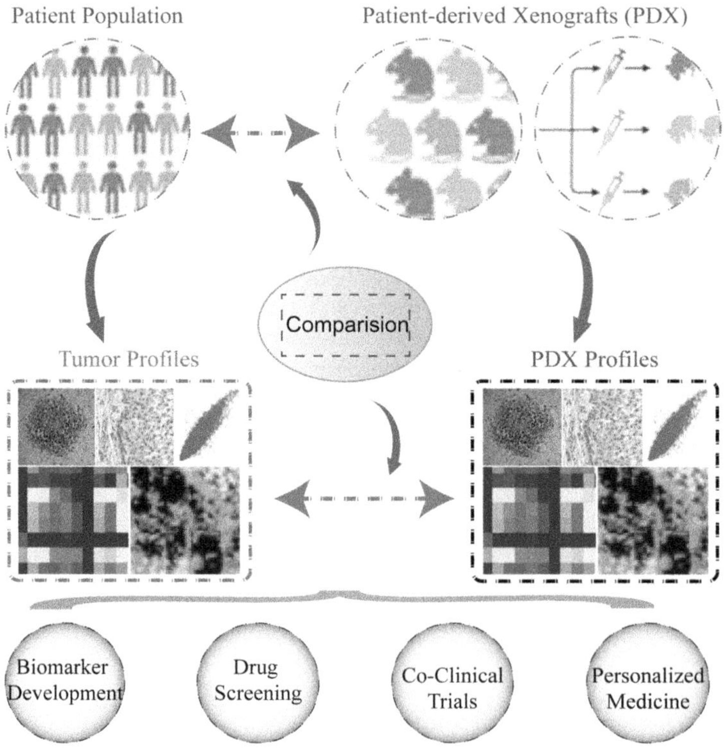

FIGURE 11.1 A schematic depicting the "one animal per model per treatment or PDX" approach in precision medicine. (Adapted from Yao et al., 2017.)

showcasing the potential for improved treatment outcomes (Shastri et al., 2021; Peng et al., 2021). Nanomedicine, which utilizes nanoparticles for diagnosis and treatment, offers a promising avenue for personalized therapies by matching treatments with patient-specific biomarkers (Shrestha et al., 2022). The development of nanocarrier formulations for optimal delivery of active molecules to targeted cells while minimizing side effects highlights the innovative approaches in nanomedicine for personalized patient treatments, paving the way for more effective and tailored therapies across various diseases. Nanomedicine reduces off-target toxicity, especially in diseases like cancer (Shrestha et al., 2022). In the era of evolving healthcare and pharmaceutical research, personalized therapy stands as a beacon of hope for tailoring treatments to individual characteristics, ultimately revolutionizing disease management and patient care. Certain disease examples that further emphasize the feasibility associated with personalized therapies that are under development are as under:

1. *Cancer*: Personalized cancer therapy involves analyzing the genetic mutations and molecular characteristics of tumors to identify targeted therapies. This includes drugs that specifically target mutations such as epidermal growth factor receptor (EGFR) inhibitors in lung cancer or BRAF inhibitors in melanoma. Additionally, immunotherapies like checkpoint inhibitors and chimeric antigen receptor (CAR)-T-cell therapy are tailored to activate the immune system against cancer cells. Recently, Government of India has cleared an indigenous CAR-T cell therapy (NexCAR19) for B-cell lymphomas and leukemia under the company name of ImmunoAct, a spin-off from IIT Bombay (H. Jain et al., 2022).
2. *Cardiovascular Diseases*: In cardiovascular diseases, personalized therapies may involve genetic testing to identify inherited conditions like familial hypercholesterolemia or Long QT syndrome. Treatment strategies can then be tailored based on genetic predispositions, lifestyle factors, and disease severity, including medication selection, lifestyle modifications, and interventional procedures.
3. *Neurological Disorders*: Personalized therapies for neurological disorders such as Alzheimer's disease, Parkinson's disease, and multiple sclerosis may involve genetic testing, biomarker analysis, and neuroimaging techniques. This information helps in predicting disease progression, guiding treatment decisions, and identifying individuals who may benefit from specific interventions or clinical trials.
4. *Genetic Disorders*: For genetic disorders like cystic fibrosis, sickle cell disease, or Duchenne muscular dystrophy, personalized therapies may involve gene therapy, gene editing (e.g., CRISPR-Cas9), or small molecule drugs targeting specific genetic mutations. These treatments aim to correct or mitigate the underlying genetic defect, offering potential cures or disease-modifying effects.
5. *Infectious Diseases*: Personalized therapies in infectious diseases may involve identifying microbial genotypes or drug resistance profiles to guide antimicrobial selection. In the case of viral infections like HIV or hepatitis C, personalized treatment regimens are tailored based on viral genotype, patient comorbidities, and drug tolerability.

Similarly, for autoimmune disorders, psychiatric disorders, and others, personalized medicine can help significantly to improve the patient care by optimizing the treatment outcomes.

11.3.2 Nano-MRI for Precision Medicine

Nano-MRI (nano-magnetic resonance imaging) plays a crucial role in precision medicine by offering advanced imaging capabilities at the nanometer scale, allowing for personalized diagnostic and therapeutic strategies tailored to individual patient's needs (Rahman, 2023). This technology combines the power of nanotechnology with MRI to provide detailed insights into tissues and diseases, enabling early detection, precise treatment decisions, and monitoring of therapeutic interventions at a personalized level. The use of nanoparticles in MRI has revolutionized the field of nanomedicine, offering a wide range of applications in cancer research, cardiovascular diseases, autoimmune disorders, neurological conditions, and infectious diseases, showcasing the potential for enhanced patient stratification and individualized care (Q. Wang et al., 2023). Furthermore, the integration of nanostructures and metamaterials in MRI has opened new avenues for high-performance imaging, leveraging the unique properties of these materials to enhance contrast and sensitivity in diagnostic imaging. Nano-MRI holds promise for the future of precision medicine, offering a non-invasive and highly accurate approach to disease diagnosis and treatment monitoring, paving the way for more effective and personalized healthcare interventions based on individual patient characteristics and responses to therapy. Nano-MRI has the potential to significantly alter the landscape of diagnosis, therapy, and patient outcomes through following means:

1. *High-Resolution Imaging*: Nano-MRI enables imaging at the nanoscale, allowing for the visualization of cellular structures, molecular interactions, and biomolecular processes with unprecedented detail. This high-resolution imaging capability provides insights into the underlying mechanisms of diseases at the molecular level, facilitating the development of targeted therapies.
2. *In Vivo Imaging*: Advancements in nano-MRI technology has led to the development of in vivo imaging techniques that allow for non-invasive visualization of biological processes within living organisms. In vivo nano-MRI enables longitudinal studies of disease progression, treatment response, and therapeutic interventions in animal models and clinical settings, providing valuable insights into disease mechanisms and personalized treatment strategies.
3. *Multimodal Imaging*: Nano-MRI can be integrated with other imaging modalities such as positron emission tomography (PET), computed tomography (CT), and optical imaging to provide complementary information and enhance diagnostic accuracy. Multimodal imaging approaches enable comprehensive characterization of disease phenotypes, molecular signatures, and treatment responses, guiding personalized treatment decisions and patient management.
4. *Personalized Treatment Monitoring*: Nano-MRI offers the potential for real-time monitoring of treatment response at the cellular and molecular level. By tracking changes in tissue morphology, metabolic activity, and drug distribution, nano-MRI enables clinicians to assess the efficacy of personalized treatment regimens and adjust therapy accordingly, optimizing patient outcomes.

11.3.3 Precision Immuno-Oncology

Precision immuno-oncology focuses on understanding the spatial biology of the TME to enhance treatment strategies (B. Patel et al., 2023). By utilizing hybrid multiplex panels combining RNA *in situ* hybridization and immunofluorescence, researchers can visualize the organization of cell types and identify the cellular sources of specific cytokines within tumors (Zhao et al., 2023). This approach allows for the semi-quantitative assessment of cytokine expression levels in different immune cells, aiding in correlating treatment responses, especially with checkpoint inhibitors. Furthermore, the complexity of the TME, including immune cells, fibroblasts, and vasculature, underscores the need for sophisticated models like organoids to study spatiotemporal interactions and improve precision immuno-oncology. In the realm of precision immuno-oncology, the focus extends beyond targeting immune checkpoints to harnessing immune cell therapies and overcoming treatment resistance (Obradovic, 2023; Buchbinder & Hodi, 2023). Understanding the intricate communication networks and functional contexts of immune and cancer cells within the TME is crucial for optimizing the selection of immune modulating agents and predicting therapy responses accurately. The integration of artificial intelligence in analyzing complex tumor-immune interactions and developing digital biomarkers enhances the selection of effective immune therapeutics based on spatial and contextual information from cancer tissue images. Some of the ways through which precision medicine can influence the immunological aspects of therapy are as follows:

1. *Biomarker Identification*: Precision immuno-oncology involves the identification of biomarkers that predict a patient's response to immunotherapy. Biomarkers such as programmed death-ligand 1 (PD-L1) expression, tumor mutational burden (TMB), microsatellite instability (MSI), and immune cell infiltration are used to stratify patients and guide treatment decisions.
2. *Genomic Profiling*: Genomic profiling of tumors helps identify genetic mutations and alterations that influence the tumor-immune microenvironment. Understanding the genetic landscape of tumors informs the selection of immunotherapies targeting specific pathways or antigens, such as immune checkpoint inhibitors or adoptive cell therapies.
3. *Personalized Combination Therapies*: Precision immuno-oncology involves the development of personalized combination therapies that enhance the efficacy of immunotherapy. Combinations of immune checkpoint inhibitors, targeted therapies, chemotherapy, radiation therapy, and immunomodulatory agents are tailored to individual patients based on their tumor characteristics and immune profile.
4. *Predictive Modeling*: Machine learning and computational algorithms are used to develop predictive models that identify patients likely to respond to immunotherapy and predict treatment outcomes. These models integrate clinical, genomic, and immunological data to optimize patient selection and treatment strategies, improving overall response rates and patient survival.
5. *Immune Profiling*: Immune profiling techniques such as flow cytometry, mass cytometry (CyTOF), and single-cell RNA sequencing (scRNA-seq) are used to characterize the immune landscape within the TME. Immune profiling provides insights into the composition, activation state, and functional status of immune cells, guiding the development of personalized immunotherapy approaches.
6. *Neoantigen Vaccines*: Precision immuno-oncology includes the development of neoantigen vaccines tailored to individual patients based on their tumor-specific mutations. Neoantigen vaccines stimulate the immune system to target tumor-specific antigens, eliciting a durable anti-tumor-immune response. Personalized neoantigen vaccines hold promise for improving the efficacy of cancer immunotherapy and achieving long-term disease control.

Apart from the above-mentioned avenues, precision immune-oncology is also advancing in the areas of liquid biopsies that employ circulating tumor DNA and circulating tumor cells for non-invasive real-time monitoring of tumors and microbiome modulation through dietary intervention or fecal microbiota transplantation.

11.3.4 Multi-Omics-Based Approach

A multi-omics-based approach integrates various omics data layers to gain a comprehensive understanding of complex diseases like cancer and plant responses to abiotic stresses. By combining genomics, transcriptomics, proteomics, metabolomics, and other omics techniques, researchers can explore common gene modules among different tumors, identify biomarkers associated with cancer development, and enhance plant traits for abiotic stress tolerance (Demir Karaman & Işık, 2023) (Roychowdhury et al., 2023). These integrated approaches not only improve survival prediction and therapeutic outcomes in cancer but also pave the way for developing climate-smart crops with enhanced stress tolerance mechanisms, ultimately ensuring food security under changing environmental conditions (Cominetti et al., 2023; Abdel-Wahab et al., 2023; Chikwambi et al., 2023). The multi-omics pipelines offer a wealth of opportunities in personalized medicine, enabling the identification of new gene targets, potential biomarkers, and precise treatment options across different cancer types. These approaches leverage machine learning tools, network-based models, and computational methods to analyze complex omics datasets, address translational challenges, and enhance precision medicine in treatment of cancer and other diseases. By combining tumor-informed and tumor-naïve strategies, researchers can detect circulating tumor DNA with high accuracy, demonstrating the complementarity of different omics approaches in molecular residual disease detection and monitoring across various stages of cancer (Figure 11.2).

11.3.5 Stem Cell-Based Approach for Precision Medicine

Stem cell therapy has emerged as a promising approach in various fields of medicine (Ilyas, 2023). Stem cells possess the unique ability to differentiate into specific cell types, making them valuable tools in regenerative medicine (Abdi et al., 2022). This therapy holds great potential in treating a wide range of diseases, including neurodegenerative disorders like Alzheimer's disease, spinal cord injuries, diabetes, and heart ailments. Stem cells offer a novel approach to regenerate damaged tissues, such as lung damage caused by viral infections like SARS-CoV-2, due

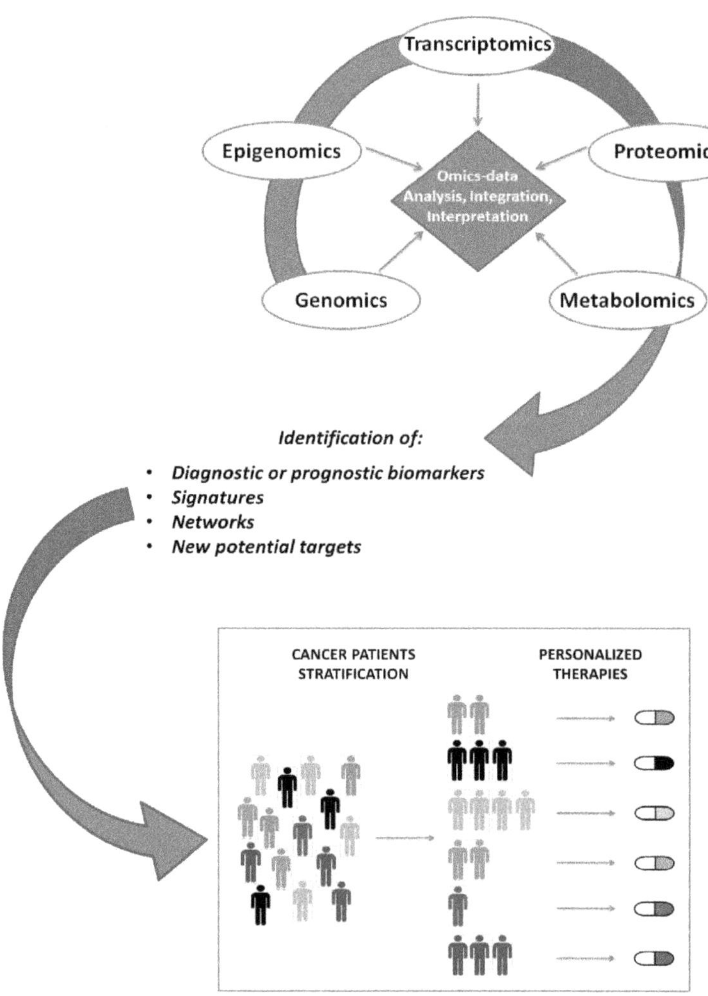

FIGURE 11.2 Scheme depicting the major steps occurring from omics data production to personalized clinical decision-making. (Adapted from Cantafio et al., 2018.)

to their regenerative, immunomodulatory, and anti-inflammatory properties (Khandelwal et al., 2023). The application of stem cells can be categorized into autotransplantation, allotransplantation, and xenotransplantation, with the latter gaining attention as a challenging yet promising avenue for research. In the realm of regenerative medicine, nanotechnology has been integrated with stem cell therapy to enhance cellular behavior and regenerative capabilities. Nanomedicine plays a crucial role in manipulating the fate of stem cells and biomaterials, offering cutting-edge strategies to engineer biological tissues. Despite the ethical and legal considerations surrounding nanotechnology applications in regenerative medicine, the field continues to evolve with a focus on developing innovative nano-based approaches to improve stem cell therapies. Stem cell therapy, coupled with nanotechnology advancements, presents a futuristic outlook in the treatment of various diseases, emphasizing the importance of ongoing research and clinical trials to harness the full potential of this innovative approach.

Stem cell-based approaches play a pivotal role in advancing precision medicine by offering personalized treatment modalities (Abdi et al., 2022). Human-induced pluripotent stem cells (hiPSCs) have revolutionized disease modeling and drug discovery, emphasizing the importance of diverse repositories reflecting different ethnicities and sexes for more inclusive research (Khandelwal et al., 2023). Stem cells, whether embryonic or nonembryonic, hold immense promise for tissue regeneration and repair, with ongoing investigations focusing on their therapeutic potential in various conditions like muscular dystrophy and cerebral infarctions (Y. Wang et al., 2023). Integrating genome profiling with in vitro human cell models derived from pluripotent stem cells enables the development of personalized treatments for diabetes, showcasing the significance of hPSC-based disease models in precision medicine. The use of induced pluripotent stem cells (iPSCs) not only aids in understanding disease pathophysiology but also allows for the creation of patient-specific therapeutic strategies, aligning with the principles of personalized medicine and optimizing treatment efficacy (Nguyen et al., 2023). In conclusion, stem cell-based approaches, particularly utilizing hiPSCs and hPSCs, offer a promising avenue for precision medicine by enabling tailored therapies, disease modeling, and drug screening based on individual genetic backgrounds and disease characteristics (S. Jain et al., 2022; Memon & Abdelalim, 2022; Leibel et al., 2022). The ability to generate patient-specific cells for diagnostic, prognostic, and therapeutic purposes underscores the potential of stem cells in advancing personalized or precision medicine. Efforts to enhance diversity in stem cell repositories and to leverage chemical engineering tools for strengthening cell functionalities further contribute to the evolution of precision medicine, emphasizing the importance of inclusive research practices and innovative technologies in advancing personalized healthcare.

11.4 REGULATORY BODY'S ROLE IN PRECISION MEDICINE

Regulatory bodies play a crucial role in advancing precision medicine by addressing key challenges and gaps in the approval and adoption of innovative technologies and personalized therapies (Adamo et al., 2020; Mol et al., 2018). These bodies are tasked with ensuring data standards, quality, and validity in the use of digital biomarkers and other advanced technologies, as highlighted in discussions from the Regulatory Science to Advance Precision Medicine Forum (Adamo et al., 2018). Moreover, regulatory considerations extend to the integration of genomics, proteomics, metabolomics, and other approaches in precision medicine, emphasizing the need for standardization of complex tests, establishing clinical validity and utility, and addressing pharmacogenomics considerations (Ali et al., 2017). The involvement of regulatory agencies like the European Medicines Agency (EMA) and the FDA is essential in facilitating the development of personalized therapies through predictive preclinical models, real-world data, and patient engagement. In the realm of precision medicine, regulatory bodies face challenges related to evidence generation, patient involvement, cost considerations, and the development of new regulatory models. These challenges underscore the importance of balancing risk tolerance, especially in early interventions for life-threatening diseases, as precision medicine continues to evolve and shape the future of healthcare. The regulation of genetic testing systems is also a critical aspect in the precision medicine landscape, emphasizing the need for quality assurance, ethical considerations, and the establishment of a federal regulatory body to oversee and address critical regulatory issues related to genetic testing. Ultimately, regulatory bodies play a pivotal role in fostering trust, ensuring safety, and driving innovation in the field of precision medicine.

11.4.1 Perspective and Policies of Regulatory Bodies

Regulatory bodies play a crucial role in shaping the perspective and policies surrounding precision medicine. Various countries have adopted different approaches to integrate precision medicine into their healthcare systems (Breckenridge et al., 2016). Some nations, like England, France, and Denmark, have implemented national strategies and invested in infrastructure for precision medicine through top-down decisions, while others, such as Sweden and Germany, have relied on bottom-up initiatives led by healthcare professionals to ensure equal access to precision medicine (Ali et al., 2017). This diversity in approaches highlights the need for sustainable governance and organization at regional, national, and international levels to effectively implement precision medicine. Additionally, ethical and legal considerations are paramount in the implementation of precision medicine, emphasizing the importance of real-world data access, clinical trials for evidence generation, improved reimbursement models, cross-disciplinary education, and patient involvement (Stenzinger et al., 2023). Furthermore, the complex legal landscape surrounding precision medicine research adds another layer of intricacy to regulatory considerations. State laws in the United States, for example, can significantly impact participant rights and protections in precision medicine studies, particularly concerning human subjects research, genetic testing, and privacy issues (Beskow et al., 2022; Verma et al., 2021). The varying perspectives on the implications of state law variations underscore the ethical and legal challenges in ensuring consistent participant protections across different jurisdictions. Addressing these challenges requires further empirical and normative work to navigate the intricate web of laws, regulations, and procedures that safeguard participants in precision medicine research.

11.4.2 Views from Regulatory Bodies on Genetic Variant-Based Companion Diagnostics

Regulatory bodies, such as the EMA, are actively involved in shaping the landscape of genetic variant-based companion diagnostics (CDx) in precision medicine. The new *In Vitro* Diagnostic Regulation (EU) 2017/746 (IVDR) introduces a risk-based classification system for in vitro diagnostic tests (IVDs) and emphasizes the importance of aligning CDx assessments with corresponding medicinal products. This regulatory framework aims to ensure the suitability of CDx for use with specific medicinal products through a consultation process involving various stakeholders, including notified bodies and medicines regulators (Hisan & Amri, 2023; Hammack et al., 2019). Furthermore, the implementation of the IVDR and CDx presents a regulatory challenge in the EU, necessitating the re-assessment of IVDs in terms of their CDx designation, especially in the context of patient stratification in clinical trials, particularly in oncology-related studies. Overall, the regulatory bodies' views underscore the importance of integrating genetic variant-based CDx into precision medicine to enhance patient care and treatment outcomes. By unifying data and concepts from rare and common disease genetics, regulatory bodies aim to promote a holistic perspective that considers diverse genetic and environmental factors in clinical decision-making (Verbaanderd et al., 2023). This approach reflects a shift toward personalized medicine, where genetic information plays a pivotal role in identifying patient subgroups that are most likely to benefit from specific treatments, emphasizing the significance of genetic variant-based CDx in advancing precision healthcare practices.

11.4.3 Role of Pharmacogenomics for Precision Medicine

Pharmacogenomics plays a crucial role in the realm of precision medicine by tailoring therapies to individual patients based on their genetic makeup, thus maximizing drug efficacy and minimizing toxicity (Wollenhaupt et al., 2023; Valla et al., 2021). This field has evolved from traditional pharmacogenetics to encompass all "-omics" fields, including proteomics, transcriptomics, metabolomics, and metagenomics, under the umbrella of pharmacogenomics (Manchia & Murri, 2023). By focusing on genetic variations in pharmacogenes, such as drug-metabolizing enzymes, drug transporters, and receptors, pharmacogenomics serves as a key tool in predicting an individual's response to medications, guiding the development of targeted therapeutics, and improving outcomes while preventing adverse effects (Turolo et al., 2023). Furthermore, pharmacogenomics not only aids in optimizing drug dosages to avoid adverse events or lack of efficacy but also enhances the understanding of drug-biomolecule interactions and their impact on treatment outcomes (Sadee et al., 2023; X. Li, 2023; Demirpolat, 2023). By leveraging genomic data to assess pharmacokinetic and pharmacodynamic parameters, pharmacogenomics contributes significantly to the personalization of medicine, taking into account factors like patient demographics, disease characteristics, and genetic variations to ensure the right drug at the right dose for each individual.

11.5 DISCUSSION AND FUTURE PROSPECTS

The integration of nanomedicine into precision medicine presents both opportunities and challenges, prompting discussions about its future benefits and drawbacks (Figure 11.3). They are as follows:

1. *Targeted Drug Delivery*: The nanoparticles can be engineered to deliver drugs specifically to diseased cells or tissues, minimizing systemic side effects and improving therapeutic efficacy.
2. *Enhanced Imaging*: Nanotechnology enables the development of contrast agents and imaging probes with higher sensitivity and specificity, facilitating earlier disease detection and more accurate diagnosis.

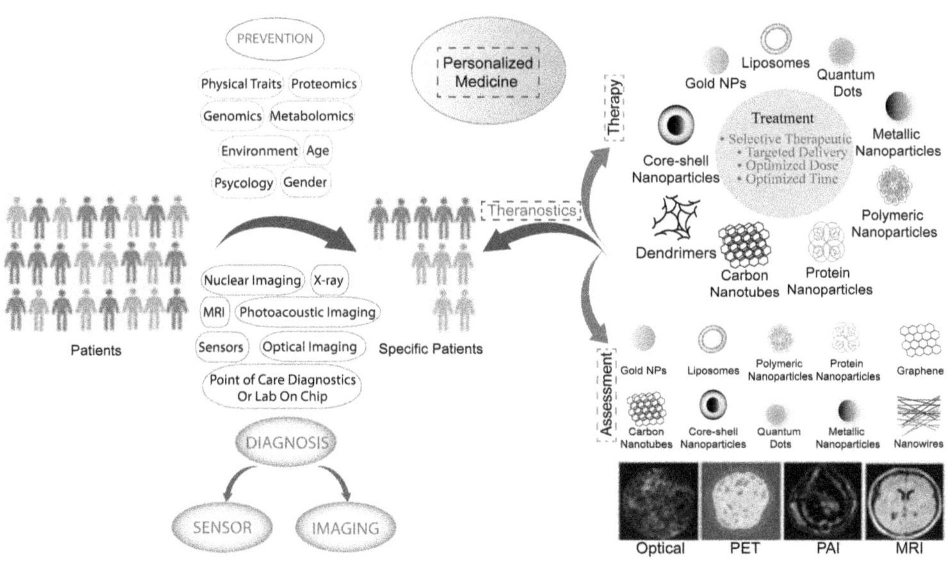

FIGURE 11.3 Schematic depicting nanomedicine's role in personalized medicine. (Taken from Shrestha et al., 2022.)

3. *Personalized Therapeutics*: Nanomedicine allows for the customization of treatment regimens based on individual patient characteristics, such as genetic makeup and disease phenotype, aligning with the principles of precision medicine.
4. *Overcoming Biological Barriers*: Nanoparticles can bypass biological barriers, such as the blood-brain barrier, to deliver therapeutics to previously inaccessible sites within the body.
5. *Safety Concerns*: The long-term safety profile of nanoparticles, particularly their potential for accumulation and toxicity in the body, requires further investigation and regulation.
6. *Cost*: The nanomedicine-based therapies may be more expensive to develop and manufacture, limiting accessibility, especially in resource-constrained healthcare settings.
7. *Regulatory Challenges*: The unique properties of nanoparticles pose challenges for regulatory approval, necessitating standardized evaluation criteria and guidelines.
8. *Ethical Considerations*: The use of nanotechnology in precision medicine raises ethical concerns regarding patient privacy, informed consent, and equitable distribution of resources.

AstraZeneca's 5Rs principle can be adapted to enhance its success and improve therapeutic efficiency in the following:

1. *Right Target*: Targeted delivery to disease sites is one of the most significant benefits of nanomedicine, as it provides the ability to precisely deliver drugs to the disease site, improving the therapeutic index. For example, nanoparticles can be designed to target cancer cells or inflamed tissues, specifically sparing healthy tissues from exposure to the drugs. Also, for crossing biological barriers, the nanomedicines can be tailored to cross biological barriers that traditional DDSs cannot, such as the blood-brain barrier in neurological diseases or the blood-tumor barrier in cancer. This ensures that the right drug reaches the right place, even in challenging diseases.
2. *Right Dose*: Nanomedicines are often designed to improve the pharmacokinetics, stability, and solubility of drugs that otherwise have poor bioavailability. The right drug in the context of nanomedicines means choosing or developing formulations that can take advantage of nanotechnology's benefits, such as better targeting and controlled release of the active pharmaceutical ingredients.
3. *Right Time*: The ability to control the timing of drug release can be crucial in diseases that evolve, such as cancer or autoimmune diseases. Nanomedicines can be designed to release their active ingredient at specific intervals or respond to specific biological triggers (pH changes, enzymes), ensuring that drugs are delivered when the disease is most vulnerable. Incorporating bioimaging moieties into the nanoformulation can further provide better functionality as it helps in real-time bioimaging of therapeutic effects.
4. *Right Route*: The route of administration can significantly impact therapeutic efficacy and patient adherence. Nanosystems are focused on developing innovative DDSs, such as extended-release formulations, subcutaneous injections, or inhalers, to enhance drug absorption and patient convenience. Patients are more likely to follow treatment protocols, improving overall therapeutic success by making drug administration more convenient and comfortable using patient-friendly forms like oral tablets, patches, or inhalers.
5. *Right Patient*: Nanomedicines can be tailored to target specific populations based on genetic, molecular, or disease characteristics. For example, nanoparticles can be surface functionalized to recognize and bind to biomarkers unique to particular cancer cells or other diseases. This ensures that only the suitable patients with the specific biomarker or disease phenotype receive the therapy, maximizing therapeutic efficacy and reducing unnecessary side effects. The ability to tailor treatments using nanotechnology allows for precision dosing and better outcomes in patients with complex diseases like cancer, neurological disorders, or rare genetic diseases (Morgan et al., 2018; Kargozar & Mozafari, 2018; Hare et al., 2017).

11.6 CONCLUSION

Nanomedicine holds great promise for advancing precision medicine through personalized therapeutics that enhances targeted drug delivery and molecular imaging. Its widespread adoption requires careful consideration of safety, cost, regulatory, and ethical implications. With continued research and collaboration, nanomedicine has the potential to significantly improve patient outcomes while addressing the complexities of individualized healthcare. Thus, nanomedicine can be definitely slated as a boon for precision medicine-based therapy and diagnostics for various diseases.

REFERENCES

Abdel-Wahab, B. A., Helmy, Y. A., & Saied, E. M. (2023). Editorial: Molecular and multi-omic approaches in understanding cancer biology and anticancer therapies: Current perspectives and new challenges. *Frontiers in Pharmacology*, 14, 1236158. https://doi.org/10.3389/fphar.2023.1236158

Abdi, S., Javanmehr, N., Ghasemi-Kasman, M., Bali, H. Y., & Pirzadeh, M. (2022). Stem cell-based therapeutic and diagnostic approaches in Alzheimer's disease. *Current Neuropharmacology*, 20(6), 1093–1115. https://doi.org/10.2174/1570159X20666211231090659

Adamo, J. E., Bienvenu II, R. V., Dolz, F., Liebman, M., Nilsen, W., & Steele, S. J. (2020). Translation of digital health technologies to advance precision medicine: Informing regulatory science. *Digital Biomarkers*, 4(1), 1–12. https://doi.org/10.1159/000505289

Adamo, J. E., Bienvenu, R. V., Fields, F. O., Ghosh, S., Jones, C. M., Liebman, M., Lowenthal, M. S., & Steele, S. J. (2018). The integration of emerging omics approaches to advance precision medicine: How can regulatory science help? *Journal of Clinical and Translational Science*, 2(5), 295–300. https://doi.org/10.1017/cts.2018.330

Ahmad, M. Z., Akhter, S., Jain, G. K., Rahman, M., Pathan, S. A., Ahmad, F. J., & Khar, R. K. (2010). Metallic nanoparticles: Technology overview & drug delivery applications in oncology. *Expert Opinion on Drug Delivery*, 7(8), 927–942. https://doi.org/10.1517/17425247.2010.498473

Alam, M. M., Ezhilan, M., Saha, S., Gopan, G., Mani, M., & Kannan, S. (2023). Design, fabrication, mechanical, and *in vitro* evaluation of 3D printed ZrO_2 reinforced polylactide scaffolds through fused deposition modeling. *Materials Chemistry Frontiers*, 7(3), 464–475. https://doi.org/10.1039/D2QM01014C

Ali, A., Hassan, A., Rehman, S., Ashraf, S. T., Naz, K., & Naz, A. (2017). Regulation of genomic testing in the era of precision medicine. In *Progress and Challenges in Precision Medicine* (pp. 129–140). Elsevier. https://doi.org/10.1016/B978-0-12-809411-2.00007-6

Appidi, T., Ravichandran, G., Mudigunda, S. V., Thomas, A., Jogdand, A. B., Kishen, S., Subramaniyam, K., Emani, N., Prabusankar, G., & Rengan, A. K. (2021). Highly fluorescent polyethylene glycol-ascorbic acid complex for imaging and antimicrobial therapeutics. *Materials Today Communications*, 29, 102987. https://doi.org/10.1016/j.mtcomm.2021.102987

Ashkarran, A. A., Sharifi, S., LaRock, C. N., & Mahmoudi, M. (2024). Improved methodology for evaluating nanomedicine antibacterial properties in biological fluids. *ACS Pharmacology & Translational Science*, 7(3), 855–862. https://doi.org/10.1021/acsptsci.3c00348

Bar-Zeev, M., Livney, Y. D., & Assaraf, Y. G. (2017). Targeted nanomedicine for cancer therapeutics: Towards precision medicine overcoming drug resistance. *Drug Resistance Updates*, 31, 15–30. https://doi.org/10.1016/j.drup.2017.05.002

Beskow, L. M., Hammack-Aviran, C., Hazel, J. W., & Wolf, L. E. (2022). Perspectives on choice of law challenges in multistate precision medicine research. *Journal of Law and the Biosciences*, 9(1), lsac010. https://doi.org/10.1093/jlb/lsac010

Breckenridge, A., Eichler, H.-G., & Jarow, J. P. (2016). Precision medicine and the changing role of regulatory agencies. *Nature Reviews Drug Discovery*, 15(12), 805–806. https://doi.org/10.1038/nrd.2016.206

Buchbinder, E. I., & Hodi, F. S. (2023). Impact of precision medicine in oncology: Immuno-oncology. *The Cancer Journal*, 29(1), 15–19. https://doi.org/10.1097/PPO.0000000000000641

Buljan, M., & Wick, P. (2022). Tailoring design of nanomaterials and systems to individualize patient treatments. *CHIMIA*, 76(3), 236. https://doi.org/10.2533/chimia.2022.236

Cantafio, M. E. G., Grillone, K., Caracciolo, D., Scionti, F., Arbitrio, M., Barbieri, V., … & Di Martino, M. T. (2018). From single level analysis to multi-omics integrative approaches: A powerful strategy towards the precision oncology. *High-throughput*, *7*(4), 33.

Chandrakala, V., Aruna, V., & Angajala, G. (2022). Review on metal nanoparticles as nanocarriers: Current challenges and perspectives in drug delivery systems. *Emergent Materials*, 5(6), 1593–1615. https://doi.org/10.1007/s42247-021-00335-x

Cherian, A. M., Joseph, J., Nair, M. B., Nair, S. V., Vijayakumar, M., & Menon, D. (2022). Coupled benefits of nanotopography and titania surface chemistry in fostering endothelialization and reducing in-stent restenosis in coronary stents. *Biomaterials Advances*, 142, 213149. https://doi.org/10.1016/j.bioadv.2022.213149

Chikwambi, Z., Hidjo, M., Chikondowa, P., Jayeoba, G., Aketch, V., Afolabi, L., Awe, O. I., & Enoma, D. (2023). *Multi-Omics Data Integration Approach Identifies Potential Biomarkers for Prostate Cancer*. https://doi.org/10.1101/2023.01.26.522643

Cominetti, O., Agarwal, S., & Oller-Moreno, S. (2023). Editorial: Advances in methods and tools for multi-omics data analysis. *Frontiers in Molecular Biosciences*, 10, 1186822. https://doi.org/10.3389/fmolb.2023.1186822

Dai, Q., Jia, R., Li, H., Yang, J., & Qin, Z. (2024). Preparation and application of sustained-release antibacterial alginate hydrogels by loading plant-mediated silver nanoparticles. *ACS Sustainable Chemistry & Engineering*, 12(4), 1388–1404. https://doi.org/10.1021/acssuschemeng.3c04907

Delpierre, C., & Lefèvre, T. (2023). Precision and personalized medicine: What their current definition says and silences about the model of health they promote. Implication for the development of personalized health. *Frontiers in Sociology*, 8, 1112159. https://doi.org/10.3389/fsoc.2023.1112159

Demir Karaman, E., & Işık, Z. (2023). Multi-omics data analysis identifies prognostic biomarkers across cancers. *Medical Sciences*, 11(3), 44. https://doi.org/10.3390/medsci11030044

Demirpolat, E. (2023). Pharmacogenetics and pharmacogenomics in precision medicine. In H. S. Tuli & M. B. Yerer Aycan (Eds.), *Oncology: Genomics, Precision Medicine and Therapeutic Targets* (pp. 151–162). Springer Nature Singapore. https://doi.org/10.1007/978-981-99-1529-3_5

Díez-Pascual, A. M. (2022). Surface engineering of nanomaterials with polymers, biomolecules, and small ligands for nanomedicine. *Materials*, 15(9), 3251. https://doi.org/10.3390/ma15093251

Ding, L., Agrawal, P., Singh, S. K., Chhonker, Y. S., Sun, J., & Murry, D. J. (2024). Polymer-Based drug delivery systems for cancer therapeutics. *Polymers*, 16(6), 843. https://doi.org/10.3390/polym16060843

Duffy, D. J. (2016a). Problems, challenges and promises: Perspectives on precision medicine. *Briefings in Bioinformatics*, 17(3), 494–504. https://doi.org/10.1093/bib/bbv060

Elzagallaai, A., Barker, C., Lewis, T., Cohn, R., & Rieder, M. (2023). Advancing precision medicine in paediatrics: Past, present and future. *Cambridge Prisms: Precision Medicine*, *1*, e11. https://doi.org/10.1017/pcm.2022.14

Espinoza, S. M., Patil, H. I., San Martin Martinez, E., Casañas Pimentel, R., & Ige, P. P. (2020). Poly-ε-caprolactone (PCL), a promising polymer for pharmaceutical and biomedical applications: Focus on nanomedicine in cancer. *International Journal of Polymeric Materials and Polymeric Biomaterials*, 69(2), 85–126. https://doi.org/10.1080/00914037.2018.1539990

Finbloom, J. A., Huynh, C., Huang, X., & Desai, T. A. (2023). Bioinspired nanotopographical design of drug delivery systems. *Nature Reviews Bioengineering*, 1(2), 139–152. https://doi.org/10.1038/s44222-022-00010-8

Gaur, N., Dharwadkar, R., & Thomas, J. (2022). Personalized therapy using deep learning advances. In R. Malviya, G. Ghinea, R. K. Dhanaraj, B. Balusamy, & S. Sundram (Eds.), *Deep Learning for Targeted Treatments* (1st ed., pp. 171–197). Wiley. https://doi.org/10.1002/9781119857983.ch6

Germain, M., Caputo, F., Metcalfe, S., Tosi, G., Spring, K., Åslund, A. K. O., Pottier, A., Schiffelers, R., Ceccaldi, A., & Schmid, R. (2020). Delivering the power of nanomedicine to patients today. *Journal of Controlled Release*, 326, 164–171. https://doi.org/10.1016/j.jconrel.2020.07.007

Ghazy, M. G. M., & Hanafy, N. A. N. (2024). Targeted therapies for breast and lung cancers by using Propolis loaded albumin protein nanoparticles. *International Journal of Biological Macromolecules*, 260, 129338. https://doi.org/10.1016/j.ijbiomac.2024.129338

Ghosh, S. (2004). Recent research and development in synthetic polymer-based drug delivery systems. *Journal of Chemical Research*, 2004(4), 241–246. https://doi.org/10.3184/0308234041209158

Golestannezhad, N., Divsalar, A., Badalkhani-Khamseh, F., Rasouli, M., Seyedarabi, A., Ghalandari, B., Ding, X., Goli, F., Bekeschus, S., Movahedi, A. A. M., & Moghadam, M. E. (2024). Oxali-palladium nanoparticle synthesis, characterization, protein binding, and apoptosis induction in colorectal cancer cells. *Journal of Materials Science: Materials in Medicine*, 35(1), 4. https://doi.org/10.1007/s10856-023-06766-8

Guo, X., Wang, L., Wei, X., & Zhou, S. (2016). Polymer-based drug delivery systems for cancer treatment: REVIEWS. *Journal of Polymer Science Part A: Polymer Chemistry*, 54(22), 3525–3550. https://doi.org/10.1002/pola.28252

Hammack, C. M., Brelsford, K. M., & Beskow, L. M. (2019). Thought leader perspectives on participant protections in precision medicine research. *Journal of Law, Medicine & Ethics*, 47(1), 134–148. https://doi.org/10.1177/1073110519840493

Han, H. S., Koo, S. Y., & Choi, K. Y. (2022). Emerging nanoformulation strategies for phytocompounds and applications from drug delivery to phototherapy to imaging. *Bioactive Materials*, 14, 182–205. https://doi.org/10.1016/j.bioactmat.2021.11.027

Hare, J. I., Lammers, T., Ashford, M. B., Puri, S., Storm, G., & Barry, S. T. (2017). Challenges and strategies in anti-cancer nanomedicine development: An industry perspective. *Advanced Drug Delivery Reviews*, 108, 25–38. https://doi.org/10.1016/j.addr.2016.04.025

He, K., Hu, C., Ding, Y.-F., Cai, W., Huang, D., Mo, L., Liu, J., & Wang, R. (2024). Renal-clearable luminescent gold nanoparticles incorporating active and bio-orthogonal tumor-targeting for drug delivery and controlled release. *Nano Today*, 56, 102245. https://doi.org/10.1016/j.nantod.2024.102245

Hisan, U. K., & Amri, M. M. (2023). Recommendation of precision medicine application in Indonesia from multiple perspective: A review. *International Journal of Public Health Science (*IJPHS*)*, 12(1), 225. https://doi.org/10.11591/ijphs.v12i1.22010

Hood, L., & Friend, S. H. (2011). Predictive, personalized, preventive, participatory (P4) cancer medicine. *Nature Reviews Clinical Oncology*, 8(3), 184–187. https://doi.org/10.1038/nrclinonc.2010.227

Ibrahim, B., Akere, T. H., Chakraborty, S., Valsami-Jones, E., & Ali-Boucetta, H. (2024). Modulation of heat shock protein expression in alveolar adenocarcinoma cells through gold nanoparticles and cisplatin treatment. *Pharmaceutics*, 16(3), 380. https://doi.org/10.3390/pharmaceutics16030380

Ilyas, S. (2023). Stem cells: DNA microarray approach. *International Journal of Ecophysiology*, 4(1), 61–70. https://doi.org/10.32734/ijoep.v4i1.11151

Jain, H., Karulkar, A., Sharma, N., Sengar, M., Jaiswal, A., Shah, S., Khan, A., Firfiray, A., Asija, S., Suvasia, P., Suvasia, P., Pendhari, J., Kalra, D., Ravikumar, S., Narula, G., Banavali, S., Poojary, M., Hiregoudar, S., Nayak, L., … Shah, N. N. (2022). Phase I trial of humanized CD19 CART-cell therapy developed in India: Safe, active and feasible for outpatient therapy. *Blood*, 140(Supplement 1), 10332–10334. https://doi.org/10.1182/blood-2022-166082

Jain, S., Singh, A. P., Kumar, A., Saluja, R., & Nema, R. (2022). Stem cells research prospects towards precision medicine. *Bratislava Medical Journal*, 123(11), 795–805. https://doi.org/10.4149/BLL_2022_128

Kargozar, S., & Mozafari, M. (2018). Nanotechnology and nanomedicine: Start small, think big. *Materials Today:* Proceedings, 5(7), 15492–15500. https://doi.org/10.1016/j.matpr.2018.04.155

Khandelwal, V., Sharma, T., Gupta, S., Singh, S., Sharma, M. K., Parashar, D., & Kashyap, V. K. (2023). Stem cell therapy: A novel approach against emerging and re-emerging viral infections with special reference to SARS-CoV-2. *Molecular Biology Reports*, 50(3), 2663–2683. https://doi.org/10.1007/s11033-022-07957-2

Kiran, N. S., Yashaswini, C., Maheshwari, R., Bhattacharya, S., & Prajapati, B. G. (2024). Advances in precision medicine approaches for colorectal cancer: From molecular profiling to targeted therapies. *ACS Pharmacology & Translational Science*, acsptsci.4c00008. https://doi.org/10.1021/acsptsci.4c00008

Leibel, S. L., McVicar, R. N., Bush, A., & Snyder, E. Y. (2022). Using human induced pluripotent stem cells to advance personalized/precision medicine. In *Current Topics in iPSCs Technology* (pp. 45–61). Elsevier. https://doi.org/10.1016/B978-0-323-99892-5.00005-0

Li, S., Li, X., Xu, Y., Fan, C., Li, Z. A., Zheng, L., Luo, B., Li, Z.-P., Lin, B., Zha, Z.-G., Zhang, H.-T., & Wang, X. (2024). Collagen fibril-like injectable hydrogels from self-assembled nanoparticles for promoting wound healing. *Bioactive Materials*, 32, 149–163. https://doi.org/10.1016/j.bioactmat.2023.09.012

Li, X. (2023). Pharmacogenomics. In *Cases in Laboratory Genetics and Genomics (LGG) Practice* (pp. 129–132). Elsevier. https://doi.org/10.1016/B978-0-323-99622-8.00009-5

Liz-Marzán, L. M., Nel, A. E., Brinker, C. J., Chan, W. C. W., Chen, C., Chen, X., Ho, D., Hu, T., Kataoka, K., Kotov, N. A., Parak, W. J., & Stevens, M. M. (2022). What do we mean when we say nanomedicine? *ACS Nano*, 16(9), 13257–13259. https://doi.org/10.1021/acsnano.2c08675

Luo, J., Gong, T., & Ma, L. (2020). Chondroitin-modified lipid nanoparticles target the Golgi to degrade extracellular matrix for liver cancer management. *Carbohydrate Polymers*, 249, 116887. https://doi.org/10.1016/j.carbpol.2020.116887

MaHam, A., Tang, Z., Wu, H., Wang, J., & Lin, Y. (2009). Protein-based nanomedicine platforms for drug delivery. *Small*, 5(15), 1706–1721. https://doi.org/10.1002/smll.200801602

Manchia, M., & Murri, M. B. (2023). The role of pharmacogenomics in precision psychiatry. *Pharmacogenomics*, 24(10), 523–527. https://doi.org/10.2217/pgs-2023-0112

Memon, B., & Abdelalim, E. M. (2022). Toward precision medicine with human pluripotent stem cells for diabetes. *Stem Cells Translational Medicine*, 11(7), 704–714. https://doi.org/10.1093/stcltm/szac030

Mitchell, M. J., Billingsley, M. M., Haley, R. M., Wechsler, M. E., Peppas, N. A., & Langer, R. (2021). Engineering precision nanoparticles for drug delivery. *Nature Reviews Drug Discovery*, 20(2), 101–124. https://doi.org/10.1038/s41573-020-0090-8

Mol, P. G. M., Thompson, A., Heerspink, H. J. L., & Leufkens, H. G. M. (2018). Precision medicine in diabetes and diabetic kidney disease: Regulatory considerations. *Diabetes, Obesity and Metabolism*, 20(S3), 19–23. https://doi.org/10.1111/dom.13453

Morgan, P., Brown, D. G., Lennard, S., Anderton, M. J., Barrett, J. C., Eriksson, U., Fidock, M., Hamrén, B., Johnson, A., March, R. E., Matcham, J., Mettetal, J., Nicholls, D. J., Platz, S., Rees, S., Snowden, M. A., & Pangalos, M. N. (2018). Impact of a five-dimensional framework on R&D productivity at AstraZeneca. *Nature Reviews Drug Discovery*, 17(3), 167–181. https://doi.org/10.1038/nrd.2017.244

Naithani, N., Sinha, S., Misra, P., Vasudevan, B., & Sahu, R. (2021). Precision medicine: Concept and tools. *Medical Journal Armed Forces India*, 77(3), 249–257. https://doi.org/10.1016/j.mjafi.2021.06.021

Nguyen, T. B., Lac, Q., Abdi, L., Banerjee, D., Deng, Y., & Zhang, Y. (2023). Harshening stem cell research and precision medicine: The states of human pluripotent cells stem cell repository diversity, and racial and sex differences in transcriptomes. *Frontiers in Cell and Developmental Biology*, 10, 1071243. https://doi.org/10.3389/fcell.2022.1071243

Obradovic, A. (2023). Precision immunotherapy. *Science (*New York, N.Y.), 379(6633), 654–655. https://doi.org/10.1126/science.adg5585

Patel, B., Dennison, B., Allen, S., Stapleton, J., Archuleta, R., Rath, M. L., Mehra, N., & Talwalkar, S. S. (2023). Precision immuno-oncology (IO) ISH/IF multiplex panel: Spatial detection of cytokines and IO biomarkers. *Journal of Clinical Oncology*, 41(16_suppl), e14654–e14654. https://doi.org/10.1200/JCO.2023.41.16_suppl.e14654

Patel, P., Garala, K., Singh, S., Prajapati, B. G., & Chittasupho, C. (2024). Lipid-based nanoparticles in delivering bioactive compounds for improving therapeutic efficacy. *Pharmaceuticals*, 17(3), 329. https://doi.org/10.3390/ph17030329

Patra, J. K., Das, G., Fraceto, L. F., Campos, E. V. R., Rodriguez-Torres, M. D. P., Acosta-Torres, L. S., Diaz-Torres, L. A., Grillo, R., Swamy, M. K., Sharma, S., Habtemariam, S., & Shin, H.-S. (2018). Nano based drug delivery systems: Recent developments and future prospects. *Journal of Nanobiotechnology*, 16(1), 71. https://doi.org/10.1186/s12951-018-0392-8

Pelaz, B., Alexiou, C., Alvarez-Puebla, R. A., Alves, F., Andrews, A. M., Ashraf, S., Balogh, L. P., Ballerini, L., Bestetti, A., Brendel, C., Bosi, S., Carril, M., Chan, W. C. W., Chen, C., Chen, X., Chen, X., Cheng, Z., Cui, D., Du, J., … Parak, W. J. (2017). Diverse applications of nanomedicine. *ACS Nano*, 11(3), 2313–2381. https://doi.org/10.1021/acsnano.6b06040

Peng, J., Jury, E. C., Dönnes, P., & Ciurtin, C. (2021). Machine learning techniques for personalised medicine approaches in immune-mediated chronic inflammatory diseases: Applications and challenges. *Frontiers in Pharmacology*, 12, 720694. https://doi.org/10.3389/fphar.2021.720694

Qi, M., Cheng, Y., Liu, K., Cai, J., Liu, T., Wu, X., Tang, H., Huang, H., Chen, Q., & Zhou, X. (2024). Recombinant human heavy chain ferritin nanoparticles serve as ROS scavengers for the treatment of ischemic stroke. *International Journal of Nanomedicine*, Volume 19, 2285–2299. https://doi.org/10.2147/IJN.S449606

Qu, S., Han, X., & Yu, Y. (2024). Protective effects of copper nanoparticles green-formulated by Ginkgo biloba leaf extract on cardiac function in obese insulin-resistant rats. *Inorganic Chemistry Communications*, 162, 112204. https://doi.org/10.1016/j.inoche.2024.112204

Rahman, M. (2023). Magnetic resonance imaging in personalized medicine. In *Metabolomics* (pp. 199–238). Elsevier. https://doi.org/10.1016/B978-0-323-99924-3.00001-7

Rizvi, A. A., Abbas, M., Verma, S., Verma, S., Khan, A., Raza, S. T., & Mahdi, F. (2022). Determinants in tailoring antidiabetic therapies: A personalized approach. *Global Medical Genetics*, 09(02), 063–071. https://doi.org/10.1055/s-0041-1741109

Roychowdhury, R., Das, S. P., Gupta, A., Parihar, P., Chandrasekhar, K., Sarker, U., Kumar, A., Ramrao, D. P., & Sudhakar, C. (2023). Multi-omics pipeline and omics-integration approach to decipher plant's abiotic stress tolerance responses. *Genes*, *14*(6), 1281. https://doi.org/10.3390/genes14061281

Sadee, W., Wang, D., Hartmann, K., & Toland, A. E. (2023). Pharmacogenomics: Driving personalized medicine. *Pharmacological Reviews*, 75(4), 789–814. https://doi.org/10.1124/pharmrev.122.000810

Saha, S., Trivedi, D., Rengan, A. K., & Yu, A. (2024). Polyurethane nanoparticles as versatile tools in nanomedicine: A review. *ACS Applied Nano Materials*, 7(6), 5729–5744. https://doi.org/10.1021/acsanm.3c06071

Sandbhor, P., Palkar, P., Bhat, S., John, G., & Goda, J. S. (2024). Nanomedicine as a multimodal therapeutic paradigm against cancer: On the way forward in advancing precision therapy. *Nanoscale*, 16(13), 6330–6364. https://doi.org/10.1039/D3NR06131K

Sevelius, J. M., Gutierrez-Mock, L., Zamudio-Haas, S., McCree, B., Ngo, A., Jackson, A., Clynes, C., Venegas, L., Salinas, A., Herrera, C., Stein, E., Operario, D., & Gamarel, K. (2020). Research with marginalized communities: Challenges to continuity during the COVID-19 pandemic. *AIDS and Behavior*, *24*(7), 2009–2012. https://doi.org/10.1007/s10461-020-02920-3

Shastri, A., Sawant, D., & Parmar, N. (2021). A Review on Personalized Therapies. *Journal of Pharmaceutical Research International*, 115–127. https://doi.org/10.9734/jpri/2021/v33i39B32188

Shaw, J., Sekalala, S., & Fiske, A. (2024). The urgent need for health data justice in precision medicine. *The American Journal of Bioethics*, 24(3), 101–103. https://doi.org/10.1080/15265161.2024.2303141

Shrestha, B., Tang, L., & Hood, R. L. (2022). Nanotechnology for personalized medicine. In N. Gu (Ed.), *Nanomedicine* (pp. 1–48). Springer Nature Singapore. https://doi.org/10.1007/978-981-13-9374-7_18-1

Singh, A. K., Malviya, R., & Verma, S. (2023). Personalized medicine: Advanced treatment strategies to revolutionize healthcare. *Current Drug Research Reviews*, 15(2), 101–104. https://doi.org/10.2174/2589977515666221104152641

Singh, R., & Lillard, J. W. (2009). Nanoparticle-based targeted drug delivery. *Experimental and Molecular Pathology*, 86(3), 215–223. https://doi.org/10.1016/j.yexmp.2008.12.004

Stenzinger, A., Moltzen, E. K., Winkler, E., Molnar-Gabor, F., Malek, N., Costescu, A., Jensen, B. N., Nowak, F., Pinto, C., Ottersen, O. P., Schirmacher, P., Nordborg, J., Seufferlein, T., Fröhling, S., Edsjö, A., Garcia-Foncillas, J., Normanno, N., Lundgren, B., Friedman, M., … Rosenquist, R. (2023). Implementation of precision medicine in healthcare—A European perspective. *Journal of Internal Medicine*, 294(4), 437–454. https://doi.org/10.1111/joim.13698

Taati, H., Sangani, H., Davoudi, A., Safabakhsh Kouchesfahani, S., Hedayati, M., Tarashandeh Hemmati, S., Ghasemipour, T., Aghajani, S., Farah Andooz, M., Amanollahi, M., Kalavari, F., & Salehzadeh, A. (2024). Silver nanoparticle functionalized by glutamine and conjugated with thiosemicarbazide induces apoptosis in colon cancer cell line. *Scientific Reports*, 14(1), 3809. https://doi.org/10.1038/s41598-024-54344-x

Takallu, S., Kakian, F., Bazargani, A., Khorshidi, H., & Mirzaei, E. (2024). Development of antibacterial collagen membranes with optimal silver nanoparticle content for periodontal regeneration. *Scientific Reports*, 14(1), 7262. https://doi.org/10.1038/s41598-024-57951-w

Thapa, R. K., & Kim, J. O. (2023). Nanomedicine-based commercial formulations: Current developments and future prospects. *Journal of Pharmaceutical Investigation*, 53(1), 19–33. https://doi.org/10.1007/s40005-022-00607-6

Turolo, S., Edefonti, A., Syren, M. L., & Montini, G. (2023). Pharmacogenomics of old and new immunosuppressive drugs for precision medicine in kidney transplantation. *Journal of Clinical Medicine*, 12(13), 4454. https://doi.org/10.3390/jcm12134454

Valla, V., Alzabin, S., Koukoura, A., Lewis, A., Nielsen, A. A., & Vassiliadis, E. (2021). Companion diagnostics: State of the art and new regulations. *Biomarker Insights*, 16, 11772719211047763. https://doi.org/10.1177/11772719211047763

Vashist, A., Vashist, A., Gupta, Y. K., & Ahmad, S. (2014). Recent advances in hydrogel based drug delivery systems for the human body. *Journal of Materials Chemistry B*, 2(2), 147–166. https://doi.org/10.1039/C3TB21016B

Verbaanderd, C., Trullás Jimeno, A., Engelbergs, J., Zander, H., Reischl, I., Moreno Oliver, A., Vamvakas, S., Vleminckx, C., Bouygues, C., Girard, T., Day, F., & Frias, Z. (2023). Biomarker-driven developments in the context of the new regulatory framework for companion diagnostics in the European Union. *Clinical Pharmacology & Therapeutics*, 114(2), 316–324. https://doi.org/10.1002/cpt.2928

Verma, S., Abbas, M., Verma, S., Abbas Rizvi, A., Khan, A., Tasleem Raza, S., & Mahdi, F. (2021). A perspective of precision medicine in the management of COVID-19. *Novel Research in Microbiology Journal*, 5(4), 1313–1324. https://doi.org/10.21608/nrmj.2021.190247

Wang, Q., Du, H., Li, F., & Ling, D. (2023). Nano-metamaterial: A state-of-the-art material for magnetic resonance imaging. *Small Science*, 3(8), 2300015. https://doi.org/10.1002/smsc.202300015

Wang, Y., Li, Z., Mo, F., Chen-Mayfield, T.-J., Saini, A., LaMere, A. M., & Hu, Q. (2023). Chemically engineering cells for precision medicine. *Chemical Society Reviews*, 52(3), 1068–1102. https://doi.org/10.1039/D2CS00142J

Wassif, R. K., Elkheshen, S. A., Shamma, R. N., Amer, M. S., Elhelw, R., & El-kayal, M. (2024). Injectable systems of chitosan in situ forming composite gel incorporating linezolid-loaded biodegradable nanoparticles for long-term treatment of bone infections. *Drug Delivery and Translational Research*, 14(1), 80–102. https://doi.org/10.1007/s13346-023-01384-x

Wollenhaupt, C., Sudhop, T., & Knoess, W. (2023). A systematic database approach to identify companion diagnostic testing in clinical trials under the new in vitro diagnostic medical devices regulation. *Diagnostics*, *13*(12), 2037. https://doi.org/10.3390/diagnostics13122037

Yao, Y. M. M., Donoho, G. P., Iversen, P. W., Zhang, Y., Van Horn, R. D., Forest, A., … & Peng, S. B. (2017). Mouse PDX trial suggests synergy of concurrent inhibition of RAF and EGFR in colorectal cancer with BRAF or KRAS mutations. *Clinical Cancer Research*, *23*(18), 5547–5560.

Zhang, C., Yan, L., Wang, X., Zhu, S., Chen, C., Gu, Z., & Zhao, Y. (2020). Progress, challenges, and future of nanomedicine. *Nano Today*, 35, 101008. https://doi.org/10.1016/j.nantod.2020.101008

Zhang, F., Zhang, S., Cui, S., Jing, X., Feng, Y., & Coseri, S. (2024). Rapid self-healing carboxymethyl chitosan/hyaluronic acid hydrogels with injectable ability for drug delivery. *Carbohydrate Polymers*, 328, 121707. https://doi.org/10.1016/j.carbpol.2023.121707

Zhang, W., Yang, Y., & Cui, B. (2021). New perspectives on the roles of nanoscale surface topography in modulating intracellular signaling. *Current Opinion in Solid State and Materials Science*, 25(1), 100873. https://doi.org/10.1016/j.cossms.2020.100873

Zhao, J., Fong, A., Seow, S. V., & Toh, H. C. (2023). Organoids as an Enabler of Precision Immuno-Oncology. *Cells*, *12*(8), 1165. https://doi.org/10.3390/cells12081165

12 Evaluation of Biocompatibility and Toxicity of Nanoparticles In Vitro and In Vivo

Navya Shet and Akshath Uchangi Satyaprasad
Department of Bio and Nanotechnology, Nitte (Deemed to be University), Nitte University Centre for Science Education and Research-NUCSER, Mangalore, India

ABBREVIATIONS

3-MPA	3-Mercaptopropionic acid
AchE	Acetylcholinesterase
Akt	Protein Kinase B (PKB)
AgNPs	Silver Nanoparticles
AuNPs	Gold Nanoparticles
BSA	Bovine Serum Albumin
CdTe QDs	Cadmium Telluride Quantum Dots
CuS	Copper Sulfide
DCFH-DA	2′,7′ Dichlorodihydrofluorescein Diacetate
ELISA	Enzyme-Linked Immunosorbent Assay
EMSAs	Electrophoretic Mobility Shift Assays
EPR	Electron Paramagnetic Resonance
FANC	Fluorescent Gold Nanoclusters Conjugated with Lipoic Acid
FDA	Food and Drug Administration
FITC	Fluorescein Isothiocyanate
GM-CSF	Granulocyte-Macrophage Colony-Stimulating Factor
GSH	Glutathione
H2DCFDA	Dichlorodihydrofluorescein Diacetate
IL	Interleukin
IL-1β	Interleukin 1 Beta
IL-6	Interleukin 6
IL-8	Interleukin 8
INT	Iodonitrotetrazolium
MAPK	Mitogen-Activated Protein Kinase
MEA	Mercaptoethylamine
MPA	Mercaptopropionic Acid
MTT	3-(4,5-Dimethylthiazol-2-yl)-2,5-Diphenyltetrazolium Bromide
NADH	Nicotinamide Adenine Dinucleotide
NF-κB	Nuclear Factor Kappa-Light-Chain-Enhancer of Activated B Cells
NLRP3	NLR Pyrin Domain Containing 3
NPs	Nanoparticles
PBMC	Peripheral Blood Mononuclear Cells
PEG	Polyethylene Glycol

DOI: 10.1201/9781003473015-12

PEI	Polyethyleneimine
PL	Photoluminescence
PLA	Polylactic Acid
PLGA	Poly(Lactic-Co-Glycolic Acid)
RT-PCR	Reverse Transcription Polymerase Chain Reaction
SEM	Scanning Electron Microscopy
SiO2 NPs	Silicon Dioxide Nanoparticles
SNPs	Single-Nucleotide Polymorphism
Src	Proto-Oncogene Tyrosine-Protein Kinase
TEM	Transmission Electron Microscopy
TGA	Thioglycolic Acid
TGF	Transforming Growth Factor
TGF-β1	Transforming Growth Factor Beta 1
TiO2 NPs	Titanium Dioxide Nanoparticles
TNF	Tumor Necrosis Factor
TNF-α	Tumor Necrosis Factor Alpha
WST-1	Water-Soluble Tetrazolium Salt
ZnCuInS/ZnS	Zinc Copper Indium Sulfide/Zinc Sulfide Quantum Dots
ZnO NPs	Zinc Oxide Nanoparticles

12.1 INTRODUCTION

Nanoparticles (NPs) are a fundamental component of nanotechnology, which typically range from 1 to 100 nm. NPs can originate both from natural sources like volcanoes, forest fires, and atmospheric gas-to-particle conversion, as well as human activities, including emissions from power plants, airplane engine metal fumes, combustion processes, and chemically synthesized NPs such as carbon nanotubes (CNTs), quantum dots (QDs), organic, and metal NPs (Srivastava, Gusain, and Sharma 2015). These synthetic NPs are prepared using various techniques, including chemical methods (top-down and bottom-up approaches) (Abid et al. 2022). NPs are generally grouped into three categories based on their composition. They can be broadly classified into three groups. The first category includes inorganic NPs, QDs, AuNPs, AgNPs, and metal oxide NPs like SiO_2NPs, TiO_2NPs, and ZnONPs. Organic NPs, such as chitosan and PLGA NPs, come under the second category. The third category comprises carbon-based NPs like CNTs and fibers (De Matteis 2017).

The unique properties of these NPs are that they have more active chemical interaction sites and are highly reactive due to their high surface area-to-volume ratio. In addition, NPs have properties that include catalytic potential, high reactivity, superior mechanical performance, surface functionalization ability, and a tunable porosity different from their parent bulk substances (Harish et al. 2022). All these properties explain why NPs are used in various sectors, including remediation of the environment, agricultural applications, food technology, biotechnology, and biomedical applications. They are used in multiple fields, such as drug delivery systems, gene therapy, cancer treatments, wastewater treatment, food additives, chemical and biological sensors, wound dressings, cosmetics, semiconductors, and catalysts (Rasouli, Barhoum, and Uludag 2018).

Due to their vast application, it is important to evaluate several factors related to NPs, such as their size, shape, dosage, route of entry, toxicity, biocompatibility, interaction with biomolecules, cellular uptake, stability in biological fluids, degradation products, byproducts, and potential for bioaccumulation (Sengul and Asmatulu 2020). It is essential to reduce the toxicity of the NPs due to their vast application, and one way to reduce toxicity is to improve biocompatibility by changing their chemical surface. These modifications can include the attachment of aptamers, proteins, ligands, oligosaccharides, or polymers such as PEG and PLGA, achieved through chemical or physical processes for specific delivery purposes (Large et al. 2019). To validate the surface modifications in NPs, characterization such as TEM, SEM, Fourier-transform infrared spectroscopy (FTIR),

Dynamic Light Scattering (DLS), and ζ-potential analysis has to be performed. Such an in-depth study must be conducted before such NPs can be used in biomedical contexts, especially in vitro and in vivo assays (Kumar and Dixit 2017).

12.2 MECHANISM OF TOXICITY

Upon administration of NPs, they interact with different cellular barriers and pass through them. They then accumulate in many body organs and interact with the cell, leading to cytotoxicity and subcellular toxicity (Raftis and Miller 2019). The level of toxicity depends on the exposure time of NPs, dosage, uptake, particle size, shape, composition, solubility, subcellular localization, aggregation, and surface characteristics of the NPs (Mo et al. 2019; Jeevanandam et al. 2018). Additionally, NPs interact with many biomolecules in the body, such as carbohydrates, proteins, and lipids, forming a protein corona. It alters the surface chemistry of the NPs and can activate the pathways of the complement system, leading to increased toxicity (Moghimi and Simberg 2017). This can cause endoplasmic reticulum (ER) stress, leading to protein unfolding and subsequent adverse effects such as loss of protein function, NP aggregation, protein fibrillation, activation of cell signaling pathways, formation of new antigenic sites, disruption of enzyme function, and development of cancer (Neagu et al. 2017). Additionally, NPs obstruct membrane receptors and ion channels, disrupting normal bodily functions (Leifert et al. 2013). This results in the generation of reactive oxygen species (ROS) and dissolution of NPs, affecting cellular function either externally or after NP internalization (Yoshida et al. 2015). The principal cause of oxidative stress is the NPs' ability to produce ROS, cell internalization, free radicals on the surfaces of NPs, and the addition of redox-active groups to functionalize NPs (Garcés et al. 2021). Furthermore, NPs can cause disruption of mitochondrial function, abnormal ROS signaling, respiratory chain dysfunction, and impairment of the detoxification system, inducing indirect oxidative stress (Gasmi et al. 2021). Various types of ROS are produced, such as peroxyl radical, organic peroxides, hydroxyl radical, superoxide anion, hydrogen peroxide, hydroxyl radical, peroxyl radical, singlet oxygen, and peroxynitrite (Garcés et al. 2021).

Most metal-based NPs generate free radicals through the Haber–Weiss and Fenton reactions by following a two-step process, where $O_2^{\bullet-}$ interacts with H_2O_2 in the presence of transition metals. In the first step, oxidized metal is reduced by $O_2^{\bullet-}$. In the second step, the Fenton reaction (a part of the Haber–Weiss reaction) reduces the metal, which interacts with hydrogen peroxide (H_2O_2) to give hydroxyl radical (Garcés et al. 2021). These radicals can trigger the complement system and hypersensitivity reaction and cause an impact on cell signaling pathways such as MAPK, NF-κB, Src, and Akt, ultimately influencing cell differentiation, proliferation, and survival (Nyga, Hart, and Tetley 2015). These processes cause the release of intracellular contents and trigger an inflammatory response (Wang et al. 2020). This will also lead to the loss of cellular function, deoxyribonucleic acid (DNA) mutations, mitochondrial damage, apoptosis, pyroptosis, and necrosis, resulting in genotoxicity and cytotoxicity (Tan et al. 2018). Due to their similarity in size to viruses, NPs can activate the immune response and defense cells such as dendritic cells and neutrophils. This activation produces proinflammatory cytokines, including TGF-β1, TNF-α, IL-6, IL-8, and IL-1β, ultimately causing severe pulmonary inflammation and fibrosis (Zhan et al. 2021).

12.3 PROPERTIES OF NPS

12.3.1 Size

NPs with smaller sizes possess a higher surface area-to-volume ratio, exposing more NPs and facilitating more extensive chemical, biological interactions and catalytic activity with cellular components (Johnston et al. 2010).

The increased interaction between smaller NPs and cellular components leads to higher cytotoxicity and easier passage through biological membrane barriers than larger NPs (Khadanga and

Mishra 2024). Consequently, smaller NPs generally exhibit more significant cytotoxicity (Huo et al. 2014), and they evade the immune system by avoiding the recognition of phagocytic cells. This allows the smaller NPs to distribute more extensively across various tissues and organs, unlike the larger NPs, which are typically taken up by phagocytic cells and transported to the liver or spleen for clearance (Sukhanova et al. 2018).

12.3.2 Shape and Aspect Ratio

NPs come in various shapes, including spherical, triangular, star, cubic, hexagonal, oval, prism, rod, and spiral forms. Their shape also influences the toxicity of NPs, as different shapes affect cellular uptake and, consequently, cytotoxicity (Awashra and Młynarz 2023). For example, due to differences in endocytosis pathways and internalization rates, cells take up star-shaped NPs more efficiently than rod-shaped or triangular NPs, nanotubes, or nanorods. This efficient binding to cellular components, which directly damages the cell, results in higher cytotoxicity for star-shaped NPs (Xie et al. 2017).

The aspect ratio (R) is referred to as the ratio of the length (L) of an NP to its diameter (d). Aspect ratio is the key parameter controlling NP sensitivity, while other factors like size, shape, composition, cross-sectional area, and initial plasmonic resonance frequency have less influence. Spherical NPs have an aspect ratio of 1, whereas nanotubes have an aspect ratio of more than 1 (Khan, Zhao, and Liu 2016).

12.3.3 Surface Charge

The interaction of NPs with cellular components depends on their surface charge. Cationic NPs can be taken up more quickly by cells, bind with DNA, and induce damage than their negatively charged counterparts or those of neutral charge (Crisponi et al. 2017). The interaction between the cationic NPs, anionic DNA, and the surface of cell components can cause disruptions in the cellular processes, affect protein function, and activate the complement system and phagocytosis. These interactions can alter the cell cycle and produce severe toxic effects. NPs adsorb proteins, which form a protein corona that changes the surface charge and aids in aggregation (Gunawan et al. 2014). For example, positively charged silica NPs generate ROS more highly than neutral and negatively charged NPs (Bhattacharjee et al. 2010).

12.3.4 Surface Coating

Surface functionalization is the coating of the surface of the NPs with organic or inorganic compounds like PEG, PLGA, proteins, and lipids. It is mainly done to reduce the toxicity of the NPs due to changes in their interaction with the biological molecules. It also helps target specific cells and improve their uptake (Sukhanova et al. 2018). This will change their physicochemical properties, like electrical, magnetic, and optical properties (Ramakrishna and Rao 2011). For example, coating of the PEG ligand decreases the toxicity of the NPs (Simpson et al. 2013). However, if the functional molecule is positively charged, like polyethyleneimine (PEI)-coated iron oxide, then it will result in increasing the uptake of NPs due to the interaction between positively charged ligand and negatively charged cell membrane, resulting in toxicity (Feng et al. 2018).

12.3.5 Agglomeration

The adhesion of the NPs by weak forces is known as aggregation. Because of the NPs' high reactivity and colloidal instability, accumulation and cluster formation will occur (Egbuna et al. 2021). This will change the size, shape, and optical characteristics of the NPs (Majumder, Saha and Choudhuri

2023), increasing their toxicity. Thus, coating NPs with protective agents will help reduce their toxicity (Bantz et al. 2014).

12.3.6 Dissolution

Dissolution of the NPs is the breakdown of NPs into their ionic solution form. Several factors are responsible for the dissolution, such as size, shape, pH, capping agents, and dissolved organic substances in the environment. Metal ions can leak into the biological environment as a result of NP disintegration, producing ROS (Egbuna et al. 2021; Benameur, Wei, and Botta 2012).

12.3.7 Composition

The toxicity of the NPs is significantly influenced by their composition (Khadanga and Mishra 2024). Based on their chemical composition, NPs cause toxicity when they dissolve. Specific NPs, especially metal NPs, release ions that can be more toxic, such as cadmium and silver, or less harmful, such as iron and zinc, since they are biologically beneficial ions. However, in higher concentrations, the toxicity will increase. Such toxicity can be reduced by coating the surface of the NPs with biocompatible organic or inorganic compounds (Soenen et al. 2015).

12.3.8 Concentration

Dosage and concentration are other essential factors that are responsible for toxicity. As the concentration of the NPs and dosage increase, the toxicity also increases. For example, higher concentrations of gold NPs generate increased cellular leakage of lactate dehydrogenase, which damages the cells. Carbon fullerenes of higher concentration lead to an increase in the malformation (Khadanga and Mishra 2024; X. Li et al. 2015).

12.3.9 Hydrophobicity

The hydrophobicity of NPs is based on the type of the core material and the surface ligands. The toxicity of NPs, uptake, and corona formation depend on the hydrophobic nature of NPs. Several reports have shown that hydrophobic NPs lead to higher cytotoxicity and internalization than hydrophilic NPs (Bai et al. 2019) (Figure 12.1).

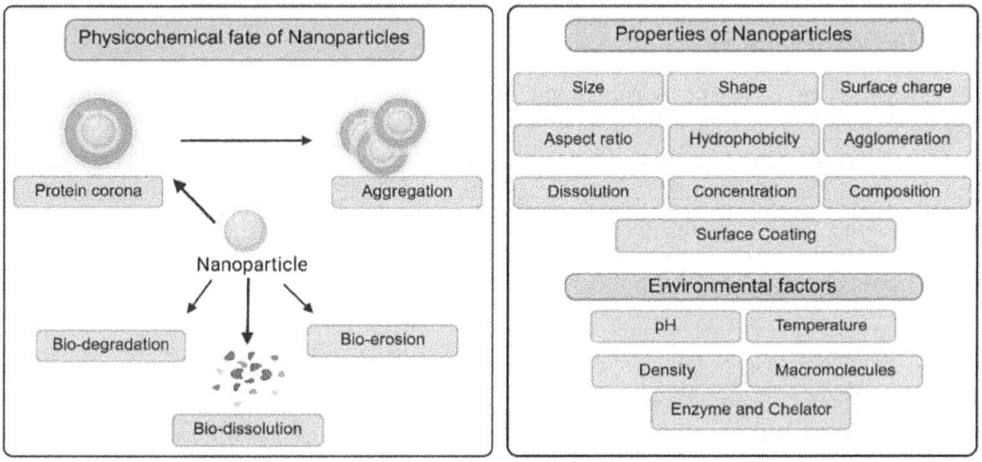

FIGURE 12.1 Schematic representation of the fate of NPs, properties and parameters influencing their stability. (Created with biorender.com.)

12.4 ROUTES OF EXPOSURE

12.4.1 Ingestion

NPs in food ingredients, supplements, and drinks enter the gastrointestinal system via oral route and reach the stomach (Braakhuis et al. 2015). The negatively charged mucus will trap the positively charged NPs; thus, negatively charged NPs can be more easily ingested than the positively charged ones (Crisponi et al. 2017). It is also possible that NPs can cross the mucosa, enter the bloodstream, and translocate into various organs, leading to organ damage (Hansson 2012). Once the NP reach the stomach, due to the low pH in gastric juice, the NPs' dissolution occurs, which leads to the release of ions. Villi and enterocytes will absorb them in the small intestine, and they can cross the intestinal epithelium by endocytosis or transcytosis. These NPs lead to inflammation and trigger ROS generation. It is seen that most of the NPs are excreted from the body through feces, and only some amounts of NPs cause damage to the organs (De Matteis 2017).

12.4.2 Inhalation

NPs in the contaminated air or aerosol enter the respiratory system by inhalation and spread all over the respiratory tract. Their impact on the lungs is determined by crucial factors such as size, concentration, rate of deposition, and elimination. Size is one of the essential factors based on which NPs settle at different respiratory tract sites (Bakand and Hayes 2016). The finest NPs with a size range of 0.1–1 μm can move by Brownian diffusion and gravitational sedimentation to the alveolar region and remain there for an extended period, interacting with the cells and causing damage to the cells, which can lead to their penetration. These small NPs can trigger ROS generation and inflammation. They can enter the blood and lymph through the damaged epithelial cells and reach various organs like heart, kidney, liver, and spleen. Larger NPs will remain either at the nasopharyngeal region (5 to 30 μm) or the tracheobronchial region (1–5 μm) (De Matteis 2017). Insoluble NPs such as carbon black and asbestos, commonly found in occupational environments, will be deposited on the lungs and removed only by alveolar macrophage phagocytosis and the mucociliary escalator. Most of the NPs will be entrapped by the mucus and reach the gastrointestinal tract, where they will undergo dissolution due to low pH. Small NPs can remain for many years, and lung tissues act against the small NPs, which causes damage to the lung tissue, asthma, and, ultimately, lung cancer (Crisponi et al. 2017).

12.4.3 Dermal Penetration

NPs in cosmetics or from the occupational area can enter the body quickly through dermal penetration (Kuwagata et al. 2017). Based on various factors such as temperature, pH, and size, the entry of the NPs will be determined. The skin cannot absorb large-sized NPs and must only enter through damaged skin (Filon et al. 2015). In contrast, small NPs can enter the stratum corneum at hair follicles. They can reach the circulatory system and reach out to various organs, which causes cellular apoptosis and DNA damage (Crisponi et al. 2017).

12.4.4 Injection

Injection is a route of exposure where NPs are injected into the circulatory system directly as a drug carrier in medical procedures. Since they enter the bloodstream, NPs can quickly move to various organs like the liver, spleen, heart, and kidney throughout the body and reach the target site quickly (Behroozi et al. 2022).

12.5 TYPES OF NPS

12.5.1 Quantum Dots

QDs are fluorescent, zero-dimensional NPs typically ranging from 1 to 10 nm in size. They are smaller than the Bohr radius of an exciton and were first identified by Alexey I. Ekimov in a glass matrix in 1981. QDs consist of a core, often coated with a shell and capped to enhance biocompatibility (Ramezani, Ghalehsardi, and Noorizadeh 2023). QDs can be classified as core-type, core-shell-type, or alloyed and can be semiconductor-based or carbon-based (Gidwani et al. 2021). They can be composed of single elements like silicon or germanium or compound elements such as cadmium selenide, cadmium telluride, indium phosphate, indium arsenide, lead sulfide, and lead selenide, typically with a zinc sulfide shell. These NPs are derived from II-VI or III-V elements of the periodic table (Park, Shin, and Yu 2021). The optical and fluorescent properties of QDs arise from their inorganic core, which is generally encapsulated by an inorganic shell with a more significant band gap and ligands that enhance optical characteristics (Reshma and Mohanan 2019). QDs are helpful for various applications due to their characteristics, which include quantum confinement, size-tunable light emission, broad absorption spectra, large strokes shift, high photostability, resistance to degradation, and high fluorescence quantum yield (Shukla 2014). Due to their unique characteristics, they are used in biosensing, imaging (such as intracellular and tissue tumor imaging), cancer detection, biomolecule identification and quantification, metal ion detection, pesticide detection, drug delivery, gene delivery, and theranostics. Specifically, ZnCuInS/ZnS and CdTe-QDs are frequently used for biosensing and imaging (Kargozar et al. 2020). QDs exhibit toxicity based on composition, surface functionalization, size and shape. For instance, cadmium sulfide capped with the dextrin and conjugated with doxorubicin showed accumulation and was distributed in the cytoplasmic and nuclear region in HeLa cells (De La Cruz et al. 2020).

12.5.2 Carbon Dots

Carbon dots (CDs) are zero-dimensional biocompatible nanomaterials characterized by their fluorescence and typically measuring less than 20 nm in size. Scrivens and colleagues first discovered it in 2004; they were termed carbon dots by Sun and colleagues in 2006 (Su et al. 2020). There are various types of CDs, including carbon QDs, carbon black dots, graphitic CDs, graphitic carbon nitride dots, polymeric dots, polymer/carbon hybrid dots, and co-doped (heteroatom) CDs. The carbon in these CDs is π-conjugated and exhibits sp^2/sp^3 hybridization (Truskewycz et al. 2022). Their distinct optical characteristics are due to π–π^* transitions of C=C bonds, resulting in strong UV absorption, high quantum yield, and significant stability with resistance to photobleaching (Wu, Liu, and Yuan 2017). CDs are biocompatible, cost-effective, environmentally friendly, highly sensitive, and easy to synthesize compared to other NPs. Due to their biocompatibility, CDs are used in various applications. They can be used for non-invasive in vitro and in vivo imaging, drug and gene delivery, biosensing, cancer, and stem cell detection, monitoring fluorescence changes in single cells, and in therapies like chemotherapy, photothermal, and photodynamic treatments. CDs are also helpful for detecting metal ions such as Zn^{2+}, Hg^{2+}, and Fe^{3+} (Liu, Li, and Yang 2020a).

However, CDs have shown varying toxicity effects on different model organisms. In ICR mice, CDs (5 to 8 nm) are primarily located in the lung and liver, where they have been shown to induce damage such as inflammation and cell death, as well as dose-dependent toxicity (Yang et al. 2018). In zebrafish, CDs were found to be minimally harmful at doses less than 150 μg/mL. Significant toxicity, including swelling of the egg yolk sac and pericardium, development retardation, mortality, decreased larval locomotor motion, dopamine levels, and various organ damage, were observed at concentrations exceeding 200 μg/mL (Liu et al. 2020b).

12.5.3 Graphene

Graphene is a two-dimensional six-membered benzene ring monolayer with a carbon atom that is sp^2 hybridized. It forms a honeycomb lattice by forming a π-bond with the p orbital electrons of the carbon atoms (Li et al. 2021a). In the carbon nanomaterial family, graphene is the basic form, and based on the functional groups, graphene-based NPs (GBNs) can be of various types such as graphene, reduced graphene oxide (rGO), graphene oxide (GO), and graphene QDs (GQDs) (Dasari Shareena et al. 2018). GBNs exhibit unique properties such as good electrical and thermal conductivity, optical properties, inert in nature, high mechanical and fracture strength, relative stability, low toxicity, high surface area, biocompatibility, and low cost (Peña-Bahamonde et al. 2018). Due to these properties, they are used in wide applications such as bioimaging, biosensing, catalysts, nano-optoelectronics, superconductors, quantum physics, drug delivery, gene and photothermal therapy, and imaging of near-infrared fluorescence (Li et al. 2021b). GO has a high physicochemical property due to the presence of functional groups on the surface, such as -COOH, -OH, -CH(O)CH, and -O- (Zhao et al. 2017). rGO is the reduced form of GO formed by thermal or chemical reduction and has a high photothermal and drug-loading ability (Li et al. 2017). In contrast, graphene also exhibits toxicity in vivo and in vitro. GO exhibited toxicity by inducing liver, lung, and spleen damage in Sprague-Dawley rats (Li et al. 2016). Apoptosis was induced by pristine graphene in murine RAW 264.7 macrophages, by disrupting mitochondrial membrane potential and activating the mitochondrial apoptotic pathway (Li et al. 2012).

12.5.4 Nanoclusters

Metal nanoclusters (MNCs) are small-sized 1–10 nm nanostructures with a core-shell structure. They show a phenomenon called quantum confinement and unique optical and catalytic characteristics (Nasrollahpour et al. 2023). They have distinct features like significant electrical properties, quantum confinement, intense PL, and nonoptical behavior (Maity, Bain, and Patra 2019). Nanoclusters (NCs) are classified into two groups: metallic and non-metallic NCs. The metal NC core can be made of homometallic like gold, silver, platinum, and copper; can be bi, tri, or tetra metallic with a few to hundreds of metal atoms; and the shell is made of the metal atom which is bridged to ligands like amino acids, DNA, dendrimers or polymers which will protect, increase their stability and quantum yield of the NCs (Lin et al. 2021). They have wide applications in bioimaging, drug/gene delivery, antibacterial agents, detecting nucleic acids, proteins, SNPs, and microRNA (Tao et al. 2015).

Although NCs have a wide range of applications, numerous reports indicate they can induce both in vivo and in vitro toxicity in cells. In zebrafish embryos, CuS NC modified with polymer (PATA3-C4@CuS) showed abnormal physical and genetic changes such as high rate of mortality, reduced head and eye size, swelling in the pericardial region, reduced hatching rates, and altered expression of certain genes involved in the gastrulation process (Zhang et al. 2022a). Bovine serum albumin (BSA) and L-histidine-modified ultra-small AuNCs accumulated in major organs such as the kidneys and lungs, but no significant damage was found in the tissue or organs of mice (Li et al. 2021a). Among AgNCs (2 nm) and TiO_2 NPs (5–15 and 30–50 nm), AgNCs showed high mutagenicity in the Ames test. TiO_2 NPs of both sizes and AgNCs showed toxicity in the chicken embryos by generating oxidative stress and lipid peroxidation (Zhang et al. 2022b).

12.5.5 Gold and Silver NPs

They are NPs with a size typically ranging from 1 to 100 nm with various shapes. The unique optical characteristics of gold NPs are surface plasmon resonance, tunable size, easy modification, and synthesis with various morphologies (Venditti 2019a). Typically, AuNPs are considered biocompatible and inert; thus, the FDA approved them for use in the biomedical field. They are highly used for

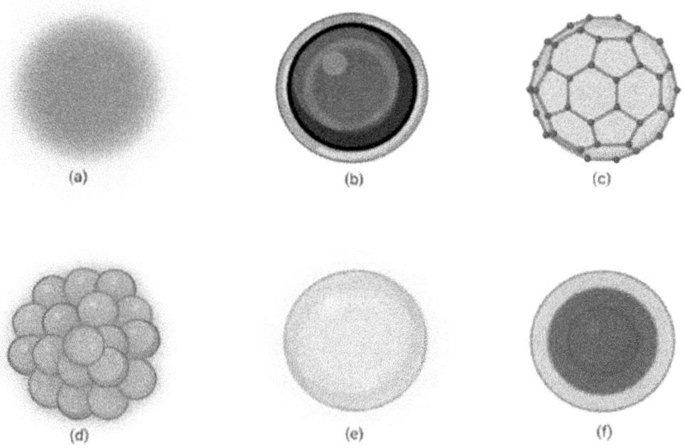

FIGURE 12.2 Schematic representation of types of NPs: (a) quantum dots, (b) carbon dots, (c) graphene, (d) nanocluster, (e) gold nanoparticles, and (f) silver nanoparticles. (Created with biorender.com.)

bioimaging, drug delivery agents, gene therapy, cancer therapy, and radiotherapy (Doren et al. 2011). The other widely used NPs are silver NPs used in the food, cosmetics, and textiles industry, and the biomedical field as biosensors, drug delivery agents, and bioimaging (Tan et al. 2021). However, they cause toxicity in cells by undergoing dissolution to form Ag^+ ions that increase the potential of the AgNPs to cause toxicity. It is vital to evaluate its in vivo and in vitro toxicity because of its vast applications (Jiravova et al. 2016). In male albino rats, the toxicity of AgNPs was found to be more significant than that of AuNPs due to their high reactivity. Moreover, both the NPs induced ROS, oxidative stress, alteration in the concentration of enzymes, inflammatory markers, and hormones (Al-Bishri 2018). AgNPs showed more in vivo toxicity than AuNPs by inducing higher ROS levels, oxidative stress, increased levels of liver enzymes, nuclear abnormalities, disruption of cells and tissue in the gill and liver of the zebrafish model (Ramachandran et al. 2018) (Figure 12.2).

12.6 BIOCOMPATIBILITY

Biocompatibility is defined as the ability of the material to show a suitable response in the host in a particular application. This material should not cause any harm or interaction between the host and the material, and it should be non-toxic, non-carcinogenic, non-allergenic, non-thrombogenic, and non-irritant to the host (Williams 2016). So, the material can be called highly biocompatible when it does not cause undesirable effects during the interaction between the host and the material. Therefore, biocompatible material will not stimulate or trigger an inflammatory reaction or the immune system (Williams 2008). The material's biocompatibility depends on its physicochemical properties, such as size, shape, and surface charge. Thus, the toxicity of NPs will be reduced by the alteration in size, shape, and modification at the surface levels (Kyriakides et al. 2021). Various artificial and natural polymers can be used for surface alteration or as carriers (Kumar et al. 2012). These biodegradable polymers have excellent biological compatibility and availability properties; they will have control over the size and surface properties of the NPs (Deirram et al. 2019). The most commonly used polymers are as follows:

Poly(D, L-lactide-co-glycolide) (PLGA): PLGA is the most extensively used polymer due to its biodegradable reaction with water to form lactic and glycolic acids (Agrawal, Patel, and Patel 2023). It is used in various applications as a delivery agent, nano-vaccines, and nanosponges. The release of encapsulated substances will depend upon the drug's dimensions and molecular mass, agents added, surface functionalization of the polymer, and the lactic to glycolic acid ratio (Mittal et al. 2007).

PLA is a biologically compatible and degradable polymer containing lactic acid units. It is an intermediate compound produced by synthesizing carbohydrates (Sreekumar, Bindhu, and Veluraja 2021).

Polycaprolactone (PCL): Compared to PLA, PCL has a slow degradation rate and undergoes hydrolysis in the biological environment at the ester linkage; hence, it is used in various long-lasting or permanent medical implants (Pranav et al. 2022).

Poly(alkyl-cyano-acrylates) (PAC) is biologically compatible and produces toxic products when esterases present in the biofluids degrade PAC, which is why using PAC is prohibited in humans. They are used in various applications and have significant advantages over the encapsulation of drugs (Sairam et al. 2023).

Chitosan is a natural biopolymer synthesized by moderate deacetylation of chitin obtained from crustaceans. They can be synthesized through ionotropic gelation, nano-emulsion, and polyelectrolyte complexation (Ambaye et al. 2022).

Gelatin is a natural biopolymer with cationic, anionic, and hydrophilic molecules and various applications. It is commonly used to encapsulate multiple molecules and medical applications due to its properties, such as the controlled delivery of encapsulated compounds (Kommareddy, Shenoy, and Amiji 2007).

Alginate is a natural biopolymer that forms cross-linkages with calcium ions through the ionotropic gelation technique to form a hydrogels. They are used to encapsulate various substances for sustained release (Severino et al. 2019).

Xanthan Gum is a natural biopolymer that is inert and used to encapsulate various substances released because of diffusion and matrix degradation (Virmani et al. 2023).

Liposomes are amphiphilic lipid nanostructures that can be functionalized with various ligands to increase their biocompatibility, stability, and retention time. They consist a phospholipid bilayer with the inner aqueous core (Musielak et al. 2021).

Dendrimers: Dendrimers are hyperbranched synthetic polymers with a core, dendrons, and multifunctional terminal groups that can be used as capping agents for metal NPs (Barman et al. 2018).

There are several methods to increase the biocompatibility of the NPs without changing their function.

12.7 STRATEGIES TO ENHANCE BIOCOMPATIBILITY

12.7.1 Size and Shape

The toxicity of the NPs can be reduced by changing the size of the NPs. By increasing the size, the cytotoxicity of the NPs can be decreased because larger NPs are more likely to be recognized by the reticuloendothelial system, which will remove the NPs from the circulation and body.

It is also seen that by changing the shape of the NPs, the toxicity of the NPs can be reduced; spherical-shaped NPs are known to cause less toxicity than other shapes due to their uniform orientation in biological systems (Breza and Šimon 2020).

12.7.2 Coating

It is the method of covering the surface of NPs with a protective layer. It helps to reduce the NPs' toxicity by acting as a physical barrier between the NPs and the external environment (Salazar-Alvarez et al. 2008). The coating helps reduce the oxidation of the NPs' metallic core, prevents the release of the hazardous substance into the biological system, and allows the functional molecules to attach to the NP surfaces (Sánchez-López et al. 2020).

There are many types of coating molecules, such as polyethylene glycol (PEG), zwitter ions, polyvinyl alcohol (PVA), polyvinyl pyrrolidone (PVP), and BSA, of which PEG is commonly used due to its advantages, such as increasing the duration of the circulation and shielding the charge of the NPs (Zhang, Xiong, and Liu 2022). This modification is usually done through noncovalent binding, which is reversible. It can also help by releasing a biocompatible molecule, which reduces the toxicity of NPs (Karakoti et al. 2008).

12.7.3 Doping

Doping is an electrochemical process of modifying the bandgap, which alters the binding properties and reduces the surface charge. The bandgap energy is the energy required by an electron to shift from the valence band region to the conduction band; it represents the stability of the NPs (Sharma et al. 2023). So, by altering the energy bandgap, ROS generation and the oxidative stress caused by the NPs can be reduced, thereby reducing the NPs toxicity. It was seen that Fe-doped titanium-NPs reduced ROS generation by modifying the energy bandgap (Hwang et al. 2012).

12.7.4 Grafting and Loading

The covalent bonding of NPs to other substances is known as grafting, and the noncovalent bonding of NPs to other substances is known as loading. These methods help reduce the toxicity of NPs by surface charge neutralization and change the toxicological profile of the NPs, especially with the metal NPs (Pounraj, Somu, and Paul 2018). Many polymers are used, such as cyclo-cages and fused rings; they have lobe channels that protect the NPs, hence reducing toxicity and stabilizing NPs, respectively (Ermis et al. 2022).

12.7.5 Ligation

Ligation refers to a process whereby several methods attach the functional group or aided moieties to specific NPs. These aided moieties help reduce the NPs' toxicity by preventing the accidental degradation of the NPs and by forming a protective shield around the NPs. They serve several purposes, such as increasing the therapeutic efficacy and bioavailability (Zangabad et al. 2017). Several ligated moieties exist, such as glutathione, vitamin E TPGS, lactoferrin, and BSA. Ligation is necessary when the NPs are sensitive to biodegradation in the body (Sharma et al. 2024).

12.7.6 Addition of an Antioxidant

Antioxidants are the compounds that neutralize the free radicals, which are produced due to the toxicity of the NPs. Thus, adding antioxidants is one strategy to reduce the NPs' toxicity (Li et al. 2013). Antioxidants can be coated on NPs by many mechanisms and can be physically or chemically bound on the surface of the NPs, including during the synthesis of the NPs. There are several antioxidants, such as curcumin, N-acetylcysteine, vitamins E and C, and glutathione. Many reports show that these antioxidants have reduced oxidative stress and the NPs associated toxicity. Antioxidants can also be administered to the environment before exposing the NPs (Kwak et al. 2003) (Figure 12.3).

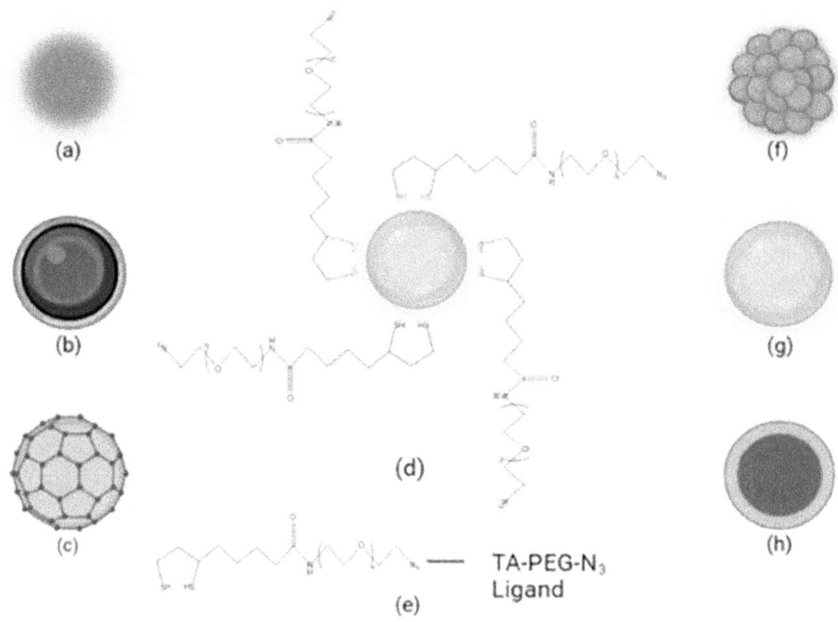

FIGURE 12.3 Schematic representation of NPs and gold NP clicked with the TA-PEG-N_3 ligand: (a) quantum dots; (b) carbon dots; (c) graphene; (d) gold NP clicked with TA-PEG-N_3 ligand; (e) structure of TA-PEG-N_3 ligand with the anchor group, hydrophilic segment, and functional azide group; (f) nanocluster; (g) gold NPs; and (h) silver NPs. (Created with biorender.com.)

12.8 BIOCOMPATIBILITY OF NPS

12.8.1 Quantum Dots

Heavy metal-containing QDs can be coated and modified using several kinds of ligands and compounds, including TGA, PEG, 3-MPA, D-penicillamine, PEG, N-acetyl-L-cysteine (NAC), polydiallydimethylammonium chloride (PDDA), carboxylic acid (CA), and amine (NH_2), to minimize their cytotoxicity (Liu and Tang 2020). QDs exhibit varying toxicity depending on the type and stability of the surface coating. CdSe/ZnS QDs without surface functionalization have been observed to exhibit cytotoxic effects by triggering liver pyroptosis and inflammation through the activation of NLRP3 inflammasomes. This results in the production of ROS and elevated calcium ion levels within the mitochondria of human hepatic LO2 cells (Lu et al. 2016), whereas QD functionalized with MPA had minimal toxicity. It was seen that, compared to MPA-functionalized QDs, PEGylated QDs produced more defective lysosomal organelles, leading to autophagy impairment (Peynshaert et al. 2017). CdTe-QDs functionalized with TGA interfered with the fluidity of the mitochondrial membrane, and they interacted with the mitochondrial permeability transition (MPT) pores in female Wistar rats. However, CdTe-QDs functionalized with MEA were biocompatible and weakly impacted membrane fluidity. CdTe-QDs coated with L-Cys demonstrated an even lesser effect on membrane fluidity (Xiang et al. 2018).

12.8.2 Carbon Dots

CDs are considered biocompatible and low-toxic because they do not ionize into toxic products or ions, and thus, they rarely cause cellular damage (Truskewycz et al. 2022). CD was found to be less toxic in mice, where only some amount of albumin and AChE activity was found in the serum, with no changes in bioassays and tissue, which was known during histology analysis (Hong et al. 2018). CDs with positively charged PEI (CDs-PEI) are known to cause more toxicity and cell damage by disrupting the phases of the cell cycle than negatively charged pristine CDs (CDs-Pri) in mouse fibroblasts (NIH/3T3). However, CDs with neutral charge are known to be more biocompatible without causing cell damage (Havrdova et al. 2016). No toxicity was seen in A549 cells, whereas in vivo toxicity varied based on the surface functional groups. Nitric acid-functionalized CDs exhibited higher toxicity than the carboxyl group during the initial days of administration in C57BL6 mice. However, this toxicity gradually decreased as the mice adapted to the treatment (Kuznietsova et al. 2023).

12.8.3 Graphene

GOs are generally modified with PEG, dextran, and amine to exhibit less toxicity and to enhance their dispersion in biological environments than the naked GO (Yang et al. 2011). PEG-functionalized GO induced low toxicity with an 80% viable rate of lymphoma cells (Du et al. 2014). Whereas in J774A.1 cell line and male BALB/c mice, polyacrylic acid showed higher biocompatibility than PEG-functionalized GO (Xu et al. 2016a). When compared with GO, rGO induced higher toxicity by generating ROS, oxidative stress, and antioxidant depletion in the Caco-2 cell line (Cebadero-Domínguez et al. 2022). Whereas rGO functionalized with PEG showed increased toxicity with increased dose, primarily through the generation of ROS and activation of an inflammatory reaction in the alveolar epithelial A549 cell line. In contrast, non-PEGylated rGO was found to exhibit toxicity at higher doses, leading to apoptosis after 24 hours of exposure (Reshma, Syama, and Mohanan 2016).

12.8.4 Nanoclusters

When modified with molecules like BSA, cytidine, dendrimers, transferrins, GSH, and mercaptopropionic acid, surface-functionalized NCs exhibit minimal toxicity, enhanced biocompatibility, and photostability. Some molecules like BSA, transferrin, and lysozyme stabilize the NC, thus reducing their toxicity (Dong et al. 2015). The study showed that BSA-AuNCs were taken up more by normal cells than tumor cells and inhibited tumor cell growth in a mouse model (Dong et al. 2015). AuNCs functionalized with MPA induced more ROS based on the uptake by exposed cells, which increased the proliferation of the cells and their metabolism than AuNCs-GSH (Tay et al. 2014). The study on FANC functionalized with α-lipoic acid found that FANC induced minimal toxicity with significant changes in body weight. However, there were no changes in animal activity and serum enzyme levels in ICR mice (Chen, Hsu, and Chung 2022).

12.8.5 Gold and Silver NPs

AuNPs and AgNPs functionalized with various molecules such as PEG, starch, gum Arabic, and citrate are known to have less toxic effects on the cells than bare NPs. When compared with starch and gum Arabic, citrate-functionalized AuNPs induced higher toxicity by reducing the viability of the MCF-7 and PC-3 cells, whereas gum Arabic exhibited minimal toxicity (Vijayakumar and Ganesan 2012). In contrast, bare AuNPs also showed biocompatibility without significant changes in body mass, organ damage, and survival rate in mice at specific concentrations (Kadhim et al. 2021).

Green-synthesized AgNPs showed varying toxicity based on the functional groups. In Sprague-Dawley rats, green-synthesized AgNPs showed negligible impact on the histology of the organs, even at greater dosages (Srisrimal et al. 2023). Further, AgNPs functionalized with PEG and BSA showed reduced ROS generation, oxidative stress, TNF-α production, and reduced cell death than bare AgNPs in PBMCs (Das et al. 2017).

12.9 IN VITRO TOXICITY OF NPS

In vitro toxicity is the study under laboratory conditions, using a particular part, such as organs, tissue, or cells, from the target organism. It reduces the time, cost, and helps to get the results within 2–3 days. Most currently used in vitro models give quantitative data in simpler terms (Shah, Bhagat, and Singh 2020).

Evaluation of cytotoxicity in vitro is done by using cell cultures. There are many assays to evaluate the cytotoxicity of NPs, and they can be grouped into five categories.

12.9.1 Multiplication and Survival of Cells

This assay is performed by examining the mitochondrial enzymes and cellular metabolism, based on the reduction of the tetrazolium salt (INT) to red-colored formazan (Kumar, Sharma, and Maitra 2017). The colorimetric assay, such as the MTT, INT, and WST-1 assay, operates on the principle that only living cells can reduce the dye via mitochondrial NADH enzymes into insoluble and soluble formazan crystals (Jo et al. 2015). Other assays, such as trypan blue, which stains explicitly dead cells, leaving viable cells unstained, neutral red dye that is retained only within the lysosomes of viable cells, and the Alamar Blue assay, undergo reduction by mitochondrial enzymes and exhibit red fluorescence in viable cells. Numerous reports of NPs have affected cell viability tests in various ways. The adsorption of mitochondrial enzymes on the surfaces of the NPs gives false results (Han et al. 2011).

12.9.2 Oxidative Stress and ROS

ROS are oxygen-containing free radicals generated by interacting with the NPs. Oxidative stress is triggered when extreme ROS are produced in the cell, leading to damage to enzymes, proteins, DNA, membranes, and organelles (He et al. 2017). There are direct methods to assess the ROS by using EPR and dyes such as DCFH-DA and H_2 DCFDA, which exhibit fluorescence when they undergo oxidation by ROS (Kalyanaraman et al. 2012). Other methods are performed by assessing the amount of antioxidants and disrupted molecules using protein carbonyl content, malondialdehyde levels, and 8-oxo-2′-deoxyguanosine (8-OdG) lesion. Other tests, such as comet, Ames, micronucleus, and chromosome aberration assays, are used to test the genomic toxicity. There are reports of NPs affecting the dye products by quenching or enhancing the dye's fluorescence.

12.9.3 Inflammatory Response

NPs-induced inflammatory response can be assessed by measuring the biomarkers such as IL, TNF-α, and GM-CSF. These biomarkers are derived from immune cells and can be measured using ELISA, EMSAs, RT-PCR, and western blotting. It has been stated that cytokines can be adsorbed on NPs, which gives false results in the above assays (Awashra and Młynarz 2023).

12.9.4 Necrosis and Apoptosis

Necrosis refers to the cell death that happens under pathological conditions, in an unprogrammed way, and apoptosis refers to programmed cell death (Kyrylkova et al. 2012). These processes can be identified based on the phosphatidylserine (PS) movement to the outer leaflet of the cellular membrane, indicating an early apoptotic state. Annexin-V protein binds to the PS present in the outer leaflet of the cellular membrane to detect apoptotic cells, and propidium iodide (PI) dye exhibits a high binding affinity for nucleic acids to detect necrotic cells. Thus, Annexin-V FITC/PI is a common assay used to differentiate between apoptotic and necrotic cells (Lakshmanan and Batra 2013).

12.9.5 Metabolomics

The conventional test, now presently used to determine cytotoxicity, cannot give information at the molecular level. The "omics" technique is a more sophisticated and recently developed method of determining the toxicity of the NPs. Metabolomics is a recent field in the omics era. It is a complete measurement of all metabolic byproducts and low-molecular-weight compounds in biomaterials such as tissues, cells, and organs (Clish 2015). The comprehensive analysis of compounds with low molecular weights can be determined via NMR or MS, along with the potent chemometric program (MetaboAnalyst), which detects the biomolecules and their derivatives (Pang et al. 2021).

12.10 CAUSES OF IN VITRO TOXICITY

12.10.1 Generation of ROS

ROS and oxidative stress induced by NPs lead to the damage of various organelles and cell death. The redox reaction in NPs, modification of NPs' surface with oxidative groups, and cellular internalization of the NPs increase the interaction between NPs and cellular components; these are three main processes that induce ROS and oxidative stress (Knaapen et al. 2004).

12.10.2 Proinflammatory Markers

NPs are taken up by macrophages via phagocytosis and stimulate the immune response for the production of the inflammatory molecules known as markers for NP toxicity. This can induce the cell to programmed cell death by activating the caspase-1 pathway (Sobota and Imlay 2011).

12.10.3 Cell Membrane Disruption

The engulfment of NPs results in the leakage of the lipid layer, perforation, disruption of the membrane integrity, and change in the hydrophobicity, asymmetry, and potential of the cell membrane (Seiffert et al. 2015).

12.10.4 Damage to the Cytoskeleton and Organelles

NPs damage the cytoskeleton by inhibiting the microfilaments and microtubules' function through depolymerization. This affects the molecule's cellular shape, stability, growth, adhesion, and transport. After internalization of NPs, they disrupt and cause leakage in mitochondria and lysosomes (Sharma et al. 2024).

12.10.5 Disruption of DNA and Signaling Pathway

Any of the paths, such as the production of ROS, activation of the signaling cascade, and organelle destruction, causes direct or indirect DNA damage (Doak and Dusinska 2017). Disruption of the signaling cascade will affect many cellular processes, such as growth and differentiation, and lead to cell death (Kheraldine et al. 2021) (Figure 12.4).

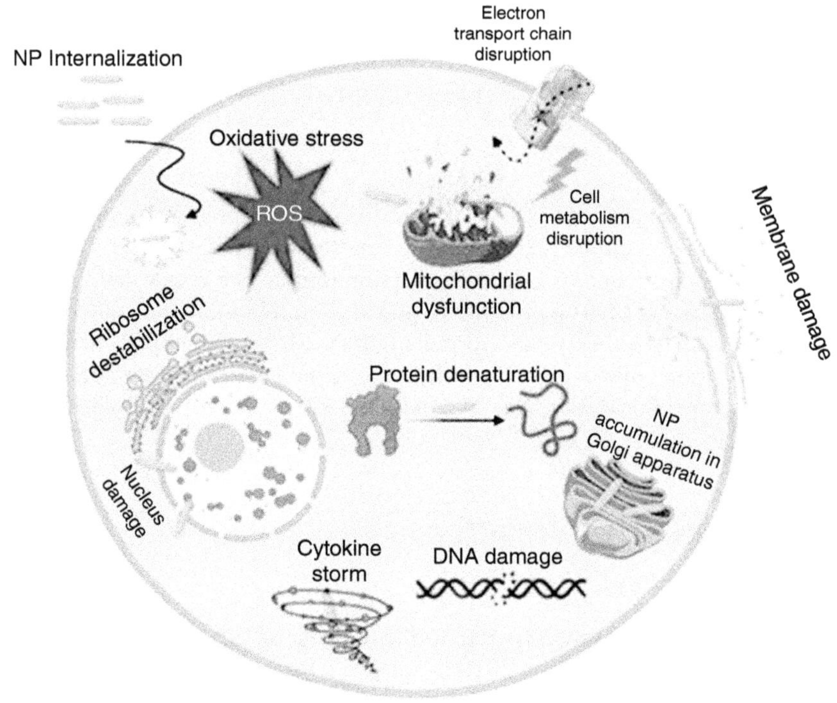

FIGURE 12.4 Schematic representation of toxicity of NPs on cells. (Reproduced and reprinted with permission from Awashra and Młynarz (2023), copyright 2023 with permission from Royal Society of Chemistry, https://creativecommons.org/licenses/by/3.0/.)

12.11 IN VITRO TOXICITY OF NPS

12.11.1 Quantum Dots

QDs have exhibited in vitro toxicity based on the size, surface functionalization, composition, and signaling pathway they activate. In the human keratinocyte cell line, QD functionalized with CA (QD 655) of 12 nm exhibited more toxicity by increasing oxidative stress and apoptosis than CA functionalization (QD 565) of 4.6 nm (Lee et al. 2017). Cytotoxicity of CdSe QDs of 2–5 nm was dose- and size-dependent. CdSe promoted oxidative stress, chromatin condensation, and disruption when exposed to the A549 cell line (Jigyasu et al. 2016). In contrast, CdTe-QDs in L929 cells resulted in an excess amount of ROS and triggered three signal pathways—Akt, JNK, and p38—leading to cellular apoptosis. This toxic effect was mitigated by treating the CDTe with H_2S, resveratrol, and thermotherapy (Wu et al. 2017).

12.11.2 Carbon Dots

The multicolor (red, green, and blue) photoluminescent CDs (o-phenylenediamine, m-phenylenediamine, and p-phenylenediamine of sizes 6, 8.2, and 10 nm, respectively) showed a low cytotoxic effect with 90% viability in MCF-7 cells (Jiang et al. 2015). Human breast cancer cell line SKBR3 and human breast epithelial cell line MCF-12A showed minimal cellular toxicity after 24 hours, with time and concentration-dependent photo-generated cellular toxicity to CDs (5 nm) (Esfandiari et al. 2019). CDs functionalized with quaternary ammonium groups showed biocompatibility despite the movement of CDs to the nuclei of the cells at 400 μg/mL in NIH/3T3 cells. In contrast, the same CDs in L929 cells, reported to be highly toxic, lead to apoptosis at the same concentration within 24 hours. This was due to higher endocytosis than NIH/3T3 cell lines (Havrdová et al. 2021).

12.11.3 Graphene

GO induced programmed necrosis, ROS, and cytoskeletal disruption in macrophages (Mouse J774A.1 and RAW 264.7 cell lines) by activating TNF-α and TLR4 signaling pathways. It altered the macrophage's phagocytic ability due to GO accumulation in the cytoplasm (Qu et al. 2013). Furthermore, the toxicity of rGO with PVP (polyvinylpyrrolidone) as a stabilizing agent was found to be more toxic than GO and GO-PVP. rGO-PVP and GO both showed an increased ROS, leading to oxidative stress in the hemocytes of mussels (Katsumiti, Tomovska, and Cajaraville 2017). Comparative studies with p-GO (pristine GO), GO-COOH, and GO-PEI (Polyethyleneimine GO) in T lymphocytes and human serum albumin (HSA), showed that p-GO and GO-COOH exhibited similar and significant toxicity at concentrations above 50 μg/mL, but GO-PEI exhibited cytotoxicity at a minimal concentration (1.6 μg/mL) (Ding et al. 2014).

12.11.4 Nanocluster

Au_{25}NCs conjugated with TAT peptide targeted the nucleus of the exposed cell (Vero, A549, and MDCK cells), and were found to generate ROS, mitochondrial dysfunction, and cell death (Zhao et al. 2014). Similarly, metal carbonyl cluster-boronic acid conjugates of ruthenium (Ru) exhibited greater cytotoxicity by inducing apoptosis in MDA-MB-231 cells than iron (Fe) and osmium (Os). Cluster (iron-molybdenum polyoxometalates) and Mo_{132} cluster (molybdenum-containing) exhibited toxic effects in normal and transformed fibroblasts, in which Mo_{132} cluster was found to be harmful, with considerable damage to organelles of ordinary and transformed fibroblasts, whereas $Mo_{72}Fe_{30}$ was non-toxic (Ostroushko et al. 2018).

12.11.5 Gold and Silver NPs

AuNPs (10, 30, or 60 nm) exhibited the size-dependent toxicity in HT-29 and HepG2 cell lines, which showed that smaller NPs showed higher ROS and DNA damage internalization than other sizes (Lopez-Chaves et al. 2018). Similarly, AuNPs in A549 cells were, found to be toxic at a dose and time-dependent manner with ROS generation, reduce the viability of cells, disrupt the potential in the mitochondrial membrane, and downregulate the PCNA (proliferating cell nuclear antigen) protein (Chairuangkitti et al. 2013). Also, AgNPs were found to cause more significant toxicity than AuNPs at high concentrations. AgNPs induced cytotoxicity by activating the *Nrf2* and *HO-1* genes and signaling pathways in Caco-2 cells (Aueviriyavit, Phummiratch, and Maniratanachote 2014). AgNPs were found to cause more genotoxic effects with DNA damage and chromosome alteration in a concentration-dependent manner than PVP-AgNPs in HepG2 cell line (Wang et al. 2019).

12.12 IN VIVO ASSAY

It is the standard method that would be used for evaluating the toxicity of the different hazardous compounds, which helps in studying the distribution, cellular uptake, metabolism, and elimination of the NPs. This method requires the administration of a minimal amount of hazardous compounds in animal models such as mice (Wen et al. 2017). Although this is very tedious and expensive, it gives more accurate readings. Consequently, this study remains the most widely accepted method for evaluating the fate of NPs (Filip et al. 2015).

12.13 TOXICOKINETICS

The toxicokinetics (TKs) of NPs are the rate of NP entry through various routes. Also, it includes the quantification, distribution, metabolism, and excretion of NPs from different organs and tissues. It is done to determine the parameters of TK and accumulation of NP in particular organs, as well as to study plasma profiles and NPs kinetics (Chen, Riviere, and Lin 2022).

12.13.1 Absorption

Absorption is the process by which NPs enter an organism from the outer environment and penetrate into the organism. NPs can enter the bloodstream via ingestion, inhalation, dermal absorption, and injection. Absorption is generally lower for extravascular routes like inhalation, ingestion, or dermal absorption, as these routes must cross multiple physiological barriers, unlike intravascular injection (Oberdörster et al. 2015). After the NPs enter, they are absorbed by the lymph nodes. Generally, NPs are absorbed into cells through simple diffusion, carrier-mediated transport, active transport, exocytosis, and endocytosis. The absorption rate varies depending on the exposure route and the physicochemical properties of the NPs, including size, chemical composition, surface charge, shape, crystallinity, and concentration (Singh 2016). The absorption rate can be determined by TK parameters such as bioavailability and the absorption rate constant (Spruill et al. 2014).

12.13.2 Distribution

After the absorption, NPs must cross the physiological barrier and reach the target tissue or organ via systemic circulation (Su et al. 2019). Distribution of the NPs to specific organs depends on the affinity of the membrane receptors, the rate of blood flow to the particular organ, and their permeability (Praetorius et al. 2014), and it is described as the "distribution coefficient" (Utembe et al. 2020). Distribution of the NPs can be identified by a quantitative method, by sacrificing the organism and quantifying the NPs by ICP-MS, or by the semi-quantitative method by evaluating the fluorescence intensity using a near-infrared reflection (NIR) fluorescence imaging system (Vats et al. 2017). NPs enter through various routes and are absorbed into lymph nodes, which are phagocytosed by the lymphocytes and macrophages and broken down partially, then enter systemic circulation by capillary lymph vessels (Fu et al. 2013). It is seen that the NP distribution in the brain is less compared to other organs due to the blood-brain barrier (BBB) in the brain. Due to the small pore size of endothelial cells, it is difficult for large-sized NPs to enter the brain, but NPs smaller than 5 nm can rarely enter the tight and normal endothelial cells (Cruz et al. 2016). NPs can quickly enter tumor tissue or inflamed areas of tissue from circulation due to their large pore size and leaky vascular nature (Hollis et al. 2013). When NPs enter the blood, the plasma proteins present in the blood will adsorb on the surface of the NPs and form a protein corona, which leads to the increased size of NPs and changes to the organ distribution (Venditti 2019b). Hydrophilic and neutral NPs can easily pass through macrophage uptake, compared to hydrophobic NPs, increasing their accumulation in the target organs and their retention time in the blood (Zhang et al. 2020). Macrophage uptake can also be escaped by surface functionalizing the NPs with biocompatible compounds such as PEG, which can increase the circulation time. Thus, the distribution of NPs strongly depends on the NPs' size, hydrophobicity, and surface functionalization (Chandran, Riviere, and Monteiro-Riviere 2017).

12.13.3 Metabolism

Metabolism is the process through which the degradation of NPs takes place, wherein NPs lose their original structure through breakdown, aggregation, and opsonization (Yuan et al. 2019). Based on the physicochemical properties of NP, they are uptaken by cells like macrophages through mechanisms like clathrin and caveolae-mediated phagocytosis and micropinocytosis, where they undergo degradation in the lysosomes (Donahue, Acar, and Wilhelm 2019). Most of the metal NPs undergo degradation by releasing their ions into the external environment due to the acidic nature of the lysosomes. These released ions can react with body molecules and undergo reduction, oxidation, or hydrolysis. They can transform into another compound that may be more toxic than the original compound (Bachler, von Goetz, and Hungerbühler 2013). Some inorganic and organic NPs get metabolized by enzymes or any other molecule; for example, CNTs undergo slow decomposition by oxidative enzymes and produce small hydrophilic molecules or metabolites, which will be excreted through bile and urine (Vlasova et al. 2016). The metabolism of NPs mainly depends on their composition. Some organic NPs will have antidegradation properties like QDs and gold, leading to long-term retention and high toxicity (Su et al. 2019). However, surface functionalization with some of the molecules like PEG is safe. But repeated exposure to such molecules will lead to the production of the anti-PEG IgM, which leads to the clearance of the NPs. Hence, the toxicity of the NPs can be reduced by changing their physicochemical property through surface functionalization, which diminishes the slow metabolism, accumulation, and toxicity (Wang et al. 2015).

12.13.4 Elimination

Elimination is the process by which NPs are removed from the body via the renal system, hepatobiliary system, or through sequestration by the mononuclear phagocyte system (MPS), mainly based on their size (Poon et al. 2019). NPs, once they enter the body, have to be excreted as soon as their purpose is fulfilled. As the NPs' retention time decreases, their toxicity decreases. Generally, the uncoated NPs are cleared by MPS and removed from circulation (Hoshyar et al. 2016). NPs are mainly excreted by the renal filtration system, which is the most effective and fastest way for excretion compared to the hepatobiliary system. The renal tubule may reabsorb the NPs larger than 8 nm and positively charged, which interact with the negatively charged glomerular capillary wall (Wang et al. 2018).

Moreover, those that are not reabsorbed will be excreted in the urine (Naeye et al. 2013). NPs smaller than 5 nm are typically cleared by the kidneys and excreted in urine. NPs larger than 5 nm may be degraded or taken up by Kupffer cells in the liver, leading to prolonged retention. If NPs escape Kupffer cells, they might traverse the liver sinusoidal endothelium and undergo hepatobiliary elimination, expelled through the bile duct into the intestines and then excreted as feces. If the NPs cannot exit the liver sinusoidal endothelium, they will re-enter the systemic circulation (Poon et al. 2019). Those NPs that exit the liver can accumulate in the kidney and can cause toxicity, such as kidney failure and fibrosis. It is seen that hepatocytes can effectively remove the NPs that are positively charged and smaller-sized NPs of 10–20 nm (Helle et al. 2013) (Figure 12.5).

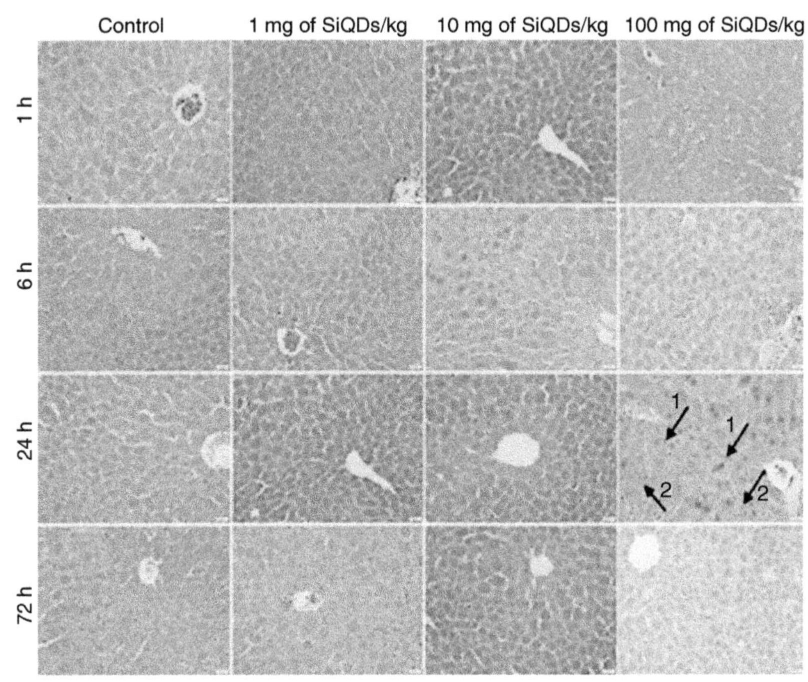

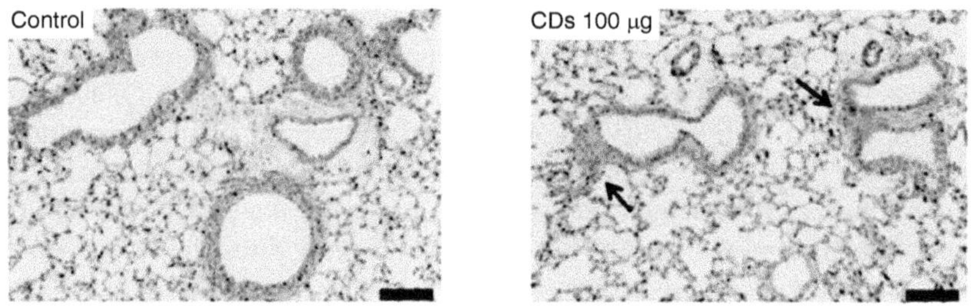

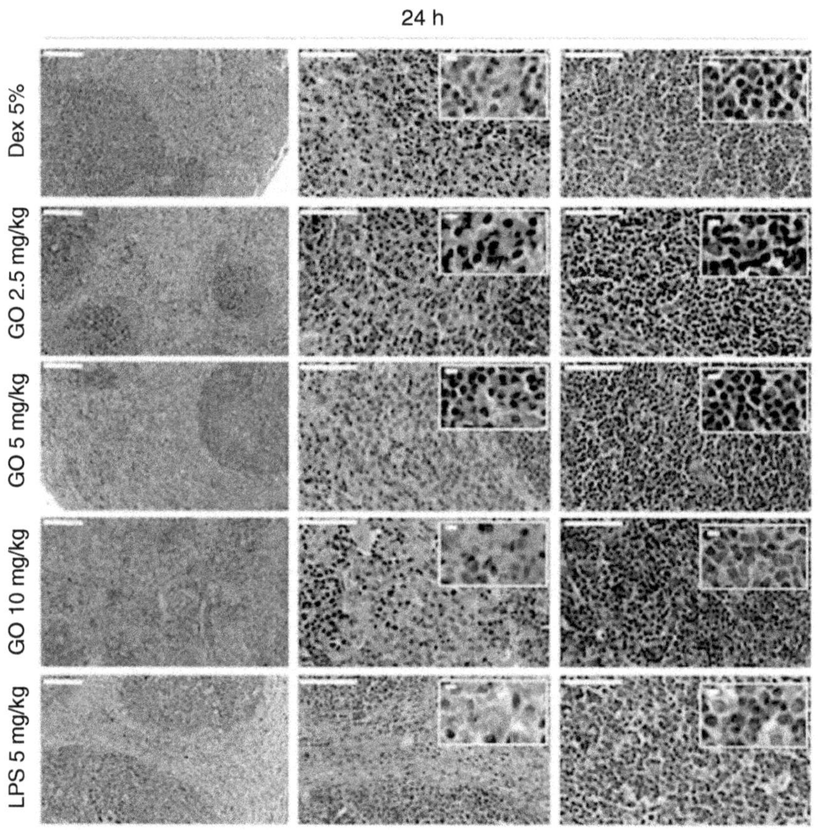

12.14 IMPACTS OF NPS ON ORGANS

12.14.1 Lungs

NPs penetrate deep into the lungs when inhaled, producing ROS, thus creating an inflammatory reaction. It creates a condition that brings about respiratory-related problems such as coughing and low lung capacity (Poh et al. 2018). It activates immune cells to release inflammatory cytokines, causing oxidative stress and lung damage. Prolonged exposure to NPs can result in severe damage and cell death through necrosis and apoptosis, loading to lesions, asthma, bronchitis, tissue damage, and dysfunction (Nabi et al. 2022). Chronic exposure to CNTs and silica NPs, particularly, can develop lung scar tissue, characteristic of pulmonary fibrosis (Ahmad et al. 2015). In vivo studies have shown that QDs induce organ-specific damage. SiQDs induced lung and spleen damage by generating ROS at a concentration above 10 mg/kg body mass in Swiss mice (Cristian, Balta, Herman, Ciceu et al. 2024), whereas in CD-1 mice, Ag_2Se QDs-MEA was

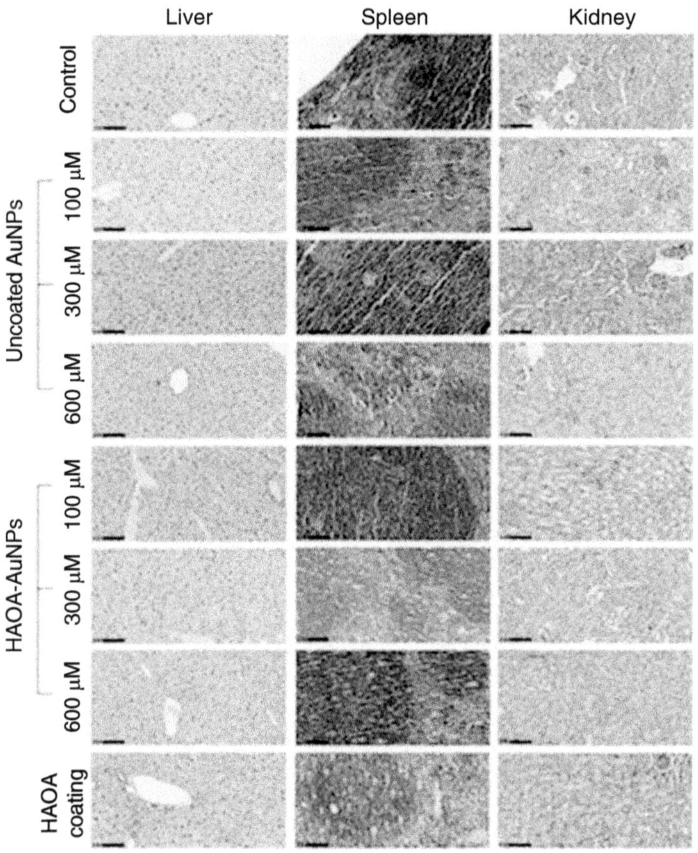

mainly accumulated in the liver, biotransformed, and induced more liver damage than Ag_2Se QDs-MPA (Tang et al. 2017). Furthermore, Cd/Se–ZnS QDs induced lung damage dependent on the strain of the mice. It was seen that A/J mice were more injured than C57BL/6 mice, with peripheral pulmonary tissue damage, increased immune cells, and lung inflammation (Scoville et al. 2018).

12.14.2 Kidney

Renal cells in the kidney will be exposed to more NPs, as this is the elimination route for NPs in the blood (Liu et al. 2013). This leads to the accumulation of the NPs in the kidney, which is known to be one of the major organs affected. These accumulated NPs lead to the generation of ROS and an inflammatory response, which leads to oxidative stress and the release of inflammatory cytokines, chemokines, and pro-apoptotic proteins, which damage the cellular components (Wu and Tang 2018). Moreover, it changes the molecular events such as activation of NF-κβ signaling and release of interleukin-6, 8, and BCL6 (Makhdoumi, Karimi, and Khazaei 2020). Acute and chronic exposure to NPs leads to extracellular matrix protein deposition and causes renal fibrosis, apoptosis, necrosis, tubular cell endocytosis, genotoxicity, and chronic renal failure (Yang et al. 2017). InP/ZnS QDs were taken up by the pronephros, which resulted in alterations in gene expression, swelling, and reduced the development and function of the kidney in zebrafish (Wang et al. 2024). SiQDs induced toxicity in liver and kidney tissue with an increased concentration of antioxidants and a change in expression of TNF-α at concentrations above 10 mg QDs/kg of body mass (Cristian, Balta, Herman, Trica, et al. 2024).

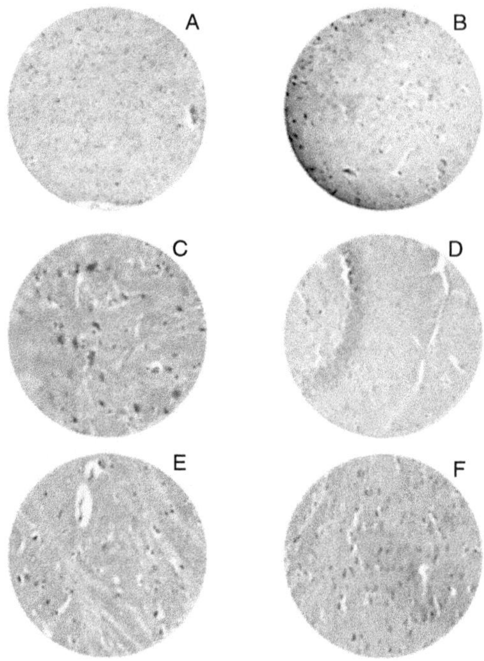

FIGURE 12.5 Images showing the toxicity of NPs on tissues in vivo. (a) Histopathological images of mice liver tissue with hematoxylin and eosin showing (1) hepatocytes swelling and (2) inflammatory infiltrates after the administration of SiQDs (1, 10, and 100 mg/kg of body weight) at 1, 6, 24, and 72 hours (Reproduced and reprinted with permission from Cristian, Balta, Herman, Ciceu et al. (2024), copyright 2024 with permission from MDPI, https://creativecommons.org/licenses/by/4.0/). (b) Histopathological images of mice lung tissue (H&E staining) of control and mice treated with 100 μg CDs (black arrow: cell infiltrate) (Reproduced and reprinted with permission from Weiss et al. (2021), copyright 2021 with permission from MDPI, https://creativecommons.org/licenses/by/4.0/). (c) Histopathological image (H&E-stained) of C57BL/6 mice spleen section after 24 hours of the treatment with GO (2.5, 5, and 10 mg/kg), Dex 5% (negative control) and LPS 5 mg/kg (positive control). The first column is composed of 20× magnification images. Scale bars represent 100 μm. The middle and last columns show 60× magnifications of red and white pulps, respectively. The scale bars represent 50 μm. The inset images show 300× magnified regions with scale bars that represent 5 μm (Reproduced and reprinted with permission from Newman et al. (2020), copyright 2020 with permission from ACS Publications https://creativecommons.org/licenses/by/4.0/). (d) Histopathological images (H&E staining) of the mice spleen, liver, and kidney tissues of different groups; control, uncoated AuNPs and HAOA (hyaluronic and oleic acids)-AuNPs (100, 300, and 600 M), and HAOA coating. (Reproduced and reprinted with permission from Lopes et al. (2023), copyright 2023 with permission from MDPI, https://creativecommons.org/licenses/by/4.0/). (e) Histopathology images of rat brain (H&E staining) of different groups. (a) Untreated rat (14th day) (-); (b) untreated rat (28th day) (-); (c) treated with Bio (biogenic)-AgNPs (14th day) (-); (d) treated with Bio-AgNPs (28th day) (-); (e) treated with Bio-AgNPs (14th day) (-); and (f) treated with Bio-AgNPs (28th day) (-), where (-) indicates no changes (Reproduced and reprinted with permission from Ashajyothi and Kelmani Chandrakanth (2019), copyright 2019 with permission from Taylor & Francis, https://creativecommons.org/licenses/by/4.0/.)

12.14.3 Brain

NPs, due to their small size, can easily cross the BBB through the bloodstream or olfactory nerves through axonal transport (Teleanu et al. 2018b). They can enter brain cells through absorption, transcytosis-mediated process, or by dissolving into the lipid layer of endothelial cells (Teleanu et al. 2018a). The protein corona formation surrounding the NPs leads to the aggregation of the NPs. It disrupts mitochondrial membrane potential, brain enzymes, neurotransmitters, and the ubiquitin-proteasome system (Zhao et al. 2020). It leads to neuroinflammation, malfunction of mitochondria, neuronal injury, protein misfolding, and neurodegenerative disorders. This results in apoptosis, brain edema, gliosis, oxidative stress, and neurological disorders (Teleanu et al. 2018b). MPA-CdTe-QDs of size 3.5 nm induced alteration in the structure of synapses and neurons in the hippocampus of rats, which was found due to the modulation of the signaling pathways like p-ERK1/2, Akt (p-Akt), and c-FOS (Wu et al. 2016), whereas CdSe/ZnS QDs (15–20 nm) showed accumulation in the brain by olfactory tract uptake, leading to microglial cell stimulation in C57BL/6 mice (Hopkins et al. 2014). Furthermore, ZnS functionalization on CdTe-QDs reduced the neurotoxicity caused by naked CdTe-QDs by reducing the translocation of the CdTe-QDs into the RME motor neurons of *Caenorhabditis elegans* (Zhao et al. 2015).

12.14.4 Liver

Due to its detoxification process, the liver is the organ where most of the NPs accumulate and affect the parenchymal and non-parenchymal cells of the liver (Tsoi et al. 2016). The hepatobiliary system takes up NPs, which are not eliminated by the renal system. Metal NP toxicity is mainly caused by the release of metal ions into the external environment and their physicochemical properties. NPs are endocytosed by liver cells and are then excreted from the duodenum (Zhang et al. 2016). It leads to lipid peroxidation, oxidative stress and inflammation, mitochondrial dysfunction, and enzyme activity change, eventually leading to hepatotoxicity like necrosis, apoptosis, liver fibrosis, and steatosis (Yao et al. 2019). CdTe-QDs (2.2 nm) in male ICR mice induced ROS generation, higher MDA expression, and modulation in *p53*, *Bcl-2*, and *Bax* gene expression. It induced apoptosis through the mitochondrial-mediated pathways (Zhang et al. 2015), whereas CdTe functionalized with QDs (15.25 nm) was shown to induce toxicity in the liver by increasing the level of AST, ALT, bilirubin, serum amyloid A, and cytokines in male BALB/c mice (Nguyen et al. 2019).

12.14.5 Spleen, Heart, and Reproductive Organs

NPs also cause toxicity in reproductive organs, which can lead to DNA damage and eventually to genotoxic effects. It also results in abnormalities in the fetus, changes in hormone levels, and altered fertility (Samrot and Noel Richard Prakash, 2023). Chronic exposure of NPs to the heart and spleen can lead to diseases such as cardiac arrest, stroke, and damage to secondary organs (Chopra et al. 2022). CdSe/ZnS QDs were accumulated in the ovaries of female mice, causing an alteration in reproductive hormones and a reduction in the formation of mature oocytes and in vitro fertilization (Xu et al. 2016b), whereas CdSe/ZnS QDs functionalized with CA also showed accumulation in the heart and significant cardiotoxicity, causing oxidative stress, an increase in serum enzymes, and oxidative damage markers in BALB/c mice (Li et al. 2019). Furthermore, black phosphorus QD (2.7 nm) in male C57BL/6 mice caused acute toxicity in the liver, but minimal damage was observed in the spleen and kidney (Mu et al. 2017) (Figure 12.6 and Table 12.1).

12.15 CONCLUSION

Advanced technology in biomedical applications and biosensors has led to the drastic development of novel NP-based applications using fluorescent NPs such as QDs, CDs, graphene, NCs, and gold and silver NPs (Medici et al. 2021). Current research trends focus on applying engineered NPs to various applications due to their unique optical property and biocompatibility. Nevertheless, the use of such NPs has been reported to have promising toxic effects on most animal models. Applying various engineered NPs on a large scale significantly affects living beings. Hence, there is a need to characterize the NPs, not only in terms of size and composition, but also in terms of their molecular effects on the biological system and their interaction, to understand their toxic effects (Egbuna et al. 2021).

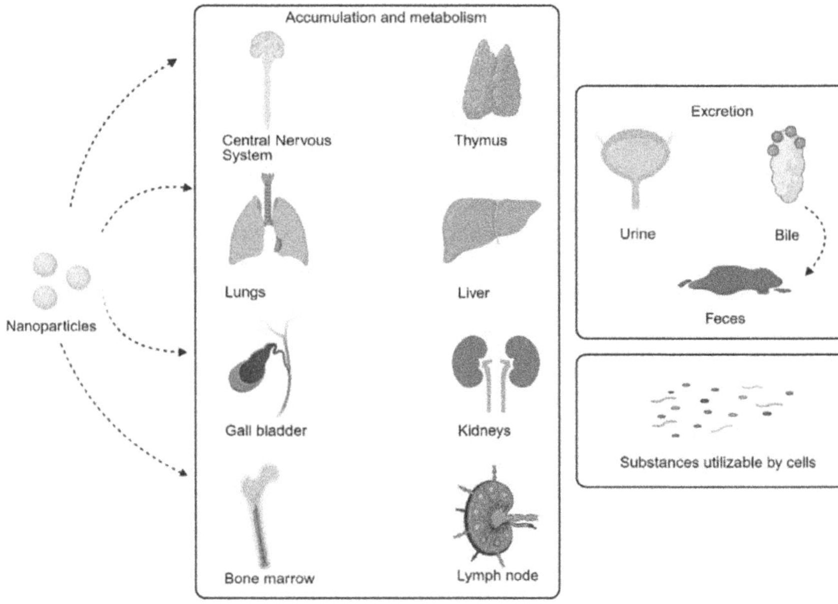

FIGURE 12.6 Schematic representation of accumulation, metabolism, and elimination of the NPs in vivo. (Created with biorender.com.)

TABLE 12.1
Nanoparticle Systems in Ongoing and Completed Clinical Trials

Intervention	Condition	Study	Status	Reference
2C-QD, Sham 2C-QD	Retinitis pigmentosa	Intravitreal Quantum Dots (QD) for Advanced Retinitis Pigmentosa (RP) (QUANTUM) (Phase-Not Applicable)	Not yet recruiting	Jackson (2023)
Quantum dots coated with veldoreotide	Breast and skin cancer, skin diseases	Topical Fluorescent Nanoparticles Conjugated Somatostatin Analog for Suppression and Bioimaging Breast Cancer (Phase 1)	Unknown status	Abdellatif (2019)
Graphene oxide	Periodontal diseases	Graphene Oxide in the Surgical Management of Intrabony Periodontal Defects (Phase-Not Applicable)	Unknown status	Khaled (2022)
Graphene-based detection system (GRIP)	COVID-19, influenza	A Study of the GRIP Influenza and SARS-CoV-2 POC Assays (Phase-Not Applicable)	Completed	Binnicker (2024)
Gold nanocrystals	Parkinson's disease	31P-MRS Imaging to Assess the Effects of CNM-Au8 on Impaired Neuronal Redox State in Parkinson's Disease (REPAIR-PD) (Phase 2)	Completed	Dewey (2024)
Gold nanocrystals	Multiple sclerosis	31P-MRS Imaging to Assess the Effects of CNM-Au8 on Impaired Neuronal Redox State in Multiple Sclerosis. (REPAIR-MS) (Phase 2)	Recruiting	Sguigna (2025)
CNM-Au8	Amyotrophic lateral sclerosis	Therapeutic Nanocatalysis to Slow Disease Progression of Amyotrophic Lateral Sclerosis (ALS) (RESCUE-ALS) (Phase 2)	Completed	**Menon** and Huynh (2024)

(Continued)

TABLE 12.1 (*Continued*)
Nanoparticle Systems in Ongoing and Completed Clinical Trials

Intervention	Condition	Study	Status	Reference
10 ppm oral silver particle, 32 ppm oral silver particle	Healthy	In Vivo Assessment of Silver Biomaterial Nano-Toxicity (Phase 1, Phase 2)	Completed	Munger (2015)
Fluor varnish with nanoparticles	Down's syndrome	Fluor Varnish With Silver Nanoparticles for Dental Remineralization in Patients With Trisomy 21 (Phase 2)	Unknown status	Pierdant-Pérez (2014)
Nanosilver fluoride	Molar-incisor hypomineralization, hypersensitivity	The Desensitising Effect of Nanosilver Fluoride in Molar-Incisor Hypomineralisation (Phase 1, Phase 2)	Active, not recruiting	Nabil (2025)

REFERENCES

Abdellatif, Ahmed A. H. 2019. *Topical Fluorescent Nanoparticles Conjugated Somatostatin Analog for Suppression and Bioimaging Breast Cancer.* Clinical trial, Al-Azhar University. ClinicalTrials.gov Identifier: NCT04138342. https://clinicaltrials.gov/ct2/show/NCT04138342 (accessed June 7, 2025).

Abid, Namra, Aqib Muhammad Khan, Sara Shujait, Kainat Chaudhary, Muhammad Ikram, Muhammad Imran, Junaid Haider, Maaz Khan, Qasim Khan, and Muhammad Maqbool. 2022. "Synthesis of Nanomaterials Using Various Top-down and Bottom-up Approaches, Influencing Factors, Advantages, and Disadvantages: A Review." *Advances in Colloid and Interface Science* 300: 102597.

Agrawal, Vikas, Rashmin Patel, and Mrunali Patel. 2023. "Design, Characterization, and Evaluation of Efinaconazole Loaded Poly (D, L-Lactide-Co-Glycolide) Nanocapsules for Targeted Treatment of Onychomycosis." *Journal of Drug Delivery Science and Technology* 80: 104157.

Ahmad, Javed, Sohail Akhter, Md Rizwanullah, Saima Amin, Mahfoozur Rahman, Mohammad Zaki Ahmad, Moshahid Alam Rizvi, Mohammad A Kamal, and Farhan Jalees Ahmad. 2015. "Nanotechnology-Based Inhalation Treatments for Lung Cancer: State of the Art." *Nanotechnology, Science and Applications*, 55–66. Taylor & Francis.

Al-Bishri, Widad M. 2018. "Toxicity Study of Gold and Silver Nanoparticles on Experimental Animals." *Pharmacophore* 9 (1–2018): 48–55.

Ambaye, Teklit Gebregiorgis, Mentore Vaccari, Shiv Prasad, Eric D van Hullebusch, and Sami Rtimi. 2022. "Preparation and Applications of Chitosan and Cellulose Composite Materials." *Journal of Environmental Management* 301: 113850.

Ashajyothi, C, and R Kelmani Chandrakanth. 2019. "A Pilot Toxicology Study of Biogenic Silver Nanoparticles: In Vivo by Intraperitoneal and Intravenous Infusion Routes in Rats." *Journal of Experimental Nanoscience* 14 (1): 89–106.

Aueviriyavit, Sasitorn, Duangkamol Phummiratch, and Rawiwan Maniratanachote. 2014. "Mechanistic Study on the Biological Effects of Silver and Gold Nanoparticles in Caco-2 Cells–Induction of the Nrf2/HO-1 Pathway by High Concentrations of Silver Nanoparticles." *Toxicology Letters* 224 (1): 73–83.

Awashra, Mohammad, and Piotr Młynarz. 2023. "The Toxicity of Nanoparticles and Their Interaction with Cells: An in Vitro Metabolomic Perspective." *Nanoscale Advances* 5 (10): 2674–2723.

Bachler, Gerald, Natalie von Goetz, and Konrad Hungerbühler. 2013. "A Physiologically Based Pharmacokinetic Model for Ionic Silver and Silver Nanoparticles." *International Journal of Nanomedicine*, 3365–82.

Bai, Xue, Shenqing Wang, Xiliang Yan, Hongyu Zhou, Jinhua Zhan, Sijin Liu, Virender K Sharma, Guibin Jiang, Hao Zhu, and Bing Yan. 2019. "Regulation of Cell Uptake and Cytotoxicity by Nanoparticle Core under the Controlled Shape, Size, and Surface Chemistries." *ACS Nano* 14 (1): 289–302.

Bakand, Shahnaz, and Amanda Hayes. 2016. "Toxicological Considerations, Toxicity Assessment, and Risk Management of Inhaled Nanoparticles." *International Journal of Molecular Sciences* 17 (6): 929.

Bantz, Christoph, Olga Koshkina, Thomas Lang, Hans-Joachim Galla, C James Kirkpatrick, Roland H Stauber, and Michael Maskos. 2014. "The Surface Properties of Nanoparticles Determine the Agglomeration State and the Size of the Particles under Physiological Conditions." *Beilstein Journal of Nanotechnology* 5 (1): 1774–86.

Barman, Snigdha Roy, Amit Nain, Saumey Jain, Nirmal Punjabi, Soumyo Mukherji, and Jitendra Satija. 2018. "Dendrimer as a Multifunctional Capping Agent for Metal Nanoparticles for Use in Bioimaging, Drug Delivery and Sensor Applications." *Journal of Materials Chemistry B* 6 (16): 2368–84.

Behroozi, Zahra, Behnaz Rahimi, Michael R Hamblin, Farinaz Nasirinezhad, Atousa Janzadeh, and Fatemeh Ramezani. 2022. "Injection of Cerium Oxide Nanoparticles to Treat Spinal Cord Injury in Rats." *Journal of Neuropathology & Experimental Neurology* 81 (8): 635–42.

Benameur, Laila, Liu Wei, and Alain Botta. 2012. "Genotoxicity of Nanoparticles." In B. Bhushan (ed.), *Encyclopedia of Nanotechnology*, 952–62. Springer, Dordrecht, Netherlands.

Bhattacharjee, Sourav, Laura H J de Haan, Nynke M Evers, Xue Jiang, Antonius T M Marcelis, Han Zuilhof, Ivonne M C M Rietjens, and Gerrit M Alink. 2010. "Role of Surface Charge and Oxidative Stress in Cytotoxicity of Organic Monolayer-Coated Silicon Nanoparticles towards Macrophage NR8383 Cells." *Particle and Fibre Toxicology* 7: 1–12.

Binnicker, Matthew J. 2024. *A Study of the GRIP Influenza and SARS-CoV-2 POC Assays.* Clinical trial, Mayo Clinic. ClinicalTrials.gov Identifier: NCT05674370. https://clinicaltrials.gov/ct2/show/NCT05674370 (accessed June 7, 2025).

Braakhuis, Hedwig M, Samantha K Kloet, Sanja Kezic, Frieke Kuper, Margriet V D Z Park, Susann Bellmann, Meike van der Zande, Séverine Le Gac, Petra Krystek, and Ruud J B Peters. 2015. "Progress and Future of in Vitro Models to Study Translocation of Nanoparticles." *Archives of Toxicology* 89: 1469–95.

Breza, Martin, and Peter Šimon. 2020. "On Shape Dependence of the Toxicity of Rutile Nanoparticles." *Journal of Nanoparticle Research* 22: 1–11.

Cebadero-Domínguez, Óscar, Concepción Medrano-Padial, María Puerto, Soraya Sánchez-Ballester, Ana María Cameán, Ángeles Jos. 2022. "In Vitro Toxicity Evaluation of Graphene Oxide and Reduced Graphene Oxide on Caco-2 Cells." *Toxicology Reports* 9: 1130–38.

Chairuangkitti, Porntipa, Somsong Lawanprasert, Sittiruk Roytrakul, Sasitorn Aueviriyavit, Duangkamol Phummiratch, Kornphimol Kulthong, Pithi Chanvorachote, and Rawiwan Maniratanachote. 2013. "Silver Nanoparticles Induce Toxicity in A549 Cells via ROS-Dependent and ROS-Independent Pathways." *Toxicology in Vitro* 27 (1): 330–38.

Chandran, Parwathy, Jim E Riviere, and Nancy A Monteiro-Riviere. 2017. "Surface Chemistry of Gold Nanoparticles Determines the Biocorona Composition Impacting Cellular Uptake, Toxicity and Gene Expression Profiles in Human Endothelial Cells." *Nanotoxicology* 11 (4): 507–19.

Chen, Qiran, Jim E Riviere, and Zhoumeng Lin. 2022. "Toxicokinetics, Dose–Response, and Risk Assessment of Nanomaterials: Methodology, Challenges, and Future Perspectives." *Wiley Interdisciplinary Reviews: Nanomedicine and Nanobiotechnology* 14 (6): e1808.

Chen, Yun-Fang, Chun-Chieh Hsu, and Ching-Hu Chung. 2022. "Acute and Subacute Toxicity of Fluorescent Gold Nanoclusters Conjugated with α-Lipoic Acid." *Nanomaterials* 12 (21): 3868.

Chopra, Hitesh, Shabana Bibi, Awdhesh Kumar Mishra, Vineet Tirth, Sree Vandana Yerramsetty, Sree Varshini Murali, Syed Umair Ahmad, Yugal Kishore Mohanta, Mohamed S Attia, and Ali Algahtani. 2022. "Nanomaterials: A Promising Therapeutic Approach for Cardiovascular Diseases." *Journal of Nanomaterials* 2022 (1): 4155729.

Clish, Clary B. 2015. "Metabolomics: An Emerging but Powerful Tool for Precision Medicine." *Molecular Case Studies* 1 (1): a000588.

Crisponi, Guido, Valeria M Nurchi, Joanna I Lachowicz, Massimiliano Peana, Serenella Medici, and Maria Antomietta Zoroddu. 2017. "Toxicity of Nanoparticles: Etiology and Mechanisms." In Alexandru Mihai Grumezescu (ed.), *Antimicrobial Nanoarchitectonics*, 511–46. Elsevier.

Cristian, Roxana-Elena, Cornel Balta, Hildegard Herman, Alina Ciceu, Bogdan Trica, Beatrice G Sbarcea, Eftimie Miutescu, Anca Hermenean, Anca Dinischiotu, and Miruna S Stan. 2024. "Exploring In Vivo Pulmonary and Splenic Toxicity Profiles of Silicon Quantum Dots in Mice." *Materials* 17 (11): 2778.

Cristian, Roxana-Elena, Cornel Balta, Hildegard Herman, Bogdan Trica, Beatrice G Sbarcea, Anca Hermenean, Anca Dinischiotu, and Miruna S Stan. 2024. "In Vivo Assessment of Hepatic and Kidney Toxicity Induced by Silicon Quantum Dots in Mice." *Nanomaterials* 14 (5): 457.

Cruz, Luis J, Marieke A Stammes, Ivo Que, Ermond R van Beek, Vicky T Knol-Blankevoort, Thomas J A Snoeks, Alan Chan, Eric L Kaijzel, and Clemens W G M Löwik. 2016. "Effect of PLGA NP Size on Efficiency to Target Traumatic Brain Injury." *Journal of Controlled Release* 223: 31–41.

Das, Balaram, Satyajit Tripathy, Jaydeep Adhikary, Sourav Chattopadhyay, Debasis Mandal, Sandeep Kumar Dash, Sabyasachi Das, Aditi Dey, Sankar Kumar Dey, and Debasis Das. 2017. "Surface Modification Minimizes the Toxicity of Silver Nanoparticles: An in Vitro and in Vivo Study." *JBIC Journal of Biological Inorganic Chemistry* 22: 893–918.

Dasari Shareena, Thabitha P, Danielle McShan, Asok K Dasmahapatra, and Paul B Tchounwou. 2018. "A Review on Graphene-Based Nanomaterials in Biomedical Applications and Risks in Environment and Health." *Nano-Micro Letters* 10: 1–34.

De La Cruz, G Gonzalez, P Rodriguez-Fragoso, A Mastache-Juarez, J Reyes-Esparza, and L Rodríguez Lourdes. 2020. "Doxorubicin-Bioconjugated Cadmium Sulfide Dextrin Quantum Dots for Imaging Cells." *Indian Journal of Pharmaceutical Sciences* 82 (2): 47–58.

De Matteis, Valeria. 2017. "Exposure to Inorganic Nanoparticles: Routes of Entry, Immune Response, Biodistribution and in Vitro/in Vivo Toxicity Evaluation." *Toxics* 5 (4): 29.

Deirram, Nayeleh, Changhe Zhang, Sarah S Kermaniyan, Angus P R Johnston, and Georgina K Such. 2019. "PH-responsive Polymer Nanoparticles for Drug Delivery." *Macromolecular Rapid Communications* 40 (10): 1800917.

Dewey, Richard. 2024. *31P-MRS Imaging to Assess the Effects of CNM-Au8 on Impaired Neuronal Redox State in Parkinson's Disease (REPAIR-PD).* Clinical trial, Clene Nanomedicine. ClinicalTrials.gov Identifier: NCT03815916. https://clinicaltrials.gov/ct2/show/NCT03815916 (accessed June 7, 2025).

Ding, Zhijia, Zhijun Zhang, Hongwei Ma, and Yanyan Chen. 2014. "In Vitro Hemocompatibility and Toxic Mechanism of Graphene Oxide on Human Peripheral Blood T Lymphocytes and Serum Albumin." *ACS Applied Materials & Interfaces* 6 (22): 19797–807.

Doak, Shareen H, and Maria Dusinska. 2017. "NanoGenotoxicology: Present and the Future." *Mutagenesis* 32 (1): 1–4.

Donahue, Nathan D, Handan Acar, and Stefan Wilhelm. 2019. "Concepts of Nanoparticle Cellular Uptake, Intracellular Trafficking, and Kinetics in Nanomedicine." *Advanced Drug Delivery Reviews* 143: 68–96.

Dong, Liyun, Mulin Li, Song Zhang, Jun Li, Guanxin Shen, Yating Tu, Jintao Zhu, and Juan Tao. 2015. "Cytotoxicity of BSA-Stabilized Gold Nanoclusters: In Vitro and In Vivo Study." *Small* 11 (21): 2571–81.

Doren, Elke A F Van, Pieter-Jan R H De Temmerman, Michel Abi Daoud Francisco, and Jan Mast. 2011. "Determination of the Volume-Specific Surface Area by Using Transmission Electron Tomography for Characterization and Definition of Nanomaterials." *Journal of Nanobiotechnology* 9: 1–8.

Du, Li, Shaoling Wu, Yanhui Li, Xindong Zhao, Xiaoyan Ju, and Yuzhen Wang. 2014. "Cytotoxicity of PEGylated Graphene Oxide on Lymphoma Cells." *Bio-Medical Materials and Engineering* 24 (6): 2135–41.

Egbuna, Chukwuebuka, Vijaykumar K Parmar, Jaison Jeevanandam, Shahira M Ezzat, Kingsley C Patrick-Iwuanyanwu, Charles Oluwaseun Adetunji, Johra Khan, Eugene N Onyeike, Chukwuemelie Zedech Uche, and Muhammad Akram. 2021. "Toxicity of Nanoparticles in Biomedical Application: Nanotoxicology." *Journal of Toxicology* 2021 (1). 9954443.

Ermis, Esra, Zeinab Bagheri, Ebrahim Behroodi, Hamid Latifi, Mahban Rahimifard, and Elham Ajorlou. 2022. "Red Emissive N–S Co-Doped Carbon Dots for Live Imaging of Tumor Spheroid in the Microfluidic Device." *Journal of Science: Advanced Materials and Devices* 7 (2): 100404.

Esfandiari, Neda, Zeinab Bagheri, Hamide Ehtesabi, Zahra Fatahi, Hossein Tavana, and Hamid Latifi. 2019. "Effect of Carbonization Degree of Carbon Dots on Cytotoxicity and Photo-Induced Toxicity to Cells." *Heliyon* 5 (12): e02940.

Feng, Qiyi, Yanping Liu, Jian Huang, Ke Chen, Jinxing Huang, and Kai Xiao. 2018. "Uptake, Distribution, Clearance, and Toxicity of Iron Oxide Nanoparticles with Different Sizes and Coatings." *Scientific Reports* 8 (1): 1–13.

Filip, Adriana, Monica Potara, Adrian Florea, Ioana Baldea, Diana Olteanu, Pompei Bolfa, Simona Clichici, Luminita David, Bianca Moldovan, and Liliana Olenic. 2015. "Comparative Evaluation by Scanning Confocal Raman Spectroscopy and Transmission Electron Microscopy of Therapeutic Effects of Noble Metal Nanoparticles in Experimental Acute Inflammation." *RSC Advances* 5 (83): 67435–48.

Filon, Francesca Larese, Marcella Mauro, Gianpiero Adami, Massimo Bovenzi, and Matteo Crosera. 2015. "Nanoparticles Skin Absorption: New Aspects for a Safety Profile Evaluation." *Regulatory Toxicology and Pharmacology* 72 (2): 310–22.

Fu, Changhui, Tianlong Liu, Linlin Li, Huiyu Liu, Dong Chen, and Fangqiong Tang. 2013. "The Absorption, Distribution, Excretion and Toxicity of Mesoporous Silica Nanoparticles in Mice Following Different Exposure Routes." *Biomaterials* 34 (10): 2565–75.

Garcés, Mariana, Lourdes Cáceres, Diego Chiappetta, Natalia Magnani, and Pablo Evelson. 2021. "Current Understanding of Nanoparticle Toxicity Mechanisms and Interactions with Biological Systems." *New Journal of Chemistry* 45 (32): 14328–44.

Gasmi, Amin, Massimiliano Peana, Maria Arshad, Monica Butnariu, Alain Menzel, and Geir Bjørklund. 2021. "Krebs Cycle: Activators, Inhibitors and Their Roles in the Modulation of Carcinogenesis." *Archives of Toxicology* 95 (4): 1161–78.

Gidwani, Bina, Varsha Sahu, Shiv Shankar Shukla, Ravindra Pandey, Veenu Joshi, Vikas Kumar Jain, and Amber Vyas. 2021. "Quantum Dots: Prospectives, Toxicity, Advances and Applications." *Journal of Drug Delivery Science and Technology* 61: 102308.

Gunawan, Cindy, May Lim, Christopher P Marquis, and Rose Amal. 2014. "Nanoparticle–Protein Corona Complexes Govern the Biological Fates and Functions of Nanoparticles." *Journal of Materials Chemistry B* 2 (15): 2060–83.

Han, Xianglu, Robert Gelein, Nancy Corson, Pamela Wade-Mercer, Jingkun Jiang, Pratim Biswas, Jacob N Finkelstein, Alison Elder, and Günter Oberdörster. 2011. "Validation of an LDH Assay for Assessing Nanoparticle Toxicity." *Toxicology* 287 (1–3): 99–104.

Hansson, Gunnar C. 2012. "Role of Mucus Layers in Gut Infection and Inflammation." *Current Opinion in Microbiology* 15 (1): 57–62.

Harish, Vancha, Devesh Tewari, Manish Gaur, Awadh Bihari Yadav, Shiv Swaroop, Mikhael Bechelany, and Ahmed Barhoum. 2022. "Review on Nanoparticles and Nanostructured Materials: Bioimaging, Biosensing, Drug Delivery, Tissue Engineering, Antimicrobial, and Agro-Food Applications." *Nanomaterials* 12 (3): 457.

Havrdová, Markéta, Iztok Urbančič, Kateřina Bartoň Tománková, Lukáš Malina, Janez Štrancar, and Athanasios B Bourlinos. 2021. "Self-Targeting of Carbon Dots into the Cell Nucleus: Diverse Mechanisms of Toxicity in NIH/3T3 and L929 Cells." *International Journal of Molecular Sciences* 22 (11): 5608.

Havrdova, Marketa, Katerina Hola, Josef Skopalik, Katerina Tomankova, Martin Petr, Klara Cepe, Katerina Polakova, Jiri Tucek, Athanasios B Bourlinos, and Radek Zboril. 2016. "Toxicity of Carbon Dots–Effect of Surface Functionalization on the Cell Viability, Reactive Oxygen Species Generation and Cell Cycle." *Carbon* 99: 238–48.

He, Long, Ting He, Shabnam Farrar, Linbao Ji, Tianyi Liu, and Xi Ma. 2017. "Antioxidants Maintain Cellular Redox Homeostasis by Elimination of Reactive Oxygen Species." *Cellular Physiology and Biochemistry* 44 (2): 532–53.

Helle, Marion, Enrico Rampazzo, Morgane Monchanin, Frederic Marchal, Francois Guillemin, Sara Bonacchi, Francesca Salis, Luca Prodi, and Lina Bezdetnaya. 2013. "Surface Chemistry Architecture of Silica Nanoparticles Determine the Efficiency of in Vivo Fluorescence Lymph Node Mapping." *ACS Nano* 7 (10): 8645–57.

Hollis, Christin P, Heidi L Weiss, Markos Leggas, B Mark Evers, Richard A Gemeinhart, and Tonglei Li. 2013. "Biodistribution and Bioimaging Studies of Hybrid Paclitaxel Nanocrystals: Lessons Learned of the EPR Effect and Image-Guided Drug Delivery." *Journal of Controlled Release* 172 (1): 12–21.

Hong, Wei, Yan Liu, Ming-Hui Li, Yue-Xiao Xing, Ting Chen, Yong-Hong Fu, Lei Jiang, He Zhao, Ai-qun Jia, and Jun-Song Wang. 2018. "In Vivo Toxicology of Carbon Dots by 1H NMR-Based Metabolomics." *Toxicology Research* 7 (5): 834–47.

Hopkins, Laurie E, Esther S Patchin, Po-Lin Chiu, Christina Brandenberger, Suzette Smiley-Jewell, and Kent E Pinkerton. 2014. "Nose-to-Brain Transport of Aerosolised Quantum Dots Following Acute Exposure." *Nanotoxicology* 8 (8): 885–93.

Hoshyar, Nazanin, Samantha Gray, Hongbin Han, and Gang Bao. 2016. "The Effect of Nanoparticle Size on in Vivo Pharmacokinetics and Cellular Interaction." *Nanomedicine* 11 (6): 673–92.

Huo, Shuaidong, Shubin Jin, Xiaowei Ma, Xiangdong Xue, Keni Yang, Anil Kumar, Paul C Wang, Jinchao Zhang, Zhongbo Hu, and Xing-Jie Liang. 2014. "Ultrasmall Gold Nanoparticles as Carriers for Nucleus-Based Gene Therapy Due to Size-Dependent Nuclear Entry." *ACS Nano* 8 (6): 5852–62.

Hwang, Huey-Min, Ray Paresh Chandra, Hongtao Yu. 2012. "Toxicology of Designer/Engineered Metallic Nanoparticles." In: Luque R, Varma RS, Clark JH, et al. (eds.), *Sustainable preparation of metal nanoparticles: methods and applications*, 190–212. Royal Society of Chemistry, Cambridge, UK.

Jackson, Timothy. 2023. *Intravitreal Quantum Dots (QD) for Advanced Retinitis Pigmentosa (RP) (QUANTUM)*. Clinical trial, 2C Tech Corp. ClinicalTrials.gov Identifier: NCT05841862. https://clinicaltrials.gov/ct2/show/NCT05841862 (accessed June 7, 2025).

Jeevanandam, Jaison, Ahmed Barhoum, Yen S Chan, Alain Dufresne, and Michael K Danquah. 2018. "Review on Nanoparticles and Nanostructured Materials: History, Sources, Toxicity and Regulations." *Beilstein Journal of Nanotechnology* 9 (1): 1050–74.

Jiang, Kai, Shan Sun, Ling Zhang, Yue Lu, Aiguo Wu, Congzhong Cai, and Hengwei Lin. 2015. "Red, Green, and Blue Luminescence by Carbon Dots: Full-color Emission Tuning and Multicolor Cellular Imaging." *Angewandte Chemie* 127 (18): 5450–53.

Jigyasu, Aditya Kumar, Sahabjada Siddiqui, Mohatashim Lohani, Irfan Ali Khan, and Md Arshad. 2016. "Chemically Synthesized CdSe Quantum Dots Inhibit Growth of Human Lung Carcinoma Cells via ROS Generation." *EXCLI Journal* 15: 54.

Jiravova, Jana, Katerina Barton Tomankova, Monika Harvanova, Lukas Malina, Jakub Malohlava, Lenka Luhova, Ales Panacek, Barbora Manisova, and Hana Kolarova. 2016. "The Effect of Silver Nanoparticles and Silver Ions on Mammalian and Plant Cells in Vitro." *Food and Chemical Toxicology* 96: 50–61.

Jo, Dong Hyun, Jin Hyoung Kim, Tae Geol Lee, and Jeong Hun Kim. 2015. "Assessing Toxicity of Nanoparticles: In Vitro and in Vivo Assays." In Mahmood Aliofkhazraei (ed.), *Handbook of Nanoparticles*, 923–40. Springer International Publishing.

Johnston, Helinor J, Gary Hutchison, Frans M Christensen, Sheona Peters, Steve Hankin, and Vicki Stone. 2010. "A Review of the in Vivo and in Vitro Toxicity of Silver and Gold Particulates: Particle Attributes and Biological Mechanisms Responsible for the Observed Toxicity." *Critical Reviews in Toxicology* 40 (4): 328–46.

Kadhim, Rua J, Esraa H Karsh, Zainab J Taqi, and Majid S Jabir. 2021. "Biocompatibility of Gold Nanoparticles: In-Vitro and In-Vivo Study." *Materials Today: Proceedings* 42: 3041–45.

Kalyanaraman, Balaraman, Victor Darley-Usmar, Kelvin J A Davies, Phyllis A Dennery, Henry Jay Forman, Matthew B Grisham, Giovanni E Mann, Kevin Moore, L Jackson Roberts II, and Harry Ischiropoulos. 2012. "Measuring Reactive Oxygen and Nitrogen Species with Fluorescent Probes: Challenges and Limitations." *Free Radical Biology and Medicine* 52 (1): 1–6.

Karakoti, Ajay S, Satyanarayana V N T Kuchibhatla, Donald R Baer, Suntharampillai Thevuthasan, Dean C Sayle, and Sudipta Seal. 2008. "Self-Assembly of Cerium Oxide Nanostructures in Ice Molds." *Small* 4 (8): 1210–16.

Kargozar, Saeid, Seyed Javad Hoseini, Peiman Brouki Milan, Sara Hooshmand, Hae-Won Kim, and Masoud Mozafari. 2020. "Quantum Dots: A Review from Concept to Clinic." *Biotechnology Journal* 15 (12): 2000117.

Katsumiti, Alberto, Radmila Tomovska, and Miren P Cajaraville. 2017. "Intracellular Localization and Toxicity of Graphene Oxide and Reduced Graphene Oxide Nanoplatelets to Mussel Hemocytes in Vitro." *Aquatic Toxicology* 188: 138–47.

Khadanga, Vidyasri, and Purna Chandra Mishra. 2024. "A Review on Toxicity Mechanism and Risk Factors of Nanoparticles in Respiratory Tract." *Toxicology* 504: 153781.

Khaled, Zeiad. 2022. *Graphene Oxide in the Surgical Management of Intrabony Periodontal Defects.* Clinical trial, Ain Shams University. ClinicalTrials.gov Identifier: NCT05341245. https://clinicaltrials.gov/ct2/show/NCT05341245 (accessed June 7, 2025).

Khan, Assad U., Shuqi Zhao, and Guoliang Liu. 2016. "Key Parameter Controlling the Sensitivity of Plasmonic Metal Nanoparticles: Aspect Ratio." *The Journal of Physical Chemistry C* 120 (34): 19353–19364.

Kheraldine, Hadeel, Ousama Rachid, Abdella M Habib, Ala-Eddin Al Moustafa, Ibrahim F Benter, and Saghir Akhtar. 2021. "Emerging Innate Biological Properties of Nano-Drug Delivery Systems: A Focus on PAMAM Dendrimers and Their Clinical Potential." *Advanced Drug Delivery Reviews* 178: 113908.

Knaapen, Ad M, Paul J A Borm, Catrin Albrecht, and Roel P F Schins. 2004. "Inhaled Particles and Lung Cancer. Part A: Mechanisms." *International Journal of Cancer* 109 (6): 799–809.

Kommareddy, Sushma, Dinesh B Shenoy, and Mansoor M Amiji. 2007. "Gelatin Nanoparticles and Their Biofunctionalization." *Nanotechnologies for the Life Sciences: Online*.

Kumar, Ajeet, and Chandra Kumar Dixit. 2017. "Methods for Characterization of Nanoparticles." In Surendra Nimesh, Ramesh Chandra and Nidhi Gupta (eds.), *Advances in Nanomedicine for the Delivery of Therapeutic Nucleic Acids*, 43–58. Woodhead Publishing.

Kumar, Sandeep, Neeraj Dilbaghi, Ruma Saharan, and Gaurav Bhanjana. 2012. "Nanotechnology as Emerging Tool for Enhancing Solubility of Poorly Water-Soluble Drugs." *Bionanoscience* 2: 227–50.

Kumar, Vinay, Neha Sharma, and S S Maitra. 2017. "In Vitro and in Vivo Toxicity Assessment of Nanoparticles." *International Nano Letters* 7 (4): 243–56.

Kuwagata, Makiko, Fumiaki Kumagai, Yoshiaki Saito, Kazuma Higashisaka, Yasuo Yoshioka, and Yasuo Tsutsumi. 2017. "Permeability of Skin to Silver Nanoparticles after Epidermal Skin Barrier Disruption in Rats." *Fundamental Toxicological Sciences* 4 (3): 109–19.

Kuznietsova, Halyna, Alain Géloën, Nataliia Dziubenko, Alexander Zaderko, Sergei Alekseev, Vladimir Lysenko, and Valeriy Skryshevsky. 2023. "In Vitro and in Vivo Toxicity of Carbon Dots with Different Chemical Compositions." *Discover Nano* 18 (1): 111.

Kwak, Mi-Kyoung, Nobunao Wakabayashi, Jennifer L Greenlaw, Masayuki Yamamoto, and Thomas W Kensler. 2003. "Antioxidants Enhance Mammalian Proteasome Expression through the Keap1-Nrf2 Signaling Pathway." *Molecular and Cellular Biology* 23 (23): 8786–94.

Kyriakides, Themis R, Arindam Raj, Tiffany H Tseng, Hugh Xiao, Ryan Nguyen, Farrah S Mohammed, Saiti Halder, Mengqing Xu, Michelle J Wu, and Shuozhen Bao. 2021. "Biocompatibility of Nanomaterials and Their Immunological Properties." *Biomedical Materials* 16 (4): 042005.

Kyrylkova, Kateryna, Sergiy Kyryachenko, Mark Leid, and Chrissa Kioussi. 2012. "Detection of Apoptosis by TUNEL Assay." In Odontogenesis*: Methods and Protocols*, 41–7. Springer.

Lakshmanan, Imayavaramban, and Surinder K Batra. 2013. "Protocol for Apoptosis Assay by Flow Cytometry Using Annexin V Staining Method." *Bio-Protocol* 3 (6): e374.

Large, Danielle E, Jonathan R Soucy, Jacob Hebert, and Debra T Auguste. 2019. "Advances in Receptor-mediated, Tumor-targeted Drug Delivery." *Advanced Therapeutics* 2 (1): 1800091.

Lee, Eun Young, Hyun Cheol Bae, Hana Lee, Yeonsue Jang, Yoon-Hee Park, Jin Hee Kim, Woo-In Ryu, Byeong Hyeok Choi, Ji Hyun Kim, and Sang Hoon Jeong. 2017. "Intracellular ROS Levels Determine the Apoptotic Potential of Keratinocyte by Quantum Dot via Blockade of AKT Phosphorylation." *Experimental Dermatology* 26 (11): 1046–52.

Leifert, Annika, Yu Pan, Anne Kinkeldey, Frank Schiefer, Julia Setzler, Olaf Scheel, Hera Lichtenbeld, Günter Schmid, Wolfgang Wenzel, and Willi Jahnen-Dechent. 2013. "Differential HERG Ion Channel Activity of Ultrasmall Gold Nanoparticles." *Proceedings of the National Academy of Sciences* 110 (20): 8004–9.

Li, Chaoqun, Jiang Wang, Xin Chen, Yingze Song, Kangjia Jiang, Hongbo Fan, Min Tang, Weitao Zhan, and Shuangquan Liao. 2017. "Structure and Properties of Reduced Graphene Oxide/Natural Rubber Latex Nanocomposites." *Journal of Nanoscience and Nanotechnology* 17 (2): 1133–39.

Li, Jie, Huamin Zeng, Zhaowu Zeng, Yiying Zeng, and Tian Xie. 2021a. "Promising Graphene-Based Nanomaterials and Their Biomedical Applications and Potential Risks: A Comprehensive Review." *ACS Biomaterials Science & Engineering* 7 (12): 5363–96.

Li, Li, Jinglin Tian, Xiaomei Wang, Gaixia Xu, Wenxiao Jiang, Zhiwen Yang, Dongmeng Liu, and Guimiao Lin. 2019. "Cardiotoxicity of Intravenously Administered CdSe/ZnS Quantum Dots in BALB/c Mice." *Frontiers in Pharmacology* 10: 1179.

Li, Na, Lina Chen, Chujie Zeng, Huanggen Yang, Silian He, and Qingmin Wei. 2021b. "Comparative Toxicity, Biodistribution and Excretion of Ultra-Small Gold Nanoclusters with Different Emission Wavelengths." *Journal of Biomedical Nanotechnology* 17 (9): 1778–87.

Li, Wei, Xiujuan Zhang, Xiaojun Hao, Jiansheng Jie, Baishun Tian, and Xiaohong Zhang. 2013. "Shape Design of High Drug Payload Nanoparticles for More Effective Cancer Therapy." *Chemical Communications* 49 (93): 10989–91.

Li, Xiaoming, Wei Liu, Lianwen Sun, Katerina E Aifantis, Bo Yu, Yubo Fan, Qingling Feng, Fuzhai Cui, and Fumio Watari. 2015. "Effects of Physicochemical Properties of Nanomaterials on Their Toxicity." *Journal of Biomedical Materials Research Part A* 103 (7): 2499–2507.

Li, Yang, Ying Liu, Yujian Fu, Taotao Wei, Laurent Le Guyader, Ge Gao, Ru-Shi Liu, Yan-Zhong Chang, and Chunying Chen. 2012. "The Triggering of Apoptosis in Macrophages by Pristine Graphene through the MAPK and TGF-Beta Signaling Pathways." *Biomaterials* 33 (2): 402–11.

Li, Yingbo, Yan Wang, Liu Tu, Di Chen, Zhi Luo, Dengyuan Liu, Zhuang Miao, Gang Feng, Li Qing, and Shali Wang. 2016. "Sub-Acute Toxicity Study of Graphene Oxide in the Sprague-Dawley Rat." *International Journal of Environmental Research and Public Health* 13 (11): 1149.

Lin, Zhenkun, Nirmal Goswami, Tiantian Xue, Osburg Jin Huang Chai, Hejie Xu, Yuxin Liu, Yu Su, and Jianping Xie. 2021. "Engineering Metal Nanoclusters for Targeted Therapeutics: From Targeting Strategies to Therapeutic Applications." *Advanced Functional Materials* 31 (51): 2105662.

Liu, Jinbin, Mengxiao Yu, Chen Zhou, and Jie Zheng. 2013. "Renal Clearable Inorganic Nanoparticles: A New Frontier of Bionanotechnology." *Materials Today* 16 (12): 477–86.

Liu, Junjun, Rui Li, and Bai Yang. 2020a. "Carbon Dots: A New Type of Carbon-Based Nanomaterial with Wide Applications." *ACS Central Science* 6 (12): 2179–95.

Liu, Na, and Meng Tang. 2020. "Toxicity of Different Types of Quantum Dots to Mammalian Cells in Vitro: An Update Review." *Journal of Hazardous Materials* 399: 122606.

Liu, Wei, Gang Huang, Xiaoying Su, Siyi Li, Qun Wang, Yuying Zhao, Yao Liu, Jingshan Luo, Ye Li, and Chuwen Li. 2020b. "Zebrafish: A Promising Model for Evaluating the Toxicity of Carbon Dot-Based Nanomaterials." *ACS Applied Materials & Interfaces* 12 (43): 49012–20.

Lopes, Joana, Tânia Ferreira-Gonçalves, Lia Ascensão, Ana S Viana, Lina Carvalho, José Catarino, Pedro Faísca, Abel Oliva, Dragana P C de Barros, and Cecília M P Rodrigues. 2023. "Safety of Gold Nanoparticles: From in Vitro to in Vivo Testing Array Checklist." *Pharmaceutics* 15 (4): 1120.

Lopez-Chaves, Carlos, Juan Soto-Alvaredo, Maria Montes-Bayon, Jörg Bettmer, Juan Llopis, and Cristina Sanchez-Gonzalez. 2018. "Gold Nanoparticles: Distribution, Bioaccumulation and Toxicity. In Vitro and in Vivo Studies." Nanomedicine*: Nanotechnology, Biology and Medicine* 14 (1): 1–12.

Lu, Yonghui, Shangcheng Xu, Haiyan Chen, Mindi He, Youcai Deng, Zhengwang Cao, Huifeng Pi, Chunhai Chen, Min Li, and Qinlong Ma. 2016. "CdSe/ZnS Quantum Dots Induce Hepatocyte Pyroptosis and Liver Inflammation via NLRP3 Inflammasome Activation." *Biomaterials* 90: 27–39.

Maity, Subarna, Dipankar Bain, and Amitava Patra. 2019. "An Overview on the Current Understanding of the Photophysical Properties of Metal Nanoclusters and Their Potential Applications." *Nanoscale* 11 (47): 22685–723.

Majumder, Surajit, Dipankar Saha, and Soumitra Kumar Choudhuri. 2023. "Nanoparticle Toxicity: A Review." *Indian Journal of Natural Sciences* 14 (80).

Makhdoumi, Pouran, Hazhir Karimi, and Mozafar Khazaei. 2020. "Review on Metal-Based Nanoparticles: Role of Reactive Oxygen Species in Renal Toxicity." *Chemical Research in Toxicology* 33 (10): 2503–14.

Medici, Serenella, Massimiliano Peana, Alessio Pelucelli, and Maria Antonietta Zoroddu. 2021. "An Updated Overview on Metal Nanoparticles Toxicity." In Seminars in Cancer Biology, 76: 17–26. Elsevier.

Menon, Parvarthi, and William Huynh. 2024. *Therapeutic Nanocatalysis to Slow Disease Progression of Amyotrophic Lateral Sclerosis (ALS) (RESCUE-ALS).* Clinical trial, Clene Nanomedicine. ClinicalTrials.gov Identifier: NCT04098406. https://clinicaltrials.gov/ct2/show/NCT04098406 (accessed June 7, 2025).

Mittal, G, D K Sahana, V Bhardwaj, and M N V Ravi Kumar. 2007. "Estradiol Loaded PLGA Nanoparticles for Oral Administration: Effect of Polymer Molecular Weight and Copolymer Composition on Release Behavior in Vitro and in Vivo." *Journal of Controlled Release* 119 (1): 77–85.

Mo, Yiqun, Mizu Jiang, Yue Zhang, Rong Wan, Jing Li, Chuan-Jian Zhong, Huangyuan Li, Shichuan Tang, and Qunwei Zhang. 2019. "Comparative Mouse Lung Injury by Nickel Nanoparticles with Differential Surface Modification." *Journal of Nanobiotechnology* 17: 1–18.

Moghimi, S M, and D Simberg. 2017. "Complement Activation Turnover on Surfaces of Nanoparticles." *Nano Today* 15: 8–10.

Mu, Xiaoyu, Jun-Ying Wang, Xueting Bai, Fujuan Xu, Haixia Liu, Jiang Yang, Yaqi Jing, Lingfang Liu, Xuhui Xue, and Haitao Dai. 2017. "Black Phosphorus Quantum Dot Induced Oxidative Stress and Toxicity in Living Cells and Mice." *ACS Applied Materials & Interfaces* 9 (24): 20399–409.

Munger, Mark A. 2015. *In Vivo Assessment of Silver Biomaterial Nano-Toxicity.* Clinical trial, University of Utah. ClinicalTrials.gov Identifier: NCT01243320. https://clinicaltrials.gov/ct2/show/NCT01243320 (accessed June 7, 2025).

Musielak, Marika, Jakub Potoczny, Agnieszka Boś-Liedke, and Maciej Kozak. 2021. "The Combination of Liposomes and Metallic Nanoparticles as Multifunctional Nanostructures in the Therapy and Medical Imaging—a Review." *International Journal of Molecular Sciences* 22 (12): 6229.

Nabi, Showkat Ul, Sofi Imtiyaz Ali, Muzafar Ahmad Rather, Wajid Mohammad Sheikh, Mehvish Altaf, Hemant Singh, Peerzada Tajamul Mumtaz, Narayan Chandra Mishra, Sheikh Uzma Nazir, and Showkeen Muzamil Bashir. 2022. "Organoids: A New Approach in Toxicity Testing of Nanotherapeutics." *Journal of Applied Toxicology* 42 (1): 52–72.

Nabil, Nouran. 2025. *The Desensitising Effect of Nanosilver Fluoride in Molar-Incisor Hypomineralisation.* Clinical trial, Alexandria University. ClinicalTrials.gov Identifier: NCT06348849. https://clinicaltrials.gov/ct2/show/NCT06348849 (accessed June 7, 2025).

Naeye, Broes, Hendrik Deschout, Vicky Caveliers, Benedicte Descamps, Kevin Braeckmans, Christian Vanhove, Jo Demeester, Tony Lahoutte, Stefaan C De Smedt, and Koen Raemdonck. 2013. "In Vivo Disassembly of IV Administered SiRNA Matrix Nanoparticles at the Renal Filtration Barrier." *Biomaterials* 34 (9): 2350–58.

Nasrollahpour, Hassan, Beatriz Jurado Sánchez, Mika Sillanpää, and Rasoul Moradi. 2023. "Metal Nanoclusters in Point-of-Care Sensing and Biosensing Applications." *ACS Applied Nano Materials* 6 (14): 12609–72.

Neagu, Monica, Zoi Piperigkou, Konstantina Karamanou, Ayse Basak Engin, Anca Oana Docea, Carolina Constantin, Carolina Negrei, Dragana Nikitovic, and Aristidis Tsatsakis. 2017. "Protein Bio-Corona: Critical Issue in Immune Nanotoxicology." *Archives of Toxicology* 91: 1031–48.

Newman, Leon, Dhifaf A Jasim, Eric Prestat, Neus Lozano, Irene De Lazaro, Yein Nam, Bakri M Assas, Joanne Pennock, Sarah J Haigh, and Cyrill Bussy. 2020. "Splenic Capture and in Vivo Intracellular Biodegradation of Biological-Grade Graphene Oxide Sheets." *Acs Nano* 14 (8): 10168–86.

Nguyen, Kathy C, Yan Zhang, Julie Todd, Kevin Kittle, Dominique Patry, Don Caldwell, Michelle Lalande, Scott Smith, Douglas Parks, and Martha Navarro. 2019. "Biodistribution and Systemic Effects in Mice Following Intravenous Administration of Cadmium Telluride Quantum Dot Nanoparticles." *Chemical Research in Toxicology* 32 (8): 1491–1503.

Nyga, Agata, Alister Hart, and Teresa D Tetley. 2015. "Importance of the HIF Pathway in Cobalt Nanoparticle-Induced Cytotoxicity and Inflammation in Human Macrophages." *Nanotoxicology* 9 (7): 905–17.

Oberdörster, Günter, Vincent Castranova, Bahman Asgharian, and Phil Sayre. 2015. "Inhalation Exposure to Carbon Nanotubes (CNT) and Carbon Nanofibers (CNF): Methodology and Dosimetry." *Journal of Toxicology and Environmental Health, Part B* 18 (3–4): 121–212.

Ostroushko, A A, M V Ulitko, M O Tonkushina, I V Zubarev, S Yu Medvedeva, I G Danilova, O V Gubaeva, I D Gagarin, and I F Gette. 2018. "Influence of Nanocluster Molybdenum Polyoxometalates on the Morphofunctional State of Fibroblasts in Culture." *Nanotechnologies in Russia* 13: 1–10.

Pang, Zhiqiang, Jasmine Chong, Guangyan Zhou, David Anderson de Lima Morais, Le Chang, Michel Barrette, Carol Gauthier, Pierre-Étienne Jacques, Shuzhao Li, and Jianguo Xia. 2021. "MetaboAnalyst 5.0: Narrowing the Gap between Raw Spectra and Functional Insights." *Nucleic Acids Research* 49 (W1): W388–96.

Park, Hyungjun, Dong Jun Shin, and Junhua Yu. 2021. "Categorization of Quantum Dots, Clusters, Nanoclusters, and Nanodots." *Journal of Chemical Education* 98 (3): 703–9.

Peña-Bahamonde, Janire, Hang N Nguyen, Sofia K Fanourakis, and Debora F Rodrigues. 2018. "Recent Advances in Graphene-Based Biosensor Technology with Applications in Life Sciences." *Journal of Nanobiotechnology* 16 (1): 75.

Peynshaert, Karen, Stefaan J Soenen, Bella B Manshian, Shareen H Doak, Kevin Braeckmans, Stefaan C De Smedt, and Katrien Remaut. 2017. "Coating of Quantum Dots Strongly Defines Their Effect on Lysosomal Health and Autophagy." *Acta Biomaterialia* 48: 195–205.

Pierdant-Pérez, Mauricio. 2014. *Fluor Varnish With Silver Nanoparticles for Dental Remineralization in Patients With Trisomy 21.* Clinical trial, Universidad Autonoma de San Luis Potosí. ClinicalTrials.gov Identifier: NCT01975545. https://clinicaltrials.gov/ct2/show/NCT01975545 (accessed June 7, 2025).

Poh, Tuang Yeow, Nur A'tikah Binte Mohamed Ali, Micheál Mac Aogáin, Mustafa Hussain Kathawala, Magdiel Inggrid Setyawati, Kee Woei Ng, and Sanjay Haresh Chotirmall. 2018. "Inhaled Nanomaterials and the Respiratory Microbiome: Clinical, Immunological and Toxicological Perspectives." *Particle and Fibre Toxicology* 15: 1–16.

Poon, Wilson, Yi-Nan Zhang, Ben Ouyang, Benjamin R Kingston, Jamie L Y Wu, Stefan Wilhelm, and Warren C W Chan. 2019. "Elimination Pathways of Nanoparticles." *ACS Nano* 13 (5): 5785–98.

Pounraj, Saranya, Prathap Somu, and Subhankar Paul. 2018. "Chitosan and Graphene Oxide Hybrid Nanocomposite Film Doped with Silver Nanoparticles Efficiently Prevents Biofouling." *Applied Surface Science* 452: 487–97.

Praetorius, Antonia, Nathalie Tufenkji, Kai-Uwe Goss, Martin Scheringer, Frank Von der Kammer, and Menachem Elimelech. 2014. "The Road to Nowhere: Equilibrium Partition Coefficients for Nanoparticles." *Environmental Science: Nano* 1 (4): 317–23.

Pranav, Upendiran, Mehak Malhotra, Shahidkhan Pathan, and Manickam Jayakannan. 2022. "Structural Engineering of Star Block Biodegradable Polymer Unimolecular Micelles for Drug Delivery in Cancer Cells." *ACS Biomaterials Science & Engineering* 9 (2): 743–59.

Qu, Guangbo, Sijin Liu, Shuping Zhang, Lei Wang, Xiaoyan Wang, Bingbing Sun, Nuoya Yin, Xiang Gao, Tian Xia, and Jane-Jane Chen. 2013. "Graphene Oxide Induces Toll-like Receptor 4 (TLR4)-Dependent Necrosis in Macrophages." *ACS Nano* 7 (7): 5732–45.

Raftis, Jennifer B, and Mark R Miller. 2019. "Nanoparticle Translocation and Multi-Organ Toxicity: A Particularly Small Problem." *Nano Today* 26: 8–12.

Ramachandran, Rajan, Chandran Krishnaraj, V K Abhay Kumar, Stacey L Harper, Thangavelu P Kalaichelvan, and Soon-Il Yun. 2018. "In Vivo Toxicity Evaluation of Biologically Synthesized Silver Nanoparticles and Gold Nanoparticles on Adult Zebrafish: A Comparative Study." *3 Biotech* 8: 1–12.

Ramakrishna, Devika, and Pragna Rao. 2011. "Nanoparticles: Is Toxicity a Concern?" *EJIFCC* 22 (4): 92.

Ramezani, Zahra, Fatemeh Kiani Ghalehsardi, and Siamak Noorizadeh. 2023. "Classifications of Quantum Dots and Their Detection Principles in Sensing." 1–36.

Rasouli, Rahimeh, Ahmed Barhoum, and Hasan Uludag. 2018. "A Review of Nanostructured Surfaces and Materials for Dental Implants: Surface Coating, Patterning and Functionalization for Improved Performance." *Biomaterials Science* 6 (6): 1312–38.

Reshma, S C, S Syama, and P V Mohanan. 2016. "Nano-Biointeractions of PEGylated and Bare Reduced Graphene Oxide on Lung Alveolar Epithelial Cells: A Comparative in Vitro Study." *Colloids and Surfaces B: Biointerfaces* 140: 104–16.

Reshma, V G, and P V Mohanan. 2019. "Quantum Dots: Applications and Safety Consequences." *Journal of Luminescence* 205: 287–98.

Sairam, Ananda Babu, Anandhavelu Sanmugam, Ashwini Pushparaj, Gaayathri Mahesh Kumar, Nithila Sundarapandian, Sulakshuna Balaji, Muthuchamy Nallal, and Kang Hyun Park. 2023. "Toxicity of Polymeric Nanodrugs as Drug Carriers." *ACS Chemical Health & Safety* 30 (5): 236–50.

Salazar-Alvarez, G, Jian Qin, V Sepelak, I Bergmann, M Vasilakaki, K N Trohidou, J D Ardisson, W A A Macedo, M Mikhaylova, and Mamoun Muhammed. 2008. "Cubic versus Spherical Magnetic Nanoparticles: The Role of Surface Anisotropy." *Journal of the American Chemical Society* 130 (40): 13234–39.

Samrot, Antony V, and Lawrence Xavier Noel Richard Prakash. 2023. "Nanoparticles Induced Oxidative Damage in Reproductive System and Role of Antioxidants on the Induced Toxicity." *Life* 13 (3): 767.

Sánchez-López, Elena, Daniela Gomes, Gerard Esteruelas, Lorena Bonilla, Ana Laura Lopez-Machado, Ruth Galindo, Amanda Cano, Marta Espina, Miren Ettcheto, and Antoni Camins. 2020. "Metal-Based Nanoparticles as Antimicrobial Agents: An Overview." *Nanomaterials* 10 (2): 292.

Scoville, David K, Collin C White, Dianne Botta, Dowon An, Zahra Afsharinejad, Theo K Bammler, Xiaohu Gao, William A Altemeier, and Terrance J Kavanagh. 2018. "Quantum Dot Induced Acute Changes in Lung Mechanics Are Mouse Strain Dependent." *Inhalation Toxicology* 30 (9–10): 397–403.

Seiffert, Joanna, Farhana Hussain, Coen Wiegman, Feng Li, Leo Bey, Warren Baker, Alexandra Porter, Mary P Ryan, Yan Chang, and Andrew Gow. 2015. "Pulmonary Toxicity of Instilled Silver Nanoparticles: Influence of Size, Coating and Rat Strain." *PLoS One* 10 (3): e0119726.

Sengul, Ayse Busra, and Eylem Asmatulu. 2020. "Toxicity of Metal and Metal Oxide Nanoparticles: A Review." *Environmental Chemistry Letters* 18 (5): 1659–83.

Severino, Patricia, Classius F da Silva, Luciana N Andrade, Daniele de Lima Oliveira, Joana Campos, and Eliana B Souto. 2019. "Alginate Nanoparticles for Drug Delivery and Targeting." *Current Pharmaceutical Design* 25 (11): 1312–34.

Sguigna, Peter. 2025. *31P-MRS Imaging to Assess the Effects of CNM-Au8 on Impaired Neuronal Redox State in Multiple Sclerosis (REPAIR-MS).* Clinical trial, Clene Nanomedicine. ClinicalTrials.gov Identifier: NCT03993171. https://clinicaltrials.gov/ct2/show/NCT03993171 (accessed June 7, 2025).

Shah, Juhi, Stuti Bhagat, and Sanjay Singh. 2020. "Standard Biological Assays to Estimate Nanoparticle Toxicity and Biodistribution." In Susai Rajendran, Anita Mukherjee, Ritesh K. Shukla (eds.), *Nanotoxicity*, 71–104. Elsevier.

Sharma, Anshul, Nitin Sharma, Sachin Singh, and Kamal Dua. 2023. "Review on Theranostic and Neuroprotective Applications of Nanotechnology in Multiple Sclerosis." *Journal of Drug Delivery Science and Technology* 81: 104220.

Sharma, Nitin, Balak Das Kurmi, Dilpreet Singh, Sidharth Mehan, Kushagra Khanna, Ritu Karwasra, Shobhit Kumar, Amit Chaudhary, Vikash Jakhmola, and Anjana Sharma. 2024. "Nanoparticles Toxicity: An Overview of Its Mechanism and Plausible Mitigation Strategies." *Journal of Drug Targeting* 32(5): 1–13.

Shukla, Samarth. 2014. "Recent Developments in Biomedical Applications of Quantum Dots." *Advanced Materials Review* 1 (1): 2–12.

Simpson, Carrie A, Kenneth J Salleng, David E Cliffel, and Daniel L Feldheim. 2013. "In Vivo Toxicity, Biodistribution, and Clearance of Glutathione-Coated Gold Nanoparticles." *Nanomedicine: Nanotechnology, Biology and Medicine* 9 (2): 257–63.

Singh, Ashok Kumar. 2016. "Chapter 6—Nanoparticle Pharmacokinetics and Toxicokinetics." 229–93. Academic Press, Boston, MA, USA.

Sobota, Jason M, and James A Imlay. 2011. "Iron Enzyme Ribulose-5-Phosphate 3-Epimerase in Escherichia Coli Is Rapidly Damaged by Hydrogen Peroxide but Can Be Protected by Manganese." *Proceedings of the National Academy of Sciences* 108 (13): 5402–7.

Soenen, Stefaan J, Wolfgang J Parak, Joanna Rejman, and Bella Manshian. 2015. "(Intra) Cellular Stability of Inorganic Nanoparticles: Effects on Cytotoxicity, Particle Functionality, and Biomedical Applications." *Chemical Reviews* 115 (5): 2109–35.

Spruill, William J, Wade, William E., DiPiro, Joseph T., Blouin, Robert A., Pruemer, Jane M. 2014. "Biopharmaceutics: Absorption." In *Concepts in Clinical Pharmacokinetics,* 6th Ed, 99–114. American Society of Health-System Pharmacists, Bethesda, MD.

Sreekumar, Kalyani, B Bindhu, and K Veluraja. 2021. "Perspectives of Polylactic Acid from Structure to Applications." *Polymers from Renewable Resources* 12 (1–2): 60–74.

Srisrimal, Deepak Abhayakumar, Darsha Kumar Dhurvas Mohandoss, Abhayakumar Srisrimal, Rashmi Dhurvas Darshakumar, S Prabhu, Shonam Tamarakar, and Yogeshkumar Murkunde. 2023. "Silver Nanoparticles: Evaluation of In Vivo Toxicity in Rats." *BioNanoScience* 13 (1): 176–85.

Srivastava, Varsha, Deepak Gusain, and Yogesh Chandra Sharma. 2015. "Critical Review on the Toxicity of Some Widely Used Engineered Nanoparticles." *Industrial & Engineering Chemistry Research* 54 (24): 6209–33.

Su, Chong, Yingze Liu, Runzhi Li, Wei Wu, John Paul Fawcett, and Jingkai Gu. 2019. "Absorption, Distribution, Metabolism and Excretion of the Biomaterials Used in Nanocarrier Drug Delivery Systems." *Advanced Drug Delivery Reviews* 143: 97–114.

Su, Wen, Hao Wu, Huimin Xu, Yang Zhang, Yunchao Li, Xiaohong Li, and Louzhen Fan. 2020. "Carbon Dots: A Booming Material for Biomedical Applications." *Materials Chemistry Frontiers* 4 (3): 821–36.

Sukhanova, Alyona, Svetlana Bozrova, Pavel Sokolov, Mikhail Berestovoy, Alexander Karaulov, and Igor Nabiev. 2018. "Dependence of Nanoparticle Toxicity on Their Physical and Chemical Properties." *Nanoscale Research Letters* 13: 1–21.

Tan, Kei X, Ahmed Barhoum, Sharadwata Pan, and Michael K Danquah. 2018. "Risks and Toxicity of Nanoparticles and Nanostructured Materials." In Abdel Salam Hamdy Makhlouf, Ahmed Barhoum (eds.), *Emerging Applications of Nanoparticles and Architecture Nanostructures*, 121–39. Elsevier.

Tan, Peng, HeSheng Li, Jian Wang, and Subash C B Gopinath. 2021. "Silver Nanoparticle in Biosensor and Bioimaging: Clinical Perspectives." *Biotechnology and Applied Biochemistry* 68 (6): 1236–42.

Tang, Huan, Sheng-Tao Yang, Da-Ming Ke, Yi-Fan Yang, Jia-Hui Liu, Xing Chen, Haifang Wang, and Yuanfang Liu. 2017. "Biological Behaviors and Chemical Fates of Ag_2Se Quantum Dots *In Vivo*: The Effect of Surface Chemistry." *Toxicology Research* 6 (5): 693–704.

Tao, Yu, Mingqiang Li, Jinsong Ren, and Xiaogang Qu. 2015. "Metal Nanoclusters: Novel Probes for Diagnostic and Therapeutic Applications." *Chemical Society Reviews* 44 (23): 8636–63.

Tay, Chor Yong, Yong Yu, Magdiel Inggrid Setyawati, Jianping Xie, and David Tai Leong. 2014. "Presentation Matters: Identity of Gold Nanocluster Capping Agent Governs Intracellular Uptake and Cell Metabolism." *Nano Research* 7: 805–15.

Teleanu, Daniel Mihai, Cristina Chircov, Alexandru Mihai Grumezescu, Adrian Volceanov, and Raluca Ioana Teleanu. 2018a. "Blood-Brain Delivery Methods Using Nanotechnology." *Pharmaceutics* 10 (4): 269.

Teleanu, Daniel Mihai, Cristina Chircov, Alexandru Mihai Grumezescu, Adrian Volceanov, and Raluca Ioana Teleanu. 2018b. "Impact of Nanoparticles on Brain Health: An up to Date Overview." *Journal of Clinical Medicine* 7 (12): 490.

Truskewycz, Adam, Hong Yin, Nils Halberg, Daniel T H Lai, Andrew S Ball, Vi Khanh Truong, Agata Marta Rybicka, and Ivan Cole. 2022. "Carbon Dot Therapeutic Platforms: Administration, Distribution, Metabolism, Excretion, Toxicity, and Therapeutic Potential." *Small* 18 (16): 2106342.

Tsoi, Kim M, Sonya A MacParland, Xue-Zhong Ma, Vinzent N Spetzler, Juan Echeverri, Ben Ouyang, Saleh M Fadel, Edward A Sykes, Nicolas Goldaracena, and Johann M Kaths. 2016. "Mechanism of Hard-Nanomaterial Clearance by the Liver." *Nature Materials* 15 (11): 1212–21.

Utembe, Wells, Harvey Clewell, Natasha Sanabria, Philip Doganis, and Mary Gulumian. 2020. "Current Approaches and Techniques in Physiologically Based Pharmacokinetic (PBPK) Modelling of Nanomaterials." *Nanomaterials* 10 (7): 1267.

Vats, Mukti, Sumit Kumar Mishra, Mahdieh Shojaei Baghini, Deepak S Chauhan, Rohit Srivastava, and Abhijit De. 2017. "Near Infrared Fluorescence Imaging in Nano-Therapeutics and Photo-Thermal Evaluation." *International Journal of Molecular Sciences* 18 (5): 924.

Venditti, Iole. 2019a. "Engineered Gold-Based Nanomaterials: Morphologies and Functionalities in Biomedical Applications. a Mini Review." *Bioengineering* 6 (2): 53.

Venditti, Iole. 2019b. "Morphologies and Functionalities of Polymeric Nanocarriers as Chemical Tools for Drug Delivery: A Review." *Journal of King Saud University-Science* 31 (3): 398–411.

Vijayakumar, Selvamani, and Sai Ganesan. 2012. "In Vitro Cytotoxicity Assay on Gold Nanoparticles with Different Stabilizing Agents." *Journal of Nanomaterials* 2012 (1): 734398.

Virmani, Tarun, Girish Kumar, Reshu Virmani, Ashwani Sharma, and Kamla Pathak. 2023. "Xanthan Gum-Based Drug Delivery Systems for Respiratory Diseases." In Harish Dureja, Jon Adams, Raimar Löbenberg, Terezinha de Jesus Andreoli Pinto, Kamal Dua (eds.), *Natural Polymeric Materials Based Drug Delivery Systems in Lung Diseases*, 279–95. Springer, Singapore.

Vlasova, Irina I, Alexandr A Kapralov, Zachary P Michael, Seth C Burkert, Michael R Shurin, Alexander Star, Anna A Shvedova, and Valerian E Kagan. 2016. "Enzymatic Oxidative Biodegradation of Nanoparticles: Mechanisms, Significance and Applications." *Toxicology and Applied Pharmacology* 299: 58–69.

Wang, Chunling, Xiaobo Cheng, Yuqing Su, Ying Pei, Yanzhi Song, Jiao Jiao, Zhenjun Huang, Yanfei Ma, Yinming Dong, and Ying Yao. 2015. "Accelerated Blood Clearance Phenomenon upon Cross-Administration of PEGylated Nanocarriers in Beagle Dogs." *International Journal of Nanomedicine*, 3533–45.

Wang, Liming, Liang Yan, Jing Liu, Chunying Chen, and Yuliang Zhao. 2018. "Quantification of Nanomaterial/Nanomedicine Trafficking in Vivo." *Analytical Chemistry* 90 (1): 589–614.

Wang, Luanjin, Cixin Liang, Naying Zheng, Chunyan Yang, Sen Yan, Xiang Wang, Zhenghong Zuo, and Chengyong He. 2024. "Kidney Injury Contributes to Edema of Zebrafish Larvae Caused by Quantum Dots." *Science of the Total Environment* 908: 168420.

Wang, Qinyang, Yupeng Wang, Jingjin Ding, Chunhong Wang, Xuehan Zhou, Wenqing Gao, Huanwei Huang, Feng Shao, and Zhibo Liu. 2020. "A Bioorthogonal System Reveals Antitumour Immune Function of Pyroptosis." *Nature* 579 (7799): 421–26.

Wang, Xiujuan, Tingzhu Li, Xuerong Su, Jiangyan Li, Wenhua Li, Junying Gan, Tianshu Wu, Lu Kong, Ting Zhang, and Meng Tang. 2019. "Genotoxic Effects of Silver Nanoparticles with/without Coating in Human Liver HepG2 Cells and in Mice." *Journal of Applied Toxicology* 39 (6): 908–18.

Weiss, Maud, Jiahui Fan, Mickaël Claudel, Luc Lebeau, Françoise Pons, and Carole Ronzani. 2021. "Combined in Vitro and in Vivo Approaches to Propose a Putative Adverse Outcome Pathway for Acute Lung Inflammation Induced by Nanoparticles: A Study on Carbon Dots." *Nanomaterials* 11 (1): 180.

Wen, Yan, Wei Zhang, Ningqiang Gong, Yi-Feng Wang, Hong-Bo Guo, Weisheng Guo, Paul C Wang, and Xing-Jie Liang. 2017. "Carrier-Free, Self-Assembled Pure Drug Nanorods Composed of 10-Hydroxycamptothecin and Chlorin E6 for Combinatorial Chemo-Photodynamic Antitumor Therapy in Vivo." *Nanoscale* 9 (38): 14347–56.

Williams, David F. 2016. "General Concepts of Biocompatibility." In Harish Dureja, Jon Adams, Raimar Löbenberg, Terezinha de Jesus Andreoli Pinto, Kamal Dua (eds.), *Handbook of Biomaterial Properties*, 563–70. Springer, Singapore.

Williams, David F. 2008. "On the Mechanisms of Biocompatibility." *Biomaterials* 29 (20): 2941–53.

Wu, Tianshu, and Meng Tang. 2018. "Review of the Effects of Manufactured Nanoparticles on Mammalian Target Organs." *Journal of Applied Toxicology* 38 (1): 25–40.

Wu, Tianshu, Keyu He, Shengjun Ang, Jiali Ying, Shihan Zhang, Ting Zhang, Yuying Xue, and Meng Tang. 2016. "Impairments of Spatial Learning and Memory Following Intrahippocampal Injection in Rats of 3-Mercaptopropionic Acid-Modified CdTe Quantum Dots and Molecular Mechanisms." *International Journal of Nanomedicine* 10: 2737–55.

Wu, Tianshu, Qingling Zhan, Ting Zhang, Shengjun Ang, Jiali Ying, Keyu He, Shihan Zhang, Yuying Xue, and Meng Tang. 2017. "The Protective Effects of Resveratrol, H_2S and Thermotherapy on the Cell Apoptosis Induced by CdTe Quantum Dots." *Toxicology in Vitro* 41: 106–13.

Wu, Zhu Lian, Ze Xi Liu, and Yun Huan Yuan. 2017. "Carbon Dots: Materials, Synthesis, Properties and Approaches to Long-Wavelength and Multicolor Emission." *Journal of Materials Chemistry B* 5 (21): 3794–3809.

Xiang, Xun, Tao Gao, Bo-Rui Zhang, Feng-Lei Jiang, and Yi Liu. 2018. "Surface Functional Groups Affect CdTe QDs Behavior at Mitochondrial Level." *Toxicology Research* 7 (6): 1071–80.

Xie, Xueping, Jinfeng Liao, Xiaoru Shao, Qianshun Li, and Yunfeng Lin. 2017. "The Effect of Shape on Cellular Uptake of Gold Nanoparticles in the Forms of Stars, Rods, and Triangles." *Scientific Reports* 7 (1): 3827.

Xu, Gaixia, Guimiao Lin, Suxia Lin, Na Wu, Yueyue Deng, Gang Feng, Qiang Chen, Junle Qu, Danni Chen, and Siping Chen. 2016a. "The Reproductive Toxicity of CdSe/ZnS Quantum Dots on the in Vivo Ovarian Function and in Vitro Fertilization." *Scientific Reports* 6 (1): 37677.

Xu, Ming, Jianqiang Zhu, Fanfan Wang, Yunjing Xiong, Yakun Wu, Qiuquan Wang, Jian Weng, Zhihong Zhang, Wei Chen, and Sijin Liu. 2016b. "Improved in Vitro and in Vivo Biocompatibility of Graphene Oxide through Surface Modification: Poly (Acrylic Acid)-Functionalization Is Superior to PEGylation." *ACS Nano* 10 (3): 3267–81.

Yang, Kai, Jianmei Wan, Shuai Zhang, Youjiu Zhang, Shuit-Tong Lee, and Zhuang Liu. 2011. "In Vivo Pharmacokinetics, Long-Term Biodistribution, and Toxicology of PEGylated Graphene in Mice." *ACS Nano* 5 (1): 516–22.

Yang, Yuan, Zhen Qin, Wei Zeng, Ting Yang, Yubin Cao, Chaorong Mei, and Yu Kuang. 2017. "Toxicity Assessment of Nanoparticles in Various Systems and Organs." *Nanotechnology Reviews* 6 (3). De Gruyter: 279–89.

Yang, Yue, Xiangling Ren, Zhenning Sun, Changhui Fu, Tianlong Liu, Xianwei Meng, and Zili Wang. 2018. "Toxicity and Bio-Distribution of Carbon Dots after Single Inhalation Exposure in Vivo." *Chinese Chemical Letters* 29 (6): 895–98.

Yao, Ying, Yiteng Zang, Jing Qu, Meng Tang, and Ting Zhang. 2019. "The Toxicity of Metallic Nanoparticles on Liver: The Subcellular Damages, Mechanisms, and Outcomes." *International Journal of Nanomedicine* 14: 8787–8804.

Yoshida, Tokuyuki, Yasuo Yoshioka, Yuki Morishita, Michihiko Aoyama, Saeko Tochigi, Toshiro Hirai, Kota Tanaka, Kazuya Nagano, Haruhiko Kamada, and Shin-ichi Tsunoda. 2015. "Protein Corona Changes Mediated by Surface Modification of Amorphous Silica Nanoparticles Suppress Acute Toxicity and Activation of Intrinsic Coagulation Cascade in Mice." *Nanotechnology* 26 (24): 245101.

Yuan, Dongfen, Hua He, Yun Wu, Jianghong Fan, and Yanguang Cao. 2019. "Physiologically Based Pharmacokinetic Modeling of Nanoparticles." *Journal of Pharmaceutical Sciences* 108 (1): 58–72.

Zangabad, Parham Sahandi, Mahdi Karimi, Fatemeh Mehdizadeh, Hedieh Malekzad, Alireza Ghasemi, Sajad Bahrami, Hossein Zare, Mohsen Moghoofei, Amin Hekmatmanesh, and Michael R Hamblin. 2017. "Nanocaged Platforms: Modification, Drug Delivery and Nanotoxicity. Opening Synthetic Cages to Release the Tiger." *Nanoscale* 9 (4): 1356–92.

Zhan, Haibing, Xuhong Chang, Xiaoxia Wang, Mengmeng Yang, Qing Gao, Han Liu, Chengyun Li, Sheng Li, and Yingbiao Sun. 2021. "LncRNA MEG3 Mediates Nickel Oxide Nanoparticles-induced Pulmonary Fibrosis via Suppressing TGF-β1 Expression and Epithelial-mesenchymal Transition Process." *Environmental Toxicology* 36 (6): 1099–1110.

Zhang, Aoxue, Kuiyu Meng, Yuda Liu, Yuanhu Pan, Wei Qu, Dongmei Chen, and Shuyu Xie. 2020. "Absorption, Distribution, Metabolism, and Excretion of Nanocarriers in Vivo and Their Influences." *Advances in Colloid and Interface Science* 284: 102261.

Zhang, Naiding, Guiya Xiong, and Zhenjie Liu. 2022. "Toxicity of Metal-Based Nanoparticles: Challenges in the Nano Era." *Frontiers in Bioengineering and Biotechnology* 10: 1001572.

Zhang, Qiuping, Lifeng Wang, Qian Gao, Xinge Zhang, Yushuang Lin, Shuhong Huang, and Dongyan Chen. 2022a. "Toxicity of Polymer-modified CuS Nanoclusters on Zebrafish Embryo Development." *Journal of Applied Toxicology* 42 (2): 295–304.

Zhang, Ting, Yuanyuan Hu, Meng Tang, Lu Kong, Jiali Ying, Tianshu Wu, Yuying Xue, and Yuepu Pu. 2015. "Liver Toxicity of Cadmium Telluride Quantum Dots (CdTe QDs) Due to Oxidative Stress in Vitro and in Vivo." *International Journal of Molecular Sciences* 16 (10): 23279–99.

Zhang, Xinwen, Jinglin Zhang, Qin Wang, Shweta Ghimire, Lei Mei, and Changqing Wu. 2022b. "Effects of Particle Size and Surface Charge on Mutagenicity and Chicken Embryonic Toxicity of New Silver Nanoclusters." *ACS Omega* 7 (21): 17703–12.

Zhang, Yi-Nan, Wilson Poon, Anthony J Tavares, Ian D McGilvray, and Warren C W Chan. 2016. "Nanoparticle–Liver Interactions: Cellular Uptake and Hepatobiliary Elimination." *Journal of Controlled Release* 240: 332–48.

Zhao, Hong, Ruihua Ding, Xin Zhao, Yiwei Li, Liangliang Qu, Hao Pei, Lara Yildirimer, Zhengwei Wu, and Weixia Zhang. 2017. "Graphene-Based Nanomaterials for Drug and/or Gene Delivery, Bioimaging, and Tissue Engineering." *Drug Discovery Today* 22 (9): 1302–17.

Zhao, Jing-Ya, Ran Cui, Zhi-Ling Zhang, Mingxi Zhang, Zhi-Xiong Xie, and Dai-Wen Pang. 2014. "Cytotoxicity of Nucleus-Targeting Fluorescent Gold Nanoclusters." *Nanoscale* 6 (21): 13126–34.

Zhao, Nanxia, Nicola L Francis, Hannah R Calvelli, and Prabhas V Moghe. 2020. "Microglia-Targeting Nanotherapeutics for Neurodegenerative Diseases." *APL Bioengineering* 4 (3): 030902.

Zhao, Yunli, Xiong Wang, Qiuli Wu, Yiping Li, and Dayong Wang. 2015. "Translocation and Neurotoxicity of CdTe Quantum Dots in RMEs Motor Neurons in Nematode Caenorhabditis Elegans." *Journal of Hazardous Materials* 283: 480–89.

13 Nanomedicine's Potential Through Regulatory and Translational Breakthroughs

Shobhona Borkotoky[1], *Supriya Bora*[1], *Lakshi Saikia*[2], *Aditya Man Borborah*[1,3], *and Madhulekha Gogoi*[1]
[1]Knowledgepie Private Limited, Bio-NEST, CSIR NEIST, Jorhat, India
[2]Coal, Energy & Material Science Division, Material Sciences Group, CSIR NEIST, Jorhat, India
[3]Department of Business Management, Assam Women's University, Jorhat, India

13.1 INTRODUCTION

The use of nanotechnology in medicine has the potential to drastically improve human health by transforming illness prevention, diagnosis, and treatment. Nanotechnology is the study of the controlling of matter on an atomic or molecular scale. A very important feature in nanomaterials to take under consideration is size. Generally, nanotechnology deals with structures sized between 1 and 100 nm in at least one dimension and involves developing or modifying materials or devices within that size. These materials include nanoparticles, nanocomposites, nanofibers, and nanotubes, and they are widely used in medicine, electronics, energy, and environmental applications.

Nanomaterials due to their unique size-dependent properties have a wide range of applications in the biological field. Due to the small size of the nanomaterial it has the ability to enhance drug delivery. By encapsulating drugs with nanoparticles its solubility and stability can be significantly improved (Soares et al. 2018). The unique size-dependent property of nanomedicine makes them different from the normal conventional medicine, as its property allows them to interact in the molecular and cellular levels. Another example is imaging, conventional imaging agents often lack specificity and require high doses of clear results, while nanomaterials such as Fe_3O_4 for magnetic resonance imaging (MRI) contrast and gold nanoparticles for imaging provide better imaging results, which helps in better and early diagnosis of diseases without leaving any toxic side effects. Nanomaterials' molecular level interaction capabilities, biocompatibility, and adjustable characteristics make them essential to current medical care.

When nanotechnology entered the pharmaceutical industry, a new field known as nanomedicine emerged. Numerous flaws of traditional medicine can be addressed by nanomedicines because of their special characteristics in terms of size, conformation, and targeted delivery. Clinical trials in nanomedicine may take longer to approve and standardize due to the intricacy of nanostructures, novel applications of nanotechnology, and inconsistent criteria (Dri et al. 2023). As the application of nanoscale formulations in medical treatments continues to grow, the unique physicochemical properties of nanomedicines, though beneficial, pose challenges in navigating regulatory pathways. Therefore, a more controlled and standardized approach to nanomedicine development is essential (Rawal et al. 2019). Characterization of nanomedicines, their future perspectives, and a better understanding of the correlation between their physicochemical properties and their pharmacokinetics need to be and are being widely investigated (Choi & Han 2018; Rawal et al. 2019;

DOI: 10.1201/9781003473015-13

Coty & Vauthier 2018; Milane & Amiji 2021). However, there is limited information on the regulatory framework and quality assessment associated with the clinical development phase of a nanomedicine or nanocarrier. By facilitating accurate drug delivery, improved diagnostics, and novel treatments for diseases including cancer, Alzheimer's, and space-related health hazards, nanomedicine is transforming healthcare. Recent developments in cytosolic delivery methods, magnetic nanodrugs, and nanocarriers are lowering adverse effects, increasing treatment efficacy, and getting past biological barriers. This chapter examines these developments and how they might revolutionize contemporary medicine.

The field of nanomedicine, encompassing nanomaterials for therapeutic and diagnostic purposes, requires rigorous safety assessment due to the distinct properties of nanomaterials and their potential biological interactions (Mendes et al. 2022; Kang et al. 2023). In the path of transformation from nanomaterial to nanomedicine it faces multiple challenges such as:

- *Lack of Standardized Definition of Nanomaterials/Nanomedicine*:
  Nanomedicine and nanomaterials are often defined based on their size (typically 1–100 nm). Different organizations such as FDA (U.S. Food and Drug Administration), EMA (European Medicines Agency), and ISO (International Organization for Standardization) consider the size, composition, and function to address nanomaterials but the definition still remains inconsistent. While some focus solely on size, others consider the unique physicochemical properties of nanomaterials. These inconsistencies in defining nanomedicine and nanomaterials create various hurdles in the field of transformation from nanomaterials to nanomedicine including difficulties in conducting clinical trials, establishing safety guidelines, and ensuring regulatory approvals across different countries.
- *Regulatory Issues*:
  The lack of internationally accepted regulations across many nations and governmental organizations makes nanomedicine's regulations still quite difficult. These regulatory problems result from uneven nanomaterial standardization because the intricate relationships between nanoparticles in biological systems necessitate specific toxicity and risk assessment procedures that are not yet globally standardized. For assessing nanomaterials, agencies including the FDA, EMA, and ISO have developed criteria, but there isn't a single, universally applicable framework. The clinical translation and commercialization of innovations in nanomedicine are slowed down by these regulatory concerns (Rosenblum et al. 2018; Zagalo et al. 2022).
- *Analytical Methods Differ for Each Nanomaterial*:
  Prior to being recognized as a "nanomedicine," the nanomaterials must pass stringent characterization procedures to guarantee a high-quality product and demonstrate its safety for usage in human bodies. Different nanomaterials necessitate distinct approaches for evaluating size, shape, surface characteristics, and stability, resulting in discrepancies in data interpretation among research. Variability in analytical methods hinders the safety of the nanomedicine, delaying clinical trials and commercialization (Đorđević et al. 2022).
- *Challenges in Maintaining Stability after Scale-Up for Manufacturing*:
  In the process of turning a nanomaterial into nanomedicine, scaling up from small laboratory batch sizes to huge industrial volumes is one of the most difficult tasks. The issue is brought on by the challenge of preserving the different characteristics of nanomaterials throughout large-scale manufacturing, including their size, shape, charge, and structure. Variations in these nanomaterials' characteristics cause stability problems for scaled-up products, which compromises their safety and effectiveness (Đorđević et al. 2022).
- *Current Toxicological Studies Fail to Fully Replicate In Vivo Complexity*:
  The properties of nanomedicine differ from laboratory research to real-world clinical application. Most of the time there lies uncertainties when in vivo studies are in

talk, as the stability of nanomaterials differs as we go from in vitro to in vivo. This struggle of in vitro studies to replicate the complex in vivo biological environments leads to significant challenges in predicting the safety and efficacy of nanomedicines in humans.

This chapter is based on addressing and highlighting key strategies for the various challenges faced by nanomedicine in the path of translation from nanomaterial to nanomedicine. Streamlining the issues of nanomedicine can substantially emulate the field of nanomedicine.

13.1.1 Lack of Standardized Definition of Nanomaterials/Nanomedicine

Multiple regulatory and scientific and economic issues exist since there is no universally acknowledged definition of nanomaterials and nanomedicine according to scholarly and institutional study. The European Commission (2011) and FDA (2013) established framework-based ways to standardize nanomaterial identification although these guidelines remain imprecise about material sources such as natural or produced chemicals and biological importance according to Nel et al. (2009) and OECD (2020).

To support responsible innovation, the European Commission introduced framework-based processes in 2011 to standardize nanomaterial identification under its sustainable development policy. The necessity for more accurate and comprehensive definitions to guarantee uniform regulation and sustainable progress in nanotechnology is highlighted by the fact that current frameworks frequently lack clarity about the origin—natural, synthetic, or incidental—of nanomaterials and their biological significance (European Commission 2011). The FDA plays a crucial role in ensuring safety, efficacy, and quality of pharmaceuticals before they reach the market. The FDA evaluates the drug's pharmacological data, manufacturing standards, labeling and risk-benefit profile before granting approval. The FDA regulates nanomedicine in accordance with the current frameworks for pharmaceuticals, biologics, and medical devices by noting the special characteristics and complexities associated with nanoscale materials. The clinical efficacy of nanomedicines may be impacted by their unique pharmacokinetic, biodistribution, and toxicity characteristics, which set them apart from traditional drugs. In view of this, the FDA assesses nanomedicine items individually, highlighting the importance of rigorous physicochemical characterization, solid safety evidence, and consistent manufacturing (U.S. Food and Drug Administration 2013). Japanese researchers Etheridge et al. (2013) contend that contradictory definitions inhibit research laboratories from creating consistent safety assessment methodologies. Tyner et al. and D'Mello et al. (2017) note that these vague definitions make it impossible to duplicate laboratory results precisely. The biological examination of nanoparticles larger than 100 nm presents intricate challenges in therapeutic evaluations and toxicity assessments, as noted by Nel et al. (2009) and Wolfram et al. (2015), while also causing delays in regulatory approvals, according to Wolfram et al. (2015). Commercial operations risk investor confusion and patent conflicts because the contradictory agency definition example between EPA and ISO generates compliance problems for developers as mentioned by Hood (2016). The world suffers trade and safety standardization barriers because of OECD (2020) and ISO/TS 80004-1:2023 (ISO 2023) paperwork which displays regulatory fragmentation issues and indicates that ISO technical specifications remain voluntary without disciplinary enforcement skills. These challenges suggest that society demands a holistic research framework which links biological truth through standardized definitions with market software development objectives and international governance mechanisms according to OECD (2020) and ISO/TS 80004-1:2023. A lack of terminology harmony poses a significant risk to constrain nanomedicine innovation by inducing terminological disagreements so stakeholders must establish collective definition standards as a fundamental basis for development.

13.1.2 Regulatory Issues

The transition of nanomedicines from laboratories to clinical practice faces difficulties because multiple regulatory systems exist alongside regional compliance standards and inadequate worldwide standardization. This part analyzes regulatory hurdles across European Union and US and Canadian and Asian jurisdictions and international platforms alongside their distinct regulations and essential recommendations and unresolved regulatory gaps.

13.1.2.1 Regulations in the European Union

The EMA rules nanomedicines through the ATMP and MDR/IVDR frameworks while regulating these products in Europe. The EMA created a 2021 reflection paper to define how nanomaterials need to be characterized physicochemically. The approval process faces significant hurdles because nanomedicines create classification ambiguity when they fit between the definitions of drugs and biologics as well as medical devices. Safety risks prompted a safety recall of iron oxide nanoparticles Ferumoxtran-10 from the market because of hypersensitivity risks even though studies showed lymph node imaging success as published by the EMA assessment report from 2017. The UK's independent operation of the Medicines and Healthcare products Regulatory Agency (MHRA) after Brexit creates new challenges because it may lead to twice the work in drug and medical device approvals. The EMA granted Onpattro® (patisiran) market approval in 2018 through its Priority Medicines scheme; however, the therapy needed extensive research on stability profiles. Hood et al.'s (2021) contribution to Pharmaceutical Research indicated that the EMA takes a cautious stance through its safety-first approach which restricts innovation but the EMA stresses the essential requirement for monitoring nanomedicines containing new excipients after market release (European Medicines Agency, 2025; European Commission 2007).

13.1.2.2 Regulations in the United States

The FDA in the United States executes nanomedicine oversight through its 2014 Guidance on Nanotechnology in Drug Products which offers voluntary tips for nanoparticle characterization of size as well as stability and surface qualities. The Emerging Technology Program of the FDA acts as a regulatory engagement tool that allows developers to work with FDA agents from early phases of new nanoplatform development. Although no enforceable standards exist, important difficulties continue since different companies file differently, hence creating regulatory uncertainty. The FDA-approved Ferumoxytol iron oxide nanoparticle that joined the market in 2009 cannot expand its use because strong hypersensitivity warnings on the black box restrict its availability to patients with chronic kidney disease anemia (U.S. Food and Drug Administration 2015). The regulatory trade-off between innovation and safety stands obvious with this case. The Moderna COVID-19 mRNA vaccine which uses lipid nanoparticles (LNPs) as its platform got emergency license by the EUA in 2020 to deal with urgent health requirements without undertaking conventional toxicological tests. According to Guillermo U. RuizEsparza (Lopez-Cantu et al. 2022), developers suffer ambiguity because the FDA employs its "enforcement discretion" policy to define long-term safety criteria. The team of researchers advises that further evaluation of LNP immunogenicity must continue beyond prior timeframes since unanticipated immune reactions may limit therapy effectiveness (Tenchov et al. 2021). The FDA must undertake a delicate operation to advance new therapeutics by addressing safety hazards that arise with nanoscale drug delivery techniques.

13.1.2.3 Regulations in Canada

The administration of nanomedicines in Canada falls under two regulatory frameworks: the Food and Drugs Act with extra control from the Vanessa's Law modifications that require post-market surveillance and safety reporting standards. The regulatory system governed by Health Canada has fewer specificity about nanomedicines compared to the FDA and EMA since it mostly focuses on precedent norms from other nations to establish its regulatory base which fails to adequately manage nanotechnology's distinctive requirements. Health Canada delays the approval of new standards which creates challenges for developers because it extends their term of working with ambiguous requirements. The small market in Canada provides limited financial options to firms which increases their hesitancy to invest in Canadian regulatory approvals therefore confining local medical progress. Treatment with Abraxane® (nab-paclitaxel)—a protein-bound nanoparticle chemotherapy—faced reimbursement challenges due to high prices despite its known therapeutic advantages after its approval in 2015.

13.1.2.4 Regulations in Asia

Asian nations utilize varied strategies to control nanomedicines throughout their areas. Nanomedicines in Japan fall under the "regenerative medical products" category of the Pharmaceuticals and Medical Devices Act (PMD Act) which requires Pharmaceutical Medical Devices Agency (PMDA) oversight as demonstrated by the approval of Onpattro® in 2019 through RNAi LNP therapy that needed additional biodistribution studies for safety assessment. The National Medical Products Administration of China established 2023 Technical Guidelines for Nanomedicines which focused on nanomedicine stability within living systems along with targeting efficiency while quality control issues continue to arise particularly with Lipusu® liposomal paclitaxel which was approved in 2008 but showed production inconsistencies due to varying particle sizes. The Central Drugs Standard Control Organization in India works without nanomedicine-specific restrictions through the usage of standard New Drug Rules (2019) (Central Drugs Standard Control Organization 2022). Lipaglyn® serves as a case in point since it represents a diabetic medicine licensed in 2013 as a nanoformulation despite lacking complete nanoparticle characterization, therefore diminishing its potential for reproducibility (Clinical Trials Arena 2022).

13.1.3 Analytical Methods Differ for Each Nanomaterial

Standardization concerns in nanomaterial analysis procedures represent a key impediment which inhibits nanomedicines in going from laboratory work to market distribution. Each nanomaterial category including lipid, metallic, polymeric, and inorganic substances requires specific analytical methods to evaluate key characteristics that include size distribution along with surface charge and stability together with drug-loading capability to guarantee reproducibility and regulatory requirements. Observational studies have shown that LNPs need fluorescence correlation spectroscopy (FCS) and ribogreen assays for encapsulation efficiency assessments because traditional UV-Vis spectroscopy does not distinguish between free mRNA and encapsulated strands (Bizmark et al. 2024). The evaluation technique for Ferumoxytol iron oxide nanoparticles needs both magnetic susceptibility assays and X-ray photoelectron spectroscopy (XPS) to assure dextran coating stability because any uneven coating can trigger hypersensitivity reactions (Shaterabadi et al. 2017). The effectiveness of gold nanoparticles for photothermal therapy requires both surface plasmon resonance (SPR) spectroscopy and transmission electron microscopy (TEM) to examine size homogeneity because aggregation affects therapeutic results (Vines et al. 2019). Silica-based nanoparticles employed in imaging and drug delivery systems need nitrogen adsorption-desorption (BET) studies to determine their porosity state since this attribute effects their drug-loading capabilities. The high-branched structures of dendrimers require to demonstrate their branching fidelity by nuclear magnetic resonance (NMR) spectroscopy to preserve targeting precision. Various dialysis methods utilized to examine drug release profiles of Doxil resulted in regulatory delays because inconsistent data production occurred when no unified protocols were established across these diverse systems (D'Souza 2014). AuroShell® became scale-challenged during cancer therapy development because DLS measurements missed batch changes until additional TEM confirmation was performed (Rastinehad et al. 2019). Proof from these investigations reveals how poor analytical standards for specific materials results in greater development expenses and delayed regulatory clearances and erroneous clinical results.

13.1.4 Challenges in Maintaining Stability after Scale-Up for Manufacturing

Transitioning from laboratory-scale synthesis to large-scale manufacturing presents significant challenges, particularly in maintaining the stability of nanomedicine, as a lot of parameters change such as particle size, which is a core property of nanomaterials on which stability is based, next is surface charge and structural integrity. Factors such as physicochemical variations, process scalability, environmental conditions, and regulatory constraints contribute to stability issues. During scale-up, changes in synthesis parameters such as mixing time, temperature, and reagent concentrations can alter nanoparticle size and morphology. Small variations in these properties can impact drug loading, release kinetics, and biodistribution, ultimately affecting therapeutic efficacy. A well-defined scale-up procedure is very necessary to ensure the quality, cost-effectiveness, and timely launch of the nanomedicine.

In order to ensure consumers that formulations are consistently of high quality from batch to batch and the finished product is suitable for its intended use, EMA has set up certain guidelines which describes all the manufacturing processes step wise which are to be followed by the manufacturers (European Medicines Agency 2025). Nanomaterials are synthesized by two processes: top-down (i.e., starting from a macro size drug powder to be reduced to smaller ones) and bottom-up processes (i.e., starting from a dissolved molecule to a precipitate). The pharmaceutical industry generally uses the top-down process to synthesize nanomedicine. This is due to various practical advantages such as scalability, reproducibility, regulatory compliance, and cost-effectiveness (Paliwal et al. 2014). While manufacturing nanomedicine in a large scale for commercialization, several parameters should be kept in mind such as selection of materials, solvent, procedures of manufacturing nanomaterials, and its cost-effectiveness. Scaling up a nanomedicine product from bench to market involves multiple critical factors. These include the material's composition and its Generally Regarded as Safe (GRAS) status, the impact of nanoparticle size and shape on toxicity, the in vivo biodegradability of nanocarriers, and the challenge of maintaining the stability of complex multicomponent systems at an industrial scale. From a scale-up perspective, choosing the right nanoparticle production method is also crucial as for large-scale production it is necessary to consider the cost of raw materials and to make sure that the synthesis process is limited to very few steps for saving time during pilot batch production. For instance, particle size distribution, drug encapsulation, efficiency, and release kinetics vary depending on the reaction conditions, solvent evaporation rates, and mixing methods used in the manufacture of PLGA (poly(lactic-co-glycolic acid))-coated nanomedicine. Even though PLGA has been approved for use in medical devices for a number of years, there is currently no nanoformulations made of PLGA polymer in the market. This is because of challenges in scaling up manufacturing, which may be related to factors like some active pharmaceutical ingredients' (API) poor drug-loading capacity, high initial burst release, the production of acidic products following polymer biodegradation, and nanotoxicology (Operti et al. 2021). The stability issue in nanomedicine can often be seen while different formulations are being prepared by different processes. Liposomes provide a good example for such issues in stability during scale-up. For instance, Desai et al. discussed the stability concerns associated with liposome production (Desai 2012). According to the study, liposomes with diverse structures such as multilamellar or unilamellar vesicles and stability profiles can be produced using a variety of production techniques. It becomes difficult to maintain constant liposome properties when scale-up occurs, which could result in aggregation because of the high surface free energy and jeopardization of stability. While going for large-scale production, inhomogeneous mixing and variable shear forces can create inconsistent vesicle sizes and bilayer structures which leads to stability issues and because of which its efficacy decreases. Because of their tendency to agglomerate and high surface free energy, each of these systems may be unstable. By lowering interfacial free energy with water and functioning as a steric barrier, the application of amphipathic polyethylene glycol on the surface can prevent liposome aggregation, increasing stability and prolonging the liposomes' half-life in vivo circulation. The FDA, in its draft guidance for liposome drug products, emphasizes the importance of strict control over the manufacturing process, noting that liposomal formulations are highly sensitive to changes in scale and production conditions (Liu et al. 2022). Another main challenge in maintaining nanomaterial stability during scale-up synthesis is transitioning from toxic organic solvents to aqueous or low-toxicity solvents. Several studies have documented stability issues during such scale-up processes, such as nanoprecipitation method; it is a simple technique which is generally adopted for preformed polymers. In order to generate nanoparticles, nanoprecipitation depends on the diffusion of an organic solvent into an aqueous phase that contains dissolved polymers or drugs (Paliwal et al. 2014). For instance, Galindo-Rodríguez et al. observed that scaling up nanoprecipitation from 60 mL to 1.5 L led to decreased particle size with increased stirring rates (Galindo-Rodríguez et al. 2005). However, this also resulted in reduced drug loading, indicating challenges in maintaining consistent encapsulation efficiency during scale-up. Switching from toxic organic solvents to environment-friendly aqueous solvents leads to stability issues in nanomaterials. Due to hydrophobic interactions and inadequate stabilization, aqueous conditions can encourage nanoparticle aggregation, which can impair colloidal stability and change the effectiveness of treatment. By addressing this issue Muthu and Singh et al. discussed that the use of toxic organic solvents like chloroform and dichloromethane poses environmental and safety concerns, leading to a shift toward safer, aqueous-based methods (Muthu & Wilson 2012). However, this transition introduces new stability challenges that must be addressed for successful industrial-scale manufacturing. The aqueous-based nanoprecipitation methods' sensitivity to process conditions is another significant issue. The size, shape, and surface characteristics of nanoparticles are greatly influenced by variables like temperature, pH, solvent-to-antisolvent ratio, and mixing speed. Achieving reproducible formulations during scale-up can be difficult since even small changes in these factors might cause batch-to-batch variability.

The synthesis of nanoparticles consists of various processes such as high-speed homogenization, sonication, milling, emulsification, centrifugation, lyophilization, etc., and in most cases organic solvents are used. During preliminary laboratory-scale synthesis itself it is essential to assess which techniques will remain feasible for large-scale production. This will help in ensuring that the final product maintains its desired attributes and functional properties throughout scale-up.

13.1.5 Current Toxicological Studies Fail to Fully Replicate In Vivo Complexity

The process of producing commercial nanomedicine confronts substantial challenges because existing toxicological exams cannot sufficiently imitate the biological systems found in living organisms. Standard in vitro laboratory studies neglect to duplicate several crucial live creature dynamics including those of the immune system and metabolic functions alongside persistent biochemical building processes. The application of animal models offers crucial discoveries although physiological and distribution variations between species and clearance differences now influence how clinical results appear (Dobrovolskaia et al. 2016). The negative nature of these limitations inhibits our power to determine correct human responses, therefore delaying regulatory authorizations and commercial availability. Researchers examine microphysiological systems (organ-on-a-chip) coupled with three-dimensional cell cultures and humanized animal models as current ways to improve preclinical toxicity assessment forecasting (Fadeel et al. 2018). Regulatory frameworks need a modification to allow incorporation of advanced models because this would boost the clinical translation of nanomedicine through safety and efficacy protocols.

13.1.6 Current Toxicological Studies Fail to Fully Replicate In Vivo Complexity

The transformative potential of nanomedicine lies in its capacity to provide tailored drug delivery, enhanced diagnostics, and innovative therapies. Nonetheless, regulatory ambiguities, safety apprehensions, challenges in characterization, and large-scale production, as well as low yield and elevated manufacturing costs, complicate its clinical translation. This chapter has identified several challenges, including the lack of standardized terminology, the distinctions across various jurisdictions at both federal and international levels, and the need for a comprehensive analytical approach to ensure reproducibility and safety.

13.2 CONCLUSION

The pain points are: harmonizing worldwide regulatory standards, enhancing toxicity assessment models, and validating characterization and stability techniques for nanomedicines. These problems must be addressed to provide a platform that embodies both patient safety and innovation through collaboration among scientists, regulators, industry stakeholders, and policymakers.

As nanomedicine advances, it will implement stringent evaluation frameworks, ethical considerations, and an interdisciplinary approach essential for successful and safe integration into contemporary medicine. These translational obstacles must be surmounted to ensure that nanomedicine becomes an effective, accessible, and sustainable healthcare solution for all individuals globally.

REFERENCES

Bizmark, Navid, Satya Nayagam, Bumjun Kim, David F. Amelemah, Dawei Zhang, Sujit S. Datta, Rodney D. Priestley, Tom Colace, Jane Wang, and Robert K. Prud'homme. 2024. "Ribogreen fluorescent assay kinetics to measure ribonucleic acid loading into lipid nanoparticle carriers". *Advanced Materials Interfaces* 11. https://doi.org/10.1002/admi.202301083.

Central Drugs Standard Control Organization. 2022. "The new drugs and clinical trials rules 2019". 227 (1): 1–233.

Choi, Young Hee, and Hyo Kyung Han. 2018. "Nanomedicines: Current status and future perspectives in aspect of drug delivery and pharmacokinetics". *Journal of Pharmaceutical Investigation* 48 (1): 43–60. https://doi.org/10.1007/s40005-017-0370-4.

Clinical Trials Arena. 2022. *Lipaglyn (Saroglitazar) for Treating Type II Diabetes*. Clinical Trials Arena. https://www.clinicaltrialsarena.com/projects/lipaglyn-saroglitazar-treating-type-ii-diabetes/?cf-view (accessed April 22, 2025)

Coty, Jean Baptiste, and Christine Vauthier. 2018. "Characterization of nanomedicines: A reflection on a field under construction needed for clinical translation success". *Journal of Controlled Release* 275: 254–268. https://doi.org/10.1016/j.jconrel.2018.02.013.

D'Mello, Sheetal R. et al. 2017. "The evolving landscape of drug products containing nanomaterials in the United States". *Nature Nanotechnology* 12 (6): 523–529. https://doi.org/10.1038/nnano.2017.67.

D'Souza, Susan. 2014. "A review of in vitro drug release test methods for nano-sized dosage forms". *Advances in Pharmaceutics* 2014: 1–12. https://doi.org/10.1155/2014/304757.

Desai, Neil. 2012. "Challenges in development of nanoparticle-based therapeutics". *AAPS Journal* 14 (2): 282–295. https://doi.org/10.1208/s12248-012-9339-4.

Dobrovolskaia, Marina A., Michael Shurin, and Anna A. Shvedova. 2016. "Current understanding of interactions between nanoparticles and the immune system". *Toxicology and Applied Pharmacology* 299: 78–89. https://doi.org/10.1016/j.taap.2015.12.022.

Đorđević, Snežana, María Medel Gonzalez, Inmaculada Conejos-Sánchez, Barbara Carreira, Sabina Pozzi, Rita C. Acúrcio, Ronit Satchi-Fainaro, Helena F. Florindo, and María J. Vicent. 2022. "Current hurdles to the translation of nanomedicines from bench to the clinic". *Drug Delivery and Translational Research* 12 (3): 500–525. https://doi.org/10.1007/s13346-021-01024-2.

Dri, Diego Alejandro, Susana Guzmán-Villanueva, Giada Ferraro, José Vicente González-Álvarez, Maria José Diez-Sales, and Maria Luisa Garcia-Garcia. 2023. "Nanomedicines and nanocarriers in clinical trials: Surfing through regulatory requirements and physico-chemical critical quality attributes". *Drug Delivery and Translational Research* 13 (3): 757–769. https://doi.org/10.1007/s13346-022-01262-y.

Etheridge, Michael L., Stephen A. Campbell, Arthur G. Erdman, Christy L. Haynes, Susan M. Wolf, and Jeffrey McCullough. 2013. "The big picture on small medicine". *Nanomedicine: Nanotechnology, Biology, and Medicine* 9 (1): 1–14. https://doi.org/10.1016/j.nano.2012.05.013.THE.

European Commission. 2007. "Medicinal products for human use". 2 (February): 1–34.

European Commission. 2011. *Sustainable Development in the European Union: 2011 Monitoring Report of the EU Sustainable Development Strategy*. Luxembourg: Publications Office of the European Union. https://ec.europa.eu/eurostat/documents/3217494/5723557/KS-32-11-956-EN.PDF (accessed April 22, 2025)

European Medicines Agency. 2025. *Nanotechnology-Based Medicinal Products for Human Use – EU-IN Horizon Scanning Report.* EMA/20989/2025. https://www.ema.europa.eu/ (accessed April 22, 2025)

Fadeel, Bengt, Lucian Farcal, Barry Hardy, Socorro Vázquez-Campos, Danail Hristozov, Antonio Marcomini, Iseult Lynch, Eugenia Valsami-Jones, Harri Alenius, and Kai Savolainen. 2018. "Advanced tools for the safety assessment of nanomaterials". *Nature Nanotechnology* 13 (7): 537–543. https://doi.org/10.1038/s41565-018-0185-0.

Galindo-Rodríguez, Sergio A., François Puel, Stephanie Briançon, Eric Allémann, Eric Doelker, and Hatem Fessi. 2005. "Comparative scale-up of three methods for producing ibuprofen-loaded nanoparticles". *European Journal of Pharmaceutical Sciences* 25 (4–5): 357–367. https://doi.org/10.1016/j.ejps.2005.03.013.

Hood, John, Ignacio Gonzalez-Garcia, Nicholas White, Leeron Marshall, Vincent FS Dubois, Paolo Vicini, and Paul G. Baverel. 2021. "Pharmacokinetic-pharmacodynamic modelling of systemic il13 blockade by monoclonal antibody therapy: A free assay disguised as total". *Pharmaceutics* 13 (4). https://doi.org/10.3390/pharmaceutics13040519.

Hood, Joshua L. 2016. "Post isolation modification of exosomes for nanomedicine applications". *Nanomedicine* 11 (13): 1745–1756. https://doi.org/10.2217/nnm-2016-0102.

ISO. 2023. *ISO 80004-1:2023 Nanotechnologies – Vocabulary*. 1. arg.

Kang, Weirong , Yuwei Liu, and Weiping Wang. 2023. "Light-responsive nanomedicine for cancer immunotherapy". *Acta Pharmaceutica Sinica B* 13 (6): 2346–2368. https://doi.org/10.1016/j.apsb.2023.05.016.

Liu, Peng, Guiliang Chen, and Jingchen Zhang. 2022. "A review of liposomes as a drug delivery system: Current". *Molecules* 27 (4): 1372.

Lopez-Cantu, Diana O., Sabrina M. Partida, Elizabeth K. Sims, and Ester Kwon. 2022. "From bench to the clinic: The path to translation of nanotechnology-enabled mRNA SARS-CoV-2 vaccines". *Nano-Micro Letters* 14. Springer Singapore. https://doi.org/10.1007/s40820-021-00771-8.

Mendes, Bárbara B., João Conniot, Aviram Avital, Dongbao Yao, Xingya Jiang, Xiang Zhou, Noga Sharf-Pauker et al. 2022. "Nanodelivery of nucleic acids". *Nature Reviews Methods Primers* 2 (1). https://doi.org/10.1038/s43586-022-00104-y.

Milane, Lara, and Mansoor Amiji. 2021. "Clinical approval of nanotechnology-based SARS-CoV-2 mRNA vaccines: Impact on translational nanomedicine". *Drug Delivery and Translational Research* 11 (4): 1309–1315. https://doi.org/10.1007/s13346-021-00911-y.

Muthu, Madaswamy S., and Barnabas Wilson. 2012. "Challenges posed by the scale-up of nanomedicines". *Nanomedicine* 7 (3): 307–309. https://doi.org/10.2217/nnm.12.3.

Nel, Andre E., Lutz Mädler, Darrell Velegol, Tian Xia, Eric MV Hoek, Ponisseril Somasundaran. 2009. "Understanding biophysicochemical interactions at the nano-bio interface". *Nature Materials* 8 (7): 543–557. https://doi.org/10.1038/nmat2442.

OECD. 2020. *Education at a Glance 2020: OECD Indicators.* OECD Publishing, Paris. https://doi.org/10.1787/69096873-en. (accessed April 22, 2025)

Operti, Maria Camilla, Alexander Bernhardt, Silko Grimm, Andrea Engel, Carl Gustav Figdor, and Oya Tagit.. 2021. "PLGA-based nanomedicines manufacturing: Technologies overview and challenges in industrial scale-up". *International Journal of Pharmaceutics* 605: 120807. https://doi.org/10.1016/j.ijpharm.2021.120807.

Paliwal, Rishi; R. Jayachandra Babu, and Srinath Palakurthi. 2014. "Nanomedicine Scale-up technologies: Feasibilities and challenges". *Ageing International* 15 (6): 1527–1534. https://doi.org/10.1208/s12249-014-0177-9.

Rastinehad, Ardeshir R., Harry Anastos, Ethan Wajswol, Jared S. Winoker, John P. Sfakianos, Sai K. Doppalapudi, Michael R. Carrick et al. 2019. "Gold nanoshell-localized photothermal ablation of prostate tumors in a clinical pilot device study". *Proceedings of the National Academy of Sciences of the United States of America* 116 (37): 18590–18596. https://doi.org/10.1073/pnas.1906929116.

Rawal, Meghana, Amit Singh, and Mansoor M. Amiji. 2019. "Quality-by-design concepts to improve nanotechnology-based drug development". *Pharmaceutical Research* 36 (11): 1–20. https://doi.org/10.1007/s11095-019-2692-6.

Rosenblum, Daniel et al. 2018. "Progress and challenges towards targeted delivery of cancer therapeutics". *Nature Communications* 9 (1). https://doi.org/10.1038/s41467-018-03705-y.

Shaterabadi, Zhila, Gholamreza Nabiyouni, and Meysam Soleymani. 2017. "High impact of in situ dextran coating on biocompatibility, stability and magnetic properties of iron oxide nanoparticles". *Materials Science & Engineering. C, Materials for Biological Applications* 75: 947–956. https://doi.org/10.1016/j.msec.2017.02.143.

Soares, Sara, Inês Sousa, Maria Carmo Pereira, and Fernando Rocha. 2018. "Nanomedicine: Principles, properties, and regulatory issues". *Frontiers in Chemistry* 6 (August): 1–15. https://doi.org/10.3389/fchem.2018.00360.

Tenchov, Rumiana, Rachna Bird, Alexey Curtze, and Qiongqiong Zhou. 2021. "Lipid nanoparticles from liposomes to mRNA vaccine delivery, a landscape of research diversity and advancement". *ACS Nano* 15 (11): 16982–17015. https://doi.org/10.1021/acsnano.1c04996.

U.S. Food and Drug Administration. 2013. "*Labeling for Human Prescription Drug and Biological Products – Implementing the PLR Content and Format Requirements: Guidance for Industry*". Silver Spring, MD: U.S. Department of Health and Human Services. https://www.fda.gov/media/84987/download. (accessed April 22, 2025)

U.S. Food and Drug Administration. 2015. *FDA Strengthens Warnings and Changes Prescribing Instructions to Decrease the Risk of Serious Allergic Reactions with Anemia Drug Feraheme (Ferumoxytol).* FDA, U.S. Food and Drug Administration: 1–4.

Vines, Jeremy B., James R. Yoon, Chang-Seon Lim, and Dong Kee Yi. 2019. "Gold nanoparticles for photothermal cancer therapy". *Frontiers in Chemistry* 7 (April): 1–16. https://doi.org/10.3389/fchem.2019.00167.

Wolfram, Joy, Motao Zhu, Yong Yang, Jianliang Shen, Emanuela Gentile, Donatella Paolino, Massimo Fresta et al. 2015. "Safety of nanoparticles in medicine". *Curr Drug Targets* 16 (14): 1671–1681.

Zagalo, Daniela M., Sérgio Simões, and João Sousa. 2022. "Regulatory science approach in pharmaceutical development of follow-on versions of non-biological complex drug products". *Journal of Pharmaceutical Sciences*. https://doi.org/10.1016/j.xphs.2022.07.015.

Index

Note: **Bold** page numbers refer to tables and *italic* page numbers refer to figures.

D

E

F

G

H

I

L

M

T

U

V

W

X

Z

For Product Safety Concerns and Information please contact our EU
representative GPSR@taylorandfrancis.com
Taylor & Francis Verlag GmbH, Kaufingerstraße 24, 80331 München, Germany

www.ingramcontent.com/pod-product-compliance
Ingram Content Group UK Ltd.
Pitfield, Milton Keynes, MK11 3LW, UK
UKHW052220190926
475702UK00006B/1117
* 9 7 8 1 0 3 2 7 5 2 3 2 7 *